Progress in Nephrology

Proceedings of the Vth Symposium of the
"Gesellschaft für Nephrologie", held in Lausanne (Switzerland)
21—23 Sept. 1967

Edited by

Georges Peters · Françoise Roch-Ramel

With 215 Figures

Springer-Verlag Berlin Heidelberg GmbH

ISBN 978-3-540-04672-1 ISBN 978-3-642-87957-9 (eBook)
DOI 10.1007/978-3-642-87957-9

Originally published by Springer-Verlag Berlin · Heidelberg in 1969
76-78289.

Preface

The present volume contains the edited proceedings of the Vth Symposium of the "Gesellschaft für Nephrologie" held in Lausanne, Switzerland, from September 21 to September 23, 1967. The manuscripts were arranged according to their contents rather than to their titles. An attempt was made to divide the allotted space between different contributors according to the apparent importance or originality of the contributions.

Most of the papers submitted were written in either German or a rather inarticulate English, and subsequently, have been translated into English by the editors and their collaborators. The editors are indebted to Mr. R. Darling, student of medicine of the Faculté de Médicine de l'Université de Lausanne, for reviewing the English translation.

Editing was limited to requirements based on form rather than on content. In a few instances, manuscripts which were inadequate in form were accepted because their contents appeared interesting or important. A very few manuscripts were either not submitted or could not be included in the present proceedings, because they did not satisfy the editorial standards. Some papers are published in the present proceedings in abstract form because they have been submitted elsewhere for full publication.

The editors' responsibility does not extend to the factual content of the manuscripts. The editors wish to apologize for the long delay in publishing these proceedings, a delay which may be attributed to difficulties in communication and cooperation with various authors.

The present volume has been printed with the help of a generous grant donated by Sharp and Dohme G.m.b.H., Munich, a subsidiary of Merck and Co. Inc., Rahway, N.J./USA. The editors wish to thank this company for their liberal assistance.

It is hoped that the present volume which gives a just picture of the status of nephrological research in the German speaking countries of Europe, will meet its aim of making this work known to nephrologists throughout the world.

Lausanne, April 1969

Georges Peters   Françoise Roch-Ramel

Table of Contents

List of Contributors

BALTZER, G., M.D., Medizinische Universitätsklinik, Mankopffstraße 1, D-355 Marburg/Lahn, Fed. Rep. of Germany

BARTH, C., M.D., II. Medizinische Universitätsklinik und Poliklinik, Landeskrankenhaus, D-665 Homburg/Saar, Fed. Rep. of Germany

BEHRENBECK, D. W., M.D., Medizinische Universitätsklinik, D-53 Bonn-Venusberg, Fed. Rep. of Germany

BLUMBERG, A., M.D., Medizinische Poliklinik der Universität Bern, Freiburgstraße 3, CH-3000 Bern, Switzerland

BOHLE, A., M.D., Professor of Pathology. Chairman: Pathologisches Institut der Universität, Liebermeisterstraße 8, D-74 Tübingen, Fed. Rep. of Germany

BONJOUR, J. PH., M.D., Department of Physiology, University of Michigan, East Medical Building, Ann Arbor (48104), Michigan, U.S.A.

BRANDIS, M., M.D., Physiologisches Institut der Freien Universität, Arnimallee 22, D-1 Berlin-Dahlem 33, Germany

BRASS, H., M.D., Medizinische Abteilung II, Technische Hochschule, Goethestraße 27—29, D-51 Aachen, Fed. Rep. of Germany

BRAUN-SCHUBERT, G., Physiologisches Institut der Freien Universität, Arnimallee 22, D-1 Berlin-Dahlem 33, Germany

BRODEHL, J., M.D., Privatdozent, Universitäts-Kinderklinik, Adenauer-Allee 119, D-53 Bonn, Fed. Rep. of Germany

BROWN, J. J., M.B. Chairman: Medical Research Council Blood Pressure Research Unit, Western, Infirmary, Glasgow, Scotland

BRUNNER, F. P., M.D., Medizinische Universitäts-Poliklinik, Inselspital, CH-3008 Bern, Switzerland

BÜCH, D., M.D., Pharmakologische Abteilung J. R. Geigy A.G., CH-4000 Basel, Switzerland

BÜNTIG, W. E., M.D., Physiologisches Institut der Universität, Pettenkoferstraße 12, D-8 München 15, Fed. Rep. of Germany

BURCK, H. C., M.D., Medizinische Universitätsklinik, Ottfried-Müller-Straße, D-74 Tübingen, Fed. Rep. of Germany

CAIN, H., M.D., Professor of Pathology. Chairman: Pathologisches Institut am Städtischen Katharinenhospital, Kriegsbergstraße 60, D-7 Stuttgart, Fed. Rep. of Germany

CAMPANACCI, L., M.D., Istituto di patologia medica dell'Università di Padova, Policlinico universitario, Via Giustiniani, I-35100 Padova, Italy

CHOMETY, FRANÇOISE, Institut de Pharmacologie de l'Université de Lausanne 21, rue du Bugnon, CH-1005 Lausanne, Switzerland

COTTIER, P., M.D., Privatdozent. Chairman: Medizinische Abteilung Bezirksspital, CH-3800 Interlaken, Switzerland

DAHLMEIM, H., Ph.D., Physiologisches Institut der Universität, Pettenkoferstraße 12, D-8 München 15, Fed. Rep. of Germany

DEETJEN, P., M.D., Privatdozent, Physiologisches Institut der Universität, Pettenkoferstraße 12, D-8 München, Fed. Rep. of Germany

DOENECKE, D., M.D., I. Medizinische Universitätsklinik, Landeskrankenhaus, D-665 Homburg/Saar, Fed. Rep. of Germany

DUBACH, U. C., M.D., Privatdozent, Medizinische Universitäts-Poliklinik, Hebelstraße 1, CH-4056 Basel, Switzerland

DÜSTERDIECK, G., Ph.D., Medical Research Council Blood Pressure Research Unit, Western Infirmary, Glasgow, Scotland

EIGLER, J., M.D., Privatdozent, Medizinische Universitäts-Poliklinik und Medizinische Klinik, Osmerheimerstraße 200, D-5 Köln-Merheim, Fed. Rep. of Germany

Eisenbach, G. M., M.D., I. Physiologisches Institut der Universität, Akademiestraße 3, D-69 Heidelberg, Fed. Rep. of Germany

Ellinghaus, K., Physiologisches Institut der Universität, Pettenkoferstraße 1a, D-8 München 15, Fed. Rep. of Germany

Enderlin, F., M.D., Chirurgische Universitätsklinik, Bürgerspital, Spitalstraße 2, CH-4056 Basel, Switzerland

Faarup, P., M.D., Institute for Experimental Medicine, University, Nørre-Allee 71, DK-2300 København, Denmark

Federlin, K., M.D., Privatdozent, Zentrum für Innere Medizin der Universität Ulm, D-79 Ulm/Donau, Fed. Rep. of Germany

Fiaschi, E., M.D., Professor of Medicine. Chairman: Istituto di patologia medica dell' Università di Padova. Policlinico universitario. Via Giustiniani 12, I-35100 Padova, Italy

Fischbach, M., M.D., Pathologisches Institut der Universität, Liebermeisterstraße 8, D-14 Tübingen, Fed. Rep. of Germany

Frey, J., M.D., Professor of Medicine. Chairman: II. Medizinische Universitätsklinik, Ludwig-Rehn-Straße 14, D-6 Frankfurt/Main Süd 70, Fed. Rep. of Germany

Frick, A., M.D., Abteilung Physiologie, Medizinische Fakultät der Technischen Hochschule Aachen, z.Z. Hermann-Herder-Straße 7, D-78 Freiburg/Breisgau, Fed. Rep. of Germany

Frick, P. G., M.D., Professor of Medicine, Medizinische Universitätsklinik, Kantonsspital, Rämistraße 100, CH-8000 Zürich, Switzerland

Friedrich, W., M.D., Prosektor, Wilhelminenspital der Stadt Wien, Montleartstraße 37, A-1170 Wien XVI, Austria

Fritz, K. W., M.D., Privatdozent, Medizinische Universitätsklinik, Richthofenstraße 63, D-53 Bonn-Venusberg, Fed. Rep. of Germany

Fülgraff, G., M.D., Privatdozent, Lehrstuhl für Pharmakologie der Medizinischen Fakultät der Technischen Hochschule Aachen, z.Z. Katharinenstraße 29, D-78 Freiburg/Breisgau, Fed. Rep. of Germany

Gammelgard, P. A., M.D., Professor of Surgery, Department of Surgery H, Gentofte Hospital Mellerup, DK 2900 København, Denmark

Gebauer, L., Ph.D., now Mrs. Reinemer, II. Medizinische Universitätsklinik, Ludwig-Rehn-Straße 14, D-6 Frankfurt/Main, Fed. Rep. of Germany

Gekle, D., M.D., Universitäts-Kinderklinik, Josef-Schneider-Straße 2, D-87 Würzburg, Fed. Rep. of Germany

Gellissen, K., M.D., St. Elisabeth-Krankenhaus, Kinderabteilung, D-5450 Neuwied, Fed. Rep. of Germany

Geltinger, A., Physiologisches Institut der Universität, Pettenkoferstraße 12, D-8 München 15, Fed. Rep. of Germany

Gertz, K. H., Ph. D., Privatdozent, Physiologisches Institut der Freien Universität, Arnimallee 22, D-1 Berlin-Dahlem 33, Germany

Gessler, U., M.D., Professor of Medicine. Chairman: 4. Medizinische Klinik der Städtischen Krankenanstalten, Kontumazgarten 14/18, D-85 Nürnberg, Fed. Rep. of Germany

Gigon, J. P., M.D., Chirurgische Universitätsklinik, Bürgerspital, Spitalstraße 21, CH-4000 Basel, Switzerland

Gloor, F., M.D., Professor of Pathology, Pathologisches Institut der Universität Basel, Hebelstraße 24, CH-4056 Basel, Switzerland

Göggel, K. H., M.D., II. Medizinische Klinik der Universität Frankfurt, Ludwig-Rehn-Straße 14, D-6 Frankfurt/Main Süd 70, Fed. Rep. of Germany

Gottesleben, A., M.D., Neurologische Klinik der Universität, v. Sieboldstraße 5, D-34 Göttingen, Fed. Rep. of Germany

Griebel, L., M.D., Medizinische Universitätsklinik, Luitpoldkrankenhaus 14, Josef-Schneider-Straße 2, D-87 Würzburg, Fed. Rep. of Germany

Grossmann, D. F., Ph.D., II. Medizinische Universitätsklinik, Ludwig-Rehn-Straße 14, D-6 Frankfurt/Main Süd 10, Fed. Rep. of Germany

Guarnieri, G. F., M.D., Istituto di chimica biologica dell' Università di Padova, Via Marpolo, I-35100 Padova, Italy

Günther, F., M.D., Medizinische Universitätsklinik, Luitpoldkrankenhaus, Josef-Schneider-Straße 2, D-87 Würzburg, Fed. Rep. of Germany

HAGGE, W., M.D., Privatdozent, Universitäts-Kinderklinik, Moorenstraße 5, D-4 Düsseldorf, Fed. Rep. of Germany

HALLAUER, W., M.D., Medizinische Universitätsklinik, Hugstetterstraße 55, D-78 Freiburg/Breisgau, Fed. Rep. of Germany

HARDT, KARIN, Physiologisches Institut der Universität, Pettenkoferstraße 12, D-8 München 15, Fed. Rep. of Germany

HEIDENREICH, D., M.D., Professor of Pharmacology. Chairman: Pharmakologisches Institut der Medizinischen Fakultät der Technischen Hochschule Aachen, z.Z. Katharinenstraße 29, D-78 Freiburg/Breisgau, Fed. Rep. of Germany

HEIDLAND, A., M.D., Univ.-Dozent, Medizinische Universitätsklinik, Luitpoldkrankenhaus, Josef-Schneider-Straße 2, D-87 Würzburg, Fed. Rep. of Germany

HEINTZ, R., M.D., Professor of Medicine. Chairman: Abteilung Innere Medizin II der Technischen Hochschule Aachen, Goethestraße 27/29, D-51 Aachen, Fed. Rep. of Germany

HEINZ, G., M.D., Abteilung für Pharmakologie der Medizinischen Fakultät der Technischen Hochschule Aachen, z.Z. Katharinenstraße 29, D-78 Freiburg/Breisgau, Fed. Rep. of Germany

HEINZE, V., M.D., Medizinische Poliklinik der Universität, Wohnhaldestraße 1—5, D-78 Freiburg/Breisgau, Fed. Rep. of Germany

HELBER, A., M.D., Pathologisches Institut, Liebermeisterstraße 8, D-74 Tübingen, Fed. Rep. of Germany

HELMCHEN, U., M.D., Pathologisches Institut der Universität, Liebermeisterstraße 8, D-74 Tübingen, Fed. Rep. of Germany

HERMS, W., M.D., Privatdozent, I. Medizinische Klinik der Universität, Moorenstraße 5, D-4 Düsseldorf, Fed. Rep. of Germany

HEROLD, I., Physiologisches Institut der Universität, Pettenkoferstraße 12, D-8 München 15, Fed. Rep. of Germany

HERZFELD, A., M.D., Abteilung für Pharmakologie der Technischen Hochschule Aachen, z.Z. Katharinenstraße 29, D-78 Freiburg/Breisgau, Fed. Rep. of Germany

HILTENBRAND, CH., M.D., Clinique Médicale, Hôpital militaire d'instruction du Val-de-Grâce, 277 bis, rue St-Jacques, F-75 Paris Ve, France

HOHENEGGER, M., M.D., Institut für experimentelle Pathologie, Währingerstraße 13, A-1090 Wien, Austria

HOLZGREVE, H., M.D., Medizinische Universitätsklinik und Medizinische Klinik, Ostmerheimerstraße 200, D-5 Köln-Merheim, Fed. Rep. of Germany

HORSTER, M., M.D., Physiologisches Institut der Universität, Pettenkoferstraße 12, D-8 München 15, Fed. Rep. of Germany

HÜBNER, K., M.D., II. Privatdozent, Pathologisches Institut der Universität, Ludwig-Rehn-Straße 14, D-6 Frankfurt/Main Süd 70, Fed. Rep. of Germany

JAENKNER, D., M.D., Medizinische Universitätsklinik, D-5 Köln-Lindenthal, Fed. Rep. of Germany

JAHN, O., M.D., II. Medizinische Universitätsklinik, Garnisongasse 13, A-1090 Wien, Austria

JUTZLER, G. A., M.D., Privatdozent, I. Medizinische Universitätsklinik des Saarlandes, D-665 Homburg/Saar, Fed. Rep. of Germany

KAMMERER, E., M.D., Rechenzentrum der Universität, D-5 Köln-Lindenthal, Fed. Rep. of Germany

KAPP, M.D., Abteilung Innere Medizin II, Technische Hochschule Aachen, Goethestraße 27 bis 29, D-51 Aachen, Fed. Rep. of Germany

KELLER, H. E., Ph.D., I. Medizinische Klinik der Universität des Saarlandes, D-665 Homburg/Saar, Fed. Rep. of Germany

KELTER, K., M.D., II. Medizinische Universitäts-Poliklinik und Medizinische Klinik, Ostmerheimerstraße 200, D-5 Köln-Merheim, Fed. Rep. of Germany

KERSTING, F., M.D., I. Medizinische Klinik der Universität, Moorenstraße 5, D-4 Düsseldorf, Fed. Rep. of Germany

KLOSE, H. J., Physiologisches Institut der Universität, Pettenkoferstraße 12, D-8 München 15, Fed. Rep. of Germany

KLUTHE, R., M.D., Privatdozent, Medizinische Poliklinik der Universität, Wohnhalde 1—5, D-78 Freiburg/Breisgau, Fed. Rep. of Germany

KLÜTSCH, K., M.D., Privatdozent, Medizinische Universitätsklinik, Luitpoldkrankenhaus, Josef-Schneider-Straße 2, D-87 Würzburg, Fed. Rep. of Germany

KONICKOVA, LIDMILA, M.D., Forschungsinstitut für Pharmazie und Biochemie, Praha 3, ČSSR

KRAMER, H. J., Ph.D., I. Medizinische Klinik der Universität des Saarlandes, D-665 Homburg/Saar, Fed. Rep. of Germany

KRAMER, K., M.D., Professor of Physiology, Physiologisches Institut der Universität, Pettenkoferstraße 12, D-8 München 15, Fed. Rep. of Germany

KRÜCK, F., M.D., Professor of Medicine, I. Medizinische Klinik und Poliklinik der Universität, Langenbeckstraße 1, D-65 Mainz, Fed. Rep. of Germany

KUNI, H., M.D., Institut für Strahlenbiologie und Medizinische Isotopenanwendung der Universität Marburg/Lahn, D-355 Marburg/Lahn, Fed. Rep. of Germany

KURTH, G., Universitäts-Kinderklinik, Josef-Schneider-Straße 2, D-87 Würzburg, Fed. Rep. of Germany

LACKENSCHWEIGER, A., M.D., Wilhelminenspital der Stadt Wien, Montleartstraße 37, A-1171 Wien XVI, Austria

LADEFOGED, J., M.D., Department of Clinical Physiology, Glastrup Hospital, DK-2900 København

LANGER, K. H., M.D., Pathologisches Institut der Universität, Luitpold-Krankenhaus, Josef-Schneider-Straße 2, D-87 Würzburg, Fed. Rep. of Germany

LAPP, H., M.D., Professor of Pathology. Pathologisches Institut der Universität, Ludwig-Rehn-Straße 14, D-6 Frankfurt/Main Süd 70, Fed. Rep. of Germany

LASSITER, W. E., M.D., Marble Scholar in Academic Medicine, Associate Professor of Medicine Department of Medicine, University of North Carolina, School of Medicine, Chapel Hill, N.C., U.S.A.

LEVER, A. F., M.B., Medical Research Council Blood Pressure Research Unit, Western Infirmary, Glasgow, Scotland

LIEBAU, G., Physiologisches Institut der Universität, Pettenkoferstraße 12, D-8 München 15, Fed. Rep. of Germany

LOESCHKE, K., M.D., Physiologisches Institut der Freien Universität, Arnimallee 22, D-1 Berlin-Dahlem 33, Germany

LOSERT, W., M.D., Abteilung für allgemeine Pharmakologie, Hauptlaboratorium, Schering AG, Sellerstraße 3—6, D-1 Berlin 85, Germany

LOSSE, H., M.D., Professor of Medicine. Chairman: Medizinische Poliklinik der Universität, Westring 3, D-44 Münster/Westf., Fed. Rep. of Germany

LUDWIG, H. J., M.D., II. Medizinische Klinik der Medizinischen Akademie, D-24 Lübeck, Fed. Rep. of Germany

MAN, N. K., M.D., Medizinische Universitätsklinik, Hugstetterstraße 55, D-78 Freiburg/Breisgau, Fed. Rep. of Germany

MASBERNARD, A., M.D., Professor of Medicine, Hôpital militaire d'instruction du Val-de-Grâce, 277 bis, rue St-Jacques, F-75 Paris Ve, France

MATHIESEN, F. R., M.D., Privatdozent, Department of Surgery H, Gentofte Hospital, DK-2900 Hellerup, Denmark

MEMIN, Y., M.D., Clinique Médicale, Hôpital militaire d'instruction du Val-de-Grâce, 277 bis, rue St-Jacques, F-75 Paris Ve, France

MERTZ, D. P., M.D., Professor of Medicine, Medizinische Poliklinik der Universität, Hermann-Herder-Straße 6, D-78 Freiburg/Breisgau, Fed. Rep. of Germany

MEYER, D., M.D., Pathologisches Institut der Universität, Liebermeisterstraße 8, D-74 Tübingen, Fed. Rep. of Germany

MITTMEYER, P. J., M.D., Pathologisches Institut der Universität, Liebermeisterstraße 8, D-74 Tübingen, Fed. Rep. of Germany

MOELLER, J., M.D., Professor of Medicine. Chairman: Medizinische Abteilung, Städtisches Krankenhaus, Weinberg 1, D-32 Hildesheim, Fed. Rep. of Germany

MOHR, H. J., M.D., Professor of Pathology. Chairman: Pathologisches Institut der Städtischen Krankenanstalten, Zeppelinallee 4—6, D-465 Gelsenkirchen, Fed. Rep. of Germany

MUEHRCKE, R. C., M.D., Director of Medical Education, West Suburban Hospital, Oak Park, Ill., U.S.A.

MULLER, A. F., M.D., Professor of Medicine. Chairman: Clinique de Médecine Interne, Université de Genève, 24 rue Micheli du Crest, CH-1200 Genève, Switzerland

MUNCK, D., M.D., Professor of Medicine. Chairman: Department of Clinical Physiology, Glastrup, Hospital, DK-2900 København, Denmark

MÜTING, D., M.D., Professor of Medicine, I. Medizinische Klinik der Universität des Saarlandes, D-665 Homburg/Saar, Fed. Rep. of Germany

NAGAND, M., M.D., Associate Professor, Dept. of Internal Medicine, Medical Academy Tokyo Jikeikai, Minatoko Nishishinbushi, Tokyo, Japan

NAGEL, W., M.D., Physiologisches Institut der Universität, Pettenkoferstraße 12, D-8 München 15, Fed. Rep. of Germany

NIEDERER, W., M.D., Chirurgische Universitätsklinik, Bürgerspital, CH-4000 Basel, Switzerland

NIETH, H., M.D., Professor, Städtische Krankenanstalten, D-64 Fulda, Fed. Rep. of Germany

NOLTE, ANNEMARIE, M.D., Pathologisches Institut der Universität, Ludwig-Rehn-Straße 14, D-6 Frankfurt/Main 70, Fed. Rep. of Germany

OKEN, D. E., M.D., Associate in Medicine, Ass. Dir., Cardiorenal Section, Dept. of Medicine, Peter Bent Brigham Hospital & Harvard Medical School, 721 Huntington Ave., Boston 02115, Mass., U.S.A.

PEDERSEN, F., M.D., Department of Clinical Physiology, Glastrup Hospital, DK-2900 København, Denmark

PETERS, G., M.D., Professor of Pharmacology. Chairman: Institut de Pharmacologie de l'Université de Lausanne, 21, rue du Bugnon, CH-1005 Lausanne, Switzerland

PETSCHAUER, K., Physiologisches Institut der Universität, Pettenkoferstraße 12, D-8 München 15, Fed. Rep. of Germany

PHILIPPSON, C., M.D., Medizinische Universitätsklinik, Karl-Marx-Universität, Johannisallee 32, X-701 Leipzig, German Democratic Republic

PINGGERA, W., M.D., II. Medizinische Universitätsklinik, Garnisongasse 13, A-1090 Wien, Austria

PITTS, R. F., M.D. Ph.D., Professor of Physiology. Chairman: Dept. of Physiology and Biophysics, Cornell University, Medical College, 1300 York Ave., New York 21, N.Y. U.S.A.

PRAT, V., M.D., Institut für Kreislaufforschung, Praha 4-Krč, Č.S.R.R,

PRILL, A., M.D., Privatdozent, Neurologische Klinik der Universität, v. Siebold-Straße 5, D-34 Göttingen, Fed. Rep. of Germany

QUELLHORST, E., M.D., Medizinische Universitätsklinik, Humboldtallee 1, D-34 Göttingen, Fed. Rep. of Germany

QUIRIN, H., M.D., Medizinische Poliklinik der Universität, Wohnhalde 1—5, D-78 Freiburg/Breisgau, Fed. Rep. of Germany

REGOLI, D., M.D., Privatdocent, Institut de Pharmacologie de l'Université de Lausanne, 21, rue du Bugnon, CH-1005 Lausanne, Switzerland

REINHARDT, H. W., M.D., Physiologisches Institut der Universität, Pettenkoferstraße 12, D-8 München 15, Fed. Rep. of Germany

RENNER, D., M.D., Abteilung für Innere Medizin II, Med. Fakultät der Technischen Hochschule Aachen, Goethestraße 27—29, D-51 Aachen, Fed. Rep. of Germany

RENNER, E., M.D., II. Medizinische Universitäts-Poliklinik und Medizinische Klinik, Ostmerheimerstraße 200, D-5 Köln-Merheim, Fed. Rep. of Germany

RENSCHLER, H., M.D., Privatdozent, I. Medizinische Universitätsklinik, Lindenburg, D-5 Köln Lindenthal, Fed. Rep. of Germany

RITZERFELD, W., M.D., Professor of Microbiology Hygiene Institut der Universität, Westring 10, D-44 Münster, Fed. Rep. of Germany

ROBERTSON, J. I. S., M.B., Medical Research Council Blood Pressure Research Unit, Western Infirmary, Glasgow, Scotland

ROCH-RAMEL, FRANÇOISE, Ph.D., Privatdocent, Institut de Pharmacologie de l'Université de Lausanne, 21, rue du Bugnon, CH-1005 Lausanne, Switzerland

ROHDE, R., M.D., Physiologisches Institut der Universität, Pettenkoferstraße 12, D-8 München 15, Fed. Rep. of Germany

ROSCHER, S., II. Medizinische Universitätsklinik und Poliklinik, Landeskrankenhaus, D-665 Homburg/Saar, Fed. Rep. of Germany

Ross, H. J., Physiologisches Institut der Universität, Akademiestraße 3, D-69 Heidelberg, Fed. Rep. of Germany

Rostock, D., M.D., Universitäts-Kinderklinik, Josef-Schneider-Straße 2, D-87 Würzburg, Red. Rep. of Germany

Rotter, W., M.D., Professor of Pathology. Chairman: Pathologisches Institut der Universität, Ludwig-Rehn-Straße 14, D-6 Frankfurt/Main Süd 70, Fed. Rep. of Germany

Sarre, H., M.D., Professor of Medicine. Chairman: Medizinische Universitäts-Poliklinik, Hermann-Herder-Straße 6, D-78 Freiburg/Breisgau, Fed. Rep. of Germany

Schaechtelin, G., M.D., Institut de Pharmacologie de l'Université de Lausanne, 21, rue du Bugnon, CH-1005 Lausanne, Switzerland

Schäfer, H. E., M.D., Privatdozent, D-492 Lemgo, Raabeweg 4, Fed. Rep. of Germany

Scheitlin, W. A., M.D., Privatdozent, Medizinische Klinik, Kantonspital, Rämistraße 100 CH-8006 Zürich, Switzerland

Scheitza, M., M.D., Medizinische Universitätsklinik, Luitpoldkrankenhaus, Josef-Schneider-Straße 2, D-87 Würzburg, Fed. Rep. of Germany

Scheler, F., M.D., Professor of Medicine, Medizinische Universitätsklinik, Humboldtallee 1, D-34 Göttingen, Fed. Rep. of Germany

Schindera, F., M.D., Universitäts-Kinderklinik, Mathildestraße 1, D-78 Freiburg/Breisgau, Fed. Rep. of Germany

Schirmeister, J., M.D., Professor of Medicine. Acting Chairman: Medizinische Universitätsklinik, Hugstetterstraße 55, D-78 Freiburg/Breisgau, Fed. Rep. of Germany

Schmidt, U., M.D., Pathologisches Institut der Universität, Liebermeisterstraße 8, D-74 Tübingen, Fed. Rep. of Germany

Schmidt, U., Privatdozent, Lecturer of Medical Statistics, University of Basle, CH-4000 Basel, Switzerland

Schmidt-Nielsen, Bodil, Ph.D., Professor of Biology, Department of Biology, Case Western Reserve University, Cleveland, Ohio (44106), U.S.A.

Schnermann, J., M.D., Physiologisches Institut der Universität, Pettenkoferstraße 12, D-8 München 15, Fed. Rep. of Germany

Schoeppe, W., M.D., Privatdozent, II. Medizinische Universitätsklinik und Poliklinik der Universität Frankfurt a.M., Ludwig-Rehn-Straße 14, D-6 Frankfurt/Main 70, Fed. Rep. of Germany

Schollmeyer, P., M.D., Privatdozent, Medizinische Universitätsklinik, Hugstetterstraße 55, D-78 Freiburg, Fed. Rep. of Germany

Scholz, A., M.D., I. Medizinische Klinik der Freien Universität, Spandauer Damm 130, D-1 Berlin 19, Germany

Schroder, E., M.D., I. Medizinische Klinik der Universität Düsseldorf, Moorenstraße 5, D-4 Düsseldorf, Fed. Rep. of Germany

Schumacher, H., M.D., Universitäts-Kinderklinik, Adenauerallee 119, D-53 Bonn, Fed. Rep. of Germany

Schürholz, J., M.D., Pathologisches Institut der Universität, Liebermeisterstraße 8, D-74 Tübingen, Fed. Rep. of Germany

Schütterle, G., M.D., Professor of Medicine, Medizinische Universitätsklinik, Klinikstraße 32b D-63 Gießen/Lahn, Fed. Rep. of Germany

Senft, G., M.D., Professor of Pharmacology. Late Chairman: Institut für Klinische Pharmakologie der Freien Universität Berlin, Germany

Siliprandi, N., Chairman: Istituto di chimica biologica dell'Università di Padova, Via Marpolo, I-35100 Padova, Italy

Sitt, R., M.D., Pharmakologisches Institut der Freien Universität, Thielallee 69/73, D-1 Berlin 33, Germany

Sorge, F., M.D., Medizinische Universitätsklinik im Krankenhaus Westend, 1000 Berlin 19, Spandauer Damm 130

Stegemann, I., M.D., Medizinische Universitätsklinik, Humboldtallee 1, D-34 Göttingen, Fed. Rep. of Germany

Steinhausen, M., M.D., Privatdozent, Physiologisches Institut der Universität, Akademiestraße 3, D-69 Heidelberg, Fed. Rep. of Germany

Tabor, M., Physiologisches Institut der Universität, Pettenkoferstraße 12, D-8 München 15, Fed. Rep. of Germany

Takuma, T., M.D., Medizinische Universitätsklinik, Luitpoldkrankenhaus, Josef-Schneider-Straße 2, D-87 Würzburg, Fed. Rep. of Germany

Thiele, K. G., M.D., Medizinische Universitäts-Poliklinik, 5 Köln, Josef-Stelzmann-Straße 9, Fed. Rep. of Germany

Thoenes, W., M.D., Univ.-Dozent, Pathologisches Institut der Universität, Josef-Schneider-Straße 2, D-87 Würzburg, Fed. Rep. of Germany

Thoma, R., M.D., Medizinische Universitätsklinik, Osterheimerstraße 200, D-5 Köln-Lindenthal, Fed. Rep. of Germany

Thurau, K., M.D., Professor of Physiology, Physiologisches Institut der Universität, Pettenkoferstraße 12, D-8 München 15, Fed. Rep. of Germany

Tourkantonis, A., M.D., Medizinische Universitäts-Poliklinik, Wohnhaldestraße 1—5, D-78 Freiburg/Breisgau, Fed. Rep. of Germany

Traut, G., M.D., I. Medizinische Universitätsklinik des Saarlandes, D-665 Homburg/Saar, Fed. Rep. of Germany

Truniger, B., M.D., Medizinische Universitätsklinik, Inselspital, Freiburger Straße, CH-3008 Bern, Switzerland

Ullrich, K. J., M.D., Professor of Physiology. Chairman: Max-Planck-Institut für Biophysik, Kennedyallee 70, D-6 Frankfurt/Main, Fed. Rep. of Germany

Valtin, H., M.D. Ph.D., Ass. Professor of Physiology, Dartmouth Medical School, Hanover, New Hampshire, 03755 U.S.A.

Vecsei, P., M.D., II. Medizinische Universitätsklinik und Poliklinik, Landeskrankenhaus, D-665 Homburg/Saar, Fed. Rep. of Germany

Volles, E., M.D., Neurologische Klinik der Universität, v. Sieboldstraße 5, D-34 Göttingen, Fed. Rep. of Germany

v. Bergmann, K., M.D., Pharmakologisches Institut der Freien Universität, Thielallee 69—73, D-1 Berlin 33, Germany

Walther, D., M.D., Privatdozent, Pathologisches Institut der Universität Frankfurt, Ludwig-Rehn-Straße 14, D-6 Frankfurt/Main 70, Fed. Rep. of Germany

Warning, A., M.D., Pathologisches Institut der Universität, Luitpoldkrankenhaus, Josef-Schneider-Straße 2, D-87 Würzburg, Fed. Rep. of Germany

Watschinger, B., M.D., Privatdozent. Chairman: Medizinische Abteilung des Elisabethinen-krankenhauses, Bethlehemstraße 19, A-4020 Linz/Donau, Austria

Weber, P., Physiologisches Institut der Universität, Pettenkoferstraße 12, D-8 München 15, Fed. Rep. of Germany

Weidinger, H., M.D., Privatdozent, Physiologisches Institut der Universität, Akademiestraße 3, D-69 Heidelberg, Fed. Rep. of Germany

Weissel, W., M.D., Professor of Medicine. Chairman: III. Medizinische Abteilung, Wilhelminenspital der Stadt Wien, Montleartstraße 37, A-1171 Wien XVI, Austria

Wiederholt, M., M.D., Physiologisches Institut der Freien Universität, Arnimalle 22, D-1 Berlin-Dahlem 33, Germany

Wirz, H. M.D., Professor of Physiology. Director: Pharmakologische Abteilung, J. R. Geigy, A.G., CH-4000 Basel, Switzerland

Wolff, G., M.D., Chirurgische Universitätsklinik, Bürgerspital, Spitalstraße 21, CH-4000 Basel, Switzerland

Wolff, H., M.D., Professor of Medicine. Chairman: I. Medizinische Universitätsklinik und Poliklinik, Langenbeckstraße 1, D-65 Mainz, Fed. Rep. of Germany

Zesch, A., M.D., D-1 Berlin 33, Germany

Zimmermann, E., M.D., III. Medizinische Abteilung Wilhelminenspital der Stadt Wien, Montlearstraße 37, A-11971 Wien XVI, Austria

Zollinger, H. U., M.D., Professor of Pathology. Former Chairman: Ludwig-Aschoff-Haus, Pathologisches Institut der Universität, D-78 Freiburg/Breisgau, Fed. Rep. of Germany. Chairman: Pathologisches Institut der Universität, Hebelstraße 24, CH-4000 Basel, Switzerland

Zöllner, N., M.D., Professor of Medicine, Medizinische Poliklinik der Universität München, D-8 München 15, Fed. Rep. of Germany

1. The Renal Excretion of Nitrogen Containing Metabolites

1.1. Urea

1.1.1. Comparative Physiology of Urea Excretion

BODIL SCHMIDT-NIELSEN[1]

With 10 Figures

Urea accumulates in the renal papilla of mammals. This accumulation plays a decisive role in the concentrating mechanism of the kidney. In our attempts to understand the mechanism through which urea accumulates in the papilla, we have found that nature has provided us with two tools, with which this mechanism can be investigated. One is that the urea concentration and distribution in the renal papilla in many mammals changes with the nitrogen content of the diet. The other is that there are two groups of mammals which behave quite differently in this respect. In the first group the amount of urea excreted in the urine relative to electrolytes has a pronounced effect upon the concentrating ability of the kidney. In the other, it has little or no effect.

The maximum osmotic concentration of the urine that a mammalian kidney can produce is primarily determined by the thickness of the renal medulla, i.e. by the length of the countercurrent system. Maximum urine concentration is obtained when the animal is maintained without water from 24—48 hours. In rats, for example, it is about 3,000 to 3,300 milliosmols/kg H_2O. In the mountain beaver *(Aplodontia rufa)* it is only 600 to 700 milliosmols/kg H_2O. The mountain beaver has only an outer zone and no inner zone of the medulla. The rat kidney has a relatively long papilla and therefore a longer countercurrent system (Fig. 1). Kidneys with still longer papillae can concentrate even better. The maximum urinary concentration found in any mammal is about 6,000 milliosmols/kg H_2O [11].

The renal concentrating ability, however, is not determined solely by the length of the renal papilla; it is also determined by the nitrogen intake of the animal. GAMBLE [2] found in rats that the ability to produce a concentrated urine increased when the nitrogen intake was increased, so that a relatively larger fraction of the solute excreted in the urine was consituted by urea (Fig. 2). He found the maximum urine concentrations when urea consituted about 65% of the total solute output. In this case the maximum urine osmolality was about 3,000 milliosmols/kg H_2O, while it decreased to about 1,400 milliosmols/kg H_2O when 70 to 80% of the total solute was consituted by sodium chloride. Furthermore, he found that among a number of different small organic molecules urea was the only one that had this effect. It was later shown that nitrogen intake has the same effect upon the concentrating ability in the dog [6], in man [1], in sheep [12], in the opossum [10] etc.

[1] Department of Biology, Case Western Reserve University, Cleveland, Ohio 44106.

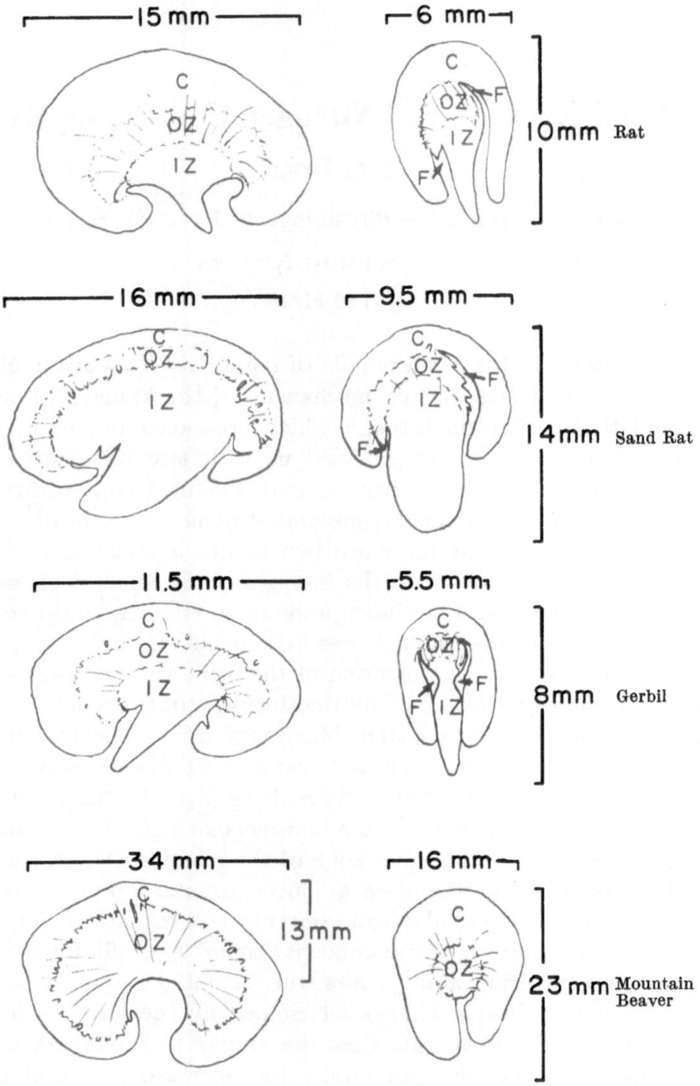

Fig. 1. *The kidneys of rat, sand rat, gerbil and mountain beaver* showing the extent of the pelvis and the relative length of outer and inner medullae. *C* cortex; *OZ* outer zone; *IZ* inner zone of the medulla; *F* fornices

Which changes in renal composition or in renal function may account for an increased concentrating ability? From micropuncture studies and from tissue slice analysis we know that the osmolality of the urine is equal to that of the tissue at the tip of the papilla [11], and that the osmotic pressure in the collecting duct fluid near the papilla is equal to that of the blood and fluid in neighboring vasa recta and loops of Henle [5, 17]. Consequently, when the osmotic concentration of the urine is increased in animals on a high nitrogen intake the osmotic concentration of the papillary tissue must also increase, and the question is which

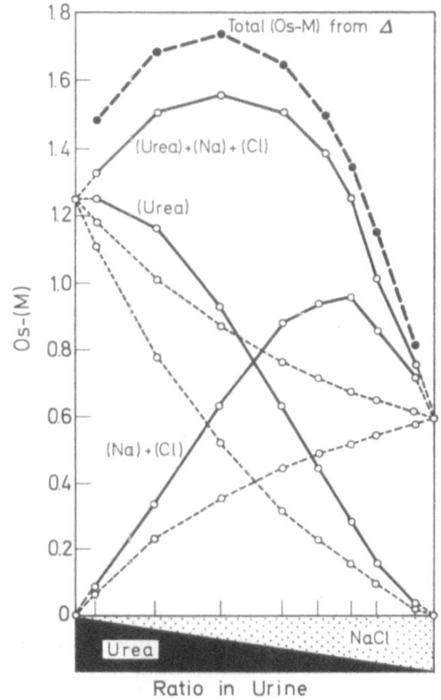

Fig. 2. *The renal concentrating ability in rats on different diets* (from GAMBLE *et al.* [2]). Diets with different relative amounts of nitrogen and NaCl were given so that the ratio of urea to NaCl in the urine could be varied over a wide range. The highest concentrating ability (urinary osmolality expressed as freezing point depression on the ordinate) was found when urea constituted about 65% of the total solute excretion

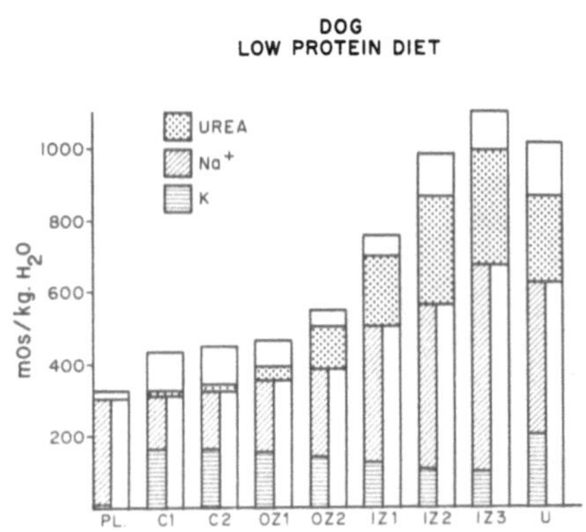

a

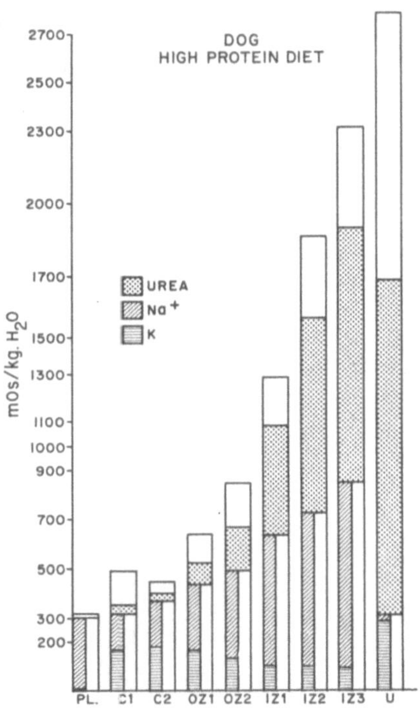

b

Fig. 3a u. b. *The solute concentrations in plasma, renal tissue and urine in dehydrated dogs on high and low protein diets.* To the low protein diet is added NaCl so that the amount of solute excreted per calorie in the diets is the same. The ability to concentrate the urine is increased in the dog on high protein diet compared to that on low protein, high salt diet. The difference in osmotic concentration of the papilla on the two diets is mainly due to a difference in the urea concentration of the papilla. *PL* plasma; *C 1*, *C 2* outer and inner layer of cortex; *OZ 1*, *OZ 2* outer and inner layer of outer zone of medulla; *IZ 1*, *IZ 2*, *IZ 3* outer, middle and inner layer of inner zone of medulla; *U* urine

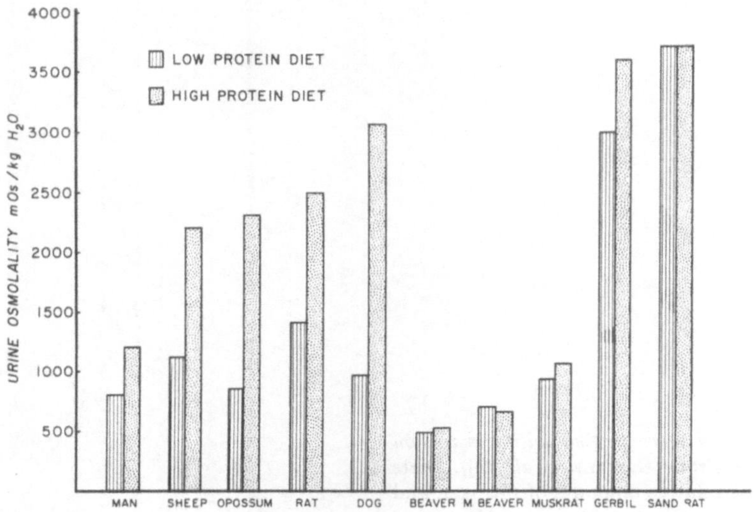

Fig. 4. *Maximum urine osmolality in the two groups of mammals on high and low protein diets.* Man [1], sheep ([12] and unpublished data), opossum [10], rat ([16] and unpublished data), and dog [14] belong to the first group in which urea profoundly affects the concentrating ability. Beaver [11], mountain beaver [13], muskrat [3], gerbil and sand rat [15], all belong to the second group, in which urea has no enhancing effect upon the concentrating ability

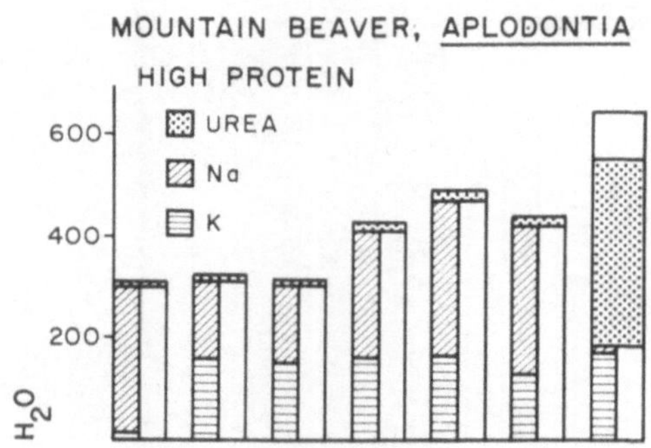

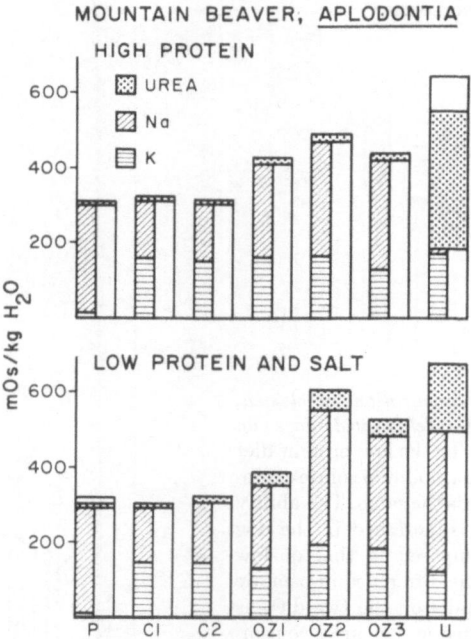

Fig. 5. *The solute concentrations in plasma, renal tissue and urine in dehydrated mountain beavers, Aplodontia rufa, on high and low protein diets.* Urea does not enhance the concentrating ability and does not accumulate in the renal tissue. Abbreviations as in Fig. 3

solutes contribute to the increased osmolality. In experiments carried out in collaboration with R. R. Robinson we performed analyses on the renal tissue of dogs maintained on high and low protein diets [14]. The composition of the diet was such that the amount of solute to be excreted per calorie of diet was the same in both cases i.e. the sodium chloride concentration in the low protein diet

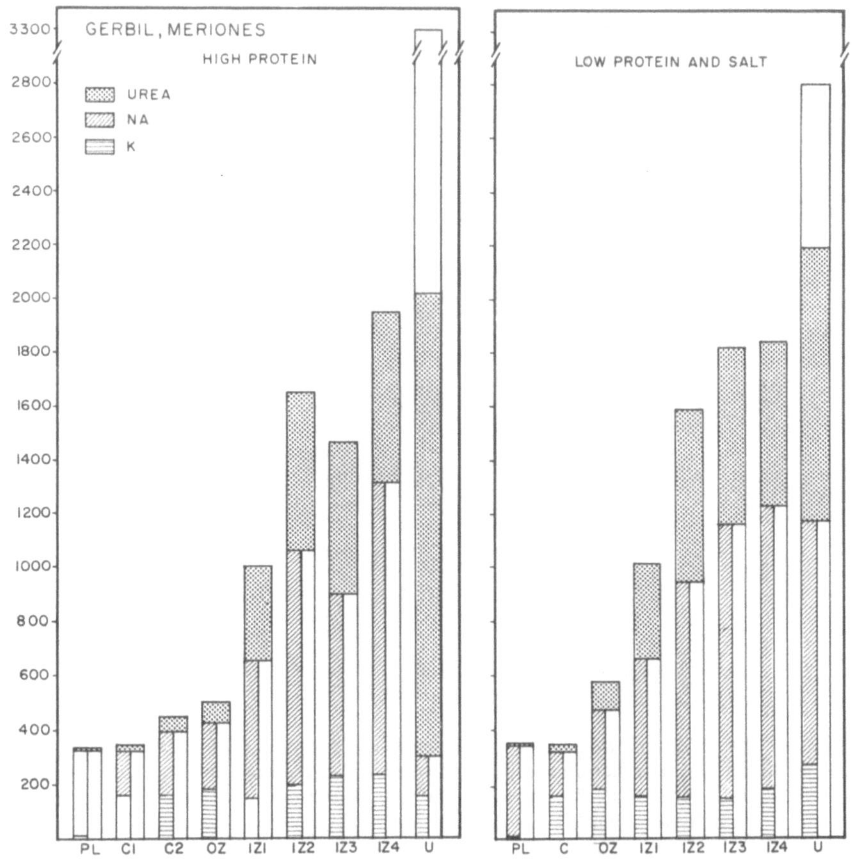

Fig. 6. *Solute concentrations in plasma, renal tissue and urine in dehydrated gerbils, Meriones unguiculatus, on high and low protein diets.* Urea does not enhance the concentrating ability, and does not accumulate any more in the high than in the low protein animal. Abbreviations as in Fig. 3

was increased [16]. In order to obtain maximum osmotic concentration of urine the animals were dehydrated before sacrifice. The results are shown in Fig. 3. The concentrating ability in the dog on high protein diet is 1,700 milliosmols/kg H_2O greater than in the dog on low protein diet. The osmotic concentration in the renal tissue is increased particularly by an increased urea concentration, and much less by an increase of electrolyte concentration. It is also seen that the urea concentration in the papilla is close to that of the urine.

As mentioned earlier, the effect of nitrogen intake on concentrating ability of the kidney is pronounced in one group of mammals (first group), while another group (2nd group) shows no such effect (Fig. 4). In Figs. 5, 6, and 7 the solute concentrations in the kidneys of three species belonging to the 2nd group, the mountain beaver [13] the gerbil *(Meriones unguiculatus)* and the sand rat *(Psammomys obesus)* on high and low protein diets are shown [15]. It is seen that very little urea accumulates in the renal papilla of the mountain beaver. In the papilla of the sand rat and gerbil there is more accumulation of urea. This could be expected since the kidneys of the gerbil and the sand rat have an inner

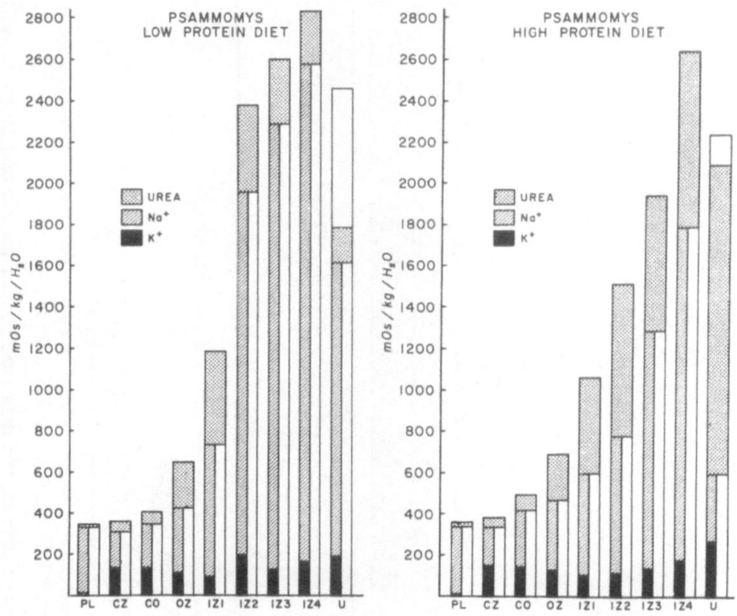

Fig. 7. *Solute concentrations in plasma, renal tissue and urine in dehydrated sand rats, Psammomys obesus, on high and low protein diets.* Urea does not enhance the concentrating ability. Urea accumulates more in the high than in the low protein animal, but this is compensated for by a higher NaCl accumulation in the low protein animal

medulla. However, compared to rat and dog the accumulation is small, and particularly there is little difference in the urea accumulation between high and low protein animals. Furthermore, the urine urea concentration may be as much as 1,500 milliosmols/kg H_2O greater than the papilla concentration. It is also seen that the papilla concentration does not increase toward the tip of the papilla.

In Fig. 8, a summary is shown of the urea concentration in the papilla compared to the urine in high and low protein diet animals in the two groups of animals. In the first group the urea concentration in the papilla is considerably higher in high protein animals than in low protein animals. In the second group the papilla urea concentration is about the same in high and low protein animals, and consequently urea does not enhance the total osmotic concentration of the papilla. Secondly, in this group the urea concentration in the urine is quite different from that of the papilla.

In order to gain a better understanding of the mechanism through which urea accumulates in the renal papilla and thereby enhances the osmotic concentration in man, dog, rat, etc. we looked for anatomical and physiological differences between the two groups that could account for this marked difference. We first believed that the difference could be explained through a difference in pelvic structure [7, 8], because GERTZ et al. [3, 4] had found that the renal

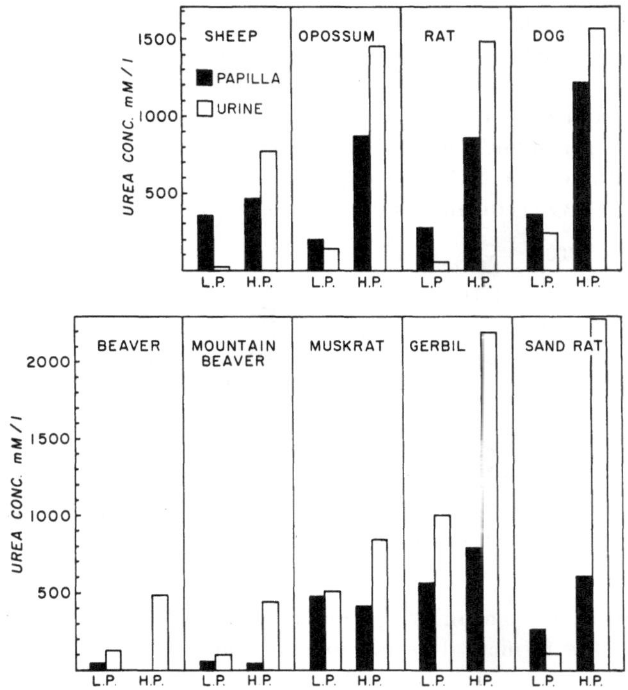

Fig. 8. *Papilla and urine urea concentrations in animals on high and low protein diets.* Upper group: animals in which urea does not enhance the concentrating ability. Lower group: animals in which urea enhances the concentrating ability. In all animals in the upper group the urea concentration in the papilla is higher in high than in low protein animals. In those in the lower group there is little or no difference between the urea concentration in the papilla, despite large differences in urine concentration on the two diets

papilla must be bathed in its own urine in order to ensure a maximum concentrating ability. When the ureter in a rat is cut so that the papilla lies free, surrounded by the peritoneal fluid, the urea concentration and the osmolality of the papilla decrease (Fig.9). A number of experiments, published [3, 4] and in preparation, that I shall not discuss further here, have shown that rinsing the papilla with different solutions changes the urea concentration of the papilla and of the urine from that kidney. The papillary tissue is particularly permeable to water and to urea, but has a relatively low permeability to sodium.

Normally, the urine which emerges from the ducts of BELLINI at the tip of the papilla does not flow directly down through the ureter but is pressed back by the pelvic contractions and flows backwards into the upper parts of the pelvis before it reverses direction and flows down through the ureter. This can be demonstrated by injecting lissamine green into the vein of a rat and observing the colored urine through the wall of the pelvis. In studies by Pfeiffer [7] it was found that the pelvis of rat, sheep, oppossum and dog is much more complicated than hitherto realized and that it extends as leaf-like structures (fornices), up between the outer zone of the medulla and the cortex. Neoprene casts of the pelves from sheep, dog and opossum ressemble those from the sand rat shown in Fig. 10. In two species from the second group, beaver and mountain beaver which have no inner medulla, no fornices could be observed. Furthermore the epithelium covering the papilla was thick (two cell layers), compared to the one in the first group. However, when studies were made on the pelvis of the gerbil and the sand rat it was found that these pelves were just as elaborate with respect to fornices as the pelves in the animals from the first group (see Fig. 1). Consequently, although fornices may play an important role

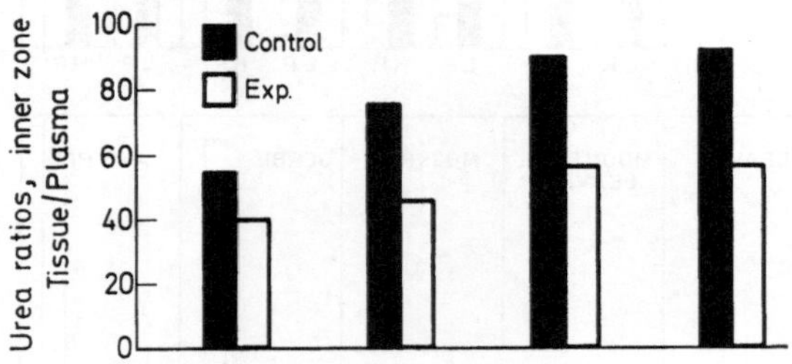

Fig. 9. *Loss of urea from the papilla of rats after the ureter has been cut.* The experimental kidney (*L*) is compared to the control kidney (*R*) [4]

in the concentrating mechanism of mammalian kidneys, a difference in the development of the fornices does not explain the difference in accumulation of urea in the two groups.

One marked physiological difference has, however, been found between the two groups. The papillas from rats and gerbils were rinsed for 10—15 minutes with a 3 M/l urea solution with added C-14 labeled urea. The specific activity in the tissue α and in the rinsing fluid β were determined and the ratio α/β calculated. In such an experiment the papilla is simultaneously perfused from the inside with non-labeled urea through the loops of Henle and the vasa recta, and rinsed from the outside with the radioactive rinsing fluid. Thus the steady state value that one will measure after a certain period of time will indicate the fraction of urea molecules which after entering the papilla through the vasa recta and loops of Henle, were exchanged against urea molecules from the superfusion solution. The results show that in the gerbil 86,2% of the urea molecules have been exchanged with molecules from the rinsing fluid, while in the rats only 41,6% have been exchanged. This means that in the rat (in which urea accumulates in the papilla) only a small percentage of the urea exchanges with the urea in the pelvis, while in the gerbil (in which urea does not accumulate) almost 100% of the urea which enters the papilla exchanges with that in the urine.

The degree of labeling of the papilla ($\alpha/\beta \cdot 100\%$), in the steady state will depend on the following movements of urea molecules:

1. J_{in}, the rate of influx from rinsing fluid to papilla.

2. J_{out}, the rate of outflux from papilla to rinsing fluid.

3. $J_{v.r.in}$, $J_{H.l.in}$, the rates of entry of urea molecules into the papilla through vasa recta and loops of HENLE.

4. $J_{v.r.out}$, $J_{H.l.out}$, $J_{u.}$ the rates of outflux through vasa recta, HENLE loops, and urine.

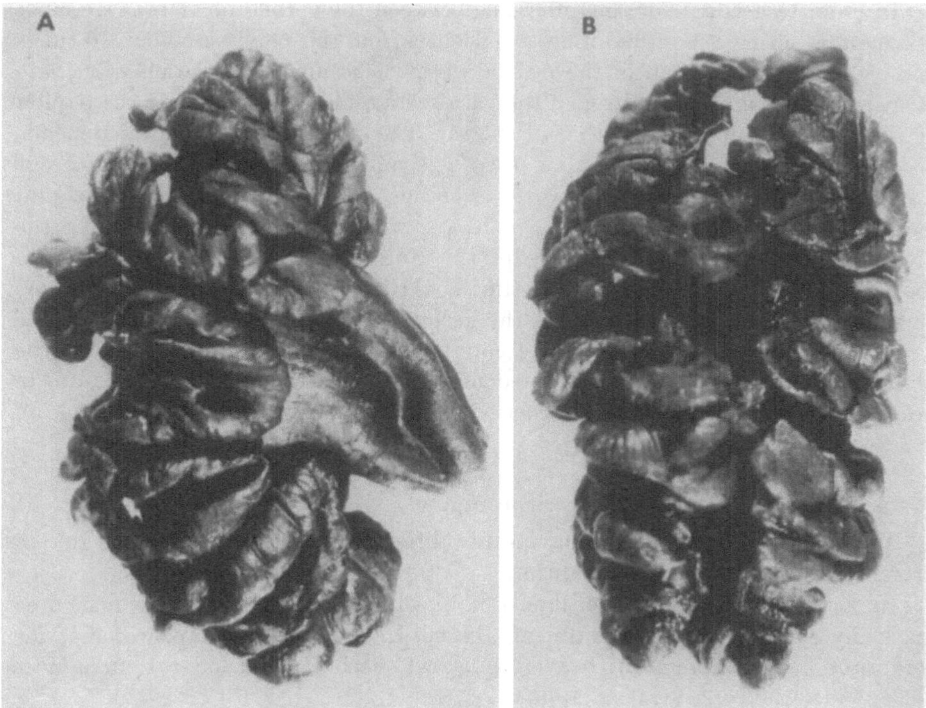

Fig. 10. *Neoprene cast of the pelvis of a sand rat* showing the pronounced fornices from the side (*A*), and from top (*B*) [15]

At steady state the rates of influx and outflux of labeled molecules must be equal. Thus we have:

$$J_{in}\beta = J_{out}\alpha + J_{v.r.out}\alpha + J_{H.l.out}\alpha + J_{u.}\alpha \quad (1)$$

and the rates of influx and outflux of unlabeled molecules must be equal:

$$J_{in} + J_{v.r.in} + J_{H.l.in} = J_{out} + J_{v.r.out} + J_{H.l.out} + J_{u.} \quad (2)$$

and hence from (1):

$$J_{in} = \frac{\alpha}{\beta}(J_{out} + J_{v.r.out} + J_{H.l.out} + J_{u.}) \, .$$

Substituting from (2):

$$J_{in} = \frac{\alpha}{\beta}(J_{in} + J_{v.r.in} + J_{H.l.in}) \, .$$

$$\frac{a}{\beta} = \frac{J_{in}}{J_{in} + J_{v.r.in} + J_{H.l.in}} \quad (3)$$

If we first make the assumption that the entry of urea through vasa recta and Henle's loop is the same in rat and gerbil we can calculate from (3) that for the ratio α/β to change from 42 to 86%, J_{in} must be 8.6 times higher in the gerbil than in the rat. If, on the other hand, we keep J_{in} the same in both animals $J_{v.r.\,in} + J_{H.l.\,in}$ would have to be decreased by a factor of 8.6 in order to account for an increase in α/β from 42 to 86%.

In order to account for the difference between the gerbil and the rat we must assume that either the influx of urea molecules from the pelvis is about 10 times greater in the gerbil than in the rat, or we must assume that the effective rate of entry of urea molecules through the vasa recta and Henle's loops to the papilla of the gerbil is only 1/10 of that of the rat. The effective rate of entry depends on the countercurrent exchange of urea. The more effective the countercurrent exchange of urea molecules between ascending and decending vasa recta and loops of HENLE, the smaller $J_{v.r.\,in} + J_{H.l.\,in}$ will be, because a fraction of the urea molecules entering at the top of the countercurrent system will by-pass the loops. The experimental results thus could indicate a less effective countercurrent exchange in the rat than in the gerbil. This result is surprising since one would guess that the more effective countercurrent exchange system would be found in the rat which accummulated more urea. Further investigations are in progress in order to compare the permeability and countercurrent exchange in the two groups of mammals.

Summary

Two groups of mammals behave quite differently with respect to the role of urea in the concentrating mechanism.

In the first group, to which man, dog, sheep, oppossum, and rat belong, urea markedly enhances the concentrating ability. In the second group, which so far comprises beaver, mountain beaver, muskrat, gerbil, and sand rat, urea does not enhance the concentrating ability.

In the first group urea accumulates in the papilla in proportion to the amount in the urine. In the second group the urea concentration in the papilla is independent of the urine urea concentration.

So far no anatomical differences have been found that can account for this difference. Both groups include animals with long inner medullas, and in both groups are found animals with well developed pelvic fornices. Pelvic perfusion with labeled urea causes a much more pronounced labeling of the papilla in the gerbil (second group) than in the rat (first group). This may indicate a difference between the two groups in permeability to urea of the outer surface of the papilla or in the efficiency of the urea countercurrent exchange system.

References

1. EPSTEIN, F. H.: Alterations in renal concentrating ability produced by diet. Clin. Res. Proc. 4, 137—138 (1956).
2. GAMBLE, J. L., C. F. MCKHANN, A. M. BUTLER, and E. TUTHILL: An economy of water in renal function referable to urea. Amer. J. Physiol. **109**, 139—154 (1934).
3. GERTZ, K. H., B. SCHMIDT-NIELSEN, and H. D. PAGEL: Exchange of water, urea and salt between the mammalian renal papilla and the surrounding urine. Fed. Proc. **25**, 327 (1966).

GERTZ, K. H., B. SCHMIDT-NIELSEN, and H. D. PAGEL: The exchange of solutes and water between renal papillary tissue and the pelvic urine. Abstr. Internat. Cong. Neph. II, 197 (1966).
5. GOTTSCHALK, C. W., W. E. LASSITER, M. MYLLE, K. ULLRICH, B. SCHMIDT-NIELSEN, R. O'DELL, and G. PEHLING: Micropuncture study of composition of loop of Henle fluid in desert rodents. Amer. J. Physiol. **204**, 532—535 (1963).
6. LEVINSKY, N. G., and R. W. BERLINER: The role of urea in the urine concentrating mechanism. J. clin. Invest. **38**, 741—748 (1959).
7. PFEIFFER, E. W.: Comparative anatomical observations of the mammalian renal pelvis and medulla. J. Anat. (Lond.) **102**, 321—331 (1968).
8. — B. SCHMIDT-NIELSEN, K. H. GERTZ, and J. R. WHEATLEY, JR.: Comparative anatomy of mammalian renal pelvis and medulla. Abstr. Internat. Cong. Neph. II, 254 (1966).
9. —, and T. ZAHN: Effect of protein intake on maximum urine and renal tissue solute concentrations in the muskrat. Abstr. Amer. Physiol. Soc. Proc. **10**, 276 (1967).
10. PLAKKE, R. K., and E. W. PFEIFFER: Influence of plasma urea on urine concentration in the opossum (*Didelphis marsupialis virginiara*). Nature (Lond.) **207**, 866—867 (1965).
11. SCHMIDT-NIELSEN, B., R. O'DELL, and H. OSAKI: Interdependence of urea and electrolytes in production of a concentrated urine. Amer. J. Physiol. **200**, 1125—1132 (1961).
12. — H. OSAKI, H. V. MURDAUGH, JR., and R. O'DELL: Renal regulation of urea excretion in sheep. Amer. J. Physiol. **194**, 221—228 (1958).
13. —, and E. W. PFEIFFER: The role of urea in the concentrating mechanism of the mountain beaver *Aplodontia rufa*). (In prep.).
14. —, and R. R. ROBINSON: The role of urea in the distribution of solutes and the osmolality of the renal tissue of dogs. (In prep.).
15. TRIMBLE, M. E., and B. SCHMIDT-NIELSEN. (In prep.)
16. TRUNIGER, B., and B. SCHMIDT-NIELSEN: Intrarenal distribution of urea and related compounds-effects of nitrogen intake. Amer. J. Physiol. **207**, 971—879 (1964).
17. WIRZ, H. v., B. HARGITARY u. W. KUHN: Lokalisation des Konzentrierungsprozesses in der Niere durch direkte Kryoskopie. Helv. physiol. pharmacol. Acta **9**, 196—207 (1951).

Discussion

STEINHAUSEN:

Did you attempt to measure, in gerbils, the frequency or the force of the rhythmic contractions of the papillary muscle bundles? I observed, in golden hamsters, rhythmic contractions of these bundles, which actually "milk" the papilla and interrupt completely the papillary blood-circulation at intervals of approximately 6 sec. Could the difference between the two groups of mammals be due to a different type of "milking" in the gerbil?

SCHMIDT-NIELSEN:

In the rat the average number of contractions per min is 34, and it does not change significantly with urine flow rate. However, the amount of urine pushed down the ureter with each peristaltic movement increases with increasing urine flow. In the gerbil the contraction rate is lower than in the rat (about 15 min). If this difference would influence the accummulation of urea in the papilla, I cannot say.

FREY:

In mice excreting a concentrated urine (> 1.000 mOsm/l) the papilla appears elongated and can easily be torn off from the deeper medullary layers. This phenomenon may be due to the leaf-like extensions of the renal pelvis (fornices) which you describe. In mice, in water diuresis (< 200 mOsm/l), on the other hand, the papilla appears short and thick: it cannot be severed from the medulla without resorting to scissors. Do you have any observation about the shape and the size of the fornices in water diuresis ? May they be occluded by tissue swelling ?

Schmidt-Nielsen:

Yes, it is quite possible that the occlusion of the fornices could be due to swelling. Your observation is extremely interesting and should be pursued further. It would appear to be functionally advantageous if the dilute urine did not enter the fornices.

Krück:

In man urea appears to contribute to the elaboration of a concentrated urine. In healthy subjects, in a state of antidiuresis, the contribution of urea to urinary osmolality amounts to 40—45%. In patients with renal failure (equally in antidiuresis) with an $U/P_{Osm} < 2$, the fractional contribution of urea remains the same, i.e. the decrease in osmolality may be due to a decrease of the concentration of urea.

1.1.2. The Renal Excretion of Urea

WILLIAM E. LASSITER[1,2]

With 3 Figures

Although urea is a small molecule which is freely filterable at the glomerulus, the urea clearance in mammals is almost invariably lower than the glomerular filtration rate, indicating net reabsorption of a portion of the filtered urea by the renal tubule. The renal clearance of urea, moreover, is not constant, but varies directly with the rate of urine flow. Quantitative aspects of the relationship between urea excretion and urine flow in the dog were investigated in detail some thirty years ago by SHANNON [13, 14], whose observations in a typical animal are summarized in Fig. 1.

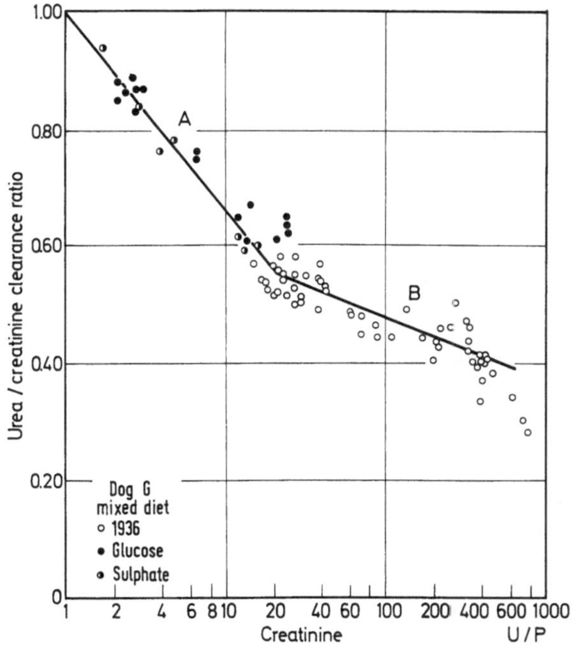

Fig. 1. The urea/creatinine clearance ratio in a typical dog, in relation to the reabsprotion of water as indicated by the U/P ratio of creatinine. The open circles represent observations at normal urine flows and during water diuresis. (SHANNON [14])

[1] Department of Medicine, University of North Carolina, School of Medicine, Chapel Hill, N.C.

[2] Markle Scholar in Academic Medicine, and recipient of U.S. Public Health Service Research Career Development Award (Number 1-KO3-AMO7234) from the National Institute of Arthritis and Metabolic Diseases.

In this figure the creatinine urine/plasma (U/P) ratio is plotted logarithmically on the abscissa, and the ratio of simultaneously measured urea and creatinine clearances on the ordinate. Since the creatinine clearance, which equals the glomerular filtration rate in female dogs, was relatively constant in these experiments, the creatinine U/P ratio was inversely proportional to the rate of urine flow, a high ratio being indicative of low urine flow, and lower ratios, larger urine flows. The urea/creatinine clearance ratio is a measure of the fraction of filtered urea which has escaped reabsorption by the renal tubule and is excreted in the urine. The open circles on the graph represent observations made at normal urine flows and during water diuresis. SHANNON observed that as urine flow increased and the creatinine U/P ratio fell, the fraction of filtered urea escaping reabsorption increased gradually to approximately 0.6 at a creatinine U/P ratio of 20, representing the maximum urine flow obtainable in water diuresis. When urine flow was further increased in osmotic diuresis, an additional and more rapid rise in the urea/creatinine clearance ratio was observed. SHANNON noted that the reabsorptive process illustrated here is distinctly divisible into two phases, indicated by the lines A and B. Since line A extrapolates to 1.0 at a creatinine U/P ratio of 1.0, indicating that there would be zero net urea reabsorption in the absence of water reabsorption, SHANNON suggested that urea reabsorption is not an active tubular process but may be due entirely to physical diffusion and hence dependent on prior or concurrent water reabsorption. The different slopes of lines A and B were interpreted as representing reabsorption of urea from segments of the nephron with differing permeabilities for urea diffusion. SHANNON identified phase A with reabsorption of urea from the proximal tubule, and phase B, that portion of urea reabsorption subject to modification by water diuresis, with reabsorption from more distal portions of the nephron.

Micropuncture techniques have made possible the direct localization of the sites of urea reabsorption in the mammalian nephron, and although observations in rats on a normal diet are compatible with the hypothesis that tubular reabsorption of urea is largely passive and dependent on concentration gradients established by water reabsorption, the pattern of urea movement in the kidney is far more complex that that originally contemplated by SHANNON. Some of our observations in anesthetized nondiuretic rats are summarized in Table 1 [8].

Table 1. *Average fluid to plasma osmolality, inulin, and urea ratios in the rat kidney*

Source	Osmolality F/P	Inulin F/P	Urea F/P	Urea ratio / Inulin ratio
Early proximal	1.0	1.0	1.0	1.0
Late proximal	1.0	3.0	1.5	0.5
Early distal	0.7	6.9	7.7	1.1
Late distal	1.0	14.9	10.5	0.7
Ureteral urine	6.4	690	90	0.13

In these and subsequent studies from our laboratory, fluid/plasma (F/P) ratios for inulin and urea were estimated using radioactively labeled compounds as tracers. The progressive increase in inulin concentration as one proceeds distally along the nephron indicates net reabsorption of water from all major segments of the nephron. The urea ratio divided by the inulin ratio at any point in the nephron is a measure of the amount of urea reaching that point relative to the amount filtered at the glomerulus. Thus, at the end of the proximal convolution the urea F/P ratio equals only one-half the inulin ratio, indicating that a quantity of urea equal to half that filtered reaches the end of the convolution. Although there is net loss of half the filtered urea from the proximal convolution, an amount at least equal to the filtered load reaches the distal convolution, indicating net addition of urea to tubular fluid in the loop of HENLE. Micropuncture studies of fluid obtained from the bend of the loop of HENLE in hamsters have revealed a high urea concentration at this locus, suggesting that the transtubular movement of urea into the loop occurs primarily in its descending limb. Some urea is lost from the distal convolution, and a comparison of the urea content of late distal convolutions and ureteral urine indicates that under these nondiuretic conditions a large amount of urea is reabsorbed by the collecting ducts. KLÜMPER, ULLRICH and HILGER [7] in 1958 demonstrated by a microcatheterization technique that the collecting duct is an important site of urea reabsorption in the nondiuretic hamster. Our observations in rats confirmed this, and indicated in addition that much of the urea reabsorbed from collecting ducts apparently diffuses ultimately into loops of HENLE and is recirculated through the distal portions of the nephron.

It is of further interest to note that significant urea reabsorption occurs in the proximal convolution despite the fact that the concentration gradient favoring diffusion of urea out of this portion of the nephron is relatively small. Urea loss from the distal convolution is no greater despite the much larger concentration gradient. These observations suggest that the distal convolution is much less permeable to urea than is the proximal tubule. This has been directly confirmed by ČAPEK, FUCHS, RUMRICH and ULLRICH [2], who have determined the diffusion permeability to urea of the proximal and distal convolutions in the rat by microperfusion of selected surface tubules of the kidney in situ. They calculated that the permeability to urea of the distal convolution is approximately 20 times smaller than that of the proximal. They also observed that, despite the fact that antidiuretic hormone (ADH) increases the water permeability of the distal convolution, it had no effect on its permeability to urea. Likewise, GRANTHAM and BURG [6] found that ADH had no effect on the urea permeability of isolated perfused collecting ducts from rabbit kidneys. These observations suggest that the alterations in urea excretion noted by SHANNON in graded water diuresis are secondary to changes in urea concentration and contact time in the distal convolutions and collecting ducts, and not to any direct effect of ADH on urea permeability or transport per se.

If tubular reabsorption of urea in the normal rat is largely passive, alteration of transtubular concentration gradients for urea should lead to predictable changes in the pattern of urea reabsorption. When rats are infused with 5% NaCl a massive solute diuresis ensues, but in spite of the increased glomerular filtration rate and increased sodium load, reabsorption of sodium in the proximal tubule increases proportionately, and therefore fractional reabsorption of water does not change. Since fractional water reabsorption is unchanged, the increase in urea concentration in proximal tubular fluid secondary to water reabsorption should be similar to that in the nondiuretic animal. On the other hand, fractional water reabsorption in the distal convolutions and collecting ducts is decreased in NaCl diuresis, and one should therefore expect to find lower urea concentrations at these sites in diuretic than in nondiuretic animals.

The patterns of urea reabsorption which we have observed [9] in diuretic and nondiuretic rats are compared in Table 2. Although fractional urea reabsorption in the proximal tubule is similar in the two groups, little further reabsorption of urea occurs in more distal portions of the nephron in the diuretic animals, and the recirculation of urea from collecting ducts to loops of HENLE, which is such a prominent feature of urea reabsorption in nondiuretic animals, cannot be detected in the diuretic group. These results are as one would predict if trans-

Table 2. *Urea remaining in tubule (fraction of amount filtered)*

	Nondiuretic	5% NaCl diuresis
Glomerulus	1.0	1.0
Late proximal	0.5	0.6
Early distal	1.1	0.6
Late distal	0.7	—
Ureteral urine	0.1	0.6

tubular movement of urea in the mammalian kidney were largely passive. Since fractional water reabsorption in the proximal tubule is unchanged in hypertonic saline diuresis, the increase in urea concentration secondary to water loss is also unaltered, and fractional urea reabsorption in the proximal tubule should be similar to that in nondiuretic animals. On the other hand, the intratubular concentration of urea in more distal parts of the nephron is much lower in the diuretic animals than in normals, and the transit time through the tubules is greatly shortened, thus offering less opportunity for urea loss through diffusion. The differences in transit time are most marked in the collecting ducts, a major site of urea loss in nondiuretic animals. Although these results of course do not exclude active transport, they suggest that under the conditions of these experiments most of the transtubular movement of urea in the rat kidney is passive.

Active Transport of Urea

I should like now to consider the controversial question of active urea transport.

Although available evidence indicates that under ordinary circumstances most transtubular transfer of urea in the mammalian kidney is in the direction of diffusional gradients, there is reason to believe that active transport may also occur, at least under certain circumstances. Active urea transport has long been recognized to exist in certain lower animal species. Urea secretion, for instance, apparently occurs in the frog [4], and the ability of elasmobranch fishes to maintain a high blood urea concentration through active tubular reabsorption of urea is well known [15, 16]. Dr. BODIL SCHMIDT-NIELSEN [11] several years ago suggested the possibility of active urea reabsorption in the mammalian kidney and pointed out that tubular regulation of urea excretion, in response to variations in the dietary intake of protein, appears to exist in a variety of mammals, most notably in ruminants and rodents. She also observed [12] in sheep maintained on a low protein diet that the concentration of urea in tissue water of the renal medulla may at times be higher than the urea concentration in urine obtained immediately before removal of the kidney. A similar phenomenon in rats was demonstrated by BRAY and PRESTON [1], who showed that under certain circumstances the concentration of urea was lower in urine than in tissue water of the renal papilla.

This they observed, not only in rats on a low protein diet, but also in rats on a normal diet if the urine urea concentration were sufficiently reduced in sustained osmotic diuresis. Although these observations on tissue slices are all compatible with active transport of urea out of collecting ducts, other possibilities, such as urea binding to tissue proteins, could not be readily excluded.

We attempted to circumvent some of the difficulties inherent in the interpretation of slice studies by comparing the urea concentration in collecting duct urine with that in plasma obtained from adjacent vasa recta, where it is possible to evaluate the contribution of protein binding [10]. Similar studies were performed in rats on protein deficient and normal diets. Rats on the low protein diet differed from those on a normal diet in several respects. Their growth was markedly retarded, and their blood urea concentration was only about half normal. Urinary concentrating ability was strikingly diminished by protein restriction, apparently because of markedly reduced urea excretion. Normal rats, after anesthesia and preparation for micropuncture, excrete 10 to 15% of the filtered urea; only 2 to 3% was excreted by the protein deficient rats.

Mean urea concentrations in collecting duct urine and in the plasma water of adjacent vasa recta in rats on the low protein diet are recorded in Table 3.

Table 3. *Average F/P urea ratios in vasa recta and collecting ducts in rats (low-protein diet)*

Rat, Wt, g	F/P Urea		
	vasa recta	collecting ducts	VR/CD
No infusion			
60	5.8	5.3	1.09
60	4.5	2.7	1.67
50	4.8	4.4	1.09
2.5% NaCl infusion			
40	6.9	6.7	1.03
60	6.6	6.3	1.05
70	7.4	6.1	1.21
55	6.5	6.0	1.08
40	3.8	3.2	1.19
Mean	5.8	5.1	1.14
	$0.01 < P < 0.02$		

The concentration of urea averaged 14% higher in vasa recta than in collecting ducts. The difference, although small, is nonetheless statistically significant ($P < 0.02$). Qualitatively similar results were obtained in animals on a normal diet made diuretic with either hypertonic NaCl or mannitol, but the difference was smaller and not statistically significant. These findings are most readily explained by active urea transport out of collecting ducts, but alternative possibilities must be considered.

Binding of urea to tissue protein has been suggested as a possible partial explanation of the high urea concentrations observed in renal papillary tissue, but it is unlikely that protein binding alone can account for the observations summarized in this table. The concentration of urea in glomerular filtrate is not measurably different from that in plasma water from the inferior vena cava, indicating the absence of significant protein binding in the glomerular capillaries. Since the concentration of protein in vasa recta is increased, we dialyzed rat plasma in which the protein concentration was increased up to 1.5 times by evaporation. Even at these elevated protein concentrations, urea binding of a significant degree was not detected.

The question of urea synthesis in the renal medulla has been evaluated by Truniger and Schmidt-Nielsen [17] in rats given C^{14}-labeled urea. They observed that after a period of equilibration the urea specific activity of papillary tissue was virtually identical to plasma, and they therefore concluded that intrarenal urea synthesis was not of sufficient magnitude to account for the high urea concentration in the renal papilla.

A third possibility is that, under circumstances in which the urine urea is greatly reduced, net reabsorption from collecting ducts ceases, and urea diffuses down its concentration gradient from the medullary interstitium into the urine. Indeed, this probably does occur acutely with rising urine flow, and Ullrich and Jarausch [18] have offered this as an explanation for the phenomenon of exaltation. For this to persist in the steady state, however, there must be a continued delivery of urea to the interstitium from some other source, presumably loops of Henle. Thus, in contrast to the usual situation in normal nondiuretic animals, in which urea moves out of collecting ducts and into loops of Henle, passive movement of urea in the reverse direction, from loop to collecting duct, might occur in protein depletion or during sustained osmotic diuresis. It is unlikely that this is the case, however. We did not find the concentration of urea in loops of Henle of protein depleted animals to be higher than in adjacent collecting ducts. Moreover, there is evidence that despite the unfavorable concentration gradient, net urea reabsorption from the collecting ducts occurs in the protein depleted rats.

As is shown in Table 4, a comparison of urea and inulin ratios in distal convolutions and in collecting ducts indicates that in diuretic protein depleted rats, urea is not added to the collecting duct urine, but to the contrary, in contrast

Table 4. *Urea remaining in tubule (fraction of amount filtered). Diuretic: 5% NaCl or Mannitol + 1% NaCl*

	Distal convolution	Collecting duct	P
Low protein diet	0.7	0.5	< 0.001
Normal diet	0.6	0.6	N.S.

to normal rats during diuresis, a significant fraction of the urea delivered to the collecting ducts from the distal convolutions is reabsorbed. In this circumstance, urea is reabsorbed from collecting ducts against its concentration gradient. This does not in itself necessarily imply active transport, since at the same time water is being reabsorbed, and a solvent drag effect cannot be excluded. However, Clapp [3] has obtained qualitatively similar evidence of urea reabsorption in collecting ducts of protein depleted rats undergoing a more intense diuresis induced by mannitol, and in his studies not only was there evidence of net urea reabsorption, but the urea concentration in the final urine was lower than that in distal convolutions. This observation suggests that solvent drag is not the mechanism responsible for the reabsorption of urea against its concentration gradient.

Additional evidence suggesting the existence of active urea transport in the mammalian kidney has recently been reported. GOLDBERG and his associates

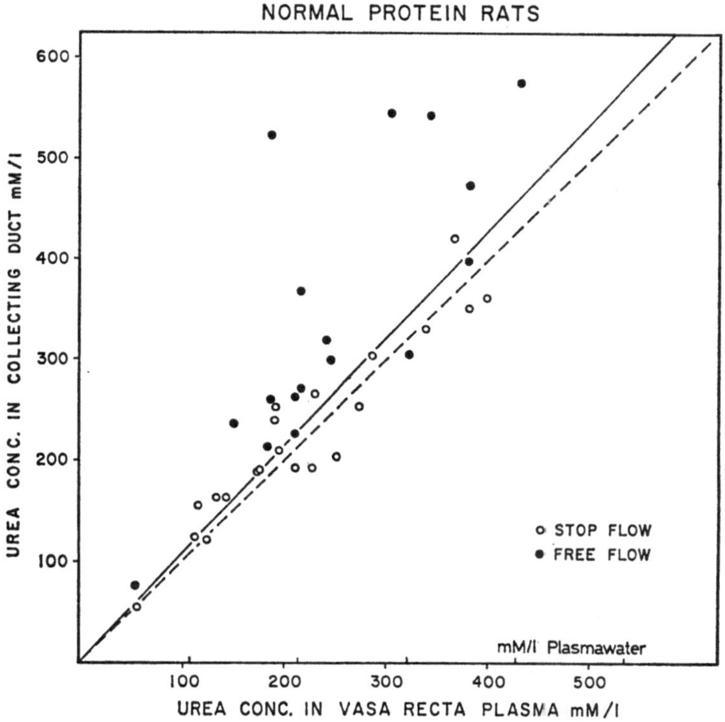

Fig. 2. Urea concentration in collecting duct plotted against urea concentration in vasa recta plasma in rats on a normal diet. Open circles represent determinations on samples obtained by stop flow perfusion of collecting ducts. (ULLRICH et al. [19])

in Philadelphia [5] compared the urea concentration in the tip of the renal papilla with that in urine from dogs in which the medullary electrolyte gradient was obliterated by a sustained ethacrynic acid diuresis. They found that the urea concentration in the papillary tip in every case exceeded that in the urine, regardless of the previous diet of the dog. It was also observed that the uphill urea gradient was markedly reduced by infusion into the renal artery of iodo-acetate, an inhibitor of anaerobic glycolysis, or of acetamide, an analogue of urea which might be expected to display competitive inhibition of any carrier mediated process of urea transfer. GOLDBERG believes that these observations in the dog point to active urea trasport in the medullary collecting ducts, with anaerobic glycolysis the source of energy.

Further evidence that the medullary collecting ducts are capable of actively transporting urea under certain circumstances has been presented by ULLRICH,

Rumrich and Schmidt-Nielsen [19]. These investigators utilized a microperfusion technique in which a collecting duct in the exposed papilla is first filled with oil. The duct is then re-entered by transmural puncture and the oil column split by injection of an aqueous test solution containing NaCl, mannitol, and urea. After three to four minutes the aqueous sample is withdrawn and its urea concentration compared with plasma obtained shortly afterward by micropuncture from an adjacent vas rectum. Studies were done both in normal rats

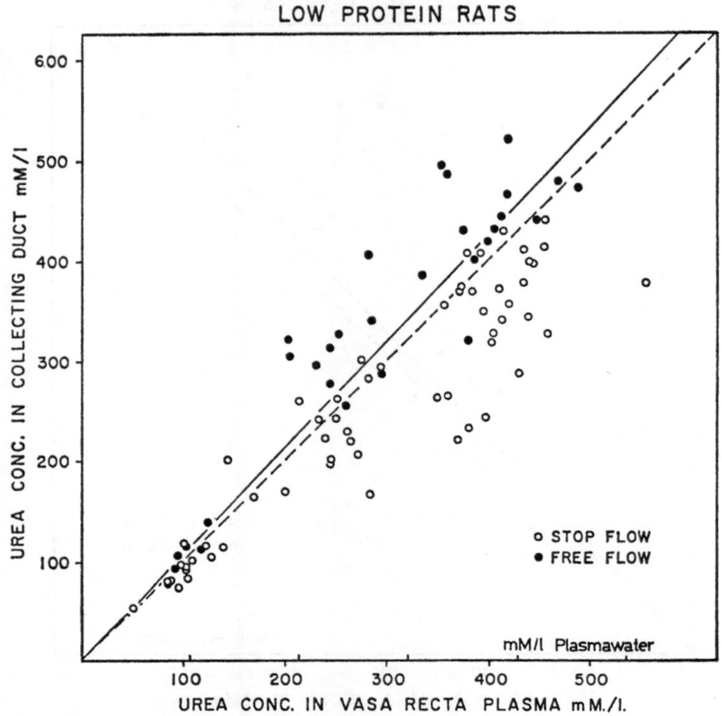

Fig. 3. Data from rats on low protein diet, plotted as in Fig. 2. (Ullrich et al. [19])

and in animals maintained for three weeks or longer on a protein deficient diet. The latter group were given a subcutaneous injection of urea shortly before the experiment to raise the urea concentration to a level comparable to that in the normal animals. Their results are summarized in Figs. 2 and 3.

In these figures the open circles represent determinations on samples obtained by the stop flow microperfusion method just described. The dotted line indicates equality between collecting duct and plasma water. As is shown in Fig. 2, in normal animals the equilibrium concentration of urea in the perfused collecting duct was not significantly different from that in plasma water from an adjacent vas rectum, and there was no evidence for active urea transport.

Results were strikingly different in protein depleted rats (Fig. 3). Here it is noted that in almost every instance the urea concentration in collecting duct fluid was lower than that in the adjacent vas rectum. If at the time of aspiration of the perfused sample net fluxes of water and all solutes were zero (and this appears to be a reasonable assumption), these observations indicate active transport of urea out of the collecting ducts in the protein deficient rats. In other experiments these investigators added C^{14}-labeled urea to the aqueous perfusate and noted that the unidirectional efflux of urea in rats on a low protein diet was higher than in rats on a normal diet. ULLRICH and his colleagues concluded from these studies that active transport of urea occurs in the collecting ducts of protein depleted rats but could not be demonstrated in rats on a diet containing adequate protein.

Conclusion

In summary, the evidence now available leads almost inescapably to the conclusion that active transport of urea out of medullary collecting ducts can occur under certain conditions in the mammalian kidney. The phenomenon is most readily demonstrated in protein depleted animals, but there is also evidence to suggest that protein depletion may not be a necessary condition for its occurrence. There is no convincing evidence at the present time for active urea transport elsewhere in the mammalian nephron, although this possibility is not excluded. It is probable that under most circumstances active transport plays a relatively minor role in the overall pattern of urea reabsorption in the mammalian kidney. Although we can no longer accept as rigorously correct Shannon's suggestion of three decades ago, that physical diffusion may be tentatively accepted as the cause of urea reabsorption, there seems little reason to doubt that, except possibly under exceptional circumstances, most of the transtubular movement of urea in the mammalian kidney is passive.

References

1. BRAY, G. A., and A. S. PRESTON: Effect of urea on urine concentration in the rat. J. clin. Invest. **40**, 1952—1960 (1961).
2. ČAPEK, K., G. FUCHS, G. RUMRICH u. K. J. ULLRICH: Harnstoffpermeabilität der corticalen Tubulusabschnitte von Ratten in Antidiurese und Wasserdiurese. Pflügers Arch. ges. Physiol. **290**, 237—249 (1966).
3. CLAPP, J.: Renal tubular reabsorption of urea in normal and protein-depleted rats. Amer. J. Physiol. **210**, 1304—1308 (1966).
4. FORSTER, R.: Active cellular transport of urea by frog renal tubules. Amer. J. Physiol. **179**, 372—377 (1954).
5. GOLDBERG, M., A. M. WOJTCZAK, and M. A. RAMIREZ: Uphill transport of urea in the dog kidney: Effects of certain inhibitors. J. clin. Invest. **46**, 388—399 (1967).
6. GRANTHAM, J. J., and M. B. BURG: Effect of vasopressin and cyclic AMP on permeability of isolated collecting tubules. Amer. J. Physiol. **211**, 255—259 (1966).
7. KLÜMPER, J. D., K. J. ULLRICH u. H. H. HILGER: Das Verhalten des Harnstoffs in den Sammelrohren der Säugetierniere. Pflügers Arch. ges. Physiol. **267**, 238—243 (1958).
8. LASSITER, W. E., C. W. GOTTSCHALK, and M. MYLLE: Micropuncture study of net transtubular movement of water and urea in nondiuretic mammalian kidney. Amer. J. Physiol. **200**, 1139—1146 (1961).
9. — M. MYLLE, and C. W. GOTTSCHALK: Net transtubular movement of water and urea in saline diuresis. Amer. J. Physiol. **206**, 669—673 (1964).
10. — — — Micropuncture study of urea transport in rat renal medulla. Amer. J. Physiol. **210**, 965—970 (1966).
11. SCHMIDT-NIELSEN, B.: Urea excretion in mammals. Physiol. Rev. **38**, 139—168 (1958).
12. —, and R. O'DELL: Effect of diet on distribution of urea and electrolytes in kidneys of sheep. Amer. J. Physiol. **197**, 856—860 (1959).

13. SHANNON, J. A.: Glomerular filtration and urea excretion in relation to urine flow in the dog. Amer. J. Physiol. **117**, 206—225 (1936).
14. — Urea excretion in the normal dog during forced diuresis. Amer. J. Physiol. **122**, 782—787 (1938).
15. SMITH, H. W.: The absorption and excretion of water and salts by the elasmobranch fishes. I. Fresh water elasmobranchs. Amer. J. Physiol. **98**, 279—295 (1931).
16. — The absorption and excretion of water and salts by the elasmobranch fishes. II. Marine elasmobranchs. Amer. J. Physiol. **98**, 296—310 (1931).
17. TRUNIGER, B., and B. SCHMIDT-NIELSEN: Intrarenal distribution of urea and related compounds: effects of nitrogen intake. Amer. J. Physiol. **207**, 971—978 (1964).
18. ULLRICH, K. J., u. K. H. JARAUSCH: Untersuchungen zum Problem der Harnkonzentrierung und Harnverdünnung. Über die Verteilung von Elektrolyten (Na, K, Ca, Mg, Cl, anorganischen Phosphat), Harnstoff, Aminosäuren und exogenem Kreatinin in Rinde und Mark der Hundeniere bei verschiedenen Diuresezuständen. Pflügers Arch. ges. Physiol. **262**, 537—550 (1956).
19. — G. RUMRICH, and B. SCHMIDT-NIELSEN: Urea transport in the collecting duct of rats on normal and low protein diet. Pflügers Arch. ges. Physiol. **295**, 147—156 (1967).

1.1.3. The Fate of Urea in the Rat's Kidney, as Studied by Micropuncture and Tissue Analysis* **

FRANÇOISE ROCH-RAMEL, FRANÇOISE CHOMÉTY and G. PETERS[1]

With 1 Figure

Complete equilibration of infused C^{14}-tagged urea with the large amounts of this solute present in renal tissues (ROCH-RAMEL and PETERS, 1967) appears doubtful. Micropuncture experiments, using a chemical ultramicromethod for estimating urea (ROCH-RAMEL, 1967) and inulin (ROCH-RAMEL et al., 1968) concentrations in tubular fluid were, therefore, done in untreated non-diuretic rats and in non-diuretic rats receiving enough intravenous urea to double the plasma concentration.

The fractional reabsorption of urea from proximal tubular fluid in both groups was comparable to that measured by LASSITER et al. (1961) with C^{14}-urea in non-diuretic rats. Addition of urea to fluid running through Henle's loops, as demonstrated by a higher fraction of filtered urea in early distal as compared to late proximal tubules, occurred only in 1/4 of the nephrons, whose early distal convolutions were punctured, but was observed in the majority of all early distal samples in the experiments of LASSITER et al. (1961). High and low values for early distal urea were often found in different early distal tubules from the same rat. Recirculation of urea from collecting duct fluid to a fraction of Henle's loops remains a possible explanation of high early distal fractions of non-reabsorbed urea, even though a loss of urea from collecting duct fluid could not be demonstrated with certainty in our experiments (Table). As in LASSITER'S (1961) experiments, the rate of loss of urea from distal convolutions was somewhat smaller than from proximal convolutions, in spite of the much larger concentration gradient at the distal site (Table).

The concentration of urea in cortical tissue water was consistently much higher than in proximal tubular fluid from any proximal site of the same rats, in untreated as well as in urea-infused non-diuretic rats. Cortical urea concentration was also significantly higher than distal tubular fluid urea concentrations in the untreated, but not in the urea-infused animals (Table). Even in the latter situation distal tubular fluid cannot account for the urea concentrations found in cortical tissue water (ROCH-RAMEL and PETERS, 1967). Since there is practically no interstitial space in renal cortical tissue, and since neither the presence of tubular fluid nor of blood in the tissue specimens can account for the high cortical urea concentration, cortical tubular cells must be assumed to contain large amounts of urea. This conclusion must be concealed with the apparently diffusional

* Supported by Fonds National Suisse de la Recherche Scientifique (Grants No 2966 and 4495).

** Abstract. Full paper: ROCH-RAMEL et al., 1968.

[1] Institut de Pharmacologie de l'Université de Lausanne.

overall movement of urea through the walls of cortical proximal tubules (Fig. 1). The overall diffusional movement could in fact be the sum of active transport through the luminal membrane with a low permeability to urea and diffusional loss through a highly urea permeable contraluminal membrane Fig. 1: A). Alternatively there could be some kind of sequestration of urea in cortical tubular

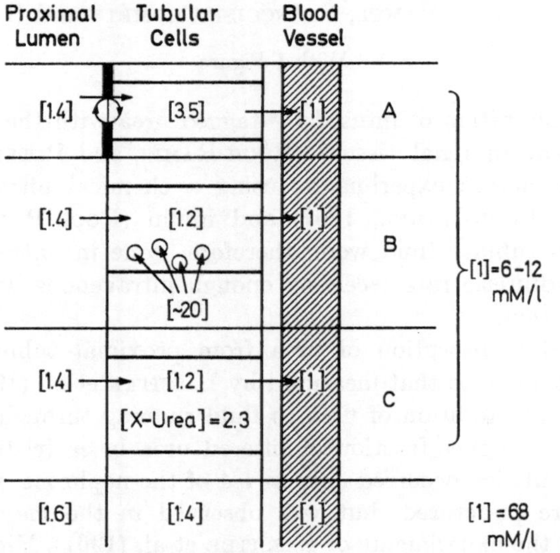

Fig. 1. Schematic representation of possible explanations for the transport of urea through proximal tubular cells containing urea in high concentrations

Table. *Non-reabsorbed fractions of filtered urea (percent). Means ± S.E.*

	Untreated non-diuretic rats (urea in plasma water 5.5 ± 0.6 mM/L)	Infusion of urea (urea in plasma water 11.8 ± 1.1 mM/L)	Values of LASSITER et al. (1961)
Late proximal (>60%)	40 ± 10	50 ± 11	50
Early distal (25—30%)	75 ± 20	69 ± 24	110
Late distal (>60%)	37 ± 7	41	70
Unteral urine	37 ± 4	40 ± 8	13

cells (Fig. 1: B and C) comparable to the sequestration observed under other circumstances in papillary tissue (ROCH-RAMEL and PETERS, 1967). Sequestration could consist in either concentration of urea in subcellular structures or in binding of urea to some type of macromolecule. If the sequestered fraction of urea becomes physico-chemically inactive, the movement of non-sequestrated urea through proximal tubular cells could still be diffusional.

References

1. LASSITER, W. E., C. W. GOTTSCHALK, and M. MYLLE: Micropuncture study of net transtubular movement of water and urea in non-diuretic mammalian kidney. Amer. J. Physiol. **200**, 1139—1196 (1961).

2. Roch-Ramel, F.: An enzymic and fluorophotometric for estimating urea concentrations in nanoliter specimens. Analyt. Biochem. **21**, 372—381 (1967).
3. —, and G. Peters: Intrarenal urea and electrolyte concentrations as influenced by water diuresis and by hydrochlorothiazide. Europ. J. Pharmacol. **1**, 124—139 (1967).
4. — F. Chométy, and G. Peters: Urea concentrations in tubular fluid and in renal tissue of non-diuretic rats. Amer. J. Physiol. **215**, 429—438 (1968).

Discussion

Wiederholt:

Did you measure proximal passage times of tubular fluid? You found inulin-TF/P ratios of 3—6 at the end of the accessible proximal convolutions. If these values were unchanged, this would mean that glomerulo-tubular balance was maintained in spite of the infusion of urea. This could be due to a change in passage time or in tubular geometry. Was the extracellular space expanded in your experiments?

Kopp:

Which amounts of urea were infused per unit of time in order to raise the plasma urea concentration to twice its normal value?

Roch-Ramel:

Passage-times for lissamine-green were measured by a procedure which differs somewhat from that used in your laboratory: we injected 1.25 ml/kg of a 2% solution of lissamine-green, within less than 0.5 sec., into a jugular vein. We then recorded the appearance of the first and of the last proximal tubule, as well as the disappearance of the first and of the last proximal tubule. The same procedure was applied to the distal tubules. There was no difference in the time of appearance of the proximal tubules between unloaded and urea-infused rats; the disappearance of lissamine-green from proximal tubular lumina started at the same time in both groups, the last proximal tubule was, however, free of lissamine-green 35.1 ± 3.3 seconds after injection in the urea-infused, as compared to 48.9 ± 4.4 seconds in the unloaded non-diuretic animals. Also the dye appeared significantly earlier in, and disappeared significantly earlier from, the distal tubules. Passage times, thus, appeared slightly shortened in the urea-infused animals. On the other hand, GFR was lower (1 ± 0.4 ml/kidney·kg·min) in the urea-infused that in the unloaded non-diuretic rats (3.1 ± 0.2 ml/kidney·kg·min). The non-reabsorbed fraction of filtered water (P/TF_{inulin}) in four specimens from late proximal (>60%) tubules of urea-infused rats was 45 ± 9% against 23 ± 5% in five late proximal specimens from unloaded rats. The difference is significant: the number of specimens analysed is, however, too small to allow conclusions.

In order to increase plasma urea concentrations, the animals were given an i.v. priming injection of 1 ml/kg of a 3.6% solution of urea in isotonic saline solution followed by an infusion at a rate of 0.05 ml/rat·min. of a solution containing 2.4% of urea + 5.6% of inulin in isotonic saline solution. This small rate of infusion may not be expected to induce an expansion of E.C.F.

1.1.4. Transtubular Movement of Urea and Related Compounds *

BRUNO TRUNIGER and BODIL SCHMIDT-NIELSEN[1]

With 2 Figures

Micropuncture and microcatheterization studies in antidiuretic rodents have shown that the amount of urea reabsorbed in the proximal and distal tubule is greater than the total urea reabsorption calculated from standard clearance experiments [2]. Furthermore the amount of urea present in the distal convolution is greater than that at the end of the proximal tubule. It has been concluded, therefore, that part of the urea reabsorbed in the collecting duct enters the loop of HENLE and recycles through the distal segments of the nephron. In antidiuresis this recycling fraction was calculated on the basis of the available micropuncture data to amount to some 5/8 of the urea reabsorbed from the collecting duct or approximately 50% of the filtered load. Since, however, the fraction of filtered urea excreted varies directly with the urine flow rate, it could be expected that changes in flow rate through the segments of the nephron permeable to urea would considerably change the intrarenal movements of urea. More recent micropuncture data tend to confirm this assumption [3]. The probable functional differences between superficial and deep nephron units still cause some difficulties as to the quantitative interpretation of the data. For this reason the intrarenal movement of urea was investigated in the rat by means of the indicator diffusion technique. Similar experiments have been performed on dogs by CHINARD [1], but without quantitative analysis of the results. Using this technique and ZIERLER's method for analysing the data [6], we have concentrated on two problems: 1. the relationship between urine flow rate and the transtubular movement of urea, 2. the influence of nitrogen intake upon transtubular movements of urea. In addition, the mode of excretion of methylurea, thiourea and acetamide, three compounds closely related chemically to urea, was studied. Our experiments, in agreement with those of CHINARD, showed a clearcut relationship between urine flow rate and the transtubular movement of urea and also demonstrated a higher permeability of the tubule to urea in rats on a low protein diet than in animals fed a normal laboratory diet.

Methods

Experiments were carried out on 26 adult Wistar rats weighing 300 to 500 g. Six animals had been fed a low protein diet (7% protein) for at least 3 weeks previously. After light Nembutal anesthesia the animal's abdomen was opened through a midline incision and both ureters were catheterized using PE 10 polyethylene tubing of equal length. The tips of the catheters were carefully placed into the kidney pelvis. A length of 20 cm PE 10 tubing was

* This work was supported by Public Health Service Grant A — 1956.

[1] Medizinische Universitätsklinik Bern and Department of Biology, Western Reserve University, Cleveland.

inserted into the aorta in a cephalad direction so that its tip was exactly at, or at most 1 mm above the origin of the left renal artery. but 3—5 mm below the right renal artery. The aorta was tied just below the origin of the left renal artery. To avoid decreased blood flow to the left renal artery due to the presence of the aortic catheter the tip of the catheter was pulled in a platinum wire coil so as to have a maximal external diameter of 0.1 mm. Urine flow rate was measured immediately before and after each experiment using calibrated polyethylene tubing. Only preparations with equal flow from both kidneys (within 5%) were used for the following experiments.

A small volume of 0.9% saline (20 to 50 µl) containing inulin-methoxy-H^3 and either C^{14}-urea, C^{14}-thiourea, C^{14}-methylurea or C^{14}-acetamide was injected within 5 seconds through the aortic catheter, and the urine from both ureteral catheters was sampled separately into counting vials at regular intervals of 1 or 2 minutes. Injections were performed in the same animal first in antidiuresis and then during mannitol diuresis (an inverted sequence did not change the results). Depending on urinary flow rate, 10 to 20 samples were taken from each catheter after the injection. The C^{14}- and H^3-activities in the urine samples were determined simultaneously using a Packard Tricarb Liquid Scintillation Counter. In order to keep all urine solutes in solution, the samples were mixed with 0.5 ml of Hyamine Hydroxide before adding the counting liquid.

Calculation of the results. As described by Chinard [1] the differences between the excretion patterns of the left and the right kidney results from passage of the compounds through the left kidney first, only the left kidney excreting the tracers immediately after injection because of the placement of the aortic catheter distal to the right renal artery. In this way the right kidney serves to correct for systemic recirculation of the isotopes. The excretion of the labelled urea and inulin by the left kidney is taken as 1 (100%). Amounts of H^3-inulin and C^{14}-urea excreted in each collection period are expressed as fractions of the total excretion observed during the first passage of the two compounds through the left kidney. Thus the frequency function of transfer times for H^3-inulin and C^{14}-urea may be determined. Inulin, a material not subject to tubular transfer, serves as an indicator of tubular transport of any other substance filtered at the glomerulus, if the urinary excretion of that substance is significantly delayed. The results were analyzed graphically: the maximum integrated difference between the frequency function of the non-diffusible (inulin) and the diffusible indicator (urea-C^{14}) corresponds closely to the "transtubular" fraction of urea and related compounds (fraction α). The transfer time of the fraction $(1-\alpha)$ is the same as that of inulin.

Results

1. *Urine flow rate and transtubular movement of urea* (Figs. 1 and 2). The fraction α is closely related to the measured urine flow rate. There is very little variation in the value of α from one animal to another when allowance is made for urine flow rate. With increasing urine flow rate due to mannitol diuresis the magnitude of fraction α decreases. However with maximum urine flow, no values lower than 0.2 were observed, i.e. not less than 20% of the excreted urea-C^{14} had left the tubule on its way from the injection site to the kidney pelvis. With decreasing urine flow rate the value of α increases and, under conditions of maximum antidiuresis, amounts to 75—80% of the total excreted C^{14}-urea.

2. *The effect of protein intake upon intrarenal movements of urea* (Fig. 2). The relationship between urine flow rate and the urea excretion pattern found in normal control animals was not changed by the magnitude of protein intake. For any given urine flow rate, however, in protein restricted animals the delayed fraction α was always higher than in rats fed the 20% protein standard laboratory diet. In maximal mannitol diuresis, the minimum values for transtubular fraction in low protein rats was 40%, whereas in antidiuresis it increased up to 95% of the excreted C^{14}-urea. Since in protein restricted animals as well as in normal

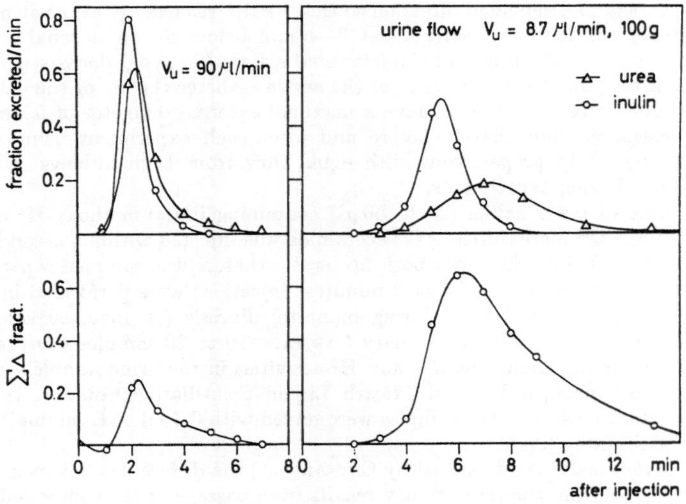

Fig. 1. Excretion patterns of H³-inulin and C¹⁴-urea after injection of the compounds into the left renal artery. Influence of urine flow rate upon the delayed fraction α. Fraction α corresponds to the maximum integrated difference between the frequency functions of labelled urea and inulin (see text)

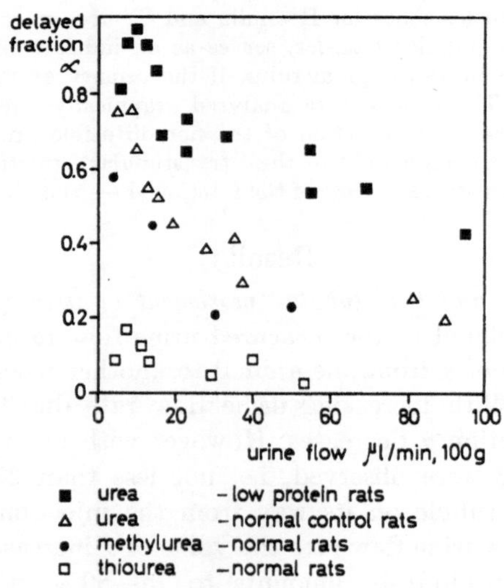

Fig. 2. Relationship between the delayed fraction α of excreted C¹⁴-urea (and related compounds) and urine flow rate. Effect of nitrogen intake

control rats the delayed fraction approaches 100% as urine flow rate decreases toward 0, the differences between normal and low protein rats increase with increasing urine flow rate.

3. *Transtubular movements of compounds chemically related to urea* (Fig. 2). Of the three additional compounds examined in the present series of experiments (thiourea, methylurea and acetamide) thiourea showed the smallest transtubular

transport value which also was little influenced by osmotic diuresis or antidiuresis. The values for methylurea were similar to those of urea. For any given urine flow, however, the transtubular fraction of methylurea was lower than that of urea. The excretion pattern of acetamide differed from that of the other compounds: whereas, with high urine flow rate, up to 40% of the excreted acetamide appeared ahead of the glomerular marker, the delayed fraction increased as urine flow decreased. The results were the same when C^{14}-methylurea, C^{14}-thiourea or C^{14}-acetamide were injected into animals previously given the respective cold compound in amounts to cause blood levels of 0.5—1.0 mM. It is concluded from this observation, that non-specific adsorption phenomena do not influence the excretion pattern of tracer amounts of the three compounds.

Discussion

The technique used in these experiments allows the separation of two fractions of excreted urea (and related compounds). Part of the filtered urea, fraction $(1-\alpha)$, escapes tubular reabsorption and, therefore, is excreted in a way kinetically similar to inulin. The complementary fraction, α, reaches the final urine only after leaving and reentering the tubular lumen. This latter fraction includes urea, that has recycled through the distal segments of the nephron. It therefore gives an index of the upper limit of the recycling process.

Using micropuncture data from antidiuretic rats [2] and rats under saline diuresis [3], the magnitude of fraction α can be predicted with the assumption, that the recycling process is the only cause for delayed excretion of C^{14}-urea. According to such calculations, the delayed fraction α would amount to 10% of excreted urea in saline diuresis and to 70—80% in maximal antidiuresis. In spite of the simplifying assumptions made in these calculations, the values are in good agreement with the results obtained in our experiments.

Previous studies concerning the influence of nitrogen intake upon the urea distribution in renal tissue [5] have shown a marked difference in the tubular handling of urea by animals on high and low protein diets. Similarly, the present experiments show, that for a given urine flow rate the delayed fraction α is considerably greater in animals on low protein diet than in normal control rats, again indicating increased transtubular movement of urea in the former animals. The experiments obviously do not allow any conclusions concerning the nature of the transport process.

Regarding the specificity of the tubular permeability and transport processes involved, our experiments with three compounds chemically related to urea are of interest. Whereas *methyl-urea* shows essentially the same excretion pattern as does urea, it differs quantitatively from urea in that for a given urine flow rate fraction α is smaller than that of urea. This finding is in good agreement with results obtained in clearance studies, and can be interpreted as a sign of lower tubular permeability to methylurea. The absolute changes in fraction α brought about by changes in urine flow rate are smaller than those found for urea. This is even more true for *thiourea*, which, under conditions of high and low urine flow, shows an excretion pattern very similar to that of the non-diffusible, glomerular indicator — again agreeing well with previous observations that the collecting duct of the rat is quite impermeable to thiourea [5]. *Acetamide* shows an excretion pattern quite different from the other three compounds. In high, as well as in low urine flow conditions a considerable fraction of acetamide preceeds the glomerular indicator. Whereas delayed excretion cannot be demonstrated at high urine flow rates, a delayed fraction appears and increases with decreasing urine flow. A similar precession over the glomerular tracer has occasionally been observed with urea and methylurea, although in much smaller amounts. These findings seem to indicate a high permeability of the tubule or some tubular segments to acetamide. The excretion patterns of the compounds tested in these experiments show an interesting correlation with findings on the enhancement of the renal concentrating ability by urea and related compounds [4]: urea increases the concentrating ability more than methylurea and methylurea enhances more than thiourea.

Summary

Micropuncture experiments in antidiuretic rats have shown, that part of the urea reabsorbed in the collecting duct enters Henle's loop and recycles through the distal segments of the tubule. The relationship between this transtubular movement of urea (and related compounds) and the urine flow rate was studied using the indicator diffusion technique. Inulin-methoxy-H^3 served as the non-diffusible, C^{14}-urea (and related compounds) as the diffusible indicator. After injection of the labelled compounds into the left renal artery, urine excretion was collected in intervals of 1 to two minutes. Fraction α was calculated as that fraction of excreted urea that appeared delayed as compared to the non-diffusible indicator. This fraction increases from 20% in mannitol diuresis to 75—80% in maximum antidiuresis. These values are in good agreement with the values predicted on the basis of available micropuncture data. For any given urine flow rate, fraction α was always higher in protein restricted animals than in normal control rats. The transtubular fraction α of excreted methylurea is always lower than that of urea when allowance for variations in urine flow rate is made. Thiourea showed the smallest values for α. The excretion pattern of acetamide indicates a high permeability of the tubule or some tubular segments to this compound.

References

1. CHINARD, F. P., and T. ENNS: Relative renal excretion patterns of sodium ion, chloride ion, urea, water and glomerular substances. Amer. J. Physiol. **182**, 247—250 (1955).
2. LASSITER, W. E., C. W. GOTTSCHALK, and M. MYLLE: Micropuncture study of net transtubular movement of water and urea in nondiuretic mammalian kidney. Amer. J. Physiol. **200**, 1139—1146 (1962).
3. — M. MYLLE, and C. W. GOTTSCHALK: Net transtubular movement of water and urea in saline diuresis. Amer. J. Physiol. **206**, 669—673 (1964).
4. RABINOWITZ, L., and R. H. KELLOGG: Enhancement of renal concentrating ability in the dog by urea and related compounds. Amer. J. Physiol. **205**, 112—116 (1963).
5. TRUNIGER, B., and BODIL SCHMIDT-NIELSEN: Intrarenal distribution of urea and related compounds: effects of nitrogen intake. Amer. J. Physiol. **207**, 971—978 (1964).
6. ZIERLER, K. L.: Theory of use of indicators to measure blood flow and extracellular volume and calculation of transcapillary movement of tracers. Circulat. Res. **12**, 464—471 (1963).

1.1.5. Chronic Overloading with Urea in Rats

D. F. Grossmann, L. Gebauer and A. Nolte[1]

With 2 Figures

It was the purpose of the present experiments to investigate the effects of chronic overloading with urea on the renal clearance and the plasma concentration of urea in rats.

Methods

The experimental animals were female Wistar rats weighing 180—200 g, with an initial serum urea concentration below 6.6 mM/l. Urea was added to the drinking water in concentrations from 0.25 to 2 M. Rat pellets (Hope Farms, containing 14% protein) and drinking fluid were given ad lib. The experimental animals were divided into 7 groups receiving drinking fluid containing different concentrations of urea for different times. Each experimental group comprised 15—20 overloaded or control rats.

Urea concentrations were assayed by enzymic cleavage and photometric measurement of NH_4^+ concentrations with 5-indophenol according to Berthelot's method [1] modified according to [2], in serum (25 µl) or urine [3]. Ammonia concentrations were measured by the same method. Na^+ and K^+ concentrations in serum, urine and homogenates of the kidneys, the liver, the spleen, the heart and the brain were measured by flame photometry. Chloride concentrations in serum, urine and tissue homogenates were measured by automatized potentiometric titration with Ag^+ (Tritrimeter and automatic burette made by Radiometer, Copenhagen). Hemoglobin was assayed photometrically as HbCN. Inulin concentrations in serum and in urine were determined according to [3].

The urinary clearance of urea was measured either (a) in metabolic cages for periods of at least 2, but usually 24 hours, or (b) with clearance periods of 30 min during 2 hours' i.v. infusion of a urea containing solution. The latter solution contained 1.0—2.0 M urea dissolved in 0.9% NaCl and was infused at rates between 0.1 and 0.2 ml/min after a priming injection of 0.5—2.0 ml of the same solution. The urinary clearance of inulin was always measured simultaneously with the clearance of urea in experimental as well as in control animals. Inulin was added to the i.v. solution at a concentration of 50 mg/100 ml.

Histologic and electron-microscopic investigations of the kidneys or liver tissue were done on tissues fixed in glutaric dialdehyde or in glutaric dialdehyde/osmium tetroxide. In a few experiments, superficial cortical tissue was fixed intravitally by applying a few drops of the fixing solution to the surface. All values are given as means ±S.D.

---

[1] II. Med. Univ.-Klinik und Pathologisches Institut der Universität Frankfurt/Main, West Germany.

Results

In the urea-loaded animals, the urinary clearance of urea rose above the initial normal value of 45 ±10 ml/h to values as high as 200 ml/h. Urea-clearances measured in metabolic cages did not differ significantly from those measured during the 1st and the 2nd 30 min periods of intravenous infusion of urea, while the 3rd and 4th 30 min period clearances with i.v. infusions were usually 20—30% lower. In the first days after overloading with urea via the drinking fluid, or after increasing the concentration of urea in the drinking fluid, the urinary clearance of urea usually rose to very high values which subsequently fell back

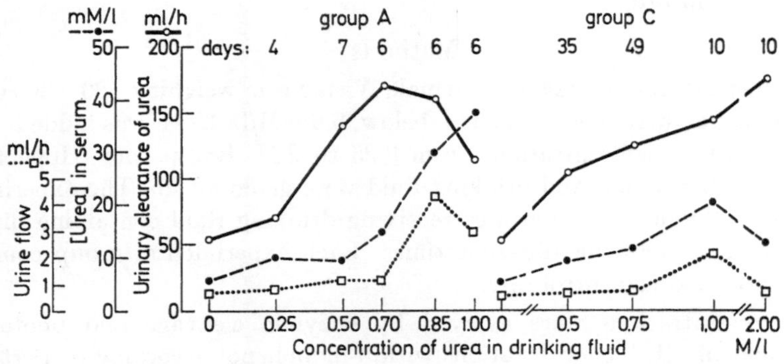

Fig. 1. Two groups of experimental animals loaded with urea in the drinking fluid at different concentrations for different times. The values shown in group A are those of the last days of the administration of a given concentration of urea. The values shown for group C refer to steady state values reached after 10 to 14 days. All values are means from groups of 20 rats. The standard deviations of these values were the following: clearance of urea ±16%, urea concentration in serum: ±10%, urine flow ±25%. Clearances of urea were measured in metabolic cages for periods of 2—24 hours, or else in 2×30 min periods in the course of an i.v. infusion of urea. The urine flows shown were measured in metabolic cages and not in the course of i.v. infusion of fluid

to steady state values. With concentrations of urea of 0.25—0.35 M in the drinking fluid, the renal clearance of urea did not rise significantly, while the plasma urea concentration reached twice its normal value. The highest clearances of urea, up to 200 ml/h, were observed in animals initially loaded with urea solutions containing less than 0.7 M urea, with subsequent increases by 0.25 M at 10 day intervals. After preloading with 0.7—0.8 M urea solutions, and after a 10 day interval on a 1.0 M urea solution, the animals may be given a 2.0 M urea solution without further intermediary steps. When rats not preloaded with urea were given drinking fluid containing more than the critical concentration of 0.7—0.8 M, half of the animals died within 2 weeks. Until death, the urinary clearance of urea in these animals did not rise above 110 ml/h. Fig. 1 shows the renal clearance of urea, plasma urea concentrations and the average urine flow in 2 groups of experimental animals which were started on different concentrations of urea in drinking fluid and overloaded for different times. In group A, the drinking fluid urea concentration was increased too rapidly: at higher concentrations, therefore, the plasma concentration of urea rose and the renal clearance fell. In group C, a progressive increase in the drinking fluid urea concentration resulted in a progressive increase in the renal clearance of urea.

In a fraction of the animals progressively adapted to a 1.0 M concentration of urea in drinking fluid, the renal clearance of urea, after an initial rise, fell progressively with a simultaneous rise of the serum-urea concentration up to 100 and death of the animals. This sequence of events occurred in 1/5 to 1/3 of all experimental animals of different groups, overloaded for periods of 3 months

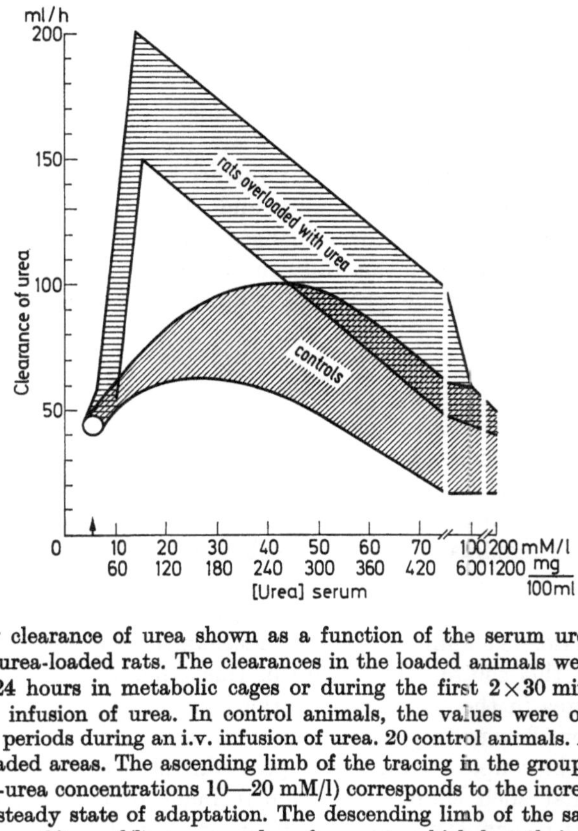

Fig. 2. Urinary clearance of urea shown as a function of the serum urea concentration in control and in urea-loaded rats. The clearances in the loaded animals were measured during periods of 2—24 hours in metabolic cages or during the first 2×30 min clearance periods during the i.v. infusion of urea. In control animals, the values were obtained during the first 2×30 min periods during an i.v. infusion of urea. 20 control animals. All measured values fell into the shaded areas. The ascending limb of the tracing in the group of the urea loaded animals (serum-urea concentrations 10—20 mM/l) corresponds to the increase of the clearance of urea in the steady state of adaptation. The descending limb of the same tracing (serum-urea values above 20 mmol/l) groups values from rats which lost their adaptation of urea excretion during a chronic overloading and showed falling values of the clearance of urea together with rising values of the plasma-urea concentrations

or longer. A progressive decrease of the urinary clearance of urea, after an initial adaptation, was regularly observed in animals whose serum-urea concentration was above 30 mM/l for more than 7 days.

When normal, not pretreated rats were overloaded with urea by the i.v. route, the serum-urea concentration rose to variable extents, while the clearance of urea rose less than in the chronically overloaded rats and never exceeded twice the control value. The initial rise was usually followed by a secondary fall in spite of continued high rates of urine flow. These results are summarized in Fig. 2: the renal clearance of urea is represented as a function of the urea concentration in the serum in rats chronically overloaded by the oral route, and in animals acutely overloaded by the i.v. route.

In rats adapted to a high oral intake of urea, the clearance of inulin had a value of 85 ± 10 ml/h, compared to 90 ± 10 ml/h in control animals. In the course of infusion experiments the values of the inulin clearance in the 3rd and 4th periods decreased to the same extent as the clearance of urea, i.e. by 20—30%. Plasma inulin concentrations varied from 0.5—1.5 mg/100 ml.

The renal excretion of sodium, potassium, chloride and ammonia was slightly accelerated during adaptation to all urea loads. In the steady state of adaptation the excretion of these ions occurred at the same rate as in normal control rats.

The total hemoglobin concentration of blood increased to 4 gm/100 ml in the animals overloaded with high concentration of urea. The tissue concentrations of sodium, potassium and chloride were not influenced by overloading with urea. Morphologic investigations of the kidneys and the livers of the overloaded animals did not show any pathological changes. Measurements of the diameter of the proximal tubules fixed intravitally in the course of an i.v. infusion of urea showed a dilatation of the proximal tubules in comparison to those of control animals.

Discussion

Chronic progressive overloading with urea in rats resulted in an increase in the clearance of urea which, after 14 days, reached a high steady state level. The slowness of adaptation could be the expression of an enzymic adaptation. With the clearance of inulin as a measure of glomerular filtration rate, the clearance of urea should maximally reach the value of the clearance of inulin, but should not exceed it, if urea was excreted solely by filtration and by back-diffusion. Since we found clearances of urea higher than the clearance of inulin in chronically overloaded animals, another mechanism must contribute to the renal excretion of this solute. The nature of this other mechanism responsible for transport of urea in the secretory direction is as yet unknown. The present experiments do not allow us to postulate active transport since the transport has not been shown to be coupled to an energy providing process. It should, however, be pointed out that such coupling is often difficult to demonstrate [4]. The unknown transport mechanism appears to be impaired in the presence of plasma urea concentrations exceeding 20 mM/l.

Summary

1. Chronic overloading with urea by adding the solute to the drinking fluid induced an increase in the renal clearance of urea which in some animals exceeded the clearance of inulin.

2. In chronically overloaded animals, the increase of the renal clearance of urea occurred progressively within the time of adaptation of 10 to 14 days, after which it remained at a high level.

3. No light or electron-microscopic pathological changes were seen in the kidneys and in the livers of the experimental animals.

References

1. RICHTERICH, R.: Klinische Chemie, S. 219—222. Frankfurt 1965.
2. GROSSMANN, D. F.: Unpublished.
3. HUBBARD, R. S., and T. A. LOOMIS: The determination of inulin. J. biol. Chem. **145**, 641—645 (1942).
4. SCHLÖGL, R.: Zum Materietransport durch Porenmembranen. Habil.-Schr. Göttingen 1957.

Discussion

ROTTER:

Chronic urea loading induces renal hypertrophy. Is this hypertrophy related to the functional changes in urea excretion observed by the authors?

SCHIRMEISTER:

What methods were used for measuring the clearances of inulin and of urea? Are the values given 24 hour clearances? At what intervals were plasma concentrations measured? Were the inulin concentrations in plasma constant or did they fall during the period of observation? Do the authors think that their results prove the occurence of urea movements in the secretory direction?

SCHOLZ:

In experiments designed to measure the compartment in which 14 C-urea and THO would distribute in rats made "uremic" by overloading with urea, we made a few observations which confirm some of the conclusions of GROSSMANN et al.

All experiments were done on Sprague-Dawley rats weighing 150—200 g. One group of animals was given a molar solution of urea instead of water as a drinking fluid. Half of the animals in this group died within one week. The other half was killed by exsanguination. Blood urea-N ranged between 200 and 300 mg-%. Two other groups of rats were given either 0.5 M, or 0.75 M urea solution as drinking fluid for two weeks. After this time, both groups received a moler urea solution as drinking fluid, for 7 weeks. None of the experimental animals died within this time. The blood urea-N values one week after switching to molar urea solution ranged between 40—60 mg-%, presumably as a consequence of an increase in the renal clearance of urea.

GROSSMANN:

To ROTTER:

In our experiments we have not estimated the kidney-weights systematically. Single measurements showed no increase in kidney weight in respect to body weight (control rats compared with treated rats).

To SCHIRMEISTER:

The urea- and inulin-clearances were measured 1. by i.v.-infusion of urea- and inulin-solutions during 2-hour-periods, the plasma levels being constant, using collecting periods of 30 minutes, 2. urea-clearances were also measured in metabolic cages in periods up to 24 hours, with plasma samples taken every 2—4 hours. Taking the inulin-clearance as a measure of CFR, urea moves in the secretory direction under the conditions of our experiments.

1.1.6. Kinetics of the Movements of Urea through a Biological Membrane

D. F. GROSSMANN and K. F. KOPP[1]

With 2 Figures

When blood is dialyzed against a physiological salt solution containing a lower concentration of urea, the blood urea concentration falls stepwise rather than continuously. This particular behavior is explained by adductive n-alkyl-binding to the red blood cell membranes [4], since urea is generally known to be subject to adductive binding to n-alkyl groups [1, 2, 3]. The assumption requires that the urea concentration in red blood cell water must be higher than in plasma water and must equally change stepwise rather than continuously with changes in the plasma urea concentration. Furthermore, the rates of transport of urea should be different for plasma and red blood cells when blood is the transport vehicle for urea between two compartments. The extent of the difference should depend on urea binding steps in red blood cells in the course of the transfer.

The present experiments were undertaken in order to find experimental answers to the following questions: 1. Is the ratio of the concentrations of urea in red blood cells to that in serum more variable than expected in the case of a constant distribution between the two phases? 2. Are the urea transport rates from red blood cells to plasma constant, while the blood transports urea from tissues to the dialyzing fluid during hemodialysis?

Formulas

1. Ratio of concentrations of urea between red blood cells and serum: if the error of measurement of a concentration of urea is Δc, the error of the ratio $c_{\mathrm{RBC}}/c_{\mathrm{ser}}$ will be:

$$\frac{c_{\mathrm{RBC}}}{c_{\mathrm{ser}}} = \frac{c_{\mathrm{ser}} + c_{\mathrm{RBC}}}{c_{\mathrm{ser}}} \Delta c\,. \tag{1}$$

2. Transport of urea through blood: within a time Δt decreases of the urea concentration of RBC or of serum must be $\Delta c = \frac{g_1 - g_2}{V}$ (g_1 amount of urea leaving a phase during Δt; g_2 amount of urea entering a phase during Δt; V volume of the phase). The ratio of the influx of urea to the outflux of urea will then be:

$$\frac{\Phi 2}{\Phi 1} = \frac{g_1 - V \cdot \Delta c}{g_1}\,. \tag{2}$$

Defining:

dc_{ser} The decrease in urea concentration of serum in the course of one passage through the dialyzer considered for the period Δt;

φ_B blood flow through the dialyzer;

[1] II. Med. Univ.-Klinik, Frankfurt/Main, West Germany.

V_B blood volume;
Δc_{step} Urea concentration step in RBC when an adductive binding step of urea to an n-alkyl occurs.

One may write:

$$F = \frac{\Delta c_{\text{step}}}{\Delta c_{\text{RBC}}}, \quad f = \frac{c_{\text{RBC}}}{c_{\text{ser}}}$$

related to the volume of both phases,

$$L = \frac{dc_{\text{ser}} \cdot \varphi_B \cdot \Delta t}{\Delta c_{\text{ser}} \cdot V_B}.$$

The ratio of the ratios Φ_2/Φ_1 of RBC and serum:

$$R = \frac{(\Phi_2/\Phi_1)_{\text{RBC}}}{(\Phi_2/\Phi_1)_{\text{ser}}} = \frac{L - \frac{f+F}{f}}{L-1} \tag{3}$$

if $\Delta c_{\text{ser}} \ll dc_{\text{ser}}$.

If during the time of observation, no binding step of urea in the RBC membrane is crossed, lm/Δc step would become equal to 0 and $F=0$ and: $R=1$. In any other case $R<1$.

Methods

1. Blood samples from patients submitted to chronic hemodialysis in our hospital. Samples taken from the entrance and the exit of the dialyzer (Chron-A-Coil made by Travenol) with disposable syringes.

2. Separation of red blood cells: blood samples centrifuged at 6,000 g for 15 min. Pipetting the deposits. The RBC column contained 1% plasma as controlled by measurements of hematocrit in capillary tubes.

3. Water content of plasma and RBC measured gravimetrically by drying to constant weight at $105 \pm 1°$C in a vacuum over silicagel. Maximum error ± 0.5% as measured by fivefold determinations.

4. Urea concentrations measured in RBC and plasma (Ca-heparinate) by splitting with urease and subsequent measurement of ammonia according to Berthelot [5], modified according to [6]. Plasma samples were not deproteinized. Red blood cells were hemolyzed in distilled water, the urea was split enzymatically, the solution was deproteinized with H_2SO_4/tungstate, prior to measurement of ammonia concentrations. The maximum error of this method measured from curves for plasma and red blood cells was ± 2%.

5. The amount of urea removed according to equation [2] was found as difference in concentration at the entrance and at the exit of the dialyzer multiplied by flow of the phase considered and time. Between two values measured at intervals of 30 min, intermediate values were obtained by linear interpoliation. R was calculated by dividing Φ_2/Φ_1 for RBC and serum [Eq. (3)]. Total blood volume was assumed to be 1/12 of body weight.

6. All calculations were done on the electronic computer Programma 101 (Olivetti).

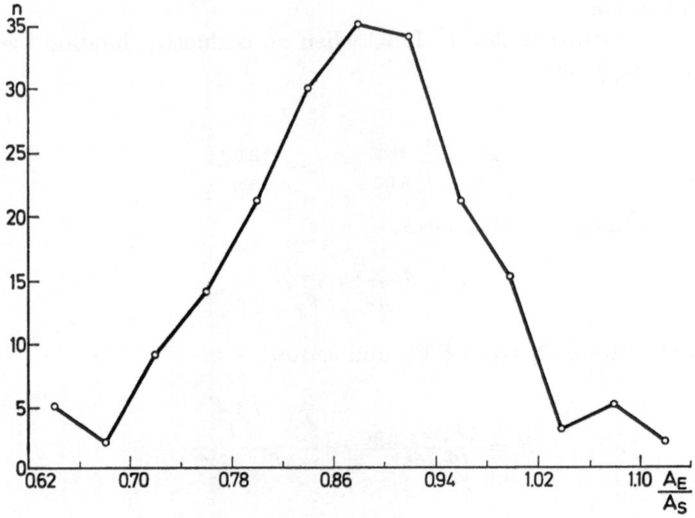

Fig. 1. Histogram of the frequency distribution of experimental ratios c_{RBC}/c_{ser} related to the phase volumes. Samples taken from the entrance to the dialyzer in 15 hemodialyses procedures (A_E = urea concentration in RBC, A_S = urea concentration in serum of these samples). n is the number of experimental A_E/A_S ratios within the intervals shown on the abscissa which correspond to 0.04 A_E/A_S. With samples obtained at the exit of the dialyzer a similar distribution is obtained

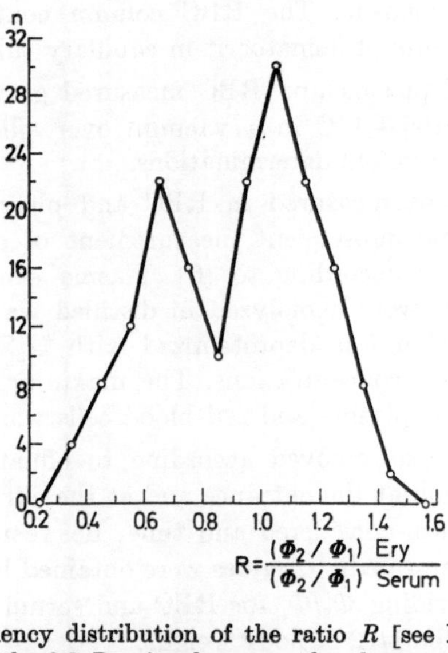

Fig. 2. Experimental frequency distribution of the ratio R [see Eq. (3)], n is the number of experimental values for the 0.1 R units shown on the abscissa. The R values shown were found during 15 hemodialysis procedures (173 observations) of 30 to 60 min. These values were obtained on the same material as the ratios c_{RBC}/c_{ser} shown on Fig. 1

Results

1. Distribution of urea between plasma and RBC: At a serum-urea concentration of 10—30 mM/l, the ratio

$$f = \frac{c_{\mathrm{RBC}}}{c_{\mathrm{ser}}} = 0.865 \pm 0.18 \text{ (SD)} .$$

The histogram of the distribution of the ratio is shown in Fig. 1. If the ratio is reported to the aqueous component of both phases, one obtains:

$$\frac{\overset{\mathrm{H_2O}}{c_{\mathrm{RBC}}}}{\underset{c_{\mathrm{ser}}}{\mathrm{H_2O}}} = 1.25 \pm 0.17 \text{ (SD)} .$$

2. Transport of urea through plasma and RBC: the histogram of the distribution of the ratio R is shown in Fig. 2. There are two peaks at $R = 1.05$ and $R = 0.65$. Each hemodialysis gives values within the slopes of both peaks. Calculating the difference in urea concentration occurring as a consequence of adductive binding in the membrane as compared to plasma [Eq. (3)], one obtains a value of 1.1 mM/l RBC (SD ± 0.2 mMl/l). This shows that any increase in plasma-urea concentration by 4.4 ± 0.9 mM/l leads from one step of adductive binding to the next.

Discussion

According to Eq. 1, the standard deviation of the ratio $c_{\mathrm{RBC}}/c_{\mathrm{ser}}$ should be 0.05. The same ratio should be found experimentally if the distribution was constant and independent of the serum-urea concentration. The experimental value being 3 times larger, the ratio $c_{\mathrm{RBC}}/c_{\mathrm{ser}}$ does not appear to be constant and could correspond to a variation as expected with several step-binding of urea in the membranes.

The 2 peaks of the histograms of R values show that the rates of transport from RBC to serum are not constant, but may be described by two different rate values. Since the condition $\Delta c_{\mathrm{ser}} \ll dc_{\mathrm{ser}}$ is well fulfilled during hemodialysis with control of removal of urea by adding urea to the dialyzing fluid [4], the ratio F in Eq. (3) would assume large values when computed over times long in comparison to the times of observation. R values, therefore, will be distinctly split into two peaks as shown in Fig. 2. The displacement of the peak at $R = 1.05$ by 0.05 from the expected value falls within the error of measurement.

Summary

The distribution of urea between RBC and serum, and the kinetics of urea transport of these 2 phases were calculated. The results are compatible with the model of adductive binding of urea to n-alkyl groups within the red blood cell unit membrane.

Discussion

BRASS:

Did you also observe a step-wise decrease instead of a continuous fall in plasma urea concentrations in patients submitted to peritoneal dialysis? This should be expected to occur, if the step-wise decrease in your observations on patients submitted to hemodialysis is due to the behavior of the red cell membrane and not to particular properties of the dialysing tubing used for hemodialysis.

PINGGERA:

What method was used for measuring the plasma urea concentration? Did you use heparinized whole blood? Did you use the auto-analyzer technique?

GROSSMANN:
To BRASS:

The stepwise decrease in plasma urea concentration is related to a critical elimination rate of urea. The elimination rates of urea during peritoneal dialysis are far beyond this critical value and a stepwise fall in plasma urea concentration is not to be expected. The urea clearances in peritoneal dialysis are also not constant with time, a condition, which makes exact measurements impossible.

To PINGGERA:

We analysed urea enzymatically in plasma and erythrocytes, collected from heparinized blood by centrifugation, We did not use the autoanalyzer technique.

1.1.7. Urine-Concentrating Mechanisms

KURT KRAMER[1]

With 2 Figures

In the animal kingdom, the ability to form a hypertonic urine appears first in mammals and is associated with the development of long loops of HENLE. The functional significance of these was not recognized by physiologists until 1951, although eight years earlier WERNER KUHN and RYFFEL had proposed the medullary loops as counter-current exchange diffusion systems [9]. In a model loop they demonstrated how concentration could occur by addition of a non-diffusible substance to the outgoing limb (Fig. 1). Since the model was not

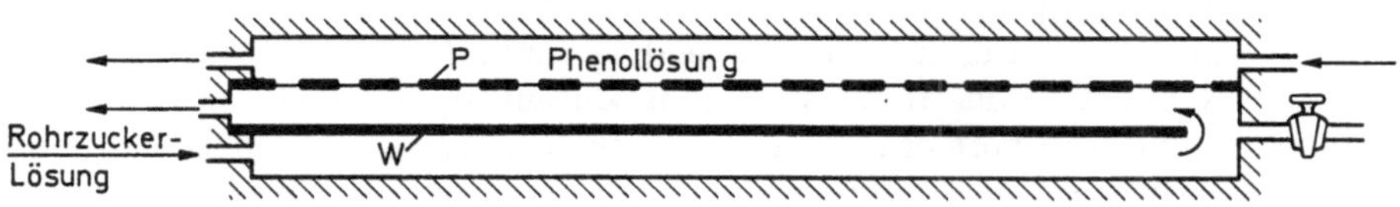

Fig. 1. Schematic drawing of Kuhn's model for concentrating sucrose utilizing the counter current principle. A phenol solution diffuses through a rubber membrane (*P*) thereby increasing molar concentration of the adjacent outflow tube of the hairpin loop. This increase leads to an osmotic water flow through the waterpermeable membrane (*W*) initiating a concentration gradient of saccharose up to the bend of the loop by counter current diffusion

strictly applicable — especially in regard to the necessary permeability characteristics of the loop-membranes — renal physiologists were slow to accept this concept which is nowadays indispensable to our understanding of the concentrating process [14].

In 1951 HARGITAY and KUHN [6] added a basically important hypothesis to the original theory: "The multiplication of a single effect" is based on the assumption that the energy for concentration is provided within the loop system itself, either by a hydrostatic pressure difference between the in and outgoing limb of the loop, or by some kind of electrochemical force driving substances from the out to the ingoing limb. By continuous repetition of such processes from the base to the tip of the loop, the single effect would be multiplied, leading to a concentration of the contents of the ingoing limb increasing from base to tip and a decreasing concentration of the outgoing limb fluid from tip to base of the loop. In an adjacent tube, more permeable to water than to solutes, the fluid could be concentrated by osmotic water loss into the loop system.

WIRZ [18] was the first physiologist to recognize the validity of KUHN's model [9] when applied to the renal medulla. He proved the existence of a counter-current multiplier system in Henle's loops by the demonstration, in the excised

[1] Physiologisches Institut der Universität München, West-Germany.

rat kidney, of decreasing freezing points of urine in loops and collecting ducts from base to tip of the renal papilla and equal freezing point values throughout slices cut perpendicularly to the papillary axis.

In a mathematical treatment of his model, Kuhn showed that the effectiveness of concentration increased with the length of the loop [9]. Indeed Peter [11] and, recently, Bodil Schmidt-Nielsen [13], in comparing the ratio of renal medulla to cortex thickness of a number of mammalian species, found a surprisingly good correlation with the ability of these animals to concentrate urine. Animals with short loops — like the beaver — are not able to concentrate urine to more than twice plasma osmolarity, while desert animals like the kangaroo rat with a high medulla-to-cortex ratio were found to produce a urine concentrated 17-fold with respect to plasma.

Kuhn's theory, in addition, requires hypotonicity of the fluid leaving the outgoing limb. Again Wirz [18] was able to show by micropuncture technique that the early distal fluid was hypotonic, a fact first observed, but not interpreted, by Walker [17]. It is, in fact, a necessary corollary to the removal of solute in excess of water from the ascending limb. Wirz suggested that this hypotonicity might be due to a low sodium concentration, which, in turn, could be due to active transport of sodium out of the ascending limb of Henle's loop. Since any active transport requires energy, Ullrich and Pehling [15] studied the O_2 uptake of kidney slices taken from cortical and medullary regions. In the outer medullary zone, but not in other layers, O_2-consumption increased with the sodium concentration of the medium, following Michaelis-Menton kinetics. This observation suggests an active transport of sodium in this location.

Ullrich and his co-workers [8] showed by catheterization of collecting ducts that urea, although becoming concentrated, leaves the duct fluid in considerable amounts. The idea of an active transport of urea back to the medullary system arose and was proved by the experiments of Ullrich and Schmidt-Nielsen [16] in rats on a low protein diet. In view of the high concentration of urea in medullary tissue, one is tempted to assign to urea an important role in concentrating urine. Whether this is accomplished by simple countercurrent exchange diffusion (see next paper of Reinhardt *et al.*) or by active transport of urea, cannot be decided at the present time.

Although the presence of a sodium transport mechanism in the *thin* limb of Henle's loops has been the subject of some controversy, Bennet and Berliner [1], applying the Sakai preparation which makes a considerable portion of the papilla accessible for micropuncture, succeeded in demonstrating osmolar differences of about 110 mosm/L between the ascending and descending limbs.

An additional mechanism operating within the concentrating process was proposed by Marsh [10] as a result of his findings in stop-flow perfusion studies on single collecting ducts of an isolated rat papilla *in vitro*. Marsh observed that the perfusion fluid decreased in volume and became hyperosmotic to both original perfusate and bath. Evidently the cells of the collecting duct are able to move a hypotonic sodium chloride solution into the interstitial space. Marsh believes that the collecting duct reabsorbate is the primary determinant of interstitial hyperosmolality. The finding of a concentrating process in a single straight tube, however, is not inconsistent with the general theory of the countercurrent system in the renal medulla, since Henle's loops and vasa recta, in Marsh's theory, act as counter-current exchangers and are still necessary for an effective concentrating process.

Whatever the mechanism of concentration may be, the inner medulla must supply the energy for the concentrating process, *i.e.*, presumably for the active transport of sodium.

How much sodium has to be pooled within the medullary tissue when, after a washout during osmotic diuresis, the concentration gradient must be built up to

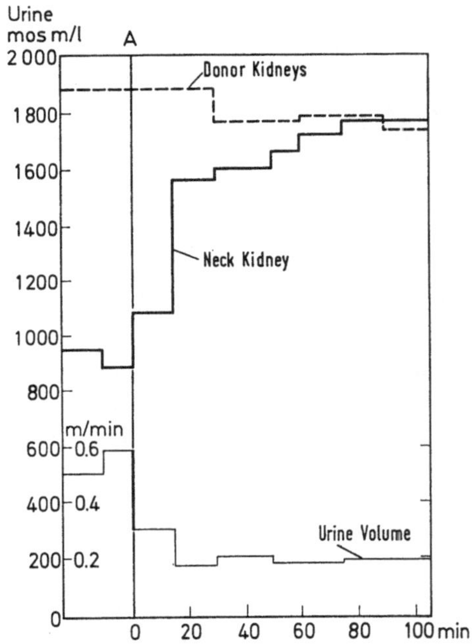

Fig. 2. Experiment on a dog anesthetized with pentobarbital, with a 3rd kidney transplanted on the neck vessels. Osmolaritics of the urine of the two kidneys in situ and of the 3rd kidney in the neck. "A"; end of a one hour mannitol infusion into the renal artery of the 3rd kidney. Note the exponential increase of urinary osmolarity, which reaches a maximum about 80 minutes after the end of the mannitol infusion

5 or 6 times the plasma value? An estimate, in terms of oxygen utilization, of the energy required to restore the medullary sodium content in the time period from the onset of antidiuresis to the return of pre-diuretic urine osmolarity (one hour, Fig. 2) becomes possible by using the slice analysis data of Boylan and Asshauer [3] and values for sodium-oxygen dependence published by Deetjen and Kramer [4].

For 10 g of inner medulla, the loss of sodium provoked by diuresis is given by the mean concentration difference for sodium in inner medullary tissue, times the water content (83%) of the inner medulla. The concentration difference for sodium was 280−150=130 mEq · Kg-1 tissue water from the antidiuretic to the diuretic state. This represents a loss of .130 × 8.3 = 1.08 mEq/10 g or about 1 mEq Na lost from the inner medulla.

To replace this 1 mEq Na in the observed restoration time for urine osmolarity would require the transport of $1/60 = 0.016$ mEq min^{-1} into the medulla.

The oxygen requirement for the transcellular transport of 1 mEq Na for the dog kidney in situ is 0.8 ml O_2. Transport at the rate necessary to restore 1 mEq in one hour would therefore require 0.016 mEq min^{-1}. 0.8 ml $= 0.0128$ ml O_2 min^{-1}. Assuming an efficiency of 20% for the net movement of sodium into the medulla, five times this amount of sodium would actually need to be transported to increase the medullary content by the required 1 mEq. This means that .064 ml of O_2 would be necessary. This is within the observed value for oxygen consumption of the inner medullary tissue of 0.06 ml O_2 min^{-1}. The observed value, however, includes basal oxygen consumption (that of the nontransporting medullary tissue). This value, believed to be exceedingly small, has been neglected in the above calculation. In view of the close agreement between observed oxygen consumption and calculated requirement, one is tempted to conclude that the main source of energy is oxydative and that the essential operation is active Na transport.

It is known since the first studies of JAENICKE [7] that intravenous infusions of urea in amounts that augment plasma urea concentration increase the papillocortical concentration gradient. As early as 1934, GAMBLE [5] had remarked upon the "unique physical properties" of urea which permitted it to be excreted with less water than was required by other substances. Urea diffuses out of the collecting duct fluid into the interstitial space and is concentrated to the tip by counter-current diffusion. This makes it possible to concentrate urea in the final urine, not only by removal of water from the collecting ducts but also by reduced back diffusion, due to an increased urea concentration in the interstitial tissue which surrounds the ducts (REINHARDT — see next paper).

In general, the permeability constant of most cell membranes for urea is high. While the loss by diffusion from proximal tubular fluid of 50% of the filtered urea load appears as a handicap for urea excretion, the high urea permeability of medullary tissue is useful in another way. It allows urea to be concentrated without water loss by osmotic diuresis. The latter, known to occur in uremic states, assumes importance only at plasma urea concentrations above 20 mM/L.

Experimental attempts to determine the role of medullary blood flow have been focused on three typical diuretic states: water, osmotic and pressure diuresis. In all three, medullary blood flow was found to be increased. However, the effect of this change in blood flow upon the other elements of the concentrating process requires careful evaluation, especially in the light of recent evidence that the glomerular filtration rate of juxtamedullary nephrons differs from that of superficial cortical nephrons and may change in the opposite direction. Moreover, mathematical treatment so far has neglected considerations implicit in the intriguing anatomical arrangements of uriniferous ducts and blood vessels.

We may say, therefore, that while there is no doubt that counter-current multiplication and exchange diffusion are the basic principles of the renal medullary concentrating process, the finer mechanisms still await precise definition.

References

1. Berliner, R. W., and C. M. Bennet: Concentration of urine in the mammalian kidney. Am. J. Med., Symposium on antidiuretic hormones **42**, 777 (1967).
2. — N. G. Levinsky, D. G. Davidson, and M. Eden: Dilution and concentration of the urine and the action of antidiuretic hormone. Amer. J. Med. **24**, 730 (1958).
3. Boylan, J. W., and E. Asshauer: Depletion and restoration of the medullary osmotic gradient in the dog kidney. Pflügers Arch. ges. Physiol. **276**, 99—116 (1962).
4. Deetjen, P., u. K. Kramer: Die Abhängigkeit des O_2-Verbrauchs der Niere von der Na-Rückresorption. Pflügers Arch. ges. Physiol. **273**, 636—650 (1961).
5. Gamble, J. L., C. F. McKhann, A. M. Butler, and E. Tuthill: An economy of water in renal function referable to urea. Amer. J. Physiol. **109**, 139 (1934).
6. Hargitay, B., u. W. Kuhn: Das Multiplikationsprinzip als Grundlage der Harnkonzentrierung in der Niere. Z. Elektrochem. **55**, 539 (1951).
7. Jaenicke, J. R.: Urea enhancement of water reabsorption in the renal medulla. Amer. J. Physiol. **199**, 1205 (1960).
8. Klümper, J. D., K. J. Ullrich u. H. H. Hilger: Das Verhalten des Harnstoffs in den Sammelrohren der Säugetierniere. Pflügers Arch. ges. Physiol. **267**, 238—243 (1958).
9. Kuhn, W., u. K. Ryffel: Herstellung konzentrierter Lösungen aus verdünnten durch bloße Membranwirkung. Ein Modellversuch zur Funktion der Niere. Hoppe-Seylers Z. physiol. Chem. **276**, 145 (1942).
10. Marsh, D. J.: Hypo-osmotic re-absorption due to active salt transport in perfused collecting ducts of the rat renal medulla. Nature (Lond.) **210**, 1179 (1966).
11. Peter, K.: Untersuchungen über Bau und Entwicklung der Niere. H. 1. Jena: Gustav Fischer 1909.
12. Sakai, F., R. L. Jamison, and R. W. Berliner: A method for exposing the rat renal medulla in vivo: micropuncture of the collecting duct. Amer. J. Physiol. **209**, 663 (1965).
13. Schmidt-Nielsen, B.: Urea excretion in mammals. Physiol. Rev. **38**, 139 (1958).
14. Ullrich, K. J., K. Kramer, and J. W. Boylan: Present knowledge of the countercurrent system in the mammalian kidney. Progr. cardiovasc. Dis. **3**, 395 (1961).
15. —, u. G. Pehling: Aktiver Natriumtransport und Sauerstoffverbrauch in der äußeren Markzone der Niere. Pflügers Arch. ges. Physiol. **267**, 207—217 (1958).
16. — G. Rumrich, and B. Schmidt-Nielsen: Urea transport in the collecting duct of rats on normal and low protein diet. Pflügers Arch. ges. Physiol. **295**, 147—156 (1967).
17. Walker, A. M., P. A. Bott, J. Oliver, and M. C. MacDowell: The collection and analysis of fluid from single nephrons of the mammalian kidney. Amer. J. Physiol. **134**, 580 (1941).
18. Wirz, H.: Der osmotische Druck in den corticalen Tubuli der Rattenniere. Helv. physiol. pharmacol. Acta **14**, 353 (1956).

1.1.8. The Role of Urea in the Renal Concentrating Operation in Dog

H. W. Reinhardt, K. Ellinghaus, H. J. Klose and P. Deetjen[1]

With 1 Figur

It is known from the experiments of several investigators [1—4, 6, 7) that intravenous infusions of urea augment the process of urine concentration. We report here experiments on anaesthetized dogs (N_2O; O_2; Halothane) in which,

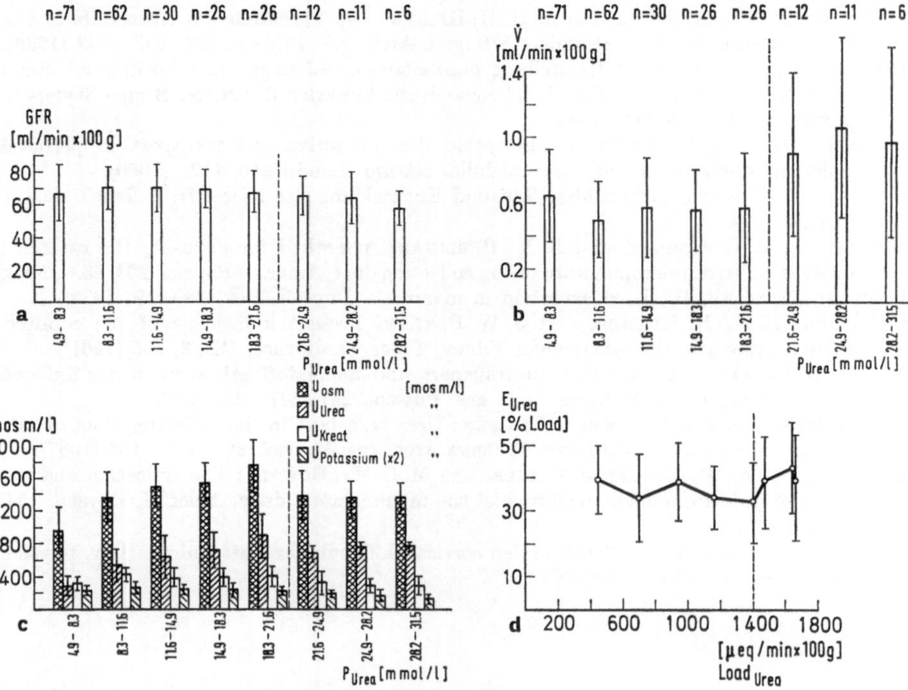

Fig. 1a—d. The effect of increasing plasma urea concentration (P_{urea}) on: a, Glomerular filtration rate. b Urine flow rate. c Total urine osmolarity and the urine concentrations of urea, creatinine and potassium. In d the percentage of filtered urea excreted is plotted against the increasing urea load

over periods of 18 hours, increasing plasma urea concentrations produced by continuous infusion of hypertonic urea (0.8—1.6 mol/L), are related to:

1. Creatinine clearances;
2. Urine volume;

[1] Physiologisches Institut der Universität München, West Germany.

3. Total urine osmolarity and osmolar concentrations of urea, creatinine, and potassium;

4. Urea excretion expressed as percentage of load.

The creatinine clearances did not change over a wide range of plasma urea concentrations (4.9—21.6 mmol/L); nor did urine volume. However, urea concentration in the urine increased linearly with plasma urea, whereas creatinine and potassium concentrations did not change significantly. The excretion of urea concentrations in percentage of filtered load was 37% and remained constant in the range of plasma urea concentrations examined. With plasma urea concentrations above 21.6 mmol/L urine flow increased to about twice the level seen with concentrations below this level. Urine osmolarity fell to a lower level and with it the concentration of all urinary constituents (Fig. 1).

In another series of experiments, a third kidney was transplanted to the neck [8] and proximal and distal tubular fluid samples were obtained from this kidney by micropuncture. The TF/P urea to TF/P inulin ratios in 32 collections from proximal tubules were found to be 0.63 ± 0.21, whether plasma urea concentration was normal or increased. In a few instances it was possible to obtain distal samples. In these, the TF/P ratios of urea to inulin were 1.0 or more. The mean value of the U/P_{urea} to $U/P_{Creatinine}$ ratio was 0.4 (Fig. 1).

Discussion

Although our micropuncture data indicate that about 37% of filtered urea leaves the proximal tubule (presumably by diffusion) the urea load delivered to the collecting ducts is equal to the filtered load. This is evidenced by the distal TF/P urea to inulin ratios of 1.0 or more.

These data confirm a recirculation of urea (from collecting ducts to Henle's loops) in the dog kidney, such as is known to exist in the rat [5].

Both of these processes appear to be independent of plasma urea concentrations over the wide range examined in these experiments.

About 60% of the urea delivered to the collecting ducts is returned to the medullary structures and enters the countercurrent system; about 40% is excreted in the urine. This fractional distribution was constant in our experiments from urea load of 0.35 to 1.4 mmol/min.

Since urine flow and GFR were constant in these experiments a similar volume of water was reabsorbed in each case and with it — one may assume — a constant fraction of the urea present at each concentration level. This reabsorbed urea, added to the countercurrent system and trapped by exchange diffusion toward the papillary tip contributes to the total medullary osmolarity in proportion to its load.

This unique characteristic of urea accounts for the rising urine urea concentration with load in the absence of progressive concentration of the other urinary constituents. In the concentrating kidneys of dehydrated animals, on the other hand, all urinary solutes share in the concentrating process.

References

1. Goldberg, M., A. M. Wojtczak, and M. A. Ramirez: Uphill transport of urea in the dog kidney. Effects of certain inhibitors. J. clin. Invest. **46**, No 3, 388 (1967).

2. JAENIKE, J. R.: Urea enhancement of water reabsorption in the renal medulla. Amer. J. Physiol. **199** (6), 1205—1210 (1960).
3. KIIL, F., and K. AUKLAND: The role of urea in the renal concentration mechanism. Scand. J. clin. Lab. Invest. **12**, 290—299 (1960).
4. KOIKE, T. J., and R. H. KELLOG: Effect of urea loading on urine osmolality during osmotic diuresis in hydropenic rats. Amer. J. Physiol. **205** (5), 1053—1057 (1963).
5. LASSITER, W. E., C. W. GOTTSCHALK, and M. MYLLE: Micropunction study of not transtibular movement of water and urea in nondiuretica mammalian kidney. Amer. J. Physiol. **200**, 1139—1146 (1961).
6. LEVINSKY, N. G., and R. W. BERLINER: The role of urea in the urine concentrating mechanism. J. clin. Invest. **38**, 741 (1959).
7. RABINOWITZ, L., and R. H. KELLOG: Enhancement of renal concentrating ability in the dog by urea and related compounds. Amer. J. Physiol. **205** (1), 112—116 (1963).
8. REINHARDT, H. W., H. J. KLOSE, K. ELLINGHAUS, H. BRECHTELSBAUER u. D. W. BEHRENBECK: Ein Nierenpräparat (sog. Halsniere) zur Erleichterung komplizierter Funktionsuntersuchungen (Homotransplantat am narkotisierten Hund). Pflügers Arch. ges. Physiol. **297**, 71—88 (1967).

1.1.9. The Transepithelial Urea Transport in Different Segments of the Mammalian Nephron

K. J. ULLRICH[1]

Three processes may be involved in the transepithelial urea flux (J_u) [7, 9]:

1. *diffusion*, with Δc_u as driving force and ωRT, the urea permeability of the membrane, as proportionality factor

2. *solvent drag*, which is proportional to the transepithelial water flux J_v, to the mean concentration of urea $\bar{c}_u$ in the membrane and to $1-\sigma$. [$\bar{c}_u$ is defined as the logarithmic mean of the urea concentration: $\bar{c}_u = \Delta c_u / \Delta \ln c_u$; Δc_u is the urea concentration difference between the tubular fluid and plasma; σ is the reflection coefficient for urea].

3. *active transport*, which must be linked by a proportionality factor U to the metabolic rate J_r.

Therefore, the following equation can be written as:

$J_u = \omega RT \, \Delta c_u + (1-\sigma) \, J_v \, \bar{c}_u + U \, J_r$, which is valid only for dilute solutions.

How can we discriminate these three processes? If the experiments are so designed that a zero transtubular water flux ($J_v \rightarrow 0$) can be obtained by perfusing the tubule with equilibrium solution [6], then we have to deal only with diffusion and (possibly) active transport. If, then, the changes of J_u are directly proportional to Δc_u, one may conclude that active urea transport is not present. From such experiments it appears, that the proximal and distal convoluted tubules in the normal rat kidney lack an active urea transport process [1]. On the other hand it is possible to lower J_u to zero by letting the equilibrium solution come into contact with the membrane for an indefinitely long time. Then Δc_u should approach zero, if there is no active transport of urea. With this experimental procedure it is demonstrated, that the collecting ducts in rats on a normal diet do not transport urea actively, but rats on a low protein diet do [11].

To evaluate the influence of solvent drag is a much more difficult problem, because it is difficult to measure the reflection coefficient (σ) in a system as complicated as a living epithelial cell layer. Principally, the method of GOLDSTEIN and SOLOMON [3] is adapted and the following formula for transepithelial volume (water) flux is used. When the transepithelial hydrostatic pressure difference is zero, $J_v = L_p RT \, (\sigma_t c_t^i - \sum_{k=1}^{n} \sigma_k \, c_k^o)$.

(L_p is the filtration permeability for water, $\sum_{k=1}^{n} \sigma_k \, c_k^o$ the sum of concentrations of all substances k at the outside (o) of the membrane with the respective reflection coefficients σ_k; c_t^i is the concentration of the test substance, which is in the experiment the *only* substance at the inside (i) of the tubular membrane and σ_t is the reflection coefficient of that substance).

[1] Max-Planck-Institut für Biophysik, Frankfurt a.M., West-Germany.

Assuming that L_p and $\sum_{k=1}^{n} \sigma_k c_k^0$ remain constant, when different test substances c_t^i are used and measuring c_t^i when J_v becomes zero, one gets the formula $\sigma_{t_1} c_{t_1}^i = \sigma_{t_2} c_{t_2}^i = \sigma_{t_3} c_{t_3}^i$;
$c_{t_{1\ldots 3}}^i$ being defined as the isotonic concentration (c_{iso}) of the substance under consideration when the water flux is zero. By comparison with the non-permeant substance raffinose, which has a reflection coefficient 1.0, the reflection coefficient of urea may be calculated from the following equation: $c_{\mathrm{iso}_{\mathrm{Raff}}} = \sigma c_{\mathrm{iso}_{\mathrm{urea}}}$.

The urea transport data measured on the kidney *in situ* are listed in Table 1. The distal convoluted tubule shows the lowest urea permeability, which is only $\frac{1}{10}$ of the proximal, and $\frac{1}{5}$ of the collecting duct value. The urea permeability

Table 1. *Transport coefficients for urea in different segments of the rat kidney*

	Urea permeability $\omega RT \cdot 10^{-4}$mm/sec	Reflection coefficient σ	Active transport $10^{-5}\mu$mol/mm · sec
Proximal convolution	11.0*	0,79	[0]
Distal convolution	1.0		[0]
Collecting duct (normal diet)	4.7		0
(low protein diet)	[4.7]		5

* This value was obtained by recalculation of the data of CAPEK et al. [1] assuming that the regression line does not originate from the 100% point.

of tubular segments which are not accessible to micropuncture is unknown, with the exception of the urea permeability of the cortical collecting ducts which was measured by GRANTHAM and BURG [4] on the *in vitro* perfused isolated collecting ducts of rabbits and found to be $1.22 \cdot 10^{-4}$ mm/sec. It is likely that the cortical collecting ducts of the rat also show a urea permeability which is intermediate between that of the distal convoluted tubules and that of the lower collecting ducts.

When compared to other mammalian cell membranes and epithelial cell layers (Table 2), the reflection coefficient of the proximal convolution for urea (0.79), appears rather high [12]. This fact favors the hypothesis that the function of the kidney is not to conserve but to excrete filtered urea. Nevertheless, 50% of the filtered urea leaves the proximal tubules and flows back into the blood, as is known from free flow micropuncture experiments. The data of Table 1, together with the known increase of the urea concentration in free flowing proximal tubular fluid, allow us to estimate that approximately 20% of the filtered urea is reabsorbed by solvent drag and 30% by backdiffusion. In the distal convoluted

Table 2. *Reflection coefficients, σ, of different cell membranes (literature)*

Toad skin without ADH (9)	0,81
Toad bladder (13)	0,79
Erythrocytes (3)	0,62
Blood-brain-barrier (2)	0,44
Gut (10)	0,2

tubules a urea reflection coefficient of 0.67 was found despite a diffusion permeability of only $1 \cdot 10^{-4}$ mm/sec [12]. Here we may put a note of caution since the procedure to measure the reflection coefficient seems to be much less reliable in the distal tubules as compared to the proximal convoluted tubules.

For many years an active urea transport out of the collecting ducts of rats on low protein diet was postulated by B. Schmidt-Nielsen (Ref. see 11). Her hypothesis was recently confirmed by stop flow microperfusion [8] and micropuncture experiments [11]. However in rats on a normal diet such an active urea transport process does not seem to occur. Therefore, we must assume that the active urea transport process is induced by lack of proteins in the diet.

In summary, we may state, that the transport parameters for urea of the principle nephron segments are known and that they satisfactorily describe the backflux of filtered urea under different experimental conditions.

References

1. Capek, K., G. Fuchs, G. Rumrich u. K. J. Ullrich: Harnstoffpermeabilität der corticalen Tubulusabschnitte von Ratten in Antidiurese und Wasserdiurese. Pflügers Arch. ges. Physiol. **290**, 237—249 (1966).
2. Fenstermacher, J. P., and J. A. Johnson: Filtration and reflection coefficients of the rabbit blood brain barrier. Amer. J. Physiol. **211**, 341—346 (1966).
3. Goldstein, D. A., and A. K. Solomon: Determination of equivalent pore radius for human red cells by osmotic pressure measurements. J. gen. Physiol. **44**, 1—17 (1960).
4. Grantham, J. J., and M. B. Burg: Effect of vasopressin and cyclic AMP on permeability of isolated collecting tubules. Amer. J. Physiol. **211**, 255—259 (1966).
5. Hoshiko, T., and B. D. Lindley: Phenomenological description of active transport of salt and water. J. gen. Physiol. **50**, 729—758 (1967).
6. Kashgarian, M., H. Stöckle, C. W. Gottschalk, and K. J. Ullrich: Transtubular electrochemical potentials of sodium and chloride in proximal and distal renal tubules of rats during antidiuresis and water diuresis (Diabetes insipidus). Pflügers Arch. ges. Physiol. **277**, 89—106 (1963).
7. Kedem, O., and A. Katchalsky: Thermodynamic analysis of the permeability of biological membranes to nonelectrolytes. Biochim. biophys. Acta (Amst.) **27**, 229—246 (1958).
8. Lassiter, W. E., M. Mylle, and C. W. Gottschalk: Micropuncture study of urea transport in rat renal medulla. Amer. J. Physiol. **210**, 965—970 (1966).
9. Leaf, A., and R. M. Hays: Permeability of the isolated toad bladder to solutes and its modification by vasopressin. J. gen. Physiol. **45**, 921—932 (1962).
10. Lifson, N., and A. A. Hakim: Simple diffusive-convective model for intestinal absorption of a nonelectrolyte (urea). Amer. J. Physiol. **211**, 1137—1146 (1966).
11. Ullrich, K. J., G. Rumrich, and B. Schmidt-Nielsen: Urea transport in the collecting duct of rats on normal and low protein diet. Pflügers Arch. ges. Physiol. **295**, 147—156 (1967).
12. — Renal transport of sodium. Proc. 3rd int. Congr. Nephrol., Washington 1966, 1, 48. Basel and New York: Karger 1967.
13. Whittembury, G.: Action of antidiuretic hormone on the equivalent pore radius at both surfaces of the epithelium of the isolated toad skin. J. gen. Physiol. **46**, 117—129 (1962).

1.2. Uric Acid

1.2.1. The Renal Excretion of Uric Acid

N. Zöllner[1]

Uric acid is excreted by the kidney and the gastrointestinal tract. Of the total excretion the kidney eliminates about 80%. The uric acid excreted into the gastrointestinal tract is degraded by bacteria; only if neomycin is given, uric acid can be demonstrated in the stools.

The renal excretion of uric acid in normal human subjects amounts to about 500 mg per day. With a nomal plasma level below 6 mg-% the resulting clearance value is much lower than the glomular filtration rate. While most authors find uric acid clearance values between 5 and 10 ml/min, 9.5 ml/min is probably the best figure. If water is given, the uric acid excretion increases with urine flow up to a limiting value. The uric acid clearance for the whole day is smaller than the clearance calculated from determinations done in the morning.

Some have considered the rather low uric acid clearance as proof that uric acid is excreted by a simple mechanism of filtration and reabsorption. Today, it is generally assumed that the largest part of the uric acid filtered is reabsorbed, and that a considerable part of the uric acid excreted is derived from tubular secretion.

At physiological pH-values, uric acid is a univalent acid with a pK_a' of 5.8. Thus, in serum, uric acid is nearly completely dissociated, while in urine, prevalence of the ionized or non-ionized form depends on the pH. Therefore, the more general term *uric acid* is preferred in the following discussion; the term *urate* will only be used if there is no doubt about the prevalence of the ionized species.

The Mechanism of Renal Uric Acid Excretion

Glomerular Filtration of Uric Acid

The total urate in plasma is freely diffusible and ultrafiltrable [24]. Therefore, the uric acid concentration in the glomerular filtrate corresponds to that in plasma. At a plasma urate level of 5 mg-% and an inulin clearance of 120 ml/min, the amount of urate filtered would be 6 mg/min.

Morris claimed in 1948 [13], that part of the uric acid in serum is bound to albumin. However, Salteri et al. [19] could not confirm this. Since uric acid is ultrafiltrable the question is of no consequence for renal physiology.

Reabsorption of Uric Acid

Normally, uric acid excretion is about 0.35 mg per minute. Thus, by far the largest part of the amount filtered is reabsorbed. Probably the proximal tubule is the site of this reabsorption.

---

[1] Medizinische Poliklinik der Universität München, West-Germany.

The Dalmatian coach hound has lost the ability to reabsorb uric acid [5]. For this reason these animals do excrete uric acid through the kidney although their livers contain uricase.

A series of drugs inhibit the reabsorption of uric acid, a fact which is important for renal physiology as well as for the treatment of hyperuricemia. Most important are the so called uricosuric drugs, N-substituted sulfonamides, as well as derivatives of phenylbutazone. An important uricosuric action is also exerted by the antagonists of vitamin K, the coumarol as well as the phenylindandione type. Other important uricosuric drugs are salicylic acid and zoxazolamine. In addition to the compounds mentioned, a number of other drugs exert uricosuric effects. Since some of them show no similarity to the known uricosuric drugs, these effects may lead to unsuspected difficulties in clinical diagnosis.

Secretion of Uric Acid

In 1950 Wolfson et al. [22] showed that in the Dalmation coach hound the uric acid clearance may be higher than glomerular filtration rate. In the same year Praetorius and Kirk [18] found uric acid clearance values around 200 ml/min in a man who had very low plasma urate levels. In 1954, Poulsen and Praetorius [17] were able to raise the ratio of uric acid/creatinine clearance in the rabbit up to 1.77 by intravenous injection of urate. Finally, the finding in gout, a congenital metabolic disorder, that the plasma urate is elevated in the face of a normal uric acid excretion, could best be interpreted by the assumption of an inadequatic tubular secretion of uric acid [27]. Since then, man's ability to secrete uric acid has been demonstrated unequivocally by Gutman et al. [8]. When these authors combined an infusion of urate with mannitol diuresis and inhibition of uric acid reabsorption by sulfinpyrazone in patients with a low inulin clearance, they found a uric acid clearance which was 1.23 times the inulin clearance. During infusion of urate and osmotic diuresis Lathem et al. (1960) could shortly afterward demonstrate uric acid secretion in the dog.

Under experimental conditions (plasma uric acid higher than 10 mg-%) it is now certain that man secretes uric acid. At normal levels this can not yet be demonstrated. However, there is no reason to assume that the renal uric acid excretion of man is basically different from that of other mammals. Also, experiments with pyrazinamide point to an important role of tubular uric acid secretion in man (see below). Finally, the renal physiology of gout, which will be described later, can best be explanined by the assumption of a tubular uric acid secretion in normal man and its failure in this disease.

The maximum rate of uric acid secretion has so far been estimated only in the rabbit. In 1966 Möller [12] found that secretion rises with the plasma level of uric acid until this has reached approximately 30 mg-%.

In man, the relative importance of secretion can only be appreciated indirectly. Berliner et al. [2] tried to determine the T_m-value of uric acid reabsorption and found considerable variation. In the range of a load of 15 mg/min, the curve for calculated reabsorption became flat. This presumably means that in this range secretion becomes of predominant importance, particularly since this flattening of the curve is not seen in patients with gout [7].

More reliable evidence about the rate and contribution of the tubular uric acid secretion may be deduced from experiments with pyrazinamide which inhibits it. The administration of this drug reduces the clearance of uric acid to very low values. Since the reabsorption of uric acid is either not influenced or inhibited by pyrazinamide, the decrease of uric acid excretion must be a crude measure for the rate of secretion: thus, one may assume that in man about 90% of the uric acid excreted by the kidney is secreted by the tubules. (The production of hyperuricemia by saluretics is probably also due to inhibition of tubular secretion.)

The finding of an "augmentation limit" may show that uric acid transport is not confined to the proximal tubule, but that reabsorption and, or secretion occur also in the dista tubule. Early stop flow experiments, however, did not give clear-cut results. Kessler et al. [10], in mongrel dogs, found only reabsorption of uric acid. Only in the Dalmatian coach hound could they demonstrate uric acid secretion. They proposed that the Dalmatian differs from other mammals by a reversion in the direction of a general transport system for uric acid. Using the same technique, Yü et al. [26] however, found uric acid secretion in the distal tubule. Davis et al. [4] confirmed these results in 1965; they also showed that secretion is completely abolished by pyrazinamide. For the dog the question concerning direction and site of tubular uric acid transport, thus, seems, to be decided.

Combining all findings (and generalizing), the uric acid secretion of mammals (excluding the Dalmatian) may be considered as the result of glomerular filtration, nearly complete reabsorption (mainly in the proximal tubule) and secretion (mainly in the distal tubule), which — as will be shown below — depends on the plasma urate level.

Excretion of Uric Acid Into the Gastrointestinal Tract

The most important routes for the uric acid excretion into the gastrointestinal tract are saliva, gastric juice, bile, and the secretions of the pancreas and the intestine. The amounts which are secreted are estimated differently by various authors. From earlier figures we calculated the intestinal uric acid excretion to be 15% of the total excretion [28]. Wyngaarden and Stetten [23], after intravenous administration of labeled uric acid, found 25% of the isotope in the degradation products which presumably arose from enteral uricolysis. Sorensen [21] estimates that up to a third of the total uric acid is eliminated into the gut.

Examination of the uric acid excretion in saliva permits a precise measurement of a part of the gastrointestinal elimination. Because this secretion might be considered a simple model for uric acid secretion in general, possibly even permitting some conclusions with respect to the pathogenesis of gout we have studied it under various conditions [30].

The results of these experiments show that, if the salivary flow is not stimulated by lemon juice or drugs, the uric acid excretion is independant of salivary flow and is constant. If the plasma urate level is increased by the oral administration of nucleic acid the salivary excretion rises; if the plasma urate is lowered, the salivary excretion decreases. The plasma urate level, therefore, determines the rate of the salivary uric acid secretion. This correlation is very close in short term experiments in any given individual. (The findings in gout will be discussed below.)

Physiological Influences on the Renal Excretion of Uric Acid

The plasma urate level of any given subject, although not constant, is kept within rather narrow limits. Under a varying dietary purine load, plasma urate changes very little. Even in proliferative diseases of the hematopoietic system, there must be a considerable excess of uric acid formation before the plasma urate level rises above the upper limit of normal values. (Exceptions to this rule are observed in the late stages of chronic diseases such as polycythemia and myeloid metaplasia.) On the other hand, it has been known for a long time that attacks of gout, presumably precipitated by an acute rise of the plasma urate level, may occur under the influence of alcohol or acute starvation.

Influence of Plasma Urate Level on Uric Acid Excretion

In 1937 BRØCHNER-MORTENSEN [3] studied the uric acid excretion after an acute uric acid load, produced by the intravenous infusion of urate or by administering a high purine diet. He found that, in normal man, under these conditions, not only the excretion, but also the renal clearance of uric acid increases. BERLINER et al. [2] and other investigators confirmed these results.

Later, man's ability to adapt his uric acid excretion to the purine load of the body and to increase the uric acid clearance when the plasma urate level rises had been studied in chronic experiments. NUGENT and TYLER [14] found that even after several days of administration of nucleic acids the clearance of uric acid remains high. These observations have also repeatedly been confirmed by others. Recently, uric acid excretion, was again measured after several months of ingestion of ribonucleic acid. The results, once again, were the same.

Influence of Lactate and β-Hydroxybutyrate on Uric Acid Excretion

In 1923 GIBSON and DOISY [6] observed that lactate administration strongly inhibits the renal uric acid excretion; when we infused lactate we found clearance values down to 1 ml/min. "Pyruvate is said to increase uric acid excretion; however it is difficult to raise pyruvate levels without concomitant increase of lactate. The infusion of β-hydroxybutyrate also leads to a strong reduction of uric acid excretion." [20]

High plasma concentrations of lactate were found after over-indulgence in alcohol [11], in preeclampsia [9] and in glycogen storage disease of type I [1]. In all these states, high uric acid levels were also observed in the plasma. Increases of plasma concentrations of β-hydroxybutyrate were the cause of a lowered uric acid clearance and of a high plasma urate level in inadequately controlled diabetes [16] and during weight reduction [20]. In patients on a 300 Cal diet we have repeatedly seen plasma urate levels above 10 mg-%, even in young girls.

The similarity of the effects of lactate and β-hydroxybutyrate seems to indicate that the transport functions of the tubular cells depend on their redox potential, or possibly on their extramitochondrial $NADH/NAD^+$ ratio.

In agreement with this assumption, the effect of the antimetabolities of vitamin K could be explained as an inhibition of cellular oxydation in certain compartments or at a certain redox potential.

Familial Hyperuricemia (Gout)

Particularities of Renal Uric Acid Excretion

Gout, as well as the inborn error of metabolism which is its cause, has been considered as the effect of either increased uric acid production or lowered uric acid excretion. Some of the bitter arguments about these alternatives have been resolved by the demonstration that one or several new nosological entities due to disturbances of uric acid production can be separated from classical gout. On the other hand, it is generally agreed that in classical gout the amount of uric acid excreted and, therefore, also the amount synthesized is about the same as in normal subjects of comparable size, age, sex and state of nutrition. The plasma urate level, however, is higher in gouty patients than in normal subjects. This discrepancy is particularly striking if normal man's ability to excrete increased amounts of uric acid in certain disease states such as pneumonia, hemolytic disorders etc. is considered. In these states, plasma urate levels are usually not above the normal limits.

In spite of clear-cut evidence (high plasma levels at a normal rate of excretion) for disturbance of the renal excretory mechanism, the role of the kidney has long been negated, particularly by American authors. Repeatedly, uric acid clearance in gout was described as normal. A close scrutiny of the literature showed however, that in every report uric acid clearance in gouty people was lower than in the control group [28], although statistical significance could be obtained only after pooling the results of several reports.

A more precise definition of the pecularities of renal uric acid excretion in gout became possible when the uric acid excretion of normal people with an experimentally elevated uric acid level had been studied. It was found that, at identical plasma urate levels, the uric acid clearance of normal subjects is about 1.5 times larger than that of gouty patients [14]. This difference remains demonstrable after several months of nucleic acid ingestion, i.e. in normal subjects with chronic hyperuricemia [15]. Only Yü et al. [25] do not agree to this conclusion; but their group of "normals" contains subjects with hyperuricemia. If, instead of the clearance, the rate of excretion of uric acid is plotted against the plasma urate level, there is again a difference in the curves. All these results have been confirmed repeatedly. We studied the excretion of uric acid in saliva and found that gouty persons at comparable plasma levels secrete less uric acid than normal controls.

Renal Consequences of Altered Uric Acid Excretion in Familial Hyperuricemia

The easiest explanation of these findings is the assumption of a hereditary disturbance of tubular secretion of uric acid in familial hyperuricemia. If this assumption is correct, the uric acid excreted in the final urine must have flowed through the whole length of the nephron, while in normal subjects, it would partly originate from distal tubules. In sites of urinary concentration, the concentration of uric acid in the lumen and interstitium must rise. Since, under physiological conditions, the concentration of uric acid is close to the upper limit of solubility, uric acid may be precipitated, particularly in the papilla.

The occurence of typical morphological changes ("gouty kidney", "kidney in gout" or "gouty nephrosis") is the rule in familial hyperuricemia; even if bioptic controls are performed early, the renal parenchyma is rarely found to be completely normal. Clinical signs of disturbed renal functions are observed early [32]: at first proteinuria, then signs of pyelonephritis, and finally excretory deficiency and hypertension. Urolithiasis is quite common: in our own material about 40% of the patients were so affected.

References

1. Alepa, F. P., R. R. Howell, J. R. Klinenberg, and J. E. Seegmiller: Relationships between glycogen storage disease and tophaceous gout. Amer. J. Med. **42**, 58 (1967).
2. Berliner, R. W., J .G. Hilton, T. F. Yü, and T. J. Kennedy Jr.: The renal mechanism for urate excretion in man. J. clin. Invest. **29**, 396 (1950).
3. Brøchner-Mortensen, K.: Uric acid in blood and urine. Acta med. scand., Suppl. **134** (1937).
4. Davis, B. B., J. B. Field, G. P. Rodnan, and L. H. Kedes: Localization and pyrazinamide inhibition of distal transtubular movement of uric acid-2-C^{14} with a modified stop-flow-technique. J. clin. Invest. **44**, 716 (1965).
5. Friedman, M., and S. O. Byers: Observations concerning the causes of the excess excretion of uric acid in the Dalmatian dog. J. biol. Chem. **175**, 727 (1948).
6. Gibson, H. V., and E. A. Doisy: A note on the effect of some organic acids upon the uric acid excretion of man. J. biol. Chem. **55**, 605 (1923).
7. Gutman, A. B., and T. F. Yü,: Renal function in gout. Amer. J. Med. **23**, 600 (1957).
8. — —, and L. Berger: Tubular secretion of urate in man.J. clin. Invest. **38**, 1778 (1959).
9. Handler, J. S.: The role of lactic acid in the reduced excretion of uric acid in toxemia of pregnancy. J. clin. Invest. **39**, 1526 (1960).
10. Kessler, R. H., K. Hierholzer, and R. S. Gurd: Localization of urate transport in the nephron of mongrel and Dalmatin dog kidney. Amer. J. Physiol. **197**, 601 (1959).
10a Lathem, W., B. B. Davis, and G. P. Roduan: Renal tubular secretion of uric acid in the mongrel dog. Amer. J. Physiol. 199, 9 (1960).
11. Lieber, Ch., D. P. Jones, M. S. Losowsky, and C. S. Davidson: Interrelation uric acid and ethanol metabolism in man. J. clin. Invest. **41**, 1863 (1962).
12. Møller, J. V.: The excretion of urate at various plasma concentrations and during osmotic diuresis in the rabbit. Acta physiol. scand. **66**, 419 (1966).
13. Morris, J. E.: The transport of uric acid in serum. Amer. J. Med. Sci. **235**, 43 (1958).
14. Nugent, C. A., and F. H. Tyler: The renal excretion of uric acid in patients with gout and in nongouty subjects. J. clin. Invest. **38**, 1890 (1959).
15. — W. D. McDiarmid, and F. H. Tyler: Renal excretion of urate in patients with gout. Arch. intern. Med. **113**, 115 (1964).
16. Padova, J., and G. Bendersky: Hyperuricemia. In: Diabetic ketoacidosis. New Engl. J. Med. **267**, 530 (1962).
17. Poulsen, H., and E. Praetorius: Tubular excretion of uric acid in rabbits. Acta pharmacol. (Kbh.) **10**, 371 (1954).
18. Praetorius, E., and J. E. Kirk: Hypouricemia: with evidence for tubular elimination of uric acid. J. Lab. clin. Med. **35**, 865 (1950).
19. Salteri, F., E. Cirla, and A. Fasoli: Electromigration on filter papers of uric acid from serum and synovial fluid. Science **127**, 85 (1958).
20. Shapiro, J. R., J. R. Klinenberg, W. Peck, S. E. Goldfinger, and J. E. Seegmiller: Hyperuricemia associated with obesity and intensified by caloric restriction. Arthr. and Rheum. **7**, 343 (1964).
21. Sorensen, L. B.: Degradation of uric acid in man. Metabolism 8, 687 (1959).

22. WOLFSON, W. Q., C. COHN, and C. SHOVE: The renal mechanism for urate excretion in the Dalmatian coach-hound. J. exp. Med. **92**, 121 (1950).
23. WYNGAARDEN, J. B., and D. STETTEN JR.: Uricolysis in normal man. J. biol. Chem. **203**, 9 (1953).
24. —, and A. B. GUTMAN: Ultrafiltrability of plasma urate in man. Proc. Soc. exp. Biol. (N.Y.) **84**, 21 (1953).
25. — L. BERGER, and A. B. GUTMAN: Renal function in gout. II. Effect of uric acid loading on renal excretion of uric acid. Amer. J. Med. **33**, 829 (1962).
26. — — S. KUPFER, and A. B. GUTMAN: Tubular secretion of urate in the dog. Amer. J. Physiol. **199**, 1199 (1960).
27. ZÖLLNER, N.: Angeborene Stoffwechselstörungen. Dtsch. med. Wschr. **83**, 609, 688 (1958).
28. — Moderne Gichtprobleme, Ätiologie, Pathogenese, Klinik. Ergebn. inn. Med. Kinderheilk. **14**, 321—389 (1960).
29. — Der Purinstoffwechsel und seine Störungen. Verh. dtsch. Ges. Urol. **20**, 15 (1963).
30. — Eine einfache Modifikation der enzymatischen Harnsäurebestimmung. Z. klin. Chem. **1**, 178 (1963).
31. — Physiologie und Pathologie der Harnsäure. Praxis **53**, 1122—1128 (1965).
32. — Die Gichtniere. In: Handbuch der inneren Medizin. Berlin-Heidelberg-New York: Springer 1968, VIII/3.

Discussion

BOHLE:

We found precipitations of uric acid within the lumens of proximal convoluted tubules of a 12 year old patient with a clinical diagnosis of "rhumatism" and glomerulo-nephritis with renal failure. The plasma uric-acid concentration was found elevated later on. Could this case be considered as classical gout?

RENSCHLER:

What is the role of non-ionic back diffusion in the excretion of uric acid? How is the clearance of uric-acid influenced by changes in urine pH?

SCHIRMEISTER:

The common occurence of hypertension and hyperuricemia does not necessarily mean that hypertension is a consequence of gouty nephropathy. The other possibility is primary hypertension with secondary lactacidemia, which, in turn, depresses the renal excretion of uric acid. In support of this possibility, CANNON et al. [New Engl. J. of Med. **275**, 457 (1966)] found increased blood concentrations of uric acid and of lactic acid in a large number of patients with hypertension.

ZÖLLNER: To BOHLE: If the manifestations of gout occur early in life, i.e. begin before puberty, the diagnosis of classical gout is doubtful. These cases should tentatively be classified as primary, juvenile gout or as a similar syndrome, associated with choreoathetosis. (WYNGAARDEN, J. B.: Gout. In: The metabolic basis of inherited disease, 2nd edit. New York: McGraw-Hill Book Co. 1966). —

To RENSCHLER: I know of no modern study that would answer this question. —

To SCHIRMEISTER: While the association mentioned in Cannon's paper undoubtedly does occur, it is true that secondary gout is not seen in primary (essential) hypertension, unless treated with saluretic drugs. On the other hand the development of hypertension in men with manifest gout is well documented and a number of case records has already been published by Gudzent (Gicht und Rheumatismus. Berlin: Springer 1928).

1.2.2. Study on Renal and Extrarenal Factors Involved in the Hyperuricemia Induced by Furosemide

J. Schirmeister, N. K. Man and W. Hallauer[1]

With 3 Figures

Modern salidiuretics may induce hyperuricemia. Available data have shown this to be due to a renal effect, but some investigators have suggested an extrarenal effect of the drugs, either an enhanced outflow of uric acid from the body pool or an increased de novo biosynthesis [1, 9, 14]. Intravenous administration of chlorothiazide [3] or furosemide [10] causes a prompt but transient increase of renal uric acid excretion without change in serum concentration. During prolonged oral administration of furosemide to patients [7], an increase of serum uric acid (SUA) associated with a reduction of urate-clearance (C_U-) was noted in some cases. The present study was undertaken in an attempt to define further the renal and extrarenal factors by which furosemide modifies the SUA concentration.

20 normal healthy volunteers received daily morning doses of 40 mg furosemide per os during 4 weeks. After 7 days of therapy and in all subjects, the SUA increased in the average by 17%, from 4.6 ± 1.5 mg-% to 5.4 ± 1.8 mg-% (Mean $\pm$ SD). The increased SUA persisted during the time of therapy and returned to control level after the drug was discontinued. The concentration of creatinine in serum (S_{Cr}) was increased by 18%, from $0{,}93 \pm 0.15$ mg-% to 1.10 ± 0.17 mg-% (Mean $\pm$ SD). This might represent a reduction of GFR which could, by itself, account for uric acid retention. The reduction of GFR measured by means of the standard inulin clearance in 5 subjects in the same experimental conditions (average 8%) was quantitatively too small to be responsible for the marked increase of SUA (see Fig. 1). Therefore other factors must be involved in the furosemide-induced hyperuricemia [11].

In an attempt to separate two possible effects of furosemide, namely an outflow of uric acid from a body pool or an increased de novo biosynthesis, another group of subjects received daily doses of 40 mg furosemide or 400 mg allopurinol, separately or in combination. Allopurinol is a potent uricogenolytic agent which reduces uric acid production [17]. 24 h urines were collected for clearance studies.

After 4 days on furosemide therapy alone (Fig. 2, B) the SUA increased by an average of 29% and the urinary excretion of uric acid (U_U-$\cdot V$) decreased on the 2nd day by 13% from control values. The urate clearance (C_U-) was reduced on the 4th day by 30%. Thus the extent of reduction in C_U- corresponds to the increase of SUA. Calculation revealed that the initial decrease of U_U-$\cdot V$ was too small to account for the increase in SUA. When the drug was discontinued (Fig. 2, B) SUA fell sharply, associated with an overwhelming urinary excretion of uric acid which resulted in a marked increase of C_U-above control levels.

[1] Medizinische Universitätsklinik Freiburg i. Br., West-Germany.

After 4 days or allopurinol alone (Fig. 2, C), both SUA and $U_{U^-} \cdot V$ decreased simultaneously by 55%. The C_U-remained constant.

In a combined study (Fig. 2, A), the mean decrease from control values was 30% for SUA, 62% for $U_{U^-} \cdot V$ and 47% for C_{U^-}.

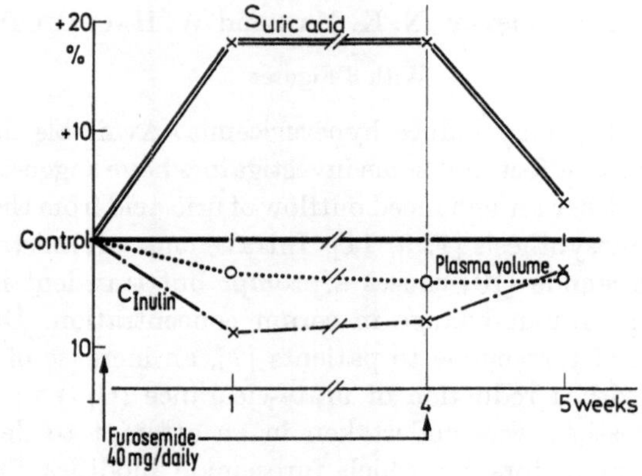

Fig. 1. *Mean change of GFR (C_{Inulin}) and plasma urate levels during treatment with furosemide*

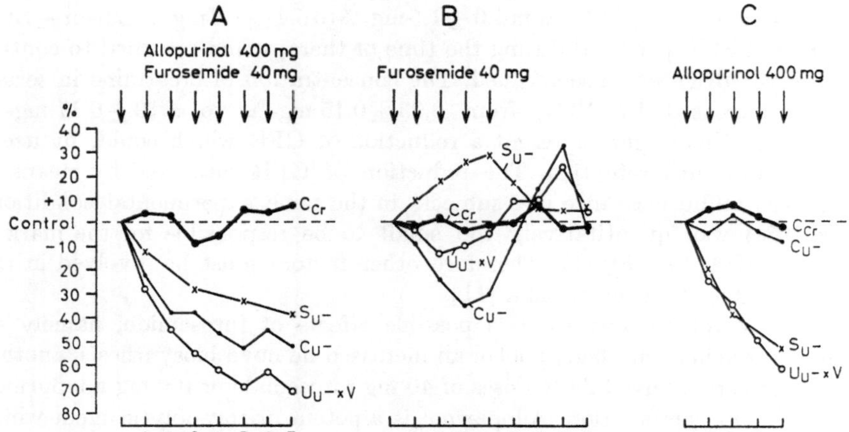

Fig. 2. *The change of urate in serum and urine during treatment with furosemide and allopurinol.* C_{Cr} = clearance of creatinine; S_{U^-} = concentration of urate in serum; $U_{U^-} \cdot V$ = urinary urate excretion/24 h; C_{U^-} = clearance of urate

The reduction of $U_{U^-} \cdot V$ on the 4th day was in the same range, both in the allopurinol study and in the furosemide-allopurinol study, but the reduction of SUA in the combined study was 20% smaller than in the allopurinol study. Thus, furosemide depressed the reduction of SUA effected by allopurinol. This could be explained only by a mobilization of urate from the miscible pool, for de novo biosynthesis was inhibited by allopurinol.

Our data show that extrarenal factors must be involved in the hyperuricemia induced by furosemide, but that the absence of an increase of urinary excretion of uric acid in the face of an increased serum level should be due to a renal effect. Yü et al. (1962) demonstrated that loading with uric acid results in an increased urinary excretion. In our furosemide study, however, the urinary excretion of uric acid failed to rise although the SUA was elevated.

After the drug was discontinued, we noted an increased renal excretion of uric acid considerably above control levels without change in GFR. This rebound effect is compatible with a renal retention of uric acid induced by furosemide.

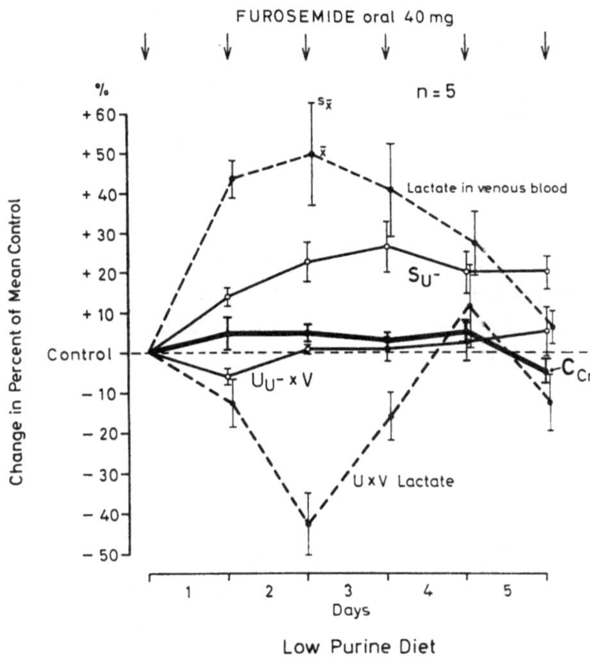

Fig. 3. *The lactacidemia and hyperuricemia induced by furosemide.* Ordinate = mean change ($\bar{x}$) in percent of control values ± standard deviation of mean ($S_{\bar{x}}$); $U \times V$ lactate = urinary lactate excretion/24 h

Since sodium lactate infusion decreases the clearance of urate [15], and an interrelationship of hyperuricemia and lactacidemia was noted in toxemia of pregnancy [4], in primary and renal hypertension [2] and in glycogen storage disease [6], we tried to find out if the furosemide hyperuricemia was effected by an increase in blood lactate.

5 healthy subjects, in another group, received during 8 days, daily doses of 40 mg furosemide without dietary restrictions. The increase of SUA (21%) was associated with a more pronounced increase of lactate (65%) in venous blood (enzymatic method: 5), but blood lactate returned to control level though SUA remained increased. The increased blood lactate could be due to either a reduced renal excretion or an increased lactate production. Therefore, the same subjects, now on a low purine diet, received again 40 mg furosemide daily and

collected their 24-h urines in plastic containers with chloroform as preservative, for clearance studies.

48 hours after initiating therapy, the blood lactate increased considerably (50%) while the urinary excretion of lactic acid decreased by 43%. Both returned to control levels during the next days, while SUA remained elevated. The initial and transient small decrease of $U_{U^-} \cdot V$ was found again. The reciprocal behavior of lactate in blood and lactate excretion in urine under furosemide suggests a renal effect. A change in GFR due to furosemide could be thought to account for the observed findings, but, during therapy, creatinine clearance was practically unchanged. Therefore variations in renal hemodynamics do not explain the changes in lactate values.

The increased lactate in blood then, could be due to an increased production. SCHULTZ et al. (1966) have shown in rats that increased blood lactate induced by diazoxide, a non-diuretic thiazide agent, resulted in an accelerated glycogenolysis in skeletal muscle, while SENFT et al. (1966) have demonstrated in rats, that furosemide did not increase the rate of glycogenolysis in skeletal muscle. Thus, the lactacidemia observed in our study in man might be the consequence of a renal effect of furosemide which could be an enhanced tubular reabsorption of lactate [8]. However, the reduction of lactate excretion was found to be insufficient to account for the extent of increase in blood lactate. The lactacidemia induced by furosemide, then, must involve metabolic effects.

Conclusion

The hyperuricemia induced by prolonged oral administration of furosemide is the result of a renal and an extrarenal effect.

As an extrarenal effect, furosemide probably causes a mobilization of urate from the urate pool. An overproduction of urate appears unlikely.

The renal effect of the drug appears to be twofold. First the initial small decrease of urinary urate excretion could be due to an increased proximal tubular reabsorption of uric acid, enhanced by an increased blood lactate. The second renal effect could be a depression of tubular secretion of urate which abolishes the increase in uric acid excretion, expected as a consequence of the augmented uric acid load.

References

1. AYVAZIAN, J. H., and L. F. AYVAZIAN: A study of the hyperuricemia induced by hydrochlorothiazide and acetazolamide separately and in combination. J. clin. Invest. **40**, 1961—1966 (1961).

2. CANNON, P. J., W. B. STASON, F. E. DEMARTINI, S. C. SOMMERS, and J. H. LARAGH: Hyperuricemia in primary and renal hypertension. New Eng. J. Med. **275**, 457—464 (1966).

3. DEMARTINI, F. E., E. A. WHEATON, L. A. HEALEY, and J. H. LARAGH: Effect of chlorothiazide on the renal excretion of uric acid. Amer. J. Med. **32**, 572—577 (1962).

4. HANDLER, J. S.: The role of lactic acid in the reduced excretion of uric acid in the toxemia of pregnancy. J. clin. Invest. **39**, 1526—1532 (1960).

5. HOHORST, H. J.: L-(+)-Lactat, Bestimmung mit Lactatdehydrogenase und DPN. In: H. U. BERGMEYER, Methoden der enzymatischen Analyse. Weinheim: Verlag Chemie 1962.

6. HOYNIGEN-HUENE, C. B. v.: Gout and glycogen storage disease in preadolescent brothers. Arch. intern. Med. **118**, 471—477 (1966).
7. KUHLBÄCK, B.: Einfluß eines neuen Diuretikums (Fursemid) auf den Harnsäurestoffwechsel. Med. Klin. **60**, 2105—2106 (1965).
8. MILLER, A. T., and J. O. MILLER: Renal excretion of lactic acid in exercise. J. appl. Physiol. **1**, 614—618 (1949).
9. REUTTER, F., u. F. SCHAUB: Harnsäurestoffwechsel und Saliduretika. Dtsch. med. Wschr. **89**, 1101—1104 (1964).
10. SCHIRMEISTER, J., u. H. WILLMANN: Über die Harnsäure- und andere Clearances nach intravenöser Gabe von Furosemid beim Menschen. Klin. Wschr. **42**, 623—628 (1964).
11. — N. K. MAN, D. WARNING u. W. HALLAUER: Zur Frage der extrarenalen Ursache einer Harnsäureretention nach Furosemid. Verh. dtsch. Ges. inn. Med. **73**, 1025—1028 (1967).
12. SCHULTZ, G., G. SENFT, W. LOSERT u. R. SITT. Biochemische Grundlagen der Diazoxid-Hyperglykämie. Naunyn-Schmiedebergs Arch. Pharmak. exp. Path. **255**, 372—387 (1966).
13. SENFT, G., W. LOSERT, G. SCHULTZ, R. SITT u. H. K. BARTELHEIMER: Ursachen der Störungen im Kohlenhydratstoffwechsel unter dem Einfluß sulfonamidierter Diuretica. Naunyn-Schmiedebergs Arch. Pharmak. exp. Path. **255**, 369—382 (1966).
14. SMILO, R. P., W. R. BEISEL, and P. H. FORSHAM: Reversal of thiazide-induced transient hyperuricemia by uricosuric agents. New Engl. J. Med. **267**, 1225—1227 (1962).
15. YÜ, T. F., J. H. SIROTA, L. BERGER, M. HALPERN, and A. B. GUTMAN: Effect of sodium lactate infusion on urate clearance in man. Proc. Soc. exp. Biol. (N.Y.) **96**, 809—813 (1957).
16. — L. BERGER, and A. B. GUTMAN: Renal function in gout. II. Effect of uric acid loading on renal excretion of uric acid. Amer. J. Med. **33**, 829—844 (1962).
17. —, and A. B. GUTMAN: Effect of allopurinol on serum and urinary uric acid in primary and secondary gout. Amer. J. Med. **37**, 885—898 (1964).

1.2.3. Renal Biopsy in Patients with Hyperuricemia

J. Moeller[1]

In collaboration with Prof. Eger, the author studied renal biopsy specimens obtained from 25 men and 1 woman with hyperuricemia. The sex distribution corresponded to that generally observed amoung patients with gout, of whom 80—90% are said to be men [3]. In six patients, the biopsy specimens were histologically normal. Three patients showed marked arterio- and arteriolosclerosis and, at the same time, the characteristic changes of intracapillary glomerulonephritis. In 13 other cases, the biopsy specimens showed only marked signs of arterio- and arteriolosclerosis, which occured independently of hypertension in most patients. Three patients had clear-cut interstitial nephritis; three others had fibrosis of the medullary tissue. In 14 of these cases, the serum creatinine concentration was near to the upper limit of normal values.

In a few patients treated with thiazide diuretics, serum urea concentration increased simultaneously with the uric acid concentration. This occured usually in subjects with high blood cholesterol, fatty liver infiltration and prediabetes or diabetes.

Arterio- and arteriolosclerosis, thus, appear to be the most characteristic renal changes in hyperuricemia. This confirms Fahr's statement, made in 1925, [1] that gouty nephritis is primarily a vascular disease. Extracapillary glomerulosclerosis in patients with gout was described by Koller and Zollinger [2].

References

1. Fahr, Th.: Handbuch der speziellen pathologischen Anatomie und Histologie (Henke-Lubarsch), Bd. VI/1, S. 156. Berlin: Springer 1925.
2. Koller, F., u. H. U. Zollinger: Gichtische Glomerulosklerose. Schweiz. med. Wschr. 75, 97 (1945).
3. Müller, H. O., u. E. Fritze: Pathophysiologie, Klinik und Therapie der Gicht. Med. Klin. 60, 735—738 (1965).

[1] Medizinische Abteilung, Städtisches Krankenhaus Hildesheim, West-Germany.

1.2.4. Benziodaron in the Long-Term Management of Gout

A. Masbernard, Ch. Hiltenbrand and Y. Mémin [1]

With 6 Figures

In patients with heart disease, treated with the coronary dilating drug ethyl-(2-iodo-3.5-hydroxy-4-benz)-cumarone = benziodaron (Amplivix Labaz) routine studies of blood chemistry showed unexpectedly low values of plasma uric acid concentrations [2]. Metabolic studies done by several investigators [1, 3—5, 8, 11, 13, 15—17, 19—21] proved that the drug lowers plasma uric acid concentrations in normal subjects as well as in patients with hyperuricemia or gout more rapidly and to a larger extent than all other known uricosuric drugs. The closely related drug, benzbromaron, (experimental drug L 2214), shares this effect, while another related drug, benzaron (Fragivix Labaz) is somewhat less potent in this respect. It should also be pointed out that benziodaron is chemically related to dicoumarol [16] which has been known for some time to lower plasma uric acid concentration [6, 10, 24].

In the present study, the uricosuric and the plasma uric acid concentration lowering effects of benziodaron were investigated in 65 patients. The clinical use of the drug in patients with gout will be discussed extensively in another paper [12].

Patients

The 65 patients investigated were 64 men aged 27—67 years (mean 49.1 years) and one 27 year old woman with renal failure. 47 patients had primary gout, 13 non-nephrogenous latent hyperuricemia, and 5 chronic renal failure with a considerable increase of the plasma uric acid concentration. In one of the latter cases, there were gout-like joint pains. In 39% of the patients with gout, tophi could be demonstrated either clinically or radiographically. One half of the patients with tophi had suffered, at one time or another, from renal colics or nephrolithiasis while such urinary symptoms occurred in only 29% of the patients without tophi. The historics of patients with primary gout ranged from a few months to 18 years.

Overweight by more than +10% of the normal weight was present in 80% of our patients, pre-diabetes or diabetes in 30%, and "essential" hypertension in 15%. None of the patients with hypertension was treated with diuretic drugs.

Some of the patients had been treated previously with orotic acid which had lost its effect and had not been continued. 8 patients were treated with benziodaron when treatment with probenecid and/or sulfinpyrazone had become unsatisfactory, or was not tolerated any more.

Most patients were treated as out-patients and were given a diet poor in purines. Repeated examinations included complete clinical investigations, i.v.

[1] Hôpital militaire d'instruction du Val-de-Grâce, Paris, France.

pyelography, tests for proteinuria, study of the urinary deposit, the pH of the urine and several renal functions.

Dosage

The usual dose was 200 mg benziodaron per day. In some cases we gave 100 or 300 mg, rarely 400 mg per day. A tablet contains 100 mg. In some patients, particularly those with frequent acute attacks and a history of urate stones, treatment was begun with low doses which were increased by 100 mg every 7 or 10 days, in order to avoid a rapid fall in plasma uric acid concentration which could result in acute attacks or in the formation of urate stones. In order to obviate the latter danger, the patients were also told to drink a lot of water and were given alcalinizing drugs. Some patients, furthermore, received one mg of colchicine per day during the first weeks of treatment in order to prevent acute attacks.

In the latter course of the treatment, the daily dose of benziodaron was decreased to 100 mg, whenever possible, but in most cases 200 mg (one tablet in the morning and one in the evening) were required. The duration of treatment ranged up to more than 1 year (Fig. 1). In only 3 cases, the drug was not well tolerated and the treatment had to be interrupted.

Results

Plasma-Uric-Acid. In all cases the concentration fell rapidly and markedly below the normal values and sometimes to very low values (Fig. 1). There was a large dose-related variation between the tracings from various patients as well as within single patients. After falling below the normal mean value, the plasma uric acid concentration never rose again above this value in the course of treatment. The average values, represented by the thick line, fell from an initial concentration of 8.3 mg-% to 3.9 mg-% on the 10th day, on the 20th day to 3.7 mg-%, on the 30th day to 3.4 mg-%, and finally stabilized at 3.3 mg-%.

The % fall of a blood uric acid did not depend on the initial value. Fig. 2 demonstrates a loose dose-response relationship. 300 mg per day were no more effective than 200 mg. Even daily doses of 25 mg could induce a fall of the plasma-uric acid concentration by 27% [19]. In patients initially treated with probenecid or sulfinpyrazon (Fig. 3), benziodaron always induced a further fall in plasma-uric acid from an average value of 5.8 mg-% to 3.7—3.9 mg-%, while the urinary clearance of uric acid rose from a mean value of 11 ml/min to 24.3 ml/min. This latter rise was significant. The comparison shows that the efficacy of benziodaron was approximately twice that of the 2 other uricosuric drugs ,and that benziodaron remained effective, when probenecid or sulfinpyrazon had lost their efficacy. The mean plasma uric acid concentration in the pretreated patients of Fig. 3 was slightly, but not significantly higher than in the non-pretreated patients shown in Fig. 1.

With maintenance treatment, plasma-uric acid concentrations did not tend to rise during the following months. The patients did not appear to become refractory to the drug. As soon as the treatment was interrupted, the plasma-uric acid concentrations rose within a few days, frequently above the initial value. Treatment, thus had to be continued permanently.

Urinary Excretion of Uric Acid. Unfortunately, in our patients, the urinary excretion of uric acid could not be measured every day. Where the measurements could be done, we found a considerable increase in the urinary excretion of uric acid, which in 9 cases exceeded 1,000 mg/day and reached 2,505 mg/day with 100 mg of benziodaron per day, and in 11 cases given 200 mg of the drug, exceeded 1,000 mg and reached values up to 2,880 mg/day. While the mean

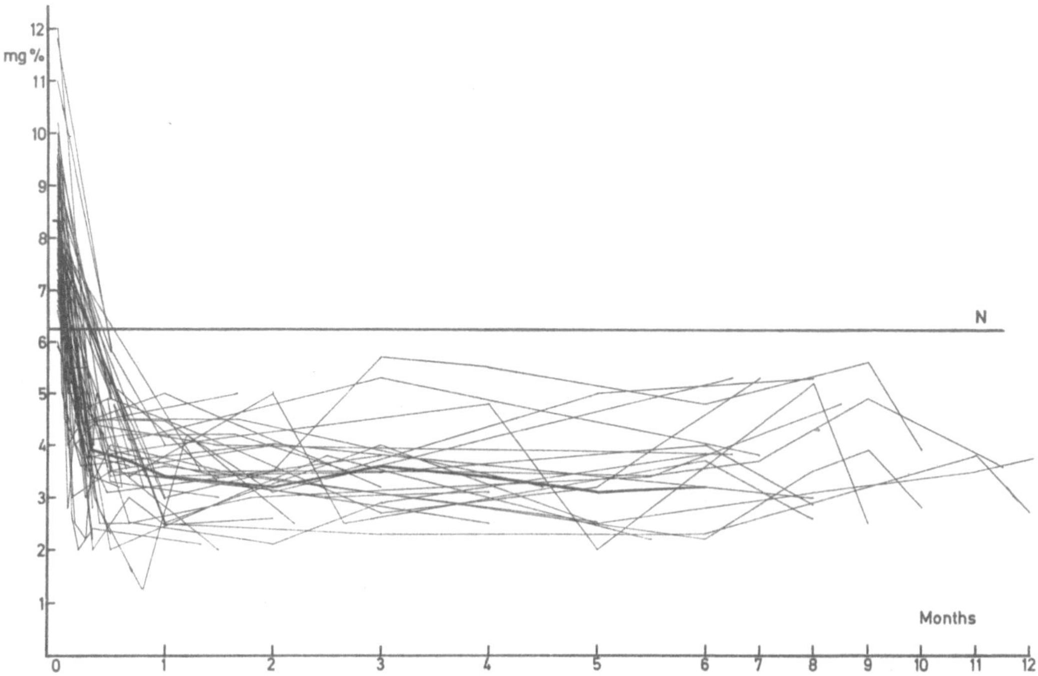

Fig. 1. The concentration of uric acid in plasma in the course of treatment with benziodaron with 100, usually 200, and rarely 300 mg/day, by the oral route, in 53 patients with gout or hyperuricemia, without severe renal failure. The patients had not been treated with uricosuric drugs previously

daily excretion of uric acid in the control periods preceding treatment was 705 mg/day, the mean excretion under 100 or 200 mg/day of benziodaron was 896 mg day and 877 mg/day respectively. As with other urisuric drugs, plasma uric acid usually decreased most rapidly in the first days of treatment, the decrease slowed down subsequently. This explains the apparently low mean daily excretion of 790 mg/day of uric acid under 300 mg of benziodaron per day. This dose, as explained above, was usually not reached earlier than after 2 to 3 weeks.

Urinary Clearance of Uric Acid. The urinary clearance was measured in 30 cases (Fig. 4). Benziodaron induced a rapid and pronounced rise of the clearance from sometimes very low values (3—11.7 ml/min, average 6.7 ml/min) to values as high as 30 or 40 ml/min, and in one case even 66 ml/min. The calculated mean values (18.3, 18.7, 18.1, 18.1, 17.0, 17.1, 18.2 ml/min) show the pronounced uricosuric effect of benziodaron. With repeatedly measured clear-

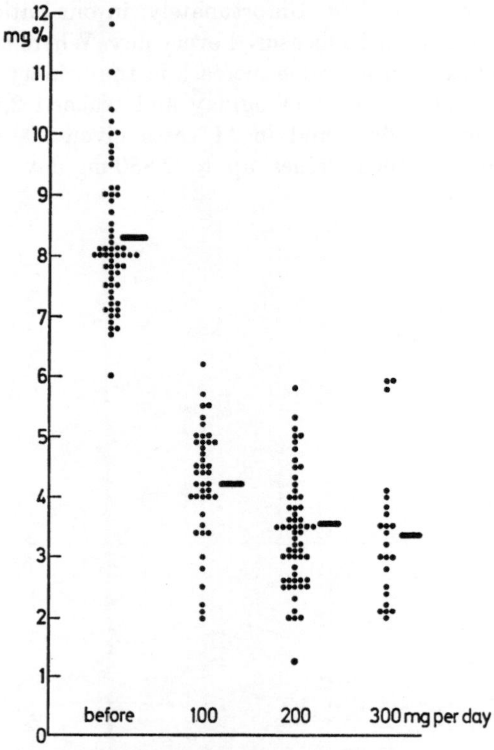

Fig. 2. Concentration of uric acid in plasma before, and in the course of, treatment with benziodaron (daily dose of 100, 200 or 300 mg) in 60 patients without severe renal failure

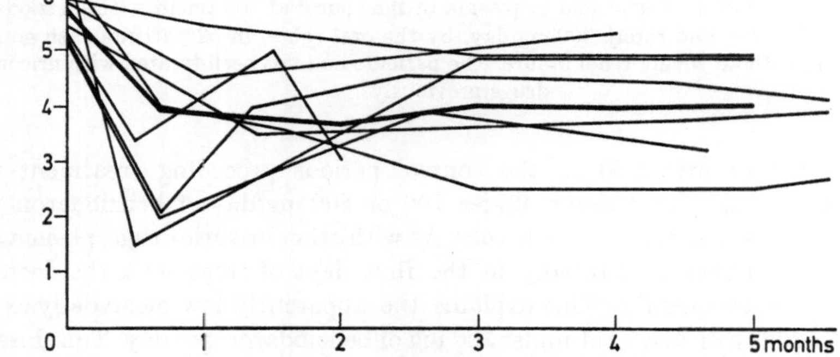

Fig. 3. Plasma-uric acid concentrations under benziodaron in 2 patients previously treated unsuccessfully with probenecid and in 6 patients treated with sulfinpyrazone

ances, there were often considerable day-to-day variations depending on the dose given and on the diet. The tracings usually showed an initial peak with a subsequent fall which rarely reached the normal value. The clearance of uric acid, under the influence of benziodaron, depended on the functional state of the

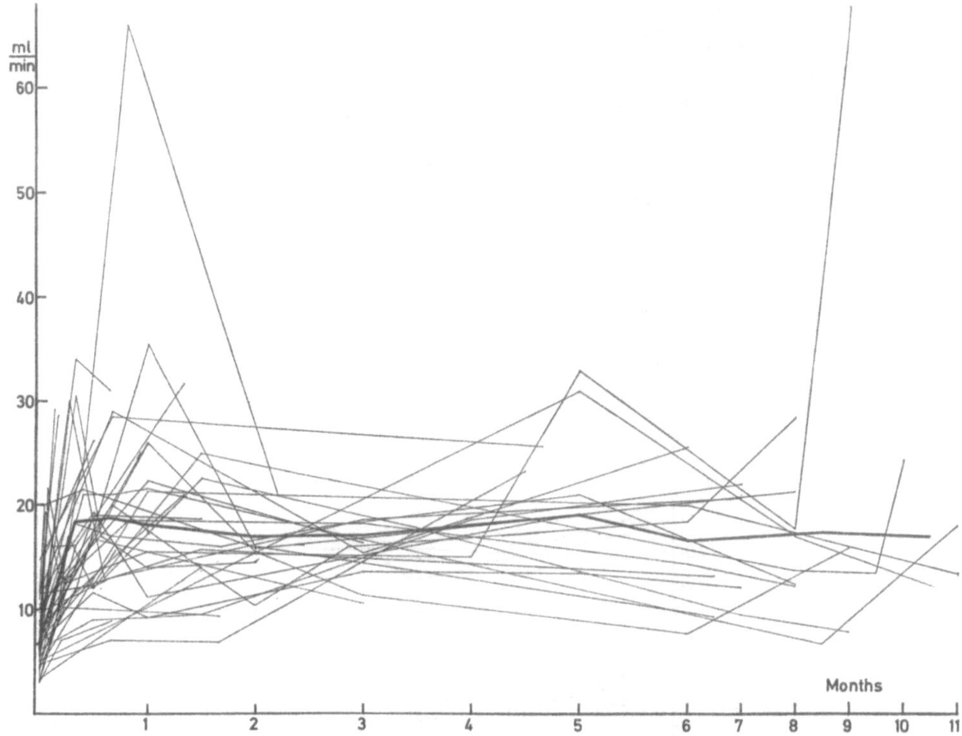

Fig. 4. Renal clearance of uric acid under benziodaron in 32 patients with gout

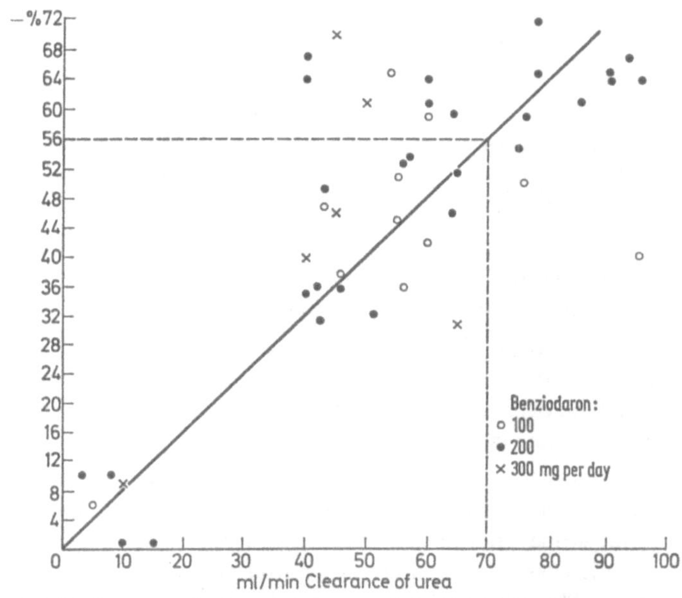

Fig. 5. Relationship between the functional state of the kidneys and the % decrease in plasma-uric acid concentration obtained under benziodaron

kidneys. Fig. 5 shows the relationship between the renal clearance of urea or creatinine and the fall in plasma-uric acid concentration obtained by giving benziodaron. At a glomerular clearance of 70 ml/min, the average fall of plasma-uric acid concentration was 56%. The individual values were distributed around the regression line shown in Fig. 5.

In severe renal failure, the drug neither lowered the plasma-uric acid concentration nor increased the clearance or the excretion of uric acid by the kidneys,

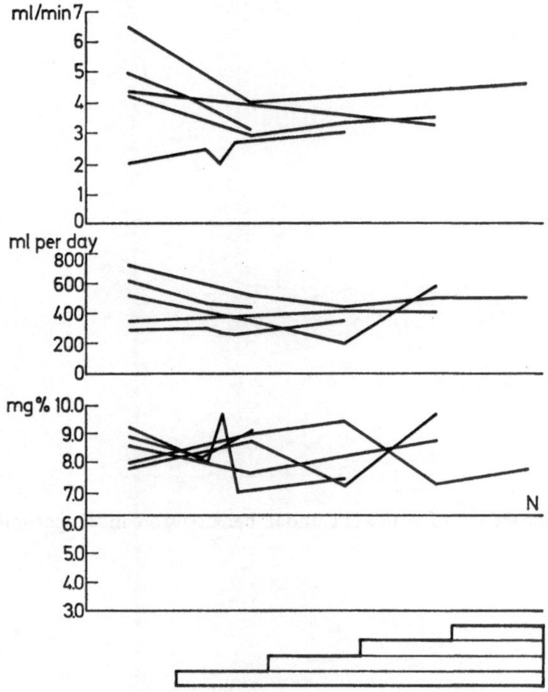

Fig. 6. Plasma concentration of uric acid, urinary excretion and renal clearance of uric acid, under the influence of progressively increasing doses of benziodaron in 5 patients with severe chronic renal failure (urea clearances below 15—20 ml/min)

although doses up to 300 mg or, in one case, up to 400 mg were given. With glomerular clearances below 20 ml/min, no effects were induced by benziodaron.

Toxicity and Side-Effects. With long-term management, we did not observe any detrimental effects of benziodaron in patients with hyperuricemia or with severe renal failure. The drug appeared to be devoid of nephrotoxicity in chronic as well as in acute experiments.

In only 3 cases were we compelled to interrupt the treatment: twice because of iodine intolerance; and once because of a renal colic with hematuria and expulsion of a renal stone on the 3rd day of treatment. No other side effects were observed. In all cases, benziodaron was well tolerated even after several months of treatment. Though the drug contains 50% of iodine, it did not appear to influence thyroid functions, though the plasma-iodine levels were very high.

The following incidents were observed in the course of treatment in 61 patients with gout:

Attacks of gout at the beginning of treatment	6
in patients not given colchicine	3
in spite of colchicine	3
as a consequence of a change of the daily dose	2
after interruption of the treatment by the patient himself	1
Renal colics at the beginning of treatment:	1
	16

In nearly 1/3 of the patients, crystals of urate or a heavy urate sediment without colics were observed in the first days and weeks of treatment. In one case, a renal colic occurred in the course of treatment by an accidental decrease in water consumption.

Clinical Efficacy. In approximately 1/3 of the cases the clinical state improved considerably under the influence of benziodaron: articular pains and stiffness decreased. In 2/3 of the cases, acute attacks disappeared or became rare. The usual dietary prescriptions were also imposed under treatment with this uricosuric drug. The time of observation was not sufficiently long to decide whether benziodaron, like other uricosuric drugs, may induce a decrease in the size of tophi or at least stabilize their size. In 2 of our cases, tophi disappeared within a few months of treatment, presumably as a consequence of the use of the drug. The biological effects of benziodaron are comparable in patients with or without tophi.

Discussion

The present results show that benziodaron has a pronounced uricosuric and plasma-uric acid concentration lowering effect in subjects whose glomerular clearances are above 20 ml/min. The effect of the drug, which can already be observed after 10 min [19], is time-limited [3, 8, 19] and cannot be ascribed to a depression of the biosynthesis of uric acid [16]. The data obtained in our patients correspond to other observations on the fall of the plasma uric acid concentrations [1, 5, 15, 20] and the enhancement of the urinary excretion of uric acid [13, 15, 20] in normal subjects [8, 19] as well as in patients with gout [3]. Benziodaron considerably increased the urinary clearance of uric acid. This increase can neither be ascribed to an increase of the glomerular filtration rate and filtered load of uric acid [8], nor to dilatation of renal blood vessels as supposed by Mudge. The mechanism of action is a depression of tubular reabsorption of uric acid, with or without an additional enhancement of tubular secretion. The effect of the experimental drug L 2214 was comparable to that of benziodaron and more pronounced than that of benzaron. A comparison of Fig. 3 with data and literature on probenecid [23], sulfinpyrazone [18], zoxazolamine or diacetural [14] shows that benziodaron is a more effective drug. Like other uricosuric drugs, benziodaron may induce acute attacks of gout or renal colic at the beginning of the treatment as a consequence of the rapid fall in plasma-uric acid concentrations. It is, therefore, recommended that a protective dose of colchicine be given with benziodaron during the first weeks of treatment and, furthermore, that large volumes of water and drugs alkalinizing the urine be prescribed. Incidents may be avoided by these measures. Continued treatment is possible because of the good tolerance and the absence of side-effects of benziodaron.

Summary

In 47 patients with gout and in 13 hyperuricemic patients without articular symptoms or signs ethyl-(2-iodo-3.5-hydroxy-4-benz)-coumarone = benziodaron (Amplivix Labaz), given at daily doses of 100, 200, or 300 mg, always induced a rapid and pronounced fall of plasma-uric acid from a mean value of 8.3 to 3.3 mg-% and a considerable enhancement of the urinary excretion and clearance of uric acid by +200% or more. In some cases, this fall was accompanied by pronounced clinical improvement. Acute attacks of gout occurred in 9 cases, renal colic in 1 case. No other side effects were observed. The present observations confirm other published reports on the superiority of benziodaron when compared to other uricosuric drugs. The treatment must be continued permanently, because the action of the drug is time-limited. In order to avoid incidents, 1 mg of colchicine per day, large doses of drinking fluid and drugs alkalinizing the urine should be given during the first weeks of treatment.

References

1. Cottet, J., et Ch. Vittu: Action de la benziodarone sur l'hyperuricémie goutteuse, Presse méd. **75**, 1355—1356 (1967).
2. Déchelotte, J.: Pers. communic.
3. Delbarre, F., C. Auscher et B. Amor: Action uricosurique de certains dérivés du benzofurane. Bull. Soc. méd. Hôp. Paris **116**, 1193—1196 (1965).
4. — — — Action uricosurique de certains dérivés du benzofurane, Presse méd. **73**, 2723—2726 (1965).
5. — C. Auscher, J. L. Olivier et A. Rose: Traitement des hyperuricémies et de la goutte par les dérivés du benzofurane; Sem. Hôp. Pricosuraris **43**, 1127—1133 (1967).
6. Dreyfuss and W. Czaczkes: The uricosuric action of bisdihydroxycoumarin (Dicoumarol). Ann. intern. Med. **102**, 389—391 (1958).
7. Gross, A., Action sur l'uricémie et sur l'uricosurie du L 2214; unpublished exper.
8. — V. Girard et J. Gaultier: Démonstration et étude de l'action uricosurique de la benziodarone. Thérapie **22**, 1097—1111 (1967).
9. Gutman, A. B.: Significance of the renal clearance of uric acid in normal and gouty man. Amer. J. Med. **37**, 833—838 (1964).
10. Hansen, O. E., and C. Holten: Uricosuric effect of Dicoumarol. Lancet **1958 I**, 1047—1048.
11. Jonio, A.: Le traitement ambulatoire des arthropathies de la goutte et de rhumatismes s'accompagnant d'hyperuricémie par la benziodarone. Gaz. Méd. de France, 15th Apr. 1967.
12. Masbernard, A., Ch. Hiltenbrand, J. Mémin et J. Déchelotte: La benziodarone dans le traitement de fond de la maladie goutteuse. C.-R. Soc. Rhum. du Sud-Ouest Nov. 1967. In: Rev. méd. Toulouse **4**, 401—424 (1968).
13. Medwedowski, J. L., et J. Marcovici: Action de la benziodarone sur l'uricosurie; Gaz. Méd. de France, 10th Jul. 1966.
14. Mugler, A.: Éffet sur l'uricémie, l'uricurie et la clearance de l'acide urique de l'acétyl-amino-2-chloro-5-benzoxazole chez 47 goutteux. Rev. Rhum. **30**, 363—369 (1963).
15. — Etude de cent goutteux traités par la benziodarone. Rev. Rhum. **34**, 197—208 (1967).
16. Nivet, M., J. Marcovici, P. Laruelle et Farah: Note préliminaire sur d'un benzofurrane sur l'uricémie. Bull. Soc. méd. Hôp. Paris **116**, 1187—1192 (1965).

17. Olmer, M., et J. Lafon: Action hypouricémiante du benziodarone dans l'insuffisance rénale chronique. Marseille-méd. **104**, 269—271 (1967).
18. Persellin, R. H., and F. R. Schmid: The use of sulfinepyrazone in the treatment of gout. Reduces uric acid level and diminishes severity of arthritic attacks with freedom from significant toxicity. J. Amer. med. Ass. **175**, 971—975 (1961).
19. Podevin, R., F. Paillard, C. Amiel et G. Richet: Action de la benziodarone sur l'excrétion rénale de l'acide urique. Rev. franç. Etud. clin. biol. **12**, 361—367 (1967).
20. Richet, G., J. Cottet, C. Amiel, C. Ledoux-Robert et R. Podevin: Traitement de l'hyperuricémie des goutteux et des insuffisants rénaux par la benziodarone. Presse méd. **74**, 1247—1249 (1966).
21. — C. Ledoux-Robert, R. Podevin et C. Amiel: Essai de traitement de l'hyperuricémie des insuffisants rénaux chroniques. Rev. franç. Etud. clin. **11**, 39—40 (1966).
22. Ryckewaert, A., J. Dry et F. Paologgi: Les hyperuricémies, I—VII. Rev. Rhum. **32**, 447—455, 783—789 (1966); **33**, 39—46, 136—144, 357—362, 580—587 (1966); **34**, 209—212 (1967).
23. Seze, S. de, A. Ryckewaert et J. D'Anglejan: Le traitement de la goutte par le Probénécide. Rev. Rhum. **30**, 93—102 (1963).
24. Soughin-Mibashan, R., and M. Horwitz: The uricosuric action of biscoumacetate. Lancet **1955 I**, 1191.

1.3. Ammonia

1.3.1. Renal Excretion of Ammonia

ROBERT F. PITTS[1]

With 9 Figures

Two-thirds or more of the non-volatile metabolic acid produced in the body is excreted in the urine neutralized by ammonia. In man phosphoric and sulfuric acids are normally generated in amounts of 40 to 80 milliequivalents per day in the oxidation of phospholipids and sulfur containing amino acids. If keto acids are formed in increased quantities, as a result of deranged metabolism of lipids, they too are excreted in large part neutralized by ammonia. Failure of renal production and excretion of ammonia to keep pace with production of acid results in acidosis.

$$NH_3 + H^+ \rightleftarrows NH_4^+$$

According to the BRØNSTED formulation, ammonia, NH_3, is a base, which in acid solution binds or buffers a hydrogen ion to form an ammonium ion, NH_4^+. Conversely the ammonium ion, NH_4^+, is an acid, which in alkaline solution dissociates a hydrogen ion to form the base ammonia. This buffer system has a number of unique properties. First, it is metabolically cheap. When demand increases, the base, NH_3, is withdrawn from the pool of excess dietary amino nitrogen which is normally excreted as the neutral waste product urea. Second, the base, NH_3, is uncharged, lipid soluble, and penetrates cell membranes readily, whereas the ammonium ion is charged, water soluble, and penetrates cell membranes slowly if at all. Third, the free base and ionic form are in equilibrium, and are rapidly interconverted in accord with the hydrogen ion concentration of the medium.

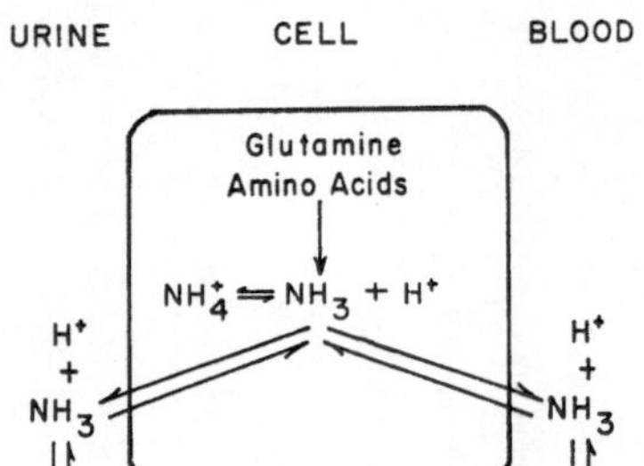

Fig. 1. Mechanism of tubular secretion of ammonia, involving intracellular synthesis from amino acids and passive non-ionic diffusion of the free base into urine and peritubular blood

These properties are basic to an understanding of the renal ammonia secreting mechanism. This mechanism is now generally conceded to be one of passive non-ionic diffusion (Fig. 1). Ammonia is formed in tubular cells from amino acids, in major part from glutamine. The base readily diffuses from cells to

[1] Department of Physiology and Biophysics, Cornell University Medial College, New York, N.Y., U.S.A.

tubular urine, where it binds hydrogen ions to form non-diffusible ammonium ions. To a lesser extent the base diffuses into peritubular capillaries and is carried out of the kidney in venous blood. No energy is expended directly in the transport of the base, only in maintaining the hydrogen ion gradient which determines the direction and magnitude of diffusion of base.

The first real proof of non-ionic diffusion as the mechanism of secretion of ammonia was provided by Dr. BALAGURA [1] in experiments illustrated by Fig. 2. Both experiments were performed on the same dog: the one on the left

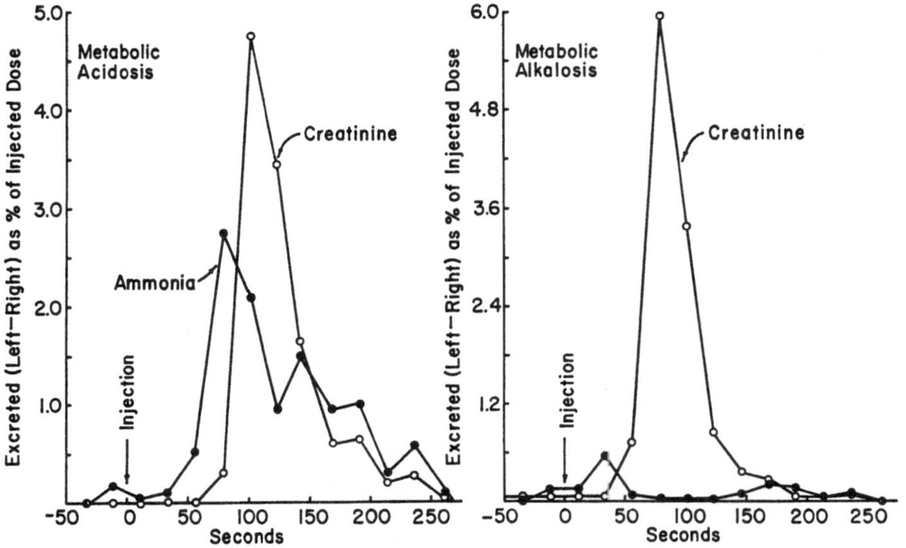

Fig. 2. Comparison of the time courses of excretion of creatinine and ammonium lactate into one renal artery of a dog. Left, dog in chronic metabolic acidosis excreting acid urine. Right, same dog in acute metabolic alkalosis excreting alkaline urine. From BALAGURA, S., and R. F. PITTS [1]

during metabolic acidosis; the one on the right, half an hour later, during metabolic alkalosis. In acidosis the urine was highly acid; in alkalosis, the urine was highly alkaline. Osmotic diuresis was induced and urine was collected separately from the two kidneys at intervals of about 20 seconds. At zero time a small volume of fluid containing creatinine and ammonium lactate was injected rapidly into one renal artery. The quantities of creatinine and ammonia excreted by the control kidney were subtracted from those excreted by the injected kidney, and the differences are plotted as per cent of the injected dose. Such subtraction corrects for recirculation.

Creatinine enters the tubule in the glomerular filtrate and must flow along the length of the nephron before appearing in the urine. In the acidotic state, shown on the left of Fig. 2, ammonia must have entered the tubular fluid downstream from the glomerulus, for it appeared in the urine significantly earlier than did creatinine. In the alkalotic state, shown on the right of Fig. 2, essentially none of the injected ammonia was excreted in the urine. Even that which entered the glomerular filtrate along with creatinine diffused back into peritubular blood.

Creatinine excretion was nearly the same in acidosis and alkalosis. These experiments demonstrate two facts: first that ammonia diffuses rapidly across the renal tubule in either direction, from blood to urine or from urine to blood; and second, that the direction of diffusion is determined by the hydrogen ion gradient. In acidosis, diffusion occurred from blood to highly acid urine. In alkalosis, diffusion occurred from highly alkaline urine to blood. Since these are the basic tenets of the theory of "non-ionic" diffusion, we can consider it established.

Dr. STONE [9] has recently shown that the base ammonia, NH_3, not only diffuses rapidly across renal tubules but also comes into diffusion equilibrium

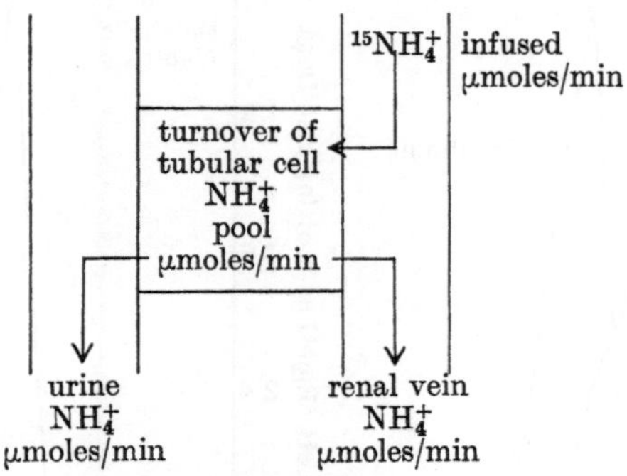

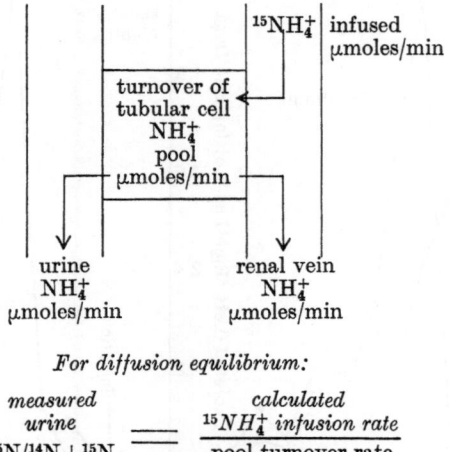

For diffusion equilibrium:

$$\text{measured urine } {}^{15}N/{}^{14}N+{}^{15}N = \frac{\text{calculated } {}^{15}NH_4^+ \text{ infusion rate}}{\text{pool turnover rate}}$$

Fig. 3. Schematic representation of the renal ammonia pool and the method of assessment of diffusion equilibrium. From STONE, W. J., S., BALAGURA, and R. F. PITTS, [9]

throughout all phases of the kidney within a period less than the transit time of blood through the kidney (see Fig. 3). The accumulation of total ammonia, base plus ammonium ion, is thus determined by the hydrogen ion concentration of the specific phase: blood, interstitial fluid, tubular cells, or tubular urine. Renal ammonia therefore exists as a single well mixed pool, mixed as a result of ready diffusion of the free base. The major fraction of this ammonia is synthesized in tubular cells from precursors delivered in arterial blood. The minor fraction is delivered to the kidney as preformed ammonia in arterial blood. The turnover of this cellular pool can be measured as the sum of the ammonia excreted in the urine and that which leaves the kidney in renal venous blood. If isotopic $^{15}NH_4Cl$ is infused at a known rate into one renal artery, it diffuses as the free base across tubular cells and into tubular urine, mixing thoroughly and completely with the ammonia produced within cells from unlabeled precursors. The dilution of the isotope in the total renal pool of ammonia can be calculated as the quotient of the rate of infusion of N^{15} ammonia and the rate of turnover of the pool. The dilution can be measured directly by quantifying the isotopic content of urine ammonia.

These principles are illustrated in an experiment on an acidotic dog shown in Table 1. Renal blood flow and renal venous ammonia concentration, and urine flow, urine ammonia concentration and the ratio of N^{15} to total urinary ammonia nitrogen were measured during infusion of N^{15} ammonium chloride into one renal artery.

Table 1. *Data illustrating the method of calculating the ammonia pool of the kidney and the attainment of diffusion equilibrium*

Ammonia			Specific activity		
venous out	urine out	pool turnover	pool	urine (L-R)	ratio of urine to pool
μmoles per min			atoms % excess ^{15}N		
Infuse $^{15}NH_4Cl$-1.85 μmoles per min					
21.2	37.6	58.8	3.16	3.30	1.04
17.4	37.7	55.1	3.36	3.35	1.00
15.1	37.2	52.3	3.45	3.44	1.00
Infuse $^{15}NH_4Cl$ — 9.27 μmoles per min					
20.4	40.0	60.4	15.35	15.39	1.00
19.1	39.0	58.1	15.95	15.85	0.99
17.0	41.3	58.3	15.90	15.91	1.00

The product of renal venous blood outflow and renal venous blood concentration of ammonia gives the ammonia leaving the kidney in the blood each min, namely 21.2 μmoles. The product of urine flow and urine ammonia concentration gives the ammonia excreted in the urine each min, namely 37.6 μmoles. The sum of venous outflow and urine excretion gives the renal ammonia pool turnover per min, namely 58.5 μmoles.

During this period, N^{15} ammonium chloride was infused at a rate of 1.85 μmoles excess N^{15} per min. The calculated pool specific activity is 1.85 μmoles N^{15} divided by 58.5 μmoles of ammonia × 100 or 3.16 atoms % excess N^{15}. The measured urine specific activity was 3.30 atoms % excess N^{15}, corrected for recirculation by subtracting the specific activity of the urine formed by the control kidney from that formed by the infused kidney. The ratio of measured to calculated specific activity was 1.04.

Increasing the rate of infusion of isotopic ammonia 5 fold to 9.27 μmoles excess N^{15} per min did not alter the ratio of measured to calculated pool specific activity. This experiment demonstrates two facts. First, N^{15} ammonia introduced into the renal artery distributes uniformly thoughout the kidney and mixes with the ammonia synthesized by the kidney in less than the transit time of blood through the kidney. Second, a five-fold increase in rate of administration of isotopic ammonia did not alter attainment of diffusion equilibrium, implying that the mechanism of distribution is one of passive non-ionic diffusion of the free base, not active transport.

Van Slyke and his associates [11] some 25 years ago provided conclusive evidence that glutamine is the major source of renal ammonia in the acidotic dog and that other unspecified amino acids constitute the minor source. Some 6 years ago, Shalhoub and his associates [8] in our laboratory and Owen and

Robinson [2] at Duke University repeated these studies on dog and man. They utilized chromatographic methods which enabled them to quantify net extraction of certain amino acids from blood and net addition of others to blood by the kidney. They observed in both dog and man that glutamine and glycine are extracted from arterial blood by the kidney and that alanine and serine are synthesized by the kidney and added to renal venous blood. The net overall extraction accounted adequately for ammonia production by the kidney [4].

We have utilized N^{15}-labeled amino acids to define more precisely the origin of urinary ammonia in the acidotic dog. Our method is illustrated in Fig. 4.

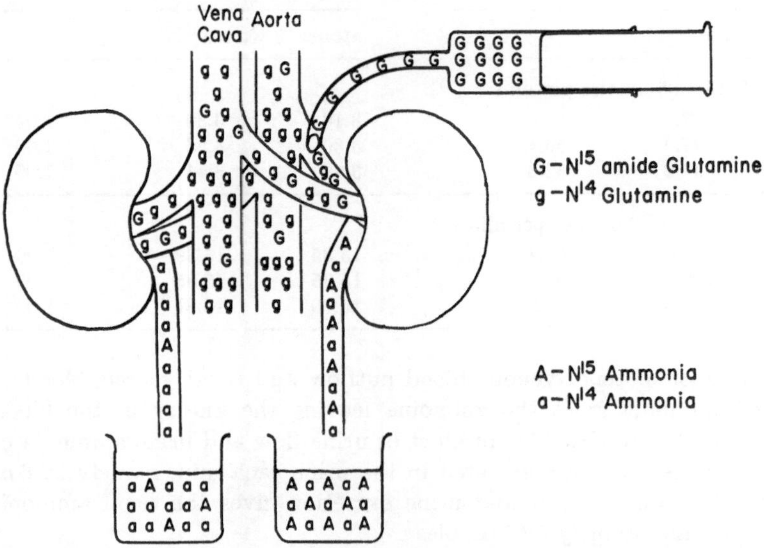

Fig. 4. Diagram illustrating the use of N^{15} labeled glutamine in the determination of the per cent of urinary ammonia derived from plasma glutamine

The ureters of an anesthetized dog are catheterized to permit collection of urine from the two kidneys separately. Through a fine needle introduced into the left renal artery, a solution of an N^{15}-labeled amino acid is infused at a constant rate in tracer amounts. In this experiment, N^{15} amide labeled glutamine was infused. This isotopic compound is represented by a capital G; the normally circulating unlabeled compound is represented by a small g. Similarly N^{15} ammonia is represented by a large A; N^{14} ammonia is represented by a small a. Ammonia containing N^{15} appears promptly and in relatively high concentration in the urine formed by the infused kidney, suggesting that the amide nitrogen of glutamine is an immediate precursor of ammonia. N^{15} also appears in much lower concentration in the ammonia excreted by the control kidney, for the labeled compound is incompletely extracted in one passage through the infused kidney, enters the general circulation, and is extracted by both kidneys. If one subtracts the atoms % excess N^{15} in the ammonia excreted by the control kidney from that excreted by the infused kidney, one corrects for this recirculation. The product of renal plasma flow and arterial concentration of glutamine gives the normal load of glutamine which perfuses the kidney. Addition of the amount of isotopic glutamine infused gives the total glutamine load. Division of rate of infusion of N^{15} by the total glutamine load gives specific activity of plasma glutamine, which like the specific activity of urine ammonia is corrected for recirculation.

Dividing specific activity of urine ammonia by specific activity of plasma glutamine and multiplying by 100, gives the percent of the urinary ammonia derived from the amide nitrogen of plasma glutamine.

A series of 36 experiments with 6 labeled compounds are summarized in Table 2. The amide nitrogen of glutamine is the source of 43.3% of the urinary

Table 2. *Percent of urinary ammonia derived from plasma precursors as determined by N^{15} labeling*

Number of	Ammonia excreted and added to renal venous blood		
experiments	Source	Mean per cent	Range per cent
9	Amide nitrogen of glutamine	43.3	35.3 —51.4
6	Amino nitrogen of glutamine	18.3	10.1 —25.5
8	Amino nitrogen of alanine	5.71	3.03— 8.41
5	Amino nitrogen of glycine	3.76	2.92— 5.55
2	Amino nitrogen of glutamate	1.88	1.43— 2.34
6	Arterial ammonia	35.0	23.0 —48.0
	Sum	108.0	

ammonia, ranging in different experiments from 35 to 51%. The amino nitrogen of glutamine is the source of some 18.3% of urinary ammonia. Thus nearly two-thirds of the urinary ammonia is derived from the two nitrogens of glutamine. The contributions of alanine, glycine and glutamate to urinary ammonia are much smaller, averaging about 6% for alanine, 4% for glycine and 2% for glutamate [6]. Arterial inflow of preformed ammonia accounts for an average of 35% of urinary ammonia [9]. The sum of the mean values for all of these potential contributors to urinary ammonia account for 108% of that excreted by the kidney. This gives us confidence that we have accounted for essentially all of the major precursors of urinary ammonia. The fact that Dr. STONE has shown that renal ammonia exists as a single well mixed pool, implies that each of these precursors contributes to the ammonia added to renal venous blood in exactly the same proportions as it does to urinary ammonia.

Glycine and alanine contribute modestly to renal ammonia production, when the plasma concentrations of these amino acids are within the range of normal [5, 7]. However, the intravenous infusion of glycine or alanine, to increase plasma concentration some five fold, greatly increases the contribution of the infused amino acid to ammonia production.

In a series of three experiments summarized in Fig. 5, plasma glycine [5] was increased in stepwise fashion from a normal value between 0.1 and 0.2 µmoles per ml to values as high as 0.6 to 0.9 µmoles per ml. In the graph on the left the per cent contribution of glycine to urinary ammonia increased linearly with plasma glycine concentration. In the graph on the right the number of µmoles of ammonia formed from glycine nitrogen similarly increased with plasma glycine concentration from about 1.0 to as much as 9.0 μmoles per min.

A series of six experiments summarized in Fig. 6 demonstrates that increasing the plasma concentration of alanine [7] similarly increases its contribution to urinary ammonia. Other experiments with N^{15} amide and amino labeled glutamines gave somewhat similar results. It is thus apparent that, if a dietary excess of one amino acid causes an increase in its plasma concentration, that

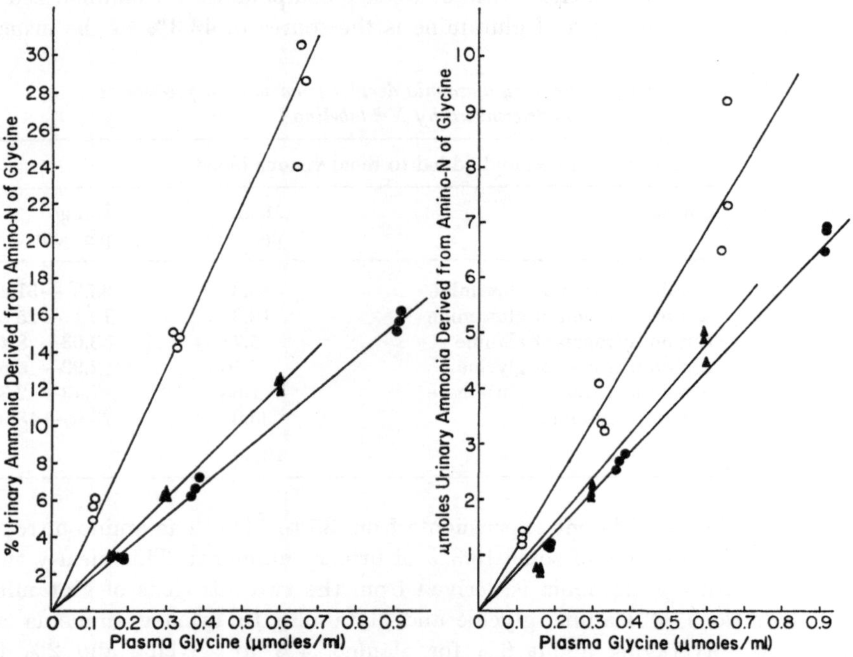

Fig. 5. Relations between plasma concentration of glycine and the per cent (left) and absolute amount (right) of urinary ammonia derived from glycine. From PITTS, R. F., and L. A. PILKINGTON, [5]

amino acid is preferentially used for ammonia formation. Some of the variability in per cent contribution of a given amino acid to ammonia formation under normal circumstances, therefore, results from normal variations in concentration of circulating plasma amino acids.

Plasma alanine is normally the precursor of some 3 to 8% of renal ammonia, implying that this amino acid is extracted from plasma and deaminated to form ammonia and pyruvic acid. However, in all of our studies in which arterio-venous differences in plasma alanine concentration have been measured, we have observed a net synthesis of alanine and its addition to renal venous plasma in the dog.

Experiments utilizing N^{15} labeled alanine have enabled us to study the simultaneous extraction of alanine from plasma, its utilization as a source of urinary ammonia, and its net renal synthesis and addition to renal venous blood. In the graph on the left of Fig. 7 are shown three experiments in which simultaneous production of alanine and utilization as a source of ammonia were studied.

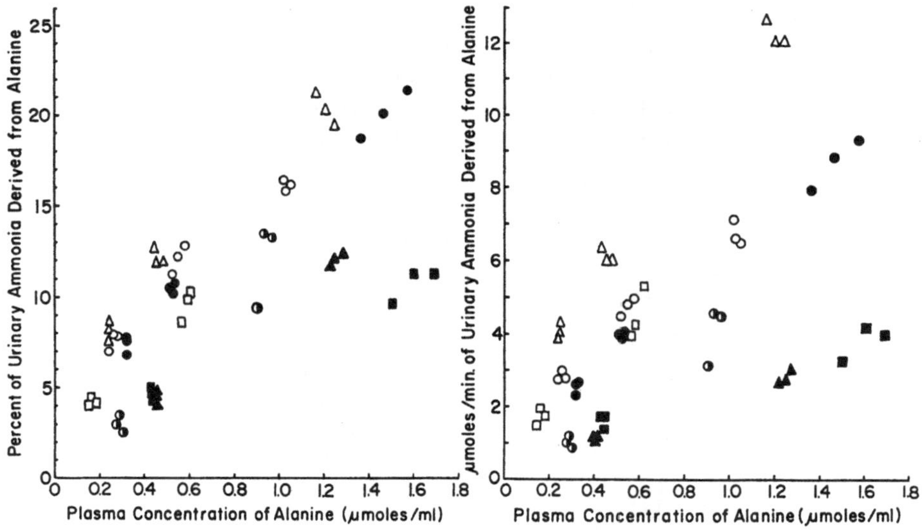

Fig. 6. Relations between plasma concentration of alanine and the per cent (left) and absolute amount (right) of urinary ammonia derived from alanine. From PITTS, R. F. and W. J. STONE [7]

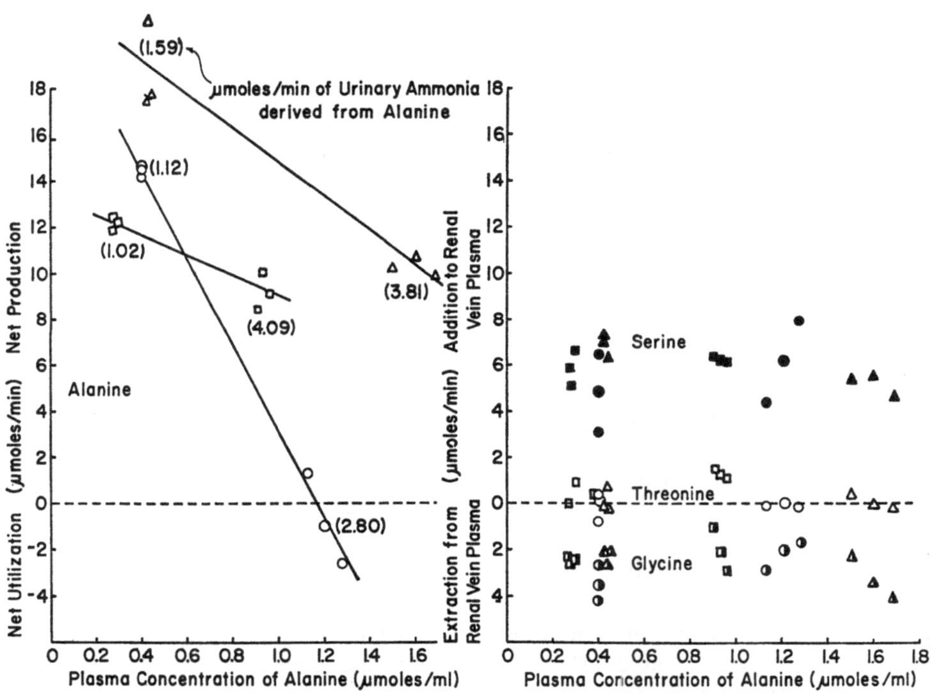

Fig. 7. Left, comparison of renal production of alanine and utilization of plasma alanine as a source of urinary ammonia at normal and elevated plasma alanine concentrations. Right, simultaneous comparison of renal production of serine, extraction of glycine and relative inertness of threonine at normal and elevated plasma alanine concentrations. From PITTS, R. F. and W. J. STONE [7]

The points to the left of this graph represent values of net production at normal plasma alanine concentrations. It is apparent at concentrations of 0.3 to 0.4 μmoles per ml, that from 12 to 18 μmoles of alanine were synthesized and added to renal venous blood each minute. Simultaneously, alanine was extracted from plasma and served as the precursor of 1.02 to 1.59 μmoles per min of urinary ammonia.

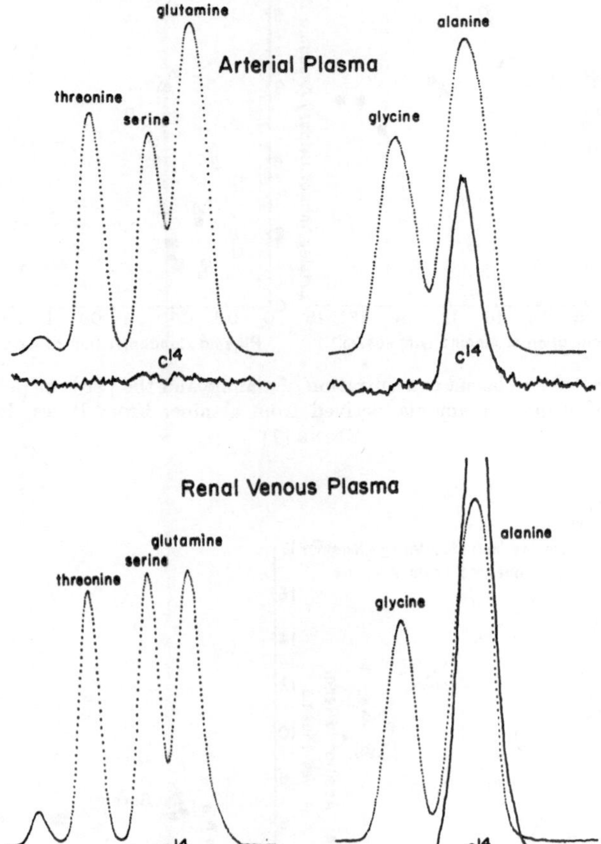

Fig. 8. Ninhydrin colorimetric and C^{14} activity chromatograms of arterial and renal venous plasmas during administration of carboxyl C^{14} pyruvate into the left renal artery. From Pitts, R. F. and W. J. Stone [7]

These values are shown in parentheses. When plasma alanine was increased 3 to 5 fold by infusing alanine intravenously, net synthesis decreased and utilization as a source of urinary ammonia increased to 2.8 to 4.09 μmoles per min. Such results suggest that synthesis of alanine and utilization of alanine as a precursor of ammonia are dependent on the reversible reactions of transamination. At normal plasma alanine concentrations, synthesis is favored; at elevated plasma alanine concentrations, utilization as a source of ammonia is favored. The data on the right of this slide were obtained in these same three experiments. They demonstrate that the net production of serine, the extraction of glycine, and the relative inertness of threonine are unaffected by increase in plasma alanine concentration. These facts add further weight to the evidence that transamination plays a major role in both production and utilization of alanine.

The production of alanine in the kidney from pyruvate and its addition to renal venous blood is demonstrated in another way in the experiment shown in Fig. 8. Results are consonant with transamination as the reaction involved. In the upper half of this figure are shown chromatograms of arterial plasma; in the lower half are shown chromatograms of renal venous plasma. The upper

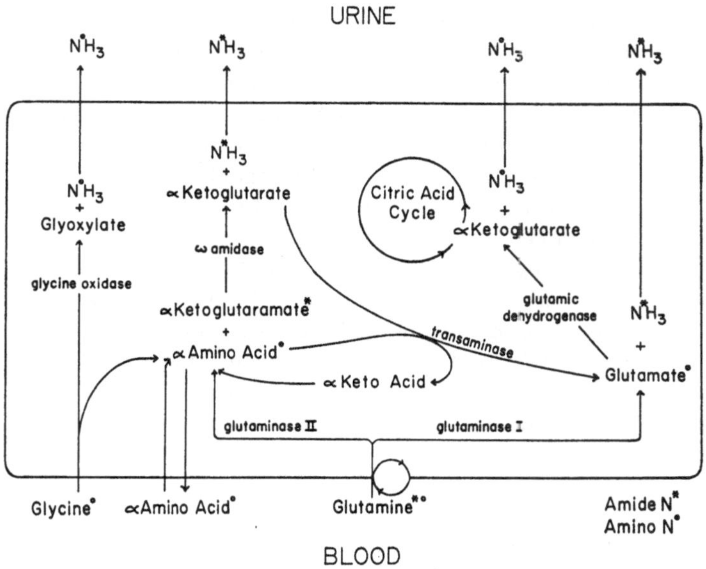

Fig. 9. Simplified scheme illustrating major metabolic pathways involved in the renal formation of ammonia and amino acids. From PITTS, R. F. [3]

trace of each pair is the colorimetric Ninhydrin curve which defines concentrations of amino acids. The lower trace is the C^{14} flow scintillation activity curve. In this experiment C^{14}-carboxyl labeled pyruvate was infused into one renal artery of a dog at a rate of 1.0 μcurie per min. Arterial blood and renal venous blood from the infused kidney were collected simultaneously, and the plasmas separated and chromatographed. It is apparent that the C^{14} of pyruvate was incorporated into the alanine which the kidney added to renal venous plasma. Thus the trace which recorded C^{14} activity was off scale for renal venous alanine in comparison with arterial alanine. None of the pyruvate-carboxyl C^{14} appeared in the other amino acids. The presence of labeled alanine in small amounts in arterial plasma is the result of recirculation of that formed by the infused kidney and added to renal venous blood.

The major pathways involved in the renal production of ammonia and in the synthesis of the alanine and serine which the kidney adds to renal venous blood are illustrated [10] in the diagram of a renal tubular cell shown as Fig. 9. Precursors are shown as entering the cell only at the antiluminal surface. Ammonia is shown as leaving the cell only at the luminal or urinary surface. This convention has been adopted arbitrarily to simplify the diagram, for obviously ammonia is added to capillary blood and precursors are reabsorbed from the glomerular filtrate. On the right of Fig. 9 is shown the glutaminase I pathway, by which glutamine is metabolized to glutamate and the amide nitrogen is liberated as ammonia. The glutamate formed in this reaction is oxidatively deaminated by glutamic dehydrogenase to form a-ketoglutarate and the amino nitrogen is liberated as ammonia. On the left of Fig. 9 is shown the glutaminase II or glutamine transaminase pathway. Glutamine transaminates a-keto acids, such as pyruvate, hydroxypyruvate and oxaloacetate to form alanine, serine and aspartate plus a-ketoglutaramate. This latter compound is immediately deamidated by tissue omega amidase to yield ammonia and a-ketoglutarate. Although the glutaminase I pathway probably plays the major role in the metabolism of glutamine, Dr. STONE has recently shown that the glutaminase II pathway may contribute significantly to the renal synthesis of alanine and aspartate [10]. In so far as it contributes to the formation of these amino acids, it contributes to ammonia formation from the amide nitrogen of glutamine. Alanine is metabolized by the a-amino acid pathway, transaminating a-ketoglutarate to glutamate which subsequently is metabolized by glutamic dehydrogenase to regenerate a-ketoglutarate and liberate ammonia. Glycine is shown at the far left, perhaps in part metabolized by glycine oxidase to glyoxalate and ammonia, possibly in part transferring its nitrogen to a-ketoglutarate by the more conventional a-amino acid pathway.

References

1. BALAGURA, S., and R. F. PITTS: Excretion of ammonia injected into renal artery. Amer. J. Physiol. **203**, 11—14 (1962).
2. OWEN, E. E., and R. R. ROBINSON: Amino acid extraction and ammonia metabolism by the human kidney during the prolonged administration of ammonium chloride. J. clin. Invest. **42**, 263—276 (1963).
3. PITTS, R. F.: Renal production and excretion of ammonia. Amer. J. Med. **36**, 720—742 (1964).
4. — J. C. M. DE HAAS, and J. KLEIN: Relation of renal amino and amide nitrogen extraction to ammonia production. Amer. J. Physiol. **204**, 187—191 (1963).
5. —, and L. A. PILKINGTON: The relation between plasma concentrations of glutamine and glycine and utilization of their nitrogens as sources of urinary ammonia. J. clin. Invest. **45**, 86—93 (1966).
6. — —, and J. C. M. DE HAAS: N^{15} tracer studies on the origin of urinary ammonia in the acidotic dog, with notes on the enzymatic synthesis of labeled glutamic acid and glutamines. J. clin. Invest. **44**, 731—745 (1965).
7. —, and W. J. STONE: Renal metabolism of alanine. J. clin. Invest. **46**, 530—538 (1967).
8. SHALHOUB, R., W. WEBBER, S. GLABMAN, M. CANESSA-FISCHER, J. KLEIN, J. DE HAAS, and R. F. PITTS: Extraction of amino acids from and their addition to renal blood plasma. Amer. J. Physiol. **204**, 181—186 (1963).
9. STONE, W. J., S. BALAGURA, and R. F. PITTS: Diffusion equilibrium for ammonia in the kidney of the acidotic dog. J. clin. Invest. **46**, 1603—1608 (1967).
10. —, and R. F. PITTS: Pathways of ammonia metabolism in the intact functioning kidney of the dog. J. clin. Invest. **46**, 1141 —1150 (1967).
11. SLYKE, D. D. VAN, R. A. PHILLIPS, P. B. HAMILTON, R. M. ARCHIBALD, P. H. FUTCHER, and A. HILLER: Glutamine as source material for urinary ammonia. J. biol. Chem. **150**, 481—482 (1943).

Discussion

MÜLLER:

Would you care to comment on the influence of potassium in renal tubular cells on ammonia excretion?

KRÜCK:

In chronic renal failure, we always find a rather close correlation between NH_4-excretion and GFR or RPF, in spite of metabolic acidosis and the excretion of an acid urine.

Would you interpret this finding as a consequence of the decrease in the amount of precursors which reach the tubular cells? Or are there other known metabolic disturbances within tubular cells which could inhibit the secretion of ammonia in renal failure?

1.4. Experimental Uremia

1.4.1. Retrograde Flow of Fluid within Superficial Tubules after Cessation of Glomerular Filtration *

M. Brandis, G. Braun-Schubert and K. H. Gertz[1]

With 1 Figure

In the literature many estimations of the amount of fluid reabsorbed out of proximal surface convolutions are available. So far, however, it appeares impossible to obtain direct information concerning fluid reabsorption in proximal convolutions of juxtamedullary nephrons, because they are not directly accessible to micropuncture. In the present experiments an attempt was made to observe the flow characteristics of surface tubules and of deep juxtamedullary tubules by inspection of the kidney surface and by inspection of the exposed papilla during aortic clamping. After cessation of glomerular filtration, the tubular epithelium continues to reabsorb the intraluminal fluid, until a complete collapse of the proximal tubular lumen results. If the rate of continuous sodium chloride and fluid reabsorption were different in surface and juxtamedullary nephrons, the longitudinal flow of tubular fluid should be affected differently in the two regions, which are connected by the distal tubular system and the upper collecting ducts. Thus we hoped to get some insight into functional differences which might exist between the two nephron populations.

Methods

The experiments were performed on rats, anesthetized with Inactin (10 mg/100 g of body weight i.p.).

The left kidney was exposed for micropuncture as originally described by Wirz [3].

First, a short column of Sudan black stained mineral oil was injected into a single proximal convolution. Subsequently, the aorta was reversibly occluded by means of a clamp, and the movement of the oil column within the tubular lumen was observed.

In a second series of experiments we injected 0.02 ml of a 10% solution of lissamine green into a jugular vein [2]. Upon filtration, a dye column, well visible from the surface, moves downstream through the nephrons. During the passage of the dye column along the proximal and distal convolution, the filtration was stopped by aortic clamping and any further movement of the dye column was observed.

In a third series of experiments intraluminal flow of lissamine green-coloured fluid columns within the long loops of Henle was observed by inspecting the trans-illuminated papilla. Such movements could be observed without cutting the ureter and the pelvis.

Results

After interruption of filtration, the oil droplet as well as the dye column in surface tubules showed a retrograde flow of the intraluminal fluid towards the glomerula.

---

* Supported by Deutsche Forschungsgemeinschaft.

[1] Physiologisches Institut der Freien Universität Berlin, Germany.

Even when the dye columns had left the proximal convolutions, so that the kidney surface had regained its usual pink colour for 5 to 7 seconds, the dye columns reappeared in the last proximal convolutions after clamping the aorta.

In the long loops of HENLE, however, no retrograde flow was observed. Quite to the contrary, the stained urine columns continued to move further downstream towards the distal parts of the nephron after clamping.

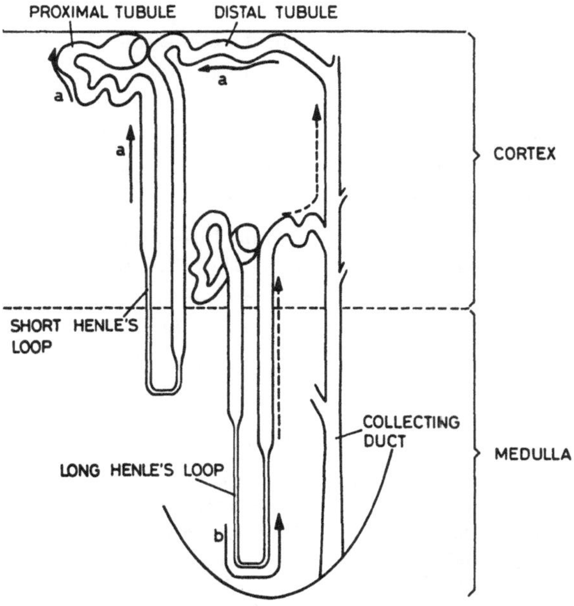

Fig. 1. Superficial and deep nephrons. *Arrow a*: Showing the retrograde flow in the superficial proximal tubules after clamping the aorta. *Arrow b*: Showing the orthograde flow in the long Henle's loops after clamping the aorta

Outflow of urine at the papillary tip stopped within a few seconds after cessation of filtration.

Fig. 1 illustrates schematically a superficial and a deep nephron. The dark arrows indicate where flow could be observed directly: i.e. the retrograde flow in kidney surface tubules (a) and the orthograde flow in the long loops of HENLE at the tip of the papilla (b).

Since after cessation of glomerular filtration, stained tubular fluid reappeared by retrograde flow in the terminal proximal convolutions, 5—7 seconds after disappearance from the kidney surface[2], a fluid volume equivalent to the capacity of the pars recta must have flowed back into the convoluted parts of the proximal tubules.

The quite different behaviour of the juxtamedullary nephrons in this time period is demonstrated by the continuous orthograde flow in the long loops. Since, at the same time, urine ceases to flow from the papillary orifice, fluid

[2] This is equivalent to 20% of the normal transit time of tubular fluid through the loop of HENLE [2].

from the juxtamedullary region cannot be drained down-stream into the collecting duct system.

We thus arrive at the assumption of a continuous flow of juxtamedullary tubular fluid through juxtamedullary distal convolutions and subsequently, in the reverse direction, through the cortical nephrons up to the cortical proximal segments. This continuous flow is illustrated by the dark (visible) and dotted (not visible) arrows in Fig. 1.

Such a movement of intratubular fluid is possible if the reabsorption from the superficial proximal convolutions is much more rapid than from any other part of the nephrons, including the proximal convolutions of juxtamedullary nephrons. From the present observations one may conclude that the relationship between filtration and rate of reabsorption is different in the deep proximal convolutions as compared with surface tubules.

An obvious implication of the retrograde flow of tubular fluid into proximal surface tubules during aortic clamping is that "*occlusion time*" [1] is an unreliable parameter for the quantitative evaluation of the transport capacity of superficial proximal convolutions, unless it be corrected by a quantitative estimation of backflow from juxtamedullary structures.

References

1. Leyssac, P. P.: Dependence of glomerular filtration rate on proximal tubular reabsorption of salt. Acta physiol. scand. 58, 236—242 (1963).
2. Steinhausen, M.: Eine Methode zur Differenzierung proximaler und distaler Tubuli der Nierenrinde von Ratten *in vivo* und ihre Anwendung zur Bestimmung tubulärer Strömungsgeschwindigkeiten. Pflügers Arch. ges. Physiol. 277, 23—35 (1963).
3. Wirz, H.: Druckmessung in Kapillaren und Tubuli durch Mikropunktion. Helv. physiol. pharmacol. Acta 13, 42—49 (1955).

Discussion

Steinhausen:

In similar experiments we observed just the contrary of your findings. With techniques similar to yours, completed by photographic recording, we found that 11 sec after injecting lissamine-green, the dye reached the lowest parts of the visible proximal convolutions. When the aorta was clamped, at this stage, above the renal arteries, the lumina of the proximal tubules collapsed, while the dye stayed in the lower parts of the proximal convolutions, which it had reached before the interruption of blood flow. There was no retrograde flow of dye in these convolutions. The apparent contradiction between your observations and ours may be due to the fact that in our experiments, the kidney was decapsulated and superfused with Tyrode solution, while in your experiments the kidney was not decapsulated, and covered by a layer of mineral oil. We recently demonstrated that the rate of reabsorption from superficial proximal tubules is depressed when the renal surface is covered with Tyrode solution. This depression may result in a decrease of the "aspiration" of fluid from collecting ducts and deeper nephrons into the superficial convolutions.

FÜLGRAFF:

Could your observations be explained by a slower rate of reabsorption in the distal as compared to the proximal convolutions of the superficial nephrons? Could the retrograde flow into the proximal convolutions originate from liquid contained in the pars recta?

BRANDIS to STEINHAUSEN: You gave the answer to your question yourself. The transit-time values under your experimental conditions were much longer than ours. This fact corresponds with depression of fluid-reabsorption from superficial proximal tubules, when the renal surface is covered by Tyrode solution instead of mineral oil. — To FÜLGRAFF: The retrograde flow in the superficial proximal and distal convolutions is possible because of a lower reabsorption rate in the juxtamedullary nephrons compared to the superficial.

1.4.2. Cellular Metabolism in Uremia

D. Renner and R. Heintz[1]

With 3 Figures

In previous investigations on the metabolism of tissues in uremia [2, 4—7], we found the following disturbances:

1. A decrease in the synthesis of coenzyme-A containing compounds.
2. Uncoupling of respiration and phosphorylations.
3. Decreased glucose utilization by brain tissue.
4. An increased utilization of amino acids and an accelerated breakdown of protein.

These findings may explain some clinical observations. As shown by Knauff [3], the concentration of amino-acids in jugular vein blood of uremic subjects is decreased while the concentration of ammonia is increased. Using the Kety-Schmidt method, Gottstein [1] found a decrease in cerebral glucose utilization with a much smaller decrease in cerebral oxygen uptake.

We previously found that the metabolic disturbances in uremia may be due to the presence in uremic serum of dialysable substances of low molecular weight. Attempts to isolate such substances from uremic serum failed, presumably because of the small amounts of serum available. We, therefore, attempted to isolate such substances from the dialysing fluid used for hemodialysis of uremic patients with a tank-kidney. We succeeded in isolating and in concentrating some fractions which, when added to the incubation medium (Krebs-Ringer-bicarbonate solution) induced changes in tissue metabolism similar to those induced by serum from uremic patients.

100 l of dialysing fluid were stirred for 12 hours with four hundred gm of activated charcoal. After setting down, the suspension was centrifuged at 12,000 g at 4°C, and the supernatant was discarded. The remaining 600 ml of moist charcoal sludge were divided into 3 portions of 200 ml each, which were brought to pH 7.0, 3.5, or 8.5 and extracted separately for 24 hours with 400 ml of freshly distilled n-butanol. Butanol extraction of each fraction was repeated twice. The butanol extracts obtained from each fraction were mixed and evaporated to dryness. We, thus, obtained 1. a "pH 7-fraction"; 2. a "pH 3.5-fraction"; and 3. a "pH 8.5-fraction". Three control fractions were obtained from unused dialysing fluid. The control fractions had no influence on the metabolic parameters measured.

The fractions were redissolved in Krebs-Ringer-bicarbonate solution and added to incubation mixtures of tissues.

Added to renal slices at a final concentration of ~ 0.1 mg/ml, the pH 7-fraction depressed, the pH 3.5-fraction did not influence, and the pH 8.5-fraction

[1] Abt. Innere Medizin II der Medizin. Fakultät der Techn. Hochschule Aachen.

increased Q_{O_2}. Pyruvate utilization was depressed by all three fractions. Gluconeogenesis was depressed by the pH 7- and the pH 3.5-fractions. With pyruvate as a substrate, in experiments with the pH 3.5- and the pH 8.5-fractions, the hydrogen accounting for the Q_{O_2} must, therefore, originate from the oxidative deamination of amino-acids contained in the tissue (Fig. 1).

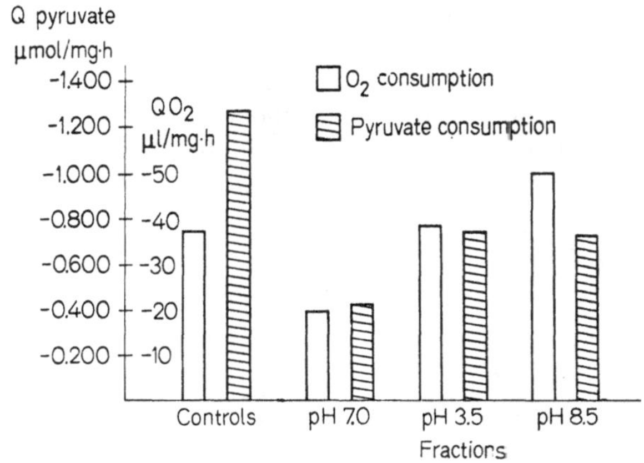

Fig. 1

With α-ketoglutarate as a substrate, the pH 7-fraction caused the same decrease in substrate utilization, while the utilization of aspartic acid and of glutamic acid was not depressed. The pH 7-fraction also depressed anaerobic glycolysis by 50%.

Added to human red blood cell suspensions, the pH 7-fraction depressed glucose degradation by aerobic glycolysis. At the same time the oxygen uptake of the RBC, as well as their glucose utilization in the presence of methylene-blue

	Q_{O_2} µL/mg·hour	$Q_{CO_2}^{O_2}$ µL/mg·hour	$Q_{CO_2}^{N_2}$ µL/mg·hour	Consumption of glucose µM/mg·hour
Renal cortex, controls			+6.7	—0.175
Renal cortex, fraction 1 added			+3.3	—0.071
R.B.C., MB, controls	—30.5			—1.270
R.B.C., MB, fraction 1 added	—42			—1.500
R.B.C., controls		+65		—1.130
R.B.C., fraction 1 added		+30		—0.860

Fig. 2. Utilization of glucose by renal cortical slices and by red blood cells. The values are means of three experiments. Fraction 1 = fraction "pH 7"

was increased. The discrepancy is presumably due to the ability of RBC to degrade glucose by the pentose-phosphate-shunt. Under the influence of the pH 7-fraction this shunt may be used to a larger extent by tissues which possess the appropriate enzymes. In brain tissue, the transfer capacities of these enzymes are quite small. The low-spontaneous oxygen consumption of RBC suspensions was increased from 2 µl to 4 µl/ml of suspension / hour by adding the pH 7-fraction. The increased oxygen consumption may serve to compensate for the loss of a source of energy by the inhibition of glycolysis.

Purification and identification of the compounds contained in the three fractions obtained from dialysis fluid was attempted by thin layer-chromatography and color reactions. The solvent used was the Partridge-mixture; the spots were stained with the Folin-Ciocalteau reagent for phenolic compounds and the Sakaguchi reagent for guanidine-bases. With all three fractions the chromatographic separation yielded four phenolic and two guanidine spots. The phenolic spots were not yet identified. The guanidine-base spots may be due to the presence of guanidine or of methylguanidine, or of dimethylguanidine. The

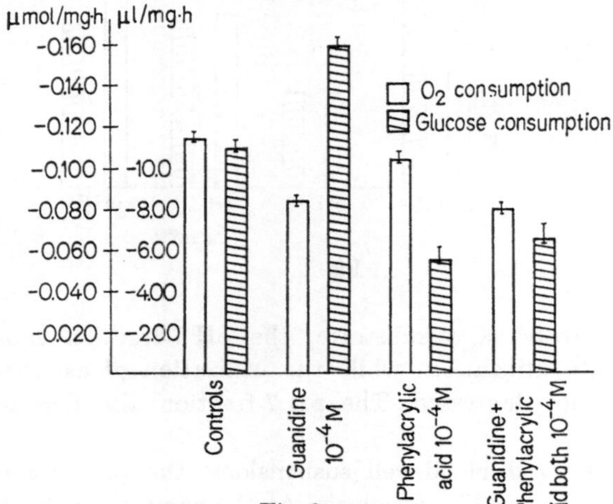

Fig. 3

presence of arginine, which would give a similare action, is excluded by the absence of CO_2-formation in the presence of ninhydrine, which should occur if the fractions contained amino-acids.

Since the fractions, thus, contained phenolic compounds and derivatives of guanidine and since other investigators [8] found that a number of phenolic compounds alter the respiration of brain homogenates, we investigated the effects of two model drugs, guanidine and phenylacrylic acid, on the metabolism of brain and kidney slices.

As shown in Fig. 3, phenylacrylic acid clearly depressed glucose utilization without depressing Q_{O_2}. This observation is similar to those made with uremic serum.

While analogous effects of this type do not prove that the effects of uremic serum or fractions isolated therefrom are due to the presence of a given substance, they may orient further research in this field.

References

1. HEINTZ, R., u. D. RENNER: Über Hemmwirkungen des Serums von Kranken mit hepatorenalem Syndrom und mit chronischer Urämie auf Sauerstoffverbrauch und Kohlenhydratstoffwechsel von Nieren- und Hirngewebe der Ratte. Klin. Wschr. 43, 1167—1173 (1965).

2. RENNER, D., and R. HEINTZ: Metabolic changes of kidney and brain tissue incubated in sera of chronic uremic patients. 2nd Congr. of E.D.T.A. Newcastle upon Tyne 1965.
3. — — Lokalisation von Störungen des Zellstoffwechsels im urämischen Serum. 4. Symposion der Dtsch. Ges. für Nephrologie Homburg (Saar) 1965.
4. — — Der O_2-Verbrauch von Nieren- und Hirngewebe in Seren von Leber- und Nierenkranken. Verh. 3. Symposion Dtsch. Ges. für Nephrologie, Bern. Stuttgart: Huber 1965.
5. — — Untersuchungen des Zellstoffwechsels im Serum von Kranken mit Urämie. II. Mitt. Klin. Wschr. **44**, 1204—1209 (1966).
6. KNAUFF, H. G.: Diskussionsbemerkung. Verh. Med. Ges. Marburg 1965 (17. 5.).
7. GOTTSTEIN, U.: Zirkulation, Sauerstoff- und Glucosestoffwechsel des Gehirns bei Encephalopathien. Verh. Dtsch. Ges. Inn. Med. Wiesbaden, 1966, S. 185—198.
8. HICKS, J. P., J. C. WOTTON, and D. S. YOUNG: Abnormal blood constituents in acute renal failure. Clin. Chim. Acta **7**, 623—633, 1962.

Discussion

SCHÜTTERLE:

Did you find any correlation between the metabolic effects of uremic serum and the concentration of NPN, urea, uric acid or other nitrogen-containing metabolites? Did you find any difference between the metabolic effects of serum from patients with acute or chronic uremia?

Did you also investigate the xanthoprotein reaction in your sera? Xanthoprotein-positive substances are usually present in higher concentrations in chronic than in acute uremia. Was there any correlation between the concentration of xanthoprotein-positive substances and metabolic effects?

1.4.3. Intratubular Pressure, Glomerular Capillary Pressure and Tubular Passage-Time in Rats with Masugi-Nephritis*

W. SCHOEPPE, K. FEDERLIN and F. SORGE[1]

With 2 Figures

A method for measuring glomerular capillary pressure in micropuncture experiments in rats was described by GERTZ and MANGOS in 1965 [1]. After blocking urine flow in a proximal tubule by injecting oil into its lower part, the pressure in the convolutions between the glomerulus and the oil block increases, and reaches an stable steady maximal value. When this value is reached and

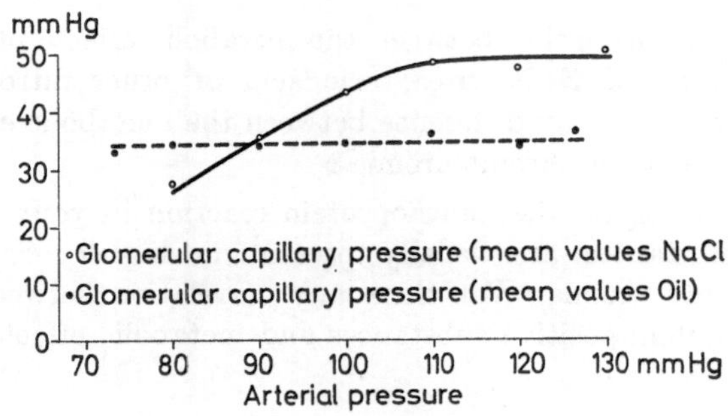

Fig. 1

glomerular filtration has stopped, this pressure equals the glomerular filtration pressure, which was found by GERTZ and MANGOS to vary around 63 mm Hg in normal rats. OCHWADT et al. [3] showed that the glomerular capillary pressure (stop-pressure), measured according to GERTZ and MANGOS, may vary in the physiological range of blood pressures. These investigators found an increase in stop-pressure after furosemide. The normal mean value was 52 mm Hg, and thus somewhat lower than the value reported by GERTZ and MANGOS.

We found still lower values of stop-pressure, using GERTZ and MANGOS' technique under different experimental conditions. Furthermore, the stop-pressure appeared to depend on the temperature as well as on the composition of the fluid covering the surface of the kidney during measurements. As shown in Fig. 1, the stop-pressure increased with arterial pressure between 80 and 110 mm Hg, when the kidney was covered with mineral oil, and reached stable values with higher blood pressures. When the kidney surface was covered with a 0.9% NaCl-solution, the stop-pressure was lower and did not increase with

* Supported by Deutsche Forschungsgemeinschaft.

[1] II. Medizinische Klinik und Medizinische Poliklinik der Universität Frankfurt a. M. und Klinischer Bereich des Zentrums für Innere Medizin der Universität Ulm, West-Germany.

changes in systemic blood pressure within the range of auto-regulation. Thus, arterial resistance, appears to be influenced by the medium covering the surface as well as by blood pressure.

Measurements of glomerular filtration pressure in nephrotoxic nephritis have not been reported hitherto. The so-called needle-pressure was found elevated in Masugi-nephritis by REUBI [4]. Inasfar as nephrotoxic nephritis is analogous to human glomerulonephritis, this result supported indirect conclusions by SARRE [5], which invalidated VOLHARD's assumption of a vasospastic ischemia of the glomerular tufts in this disease.

Masugi-nephritis was induced in Sprague-Dawley rats, weighing 150 to 200 g, by an intravenous injection of 8 ml/kg b.w. of a nephrotoxic serum. The nephro-

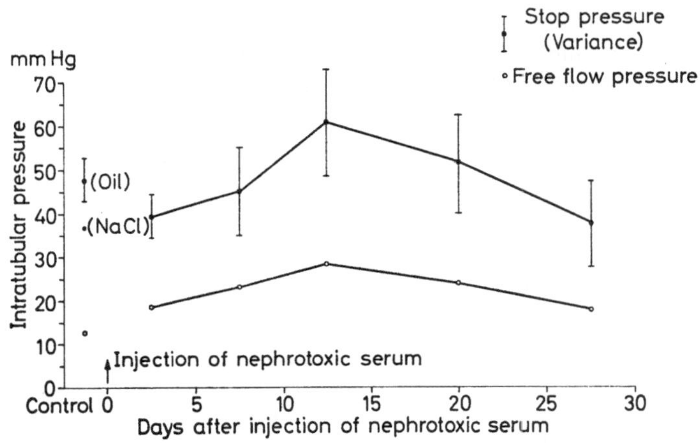

Fig. 2

toxic anti-rat kidney-serum was obtained from rabbits, and tested in other rats prior to use in the present experiments. At different intervals after injection of nephrotoxic serum, animals were anesthethized with Inactin and prepared for intratubular pressure measurements as described by WIRZ [6] and GOTTSCHALK [2]. Proximal tubular pressure was then first measured during free flow of tubular fluid, and then after injecting oil. The lissamine green-passage time was also measured. Arterial blood pressure was recorded during the whole experiment. At the end of each experiment the kidneys were removed, and stained sections studied for the presence of typical glomerulo-nephritis, i.e. splitting of the basal membrane and enlargement of the mesangium, which were present in all animals included in the present series.

Fig. 2 shows free flow-pressures and stop-pressures measured in the 30 days following the injection of nephrotoxic serum. The injection was first followed by an increase in free-flow pressure in the proximal tubule; after 10 to 14 days, the stop-pressure, i.e. the capillary filtration pressure, also increased. 4 weeks after the injection of nephrotoxic serum, both pressures decreased slightly. With the increase in free flow- and stop-pressure, the scatter of these values increased considerably: 14 days after the injection of nephrotoxic serum, free flow-pressures varied from 15 to 40 mm Hg, stop-pressures from 30 to 90 mm Hg.

Proximal lissamine green-passage time through proximal tubules increased from an initial value of 9 sec to 16 sec, 14 days after nephrotoxic serum. Passage-time through HENLE's loop remained unchanged (30 sec).

In the animals with nephrotoxic nephritis there was no difference between stop-pressures measured with the kidney surface covered with mineral oil or with 0.9% NaCl-solution.

The data, thus, show an increase in glomerular-capillary filtration-pressure and in proximal tubular pressure in the course of nephrotoxic nephritis with a large variation between different nephrons. These changes appear to be independent of changes in blood pressure. There is no reason to assume that vascular resistance in efferent arterioles changes in the course of nephrotoxic nephritis. Vascular resistance, furthermore, proved to be less dependent on changes of conditions on the surface of the kidney than in normal animals. The increase in proximal passage-time of lissamine-green may be due to a decrease in glomerular filtration rate, which was not measured in the present experiments. If this were so, the unchanged passage time through HENLE's loops would argue for a decreased fractional reabsorption in the proximal tubules, unless there was a simultaneous increase in distal tubular resistance.

References

1. GERTZ, K. H., and J. A. MANGOS: On the pressure in the glomerular capillaries of the rat kidney. In: Aktuelle Probleme der Nephrologie. IV. Symposion der Ges. für Nephrologie. Hrsg. F. KRÜCK. Berlin-Heidelberg-New York: Springer 1966.
2. GOTTSCHALK, C. W., and M. MYLLE: Micropuncture study of pressures in proximal tubules and peritubular capillaries of the rat kidney and their relation to ureteral and renal venous pressures. Amer. J. Physiol. **185**, 430—439 (1956).
3. KRAUSE, H. H., TH. DUME, K. M. KOCH u. B. OCHWADT: Intratubulärer Druck, glomerulärer Capillardruck und Glomerulumfiltrat nach Furosemid und Hydrochlorothiazid. Pflügers Arch. ges. Physiol. **295**, 80—89 (1967).
4. REUBI, F.: La signification de la pression intrarénale en pathologie médicale. Schweiz. med. Wschr. **86**, 385 (1956).
5. SARRE, H.: Die Durchblutung der Niere bei der experimentellen Glomerulonephritis. Dtsch. Arch. klin. Med. **183**, 515 (1939).
6. WIRZ, H.: Druckmessung in Kapillaren und Tubuli der Niere durch Mikropunktion. Helv. physiol. pharmacol. Acta **13**, 42—49 (1955).

1.4.4. The Pathogenesis of Experimental Ascending E. coli Pyelonephritis*

V. Prát[1], Ludmila Koníčková[1], W. Ritzerfeld and H. Losse[2]

With 4 Figures

The induction of experimental pyelonephritis by introducing pathogenic microorganisms into the urinary bladder depends on the conditions for the proliferation of the microorganisms in renal tissue, as well as on the reflux of urine from the bladder to the ureters. Normal kidneys are highly resistant against infection. Proliferation of microorganisms is favored by damage to the renal parenchyma as induced by blocking the ureters. Spontaneous vesico-ureteral reflux in rats occurs frequently under physiological conditions. In rabbits the sphincter around the ureteral ostium is more developed, therefore it is more difficult to induce the vesico-ureteral reflux.

In order to induce ascending pyelonephritis, we first damaged the left kidney by ligating its ureter 2 to 3 cm below the renal pelvis. Both ends of a thread slung around the ureter were led through the abdominal wall and the skin and tied at the surface of the skin. 20 to 30 hours after ligating the ureter in rabbits, after 6 hours in rats, the thread was cut. This reestablished urine flow through the ureter which in some instances remained slightly narrowed at the site of ligation.

In rabbits, one hour later a catheter was introduced into the bladder through which a suspension containing $6—10 \times 10^9$ E. coli was injected into the bladder in a total volume of 25 ml of isotonic saline. The large volume was needed in order to increase intravesical pressure to 35—40 cm H_2O and to induce vesico-ureteral reflux (Fig. 1). Microorganisms were found to reach both kidneys, where their number increased rapidly within a short time. The left predamaged kidney was always infected more heavily than the right intact kidney (Fig. 2). Within four to five days acute ascending pyelonephritis developed in the left kidney, where it either damaged the whole organ or showed a patchy distribution. Histologically, the inflammation originated in the renal pelvis and reached the medulla and the cortex through the papilla which was damaged by the ureteral blockade. The pyelonephritis healed spontaneously within a short time with postinflammatory scar formation.

In rats 1—1.2 ml of a suspension, containing 1.5×10^9 microorganisms per ml, were injected into the urethra. Both kidneys were infected by these injections in 90% of the animals. Ascending pyelography with a radiocontrast agent showed

* Supported by Deutsche Forschungsgemeinschaft.

[1] Recipients of awards from Deutsche Forschungsgemeinschaft.

[2] Lehrstuhl für Medizinische Poliklinik und Hygiene-Institut der Universität Münster/Westf., West-Germany.

a delayed emptying of the radiocontrast agent. Intravenous pyelography gave similar results. As shown in Fig. 3 the emptying of the left renal pelvis was still delayed after 10 days.

Our investigations, thus, showed that 18 hours after injecting microorganisms into the urinary bladder of rabbits or rats both kidneys became infected. This infection was more pronounced on the left pre-damaged side. Simultaneously

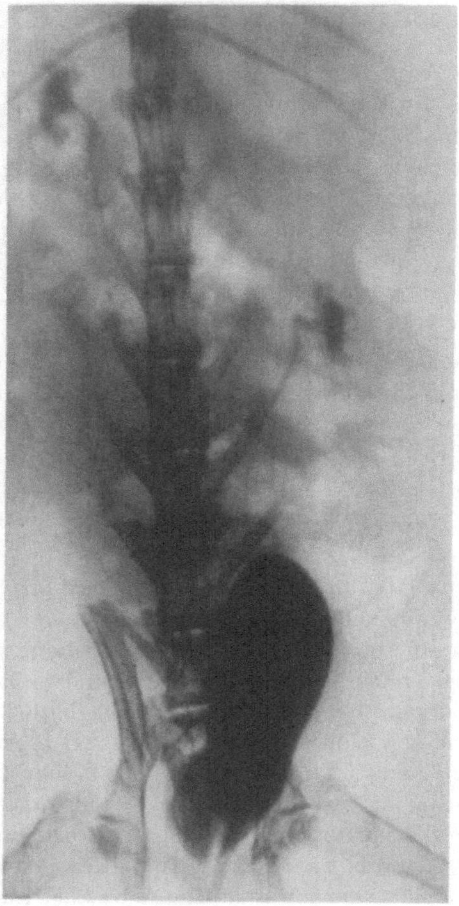

Fig. 1. Cystography in an intact rabbit. The contrast medium reaches both renal pelves

there was a bacteremia. Heptinstall suggested that renal infections after injection of microorganisms into the urinary bladder occur also by the blood stream, because in rats in which one ureter was ligated, he found microorganisms in the kidney on the ligated side within a few minutes after injecting the microorganisms into the bladder. We tried to duplicate these findings in rats in which both ureters were ligated. One hour after injecting microorganisms into the bladder, we cultured the blood and homogenates from both kidneys. We found only a very few microorganisms which were probably contaminants. In contrast to Heptinstall, we, therefore, think that microorganisms from the urinary bladder

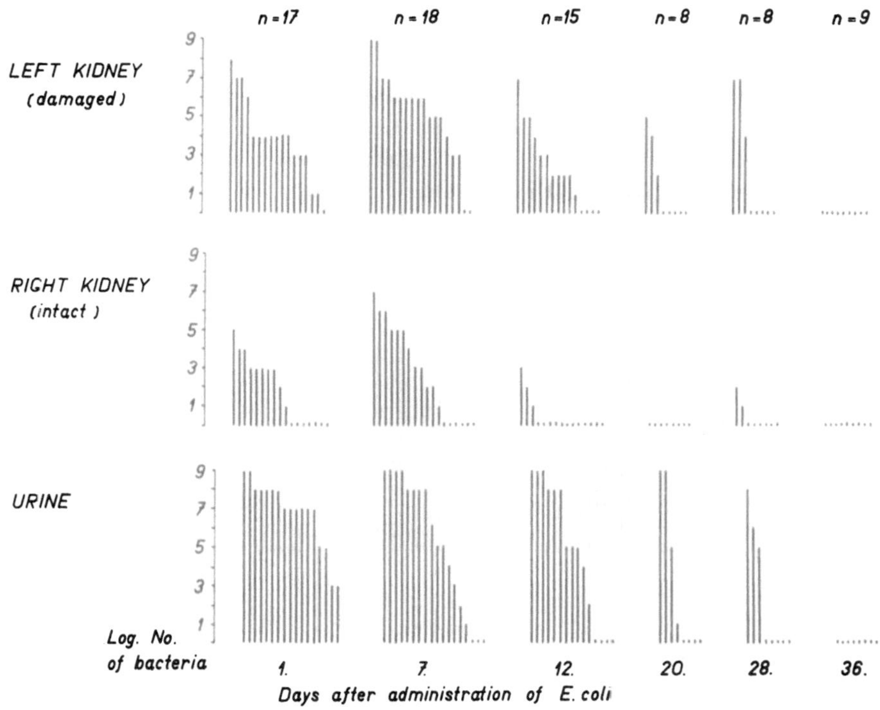

Fig. 2. Bacteriological findings in kidneys and in urine in various intervals after intravesical administration of E. coli 026 in rabbits

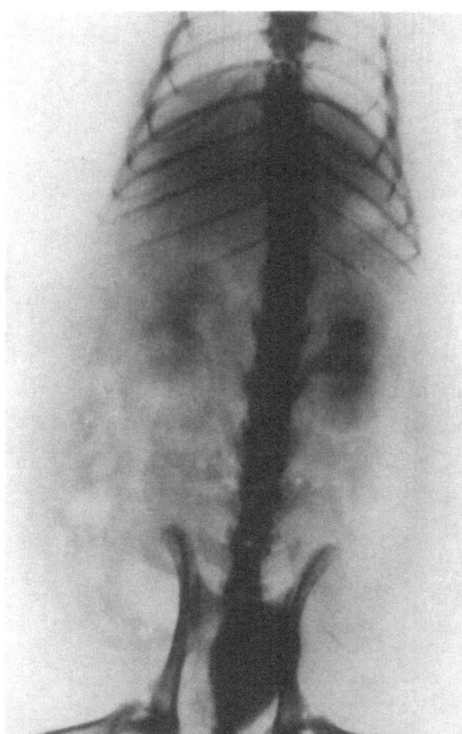

Fig. 3. Intravenous pyelography in a rat 10 days after temporary ligature of the left ureter. The left pelvis is enlarged

reach the kidney exclusively through the ureters. HEPTINSTALL'S findings may be explained by assuming that the microorganisms in his experiments, first reached the kidney with the non-ligated ureter, and from there were carried on to the opposite kidney by the blood stream.

Ascending pyelonephritis in rats usually lasts somewhat longer than in rabbits (Fig. 4).

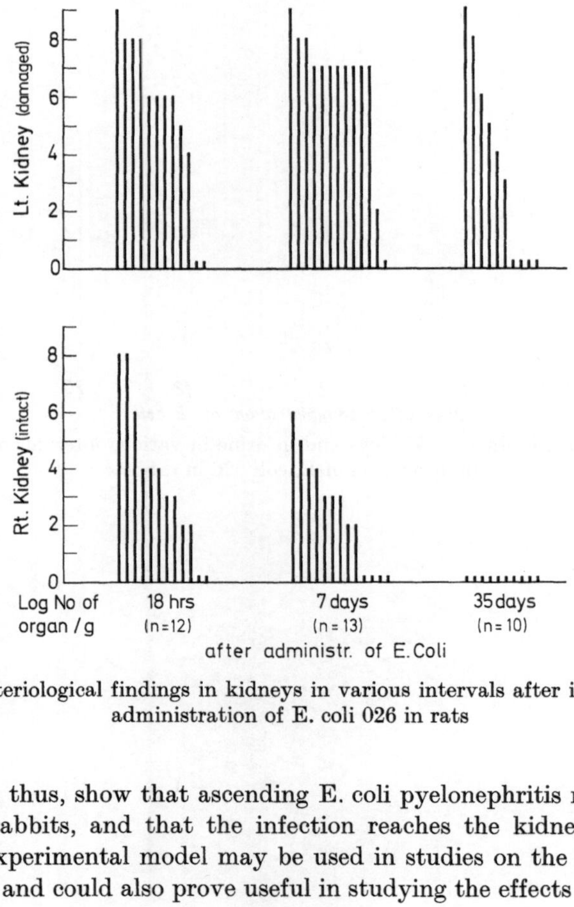

Fig. 4. Bacteriological findings in kidneys in various intervals after intraurethral administration of E. coli 026 in rats

Our results, thus, show that ascending E. coli pyelonephritis may be induced in rats or in rabbits, and that the infection reaches the kidneys through the ureters. This experimental model may be used in studies on the pathogenesis of pyelonephritis, and could also prove useful in studying the effects of antibacterial drugs.

Reference

HEPTINSTALL, R. H.: Nephron 1, 73 (1964).

1.4.5. Trials of Antibacterial Drugs in Experimental Pyelonephritis

H. Losse, V. Prát, Ludmila Koníčková and W. Ritzerfeld[1]

With 3 Figures

The pharmacological and toxicological effects of antibacterial drugs are usually tested in healthy experimental animals. Their efficacy against microorganisms is usually tested in vitro. The usefulness of an antibacterial drug in

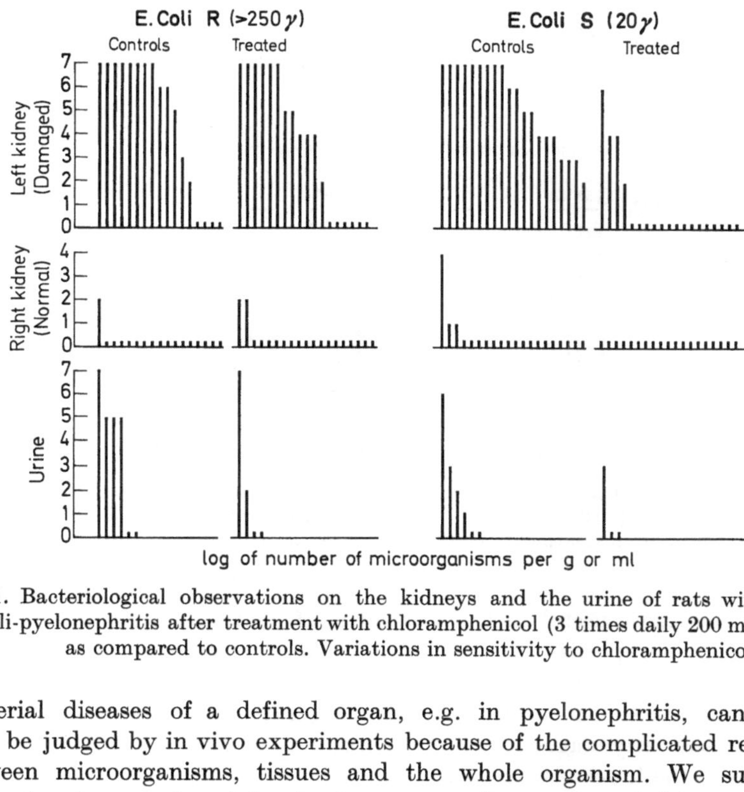

Fig. 1. Bacteriological observations on the kidneys and the urine of rats with ascending E. coli-pyelonephritis after treatment with chloramphenicol (3 times daily 200 mg/kg per os), as compared to controls. Variations in sensitivity to chloramphenicol

bacterial diseases of a defined organ, e.g. in pyelonephritis, can, however, only be judged by in vivo experiments because of the complicated relationships between microorganisms, tissues and the whole organism. We succeeded in producing, in experimental animals, an ascending pyelonephritis comparable to human E. coli-pyelonephritis. The effects of chloramphenicol, nitrofurantoin and nalidixic acid were tested in this experimental disease (Figs. 1—3).

The experimental results lead to two important conclusions:

1. The therapeutic efficacy of the chemotherapeutic drugs tested in acute experimental E. coli-pyelonephritis is correlated to the sensitivity of the microorganisms measured in vitro.

[1] Medizinische Poliklinik and Hygiene-Institut der Universität Münster/Westf., West-Germany.

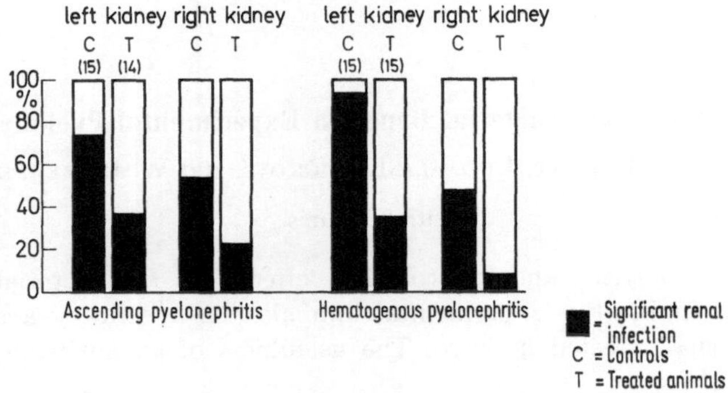

Fig. 2. Frequency of high numbers of microorganisms ($>10^2$/g of tissue) in rats with ascending or hematogenous E. coli-pyelonephritis, after treatment with nalidixic acid (3 × daily 100 mg/kg per os)

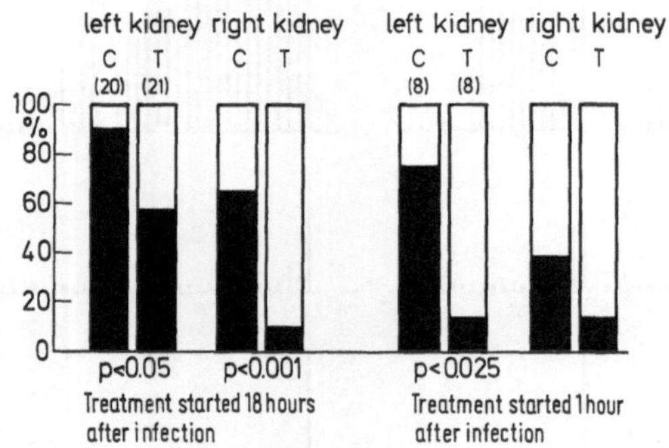

Fig. 3. The frequency of high numbers of microorganisms ($>10^2$/g of tissue) in rats with ascending E. coli-pyelonephritis, after treatment with nitrofurantoin (3 × daily 20 mg/kg). Nitrofurantoin treatment begun at variable intervals after infection

2. The drugs most useful in the treatment of acute ascending or hematogenous E. coli-pyelonephritis are those which, like chloramphenicol, reach high plasma concentrations. Drugs, like nitrofurantoin and nalidixic acid, which reach high concentration in urine, but not in plasma, may eliminate small foci of infection in the early stages of pyelonephritis, but are useful mainly in bacterial inflammation of the lower urinary tract.

1.4.6. An Experimental Investigation of the Hepatorenal Syndrome

D. Walther, K. H. Göggel, K. Hübner and W. Schoeppe[1]

With 4 Figures

Diseases of the liver are sometimes complicated by renal failure: the resulting syndrome has been called "hepatorenal syndrome".

The mechanism of the renal damage induced by liver disease is still quite unknown. We, therefore, investigated renal changes occuring in the course of experimental biliary cirrhosis of the liver, induced in the rat by ligating the bile duct.

The experiments were done on 78 female white Wistar rats. The bile duct was ligated under ether anesthesia immediately below the liver. The animals were kept up to 12 weeks in metabolic cages and were fed on rat pellets and water. For 7 weeks the daily urine volume, urinary osmolarity and specific weight, urinary sodium, potassium and urea excretions and urinary protein and bilirubin excretions were measured. At regular intervals, the concentration of urea in serum and the transminase, the leucinamino peptidase and alcaline phosphatase activities of serum were estimated. Some animals were sacrificed at regular intervals for histological studies of the liver and of the kidneys, up to 12 weeks after ligating the bile duct. The tissues were fixed in formalin immediately after sacrifice and were embedded in paraffin. Liver slices were stained with hematoxylin-eosin, van Gieson and with an iron stain. Kidney slices were stained with hematoxylin-eosin and with PAS.

During the first five weeks after ligating the bile duct, the weekly mortalities of the animals ranged between 5 and 7%. An increasing number of animals died after the 6th week. In the 7th and 8th weeks, the weekly mortality rate was 10%, in the 9th week, 15%, in the 10th week, 20%, in the 11th week 38% and in the 12th week, 80% of the survivors.

The histological picture of the liver showed changes typical for biliary cirrhosis, beginning 1 week after ligature of the bile duct. There was a marked proliferation of small bile ducts, but no notable increase of connective tissue.

In the neighborhood of the proliferating bile ducts there were isolated necrotic cells. There was little cellular infiltration, little cell icterus and little cholostasis. 5 weeks after ligature, the rearrangement of liver architecture was complete (Fig. 1). Lobular structure had disappeared as a consequence of the proliferation of bile ducts. There were focal necroses and brown cells. Even at this time, cell icterus was not pronounced, and there was little cholestasis and sparse round cell infiltration.

Serum enzyme activities (transaminase, LAP, AP) increased within 1 week after ligature with the beginning of histological changes. The activities of trans-

[1] Pathologisches Institut und II. Medizinische Klinik der Universität Frankfurt, Frankfurt (Main, West Germany).

aminases and of LAP subsequently decreased slowly but had not yet reached normal values at the end of 7 weeks. The alcaline phosphatase activity remained elevated up to the end of the 7th week (Fig. 2).

Kidney histology was normal up to the end of the 2nd week. At this time small droplets of bilirubin could be demonstrated in the cells of the proximal convoluted tubules. After the 4th week, there was increased deposition of bilirubin and many necrotic epithelial cells in proximal convoluted tubules. In the distal tubules, there were no necrotic cells, although in the lowest

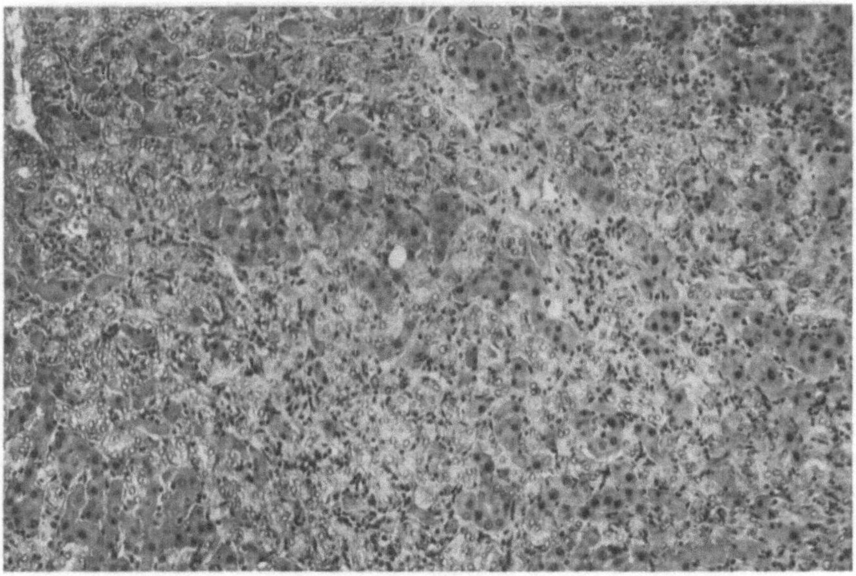

Fig. 1. Biliary cirrhosis of the liver 5 weeks after ligating the common bile duct

part of the distal tubules, the nuclei and the cell plasma appeared swollen. There is, thus, a syndrome of icteric nephrosis and tubular necrosis in the rat which occurs approximately 4 weeks after ligating the common bile duct (Fig. 3). Glomerular changes, at this time, are still inconspicuous. The only sign of an incipient "glomerulonephrosis" is a slight enlargement of the glomerular endothelial cells (ZOLLINGER [3]).

The daily urine volume increased to twice its normal value in the second week (Fig. 4). Urinary osmolarity and specific weights were unchanged or increased. The urinary excretion of sodium and of potassium increased considerably and reached a maximum in the 5th week. The renal clearance of urea fell to half of its normal value: there was a considerable increase in the urea plasma concentration. A slight proteinuria and bilirubinuria began during the 2nd week.

In summary liver damage induced by ligature of the bile duct in the rat, induces secondary functional and morphological changes of the kidneys. Ligating the bile duct induces typical biliary cirrhosis within 4 weeks. The histological changes are accompanied by increased serum enzyme activities which fall back to near-normal values at the end of the 7th week. Similar observations were

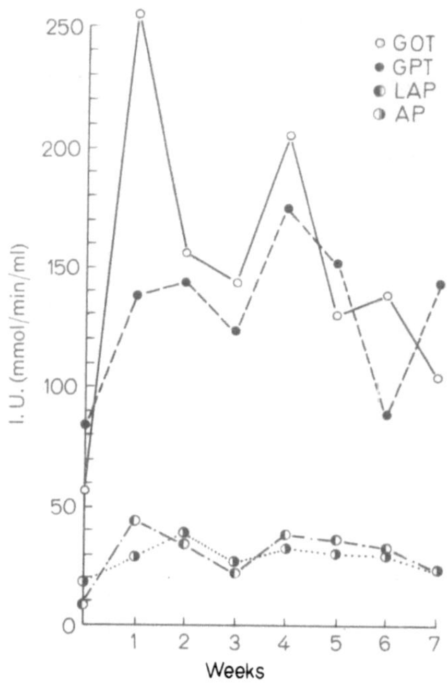

Fig. 2. Serum enzyme activities at various intervals after ligating the common bile duct

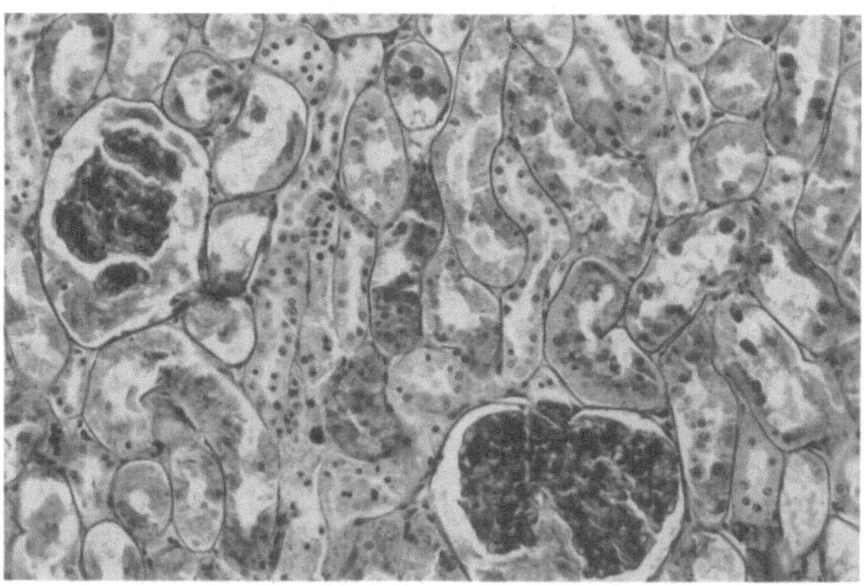

Fig. 3. "Icteric nephrosis" with (proximal) tubular necrosis 4 weeks after ligating bile duct. (Stained with H.E. enlarged 450×)

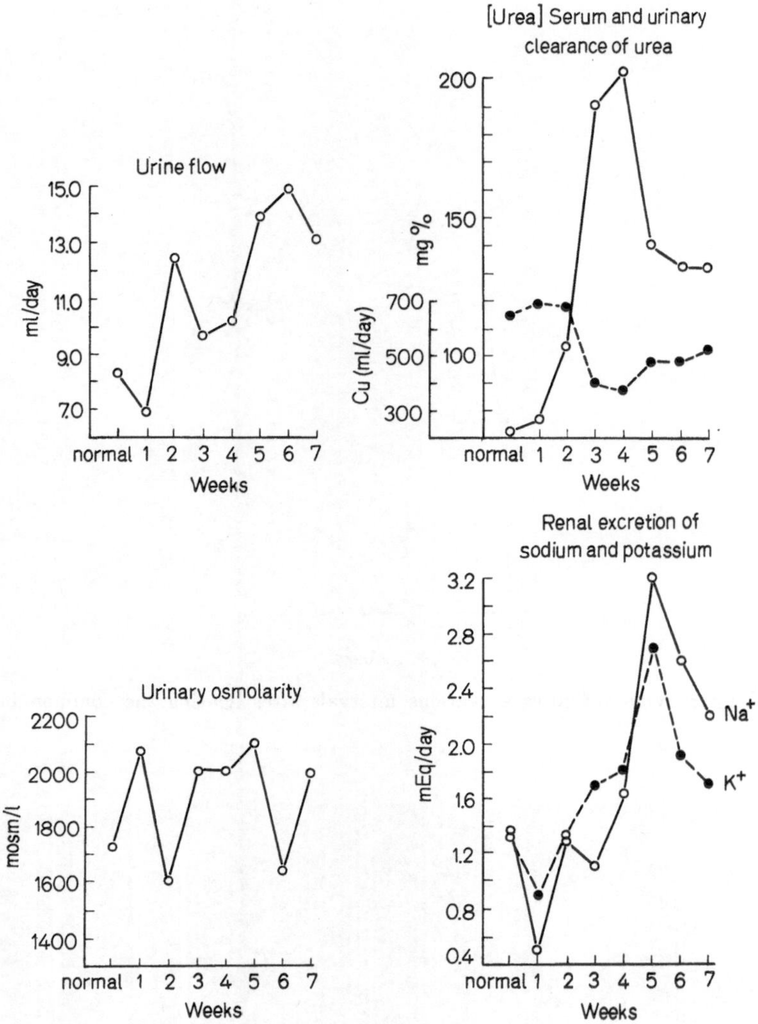

Fig. 4. Renal functions after ligating the bile duct

made by CHINSKY and SHERRY [1]. HESS [2] described increases of serum transaminase and alcaline phosphatase activities as well as of bilirubin in dogs after ligating the common bile duct.

Renal damage first is demonstrated by deposition of bilirubin in proxima tubular cells, as a first sign of "cholemic nephrosis" occuring in the 2nd week. All clinicians and pathologists agree on the occurence of this picture in patients with primary liver disease. There is, however, no agreement on the occurence of tubular necrosis and functional disturbances of the kidneys which we observed with certainty four weeks after ligating the bile duct in rats. Thus, FAJERS thinks that an icteric nephrosis accompanied by functional disturbances does not occur after ligating the common bile duct, unless there is a simultaneous decrease in renal blood flow. Our data do not confirm this opinion. Zollinger [3] points out that in patients with liver disease, tubular necrosis is extremely rare and that a wrong diagnosis of epithelial damage may be due to the propensity of the tubular cells to undergo autolytic changes. Changes observed in the present experiments could not be autolytic, since tissues were fixed immediately after sacrifice. Increased excretion of sodium and potassium, furthermore, points to a disturbance of proximal tubular sodium reabsorption. Sodium escaping proximal reabsorption may have induced a type of osmotic diuresis in the lower nephron.

Renal damage as a concequence of biliary cirrhosis may either be due to the occurrence of toxic substances of hepatic origin or to the non-detoxication of endogenous metabolites which are normally detoxicated in the liver. Circulatory disturbances do not appear to play a role, since we did not observe changes in blood pressure in some preliminary experiments.

References

1. Chinsky, M., and S. Sherry: Serum transaminase as diagnostic aid. Arch. intern. Med. **99**, 556—568 (1957).
2. Hess, B.: Enzyme im Blutplasma. Stuttgart: Georg Thieme 1966.
3. Zollinger, H. U.: Niere und ableitende Harnwege. In: W. Doerr, and E. Uehlinger, eds., Spezielle pathologische Anatomie, Bd. 3. Berlin-Heidelberg-New York: Springer 1966.

1.5. Clinical Uremia

1.5.1. Clinical and Therapeutic Considerations on Chronic Renal Failure

A. BLUMBERG[1]

The present report is concerned with a few particular clinical problems in the management of renal failure, which are either relatively unknown or have been partially clarified by recent findings.

A *disturbance of glucose utilization* occurring in renal failure is an interesting and well known metabolic disorder which often may escape detection [54]. The mechanism of the disturbance has been intensively investigated in recent years, e.g. in our department by FANKHAUSER et al. [17, 77]. As shown by several investigators, a decreased glucose tolerance may be found in uremic patients after oral glucose loads [8, 9, 17, 28, 36, 59, 77, 79]. Studies in patients with incipient renal failure who were submitted to dialysis showed that the depression of glucose tolerance is not due to malnutrition or infection, since these patients were adequately nourished and in a good clinical state [17, 28, 36]. After a glucose load, in uremic patients the blood glucose concentration rises to higher levels and for longer times than in normal subjects. A delayed fall in glucose concentration is also observed after intravenous glucose loads [28, 36]. Several investigators attempted to elucidate the mechanism of this disturbance, and contradictory findings may be due to considerable interindividual differences. Thus, tolbutamide tests were found to give normal results in some studies [76, 77, 79], while in other studies there was a delayed but extensive fall in blood glucose [8, 28]. Insulin in plasma was measured as immunoreactive insulin (IRI), or as insulin-like activity (ILA). All observers agree that after glucose loads or injection of tolbutamide, the blood insulin-like activities were normal or higher and remained elevated for a longer time than in normal subjects [8, 17, 36]. The hypoglycemic effect of intravenous insulin was either found normal or delayed [8, 59, 79] but all investigators agree that the hypoglycemia after intravenous insulin lasts longer than in normal subjects. Injection of glucagon induces the same hyperglycemia as in normal subjects; there is thus no disturbance of glycogenolysis [8, 76]. Finally it has been shown repeatedly that adequate frequent hemodialysis may improve or normalize the glucose tolerance [28, 36, 77].

Insulin deficiency may thus be excluded as a possible cause of the disturbance, because the measured blood insulin activities are large enough to maintain a normal glucose tolerance. The possibility of a disturbance of glycogenolysis is excluded by the normal effect of glucagon; it is, furthermore incompatible with the results of in vitro experiments [11]. The peripheral glucose utilization is, thus, depressed in the presence of normal blood insulin levels. As pointed out by FANKHAUSER [17], this depression is more pronounced with higher blood glucose levels: at normal

1 Medizinische Poliklinik der Universität Bern, Switzerland.

blood sugar concentrations, the results of intravenous tolbutamide or insulin tolerance tests are often normal; a normal glucose tolerance is often found after small glucose loads, while after large glucose loads the tolerance is smaller than in normal subjects. This investigator thinks that a factor, occurring in blood as a consequence of renal failure, may depress cellular glucose utilization, possibly by inhibiting enzyme systems. Other investigators, who observed a delayed fall in blood glucose after intravenous insulin or tolbutamide, favor the assumption that this factor could be an insulin antagonist [8].

Thus, the mechanism of the disturbance of carbohydrate metabolism in uremia is unknown. It is known, however, that the disturbance may be eliminated by intense treatment by hemodialysis and recurs after a few days without dialysis. When urea was added to the dialyzing fluid, the glucose tolerance was equally improved. This observation argues against the assumption that urea could be the only responsible factor. On the other hand, an increase in blood urea concentration produced by adding urea to dialyzing fluid during several weeks depresses the glucose tolerance. In any case, the substance in blood which is responsible for the decrease in glucose tolerance appears to be dialyzable.

The clinical significance of the disturbance in carbohydrate metabolism is not clear. It does not appear to have considerable bearing on the general state of the patients. In patients who were maintained by hemodialysis for some years, the disturbance never evolved into frank clinical diabetes.

Renal osteopathy is a metabolic disturbance of increasing clinical importance in cases of chronic renal failure. This disturbance is interesting from the physiopathological viewpoint and practically important, since its occurrence may annihilate the success of treatment by chronic repeated hemodialysis or by renal transplantations [30, 47, 58, 68, 80].

Bone biopsies are required for the differential diagnosis and for guiding the treatment [73]. Three mechanisms probably contribute to the pathogenesis of the disturbance:

1. Patients with chronic uremia have been shown to suffer from a depressed intestinal absorption of calcium [12, 15, 45, 75]. The lack of calcium is aggravated by the low calcium content of the usual diet which is poor in protein [58]; a massive increase of oral intake by adding 10 gm of calcium citrate may induce a positive calcium balance [45]. — 2. Target organ refractoriness against vitamin D appears to be an important component of uremic osteopathy [15,75]. The concentration of vitamin D in serum was usually found normal [12]. The doses of vitamin D required for improving or healing the bone lesions are much larger than those needed in rickets or osteomalacia. There is, therefore, a relative lack of vitamin D which is aggravated by a depressed intestinal absorption of the vitamin and an enhanced degradation of its biologically active form [2]. On the other hand, refractoriness against vitamin D effects, depresses the intestinal absorption of calcium and thus favors the development of osteomalacia. — 3. A third mechanism of renal osteopathy may be metabolic acidosis. Stanbury [75] found that correction of the acidosis by sodium bicarbonate did not induce a normal calcium balance and, therefore, concluded that acidosis does not contribute to the disturbance in calcium metabolism. Other investigators think that bone salt may act as a buffer and that acidosis may play a role in renal osteopathy. This

viewpoint is based on the following arguments: the acid balance is positive in normal subjects loaded with acids, as well as in stabilized patients with renal failure with the plasma concentration of bicarbonate remaining constant. The calcium carbonate content of bones of patients who died in renal failure decreased progressively with the duration of the disease [57]. Finally, and in contradiction to Stanbury's observations, the calcium-balance may be influenced favorably by eliminating the acidosis [44].

According to Stanbury [73, 74, 75], the sequence of events in renal osteopathy may be described in the following manner: refractoriness to vitamin D depresses the intestinal absorption of calcium and thereby induces a tendency to low plasma calcium concentrations. Low plasma-calcium, in turn, stimulates the parathyroids. Increased secretion of parathyroid hormone does not raise plasma-calcium to normal values as a consequence of the refractoriness to vitamin D. At this stage the patients have a low plasma-calcium, a moderately increased plasma-phosphate concentration and an approximately normal calcium phosphate product. The main bone lesion is inadequate mineralization i.e. osteomalacia [74]. In the second stage hypersecretion of parathyroid hormone results in a normalization of the plasma calcium concentration. The parathyroids are considerably enlarged. The occurrence of effective secondary hyperparathyroidism depends on the duration of the disease. The plasma phosphate concentration, at this stage, is increased. There is, thus, no reciprocal correlation between calcium and phosphate concentrations, as thought previously. The calcium phosphate product reaches values above 65, while the bone lesion resembles ostitis fibrosa. There is a tendency to metastatic calcification [74]. Possibly, acidosis favors demineralization of the bones. Finally, the parathyroids become "autonomous" and continue to secrete excessive amounts of parathyroid hormone, in spite of a normal plasma-calcium concentration. Autonomy of the parathyroid hypersecretion is demonstrated by a continued hyperparathyroidism after successful renal transplantation. In such cases, subtotal parathyroidectomy became necessary in order to arrest the destruction of bone and hypercalcemia [24, 47, 80].

Treatment of the condition may be successful when the stages of the disease are taken into consideration. At the stage of defective bone mineralization (osteomalacia) with a normal calcium phosphate product, the treatment of choice is high doses of vitamin D (18,000 up to more than 250,000 units per day). This treatment may heal the bone lesions and eliminate the symptoms. Regular checks of plasma calcium are necessary, when the radiological appearances are improved and the alcaline phosphatase values become normal, since, at this stage, hypercalcemia may occur. Vitamin D therapy may induce involution of the hyperplastic parathyroids [73]. At the stage of ostitis fibrosa with signs of secondary hyperparathyroidism, vitamin D, may improve the bone lesions [73], but may also precipitate extensive metastatic calcifications by further increasing the calcium phosphate product. At this stage, the logical treatment is subtotal parathyroidectomy in order to eliminate the hypersecretion of parathyroid hormone. When the plasma-calcium falls, high doses of vitamin D may be given in order to accelerate the healing of the bone lesions. After successful renal transplantation these lesions heal spontaneously as a consequence of the disappearance of the refractory state to vitamin D. In such cases, the normal vitamin D-concentrations in blood are adequate for maintaining normal bone structure.

Such treatment, based on physiological principles, not only improves the state of patients with chronic renal failure and renal osteopathy, but may also contribute to successful treatment of the growing group of patients submitted to long term-hemodialysis, or to renal transplantation.

Renal hypertension is a still ill-understood complication of chronic renal failure. The factors responsible for this complication have been extensively studied during the last years. The introduction of long term dialysis made it possible to study patients with progressive renal failure, after bilateral nephrectomy and finally after renal transplantation. A fall in blood pressure, observed in the majority of patients with renal hypertension and even in some subjects with malignant hypertension, after removal of sodium and water by hemodialysis with ultrafiltration, was a surprising finding [29], confirmed by many investigators [10, 13, 45, 58]. When measuring the extracellular space and the exchangeable sodium pool in such subjects, we found that the blood pressure falls before the ECF and the sodium pool contract below normal values [5]. It is not clear whether these observations are applicable to patients in the initial stage of renal failure and hypertension; they only favour the assumption that sodium and water retention may in some way contribute to the establishment of nephrogenous hypertension. This contribution varies from one case to the next, for in dialyzed patients, ultrafiltration does not always induce a satisfactory lowering of blood pressure. In such resistant cases, several clinicians resorted to nephrectomy and studied its influence on blood pressure. In the majority of the published cases, bilateral nephrectomy induced a fall in blood pressure [19, 35, 39, 55, 78]. After nephrectomy, patients who previously suffered from particularly severe or particularly long-lasting hypertension, became very sensitive to changes of extra-cellular volume; their blood pressure always proved lower than that observed before nephrectomy for any given size of the exchangeable sodium pool [16, 48]. The blood pressure, under these circumstances, may [27], or may not, depend on the blood volume, as found by one group of investigators [16].

An important issue is the possible role of renal pressor substances in the pathogenesis of renal hypertension. A large number of investigations on the renin-angiotensin system have been published recently. There are cases in which one is tempted to ascribe a role to the renin-angiotensin-system, as e.g. one of our own patients in whom the plasma renin activity was considerably increased and fell to non-measurable values when the blood pressure became normal after nephrectomy. In many cases of chronic renal failure with hypertension, the renin activity in the kidneys was found elevated [25, 39, 70]. On the other hand, there are certainly cases of severe hypertension in which blood pressure was lowered by nephrectomy, but neither the blood, nor the kidneys contained increased amounts of renin [35, 39, 70]. No correlation between blood renin activity and blood pressure was found by Hodler in patients of our department suffering from chronic renal diseases [32]. Normal as well as elevated values were found in patients with renal hypertension as well as in normal subjects. Similar results were published by other authors [4, 7].

I should finally like to mention renoprival hypertension, i.e. a type of hypertension which would be due to the loss of a blood pressure lowering factor of the kidneys or to non-excretion of a pressor substance normally excreted into the urine. The presence of a blood pressure lowering substance in the renal medulla has been convincingly demonstrated in experimental animals [7, 52, 53]. There is also some evidence for the occurence of renoprival hypertension in man. Thus, hypertension was not influenced by nephrectomy in some cases but was abolished after successful renal transplantation [35, 39]. It has also been found that after renal transplantation, sudden increases in plasma volume cease to cause an increase in blood pressure [16]. This finding may also argue for a blood pressure lowering effect of the healthy kidney.

All three groups of factors may contribute to the establishment of renal hypertension. In renal failure, blood pressure often responds in a very sensitive manner to changes in the water and electrolyte content of the organism. Diseased kidneys may produce one or more hypertensive substances. It appears quite doubtful, whether renin is one of them. Finally a renoprival factor in renal hypertension is demonstrated by the blood pressure lowering effect of transplanted healthy kidneys.

Treatment of hypertension in renal failure is an important practical problem. Some clinicians are reluctant to use classical antihypertensive therapy in such cases. The doctrine of our department is, however, that hypertension should be treated in patients with renal failure. It is known since a long time that severe grades of essential hypertension with eyeground changes belonging to the stage III and the stage IV of KEITH et al. [37] carry a bad prognosis. Eighty to ninty percent of patients with malignant hypertension die within one year, ninety percent or more within two years [26, 37, 38, 56, 65, 72]. Effective treatment may lower this mortality to approximately 20 per cent after one to one and a half years [33, 34, 67, 71]. Long term-effects of treating slighter grades of hypertension were the subject of discussions for a long time. Smirk has recently demonstrated on a material comprising several hundreds of patients, that in such cases the five year mortality may be lowered by treatment [71]. In hypertension of patients with chronic renal disease it is more difficult to judge the efficacy of blood pressure lowering treatment, because in contrast to essential hypertension the final result is mainly determined by the basic renal disease which usually progresses more or less rapidly. The rate of progression varies greatly from one patient ot the other, but also from one month to the next or from one year to the next within one patient. It is, therefore, nearly impossible to constitute comparable groups of patients in which the hypertension is, or is not, treated. An important argument often used against antihypertensive therapy in renal failure, is a possible depression of renal function by a fall in blood pressure [23, 33, 46, 66]. While it occurs sometimes, such a depression is by no means unavoidable [66]. The critical issue is the distinction of long term from short term-effects of antihypertensive therapy on renal function. Thus REUBI found a decrease of glomerular filtration rate by 28.6% and of the clearance of PAH by 36.5% within one and a half years in eight severe cases of untreated renal hypertension, while the decrease in a similar group submitted to antihypertensive therapy was only 7.4, and 2.7% resp. MOYER et al. [50, 51] found no decrease in renal function in 12 patients whose hypertension was treated, but a 60% deterioration in untreated patients. Wood and Blythe investigated 20 cases of malignant hypertension with blood urea-N values above 50 mg-%. They found that 45% of these patients survived from one to five years with intensive antihypertensive therapy. It appears logical to extrapolate these observations to patients with secondary hypertension in primary renal disease, since there is no reason to assume that the detrimental effect of high blood pressure observed in patients with essential hypertension should not occur in patients with primary renal disease. There is no way of foretelling the progression of the basic renal disease which may be rather slow. Finally, at the present time, a certain fraction of patients with chronic renal failure may be kept alive by hemodialysis or by renal transplantation. With these possibilities one would never be justified in taking the risk of death as a consequence of hypertension before or during the use of new therapeutic possibilities.

We, therefore, think that hypertension in patients with chronic renal failure should be treated to the same extent as essential hypertension. This statement, however, raises the question, up to which stage of the renal disease antihypertensive therapy is a practical possibility. In the latter stages of renal failure, a sudden decrease of blood pressure may induce a sudden fall of urine flow and an increase of blood urea. It is difficult to establish general rules for the limits of antihypertensive treatment in renal failure. Generally, progressive lowering of blood pressure by antihypertensive drugs is well supported by patients with a glomerular filtration rate above 15—20 ml/min. Like a few other clinicians [31], we cautiously try antihypertensive treatment in more severe cases of renal failure. The continuation of the treatment, then, depends on the reactions or the success observed: in some cases a compromise solution, i.e., lowering of blood pressure to values above normal, appears acceptable. In a few cases it may be useful to bridge the patient over the critical period of a depression of GFR and an increase of blood urea by dialysis. In a few cases of this type, renal function improved after treatment [6].

A major progress in the conservative management of renal failure in the last year is due to the introduction of diets extremely poor in protein, as recommended by Giordano, Giovannetti and Berlyne [3, 20, 22, 46, 69]. The efficacy of these diets was convincingly demonstrated to us in our own department. Their mechanism of action may be understood by recalling some principles of protein metabolism. The organism builds proteins from ingested essential and non-essential amino-acids. The proteins, thus synthesized, are subject to continuous catabolism. There are large differences between the biological half-life times of different proteins. The end product of protein catabolism is urea produced through the Krebs-Henseleit cycle. Urea, as excreted by the kidney is partially derived from the body's own protein, and partially from food protein. In healthy adults, protein anabolism and catabolism occur at equal rates i.e. the nitrogen balance is equilibrated. In patients with renal failure, the decrease in GFR induces a retention of urea and other nitrogenous waste products. Depression of renal function below certain values is accompanied by characteristic symptoms, as e.g. gastro-intestinal disturbances (anorexia, nausea, vomiting, diarrhea). These symptoms may be partly due to the formation of ammonia by bacterial decomposition of urea within the alimentary tract [43]. The gastro-intestinal disturbances interfere with nutrition; the patients may, thus, take inadequate amounts of calories and often essential amino-acids. This state of affairs, in turn, depresses the synthesis of proteins and, thus, induces a negative nitrogen balance. In this situation, an increase in protein ingestion should be expected to enhance protein syntheses. On the other hand, and without considering the difficulty of giving more protein to a nauseated patient, degradation of a fraction of the additional protein may cause a further increase in blood urea and a further deterioration of gastro-intestinal function. Lowering the protein intake, i.e. the opposite measure, in this situation is known to deplete the organism of "labile" protein, but subsequently enhances the synthesis of new body proteins, i.e. exerts an anabolic effect. As a consequence of this increased utilization of dietary protein, the amount of protein needed for maintaining a positive nitrogen balance decreases [1, 18]. A new steady state is thus reached at a lower level of protein intake. It was furthermore shown that in patients with uremia, urea not excreted by the kidneys, may be cleared by other ways [14, 64] and may be utilized in the synthesis of non-essential or even essential amino-acids and of proteins [21]. A decreased protein catabolism and re-utilization of urea must lower the total amount of urea present in the body.

Several diets poor in protein and useful in the treatment of patients with uremia were described. Among these, Giovannetti's diet appears preferable for reasons of taste. It is based on a reduction of the ingestion of biologically non-essential protein to the very low amount of 6 g a day, while biologically essential protein, i.e. protein containing all the essential amino-acids in suitable proportions is given in the form of 2 eggs per day. The total protein ingestion is thus reduced to 18 g which are supplemented by high calory non-protein material. Baked goods made from ordinary wheat flour are eliminated because of their high content of biologically non-essential proteins. They are replaced by bread and other baked goods made from starch. The patients are furthermore given butter, oil, sugar, honey, alcohol and certain kinds of fruit and vegetables. On two days of the week the eggs may be replaced by milk or by meat [49]. Giovannetti et al. usually started treatment by a basic diet containing only 6 g of protein and added eggs only after 3 weeks on the basic diet. The eggs may, however, be given from the onset [3, 69]. The labile protein pool tends to decrease in the first weeks of treatment. After this time, the nitrogen balance becomes equilibrated or positive. Without any change in renal function, the blood urea concentration falls and the general state of the patients improves, mainly by the disappearance of gastro-intestinal symptoms.

The best results are obtained in patients with a GFR above 3 ml/min, though some success has been obtained with GFR values down to 1.5 ml/min. With a GFR above 10—15 ml/min, conventional diets poor in proteins are adequate. Some patients have difficulties with the taste of the Giovannetti-type diets, which can be overcome when their state improves, the gastro-intestinal symptoms disappear and the working capacity is re-established.

Changes in serum chemistry comprise a progressive decrease in plasma urea nitrogen without any change in renal function, and a decrease in plasma phosphate concentration, while plasma uric acid concentration and acidosis are usually not influenced. Anemia may be improved in some cases [3, 22]. In patients who tend to retain salt and water, the intake of both should be limited. In patients treated by the diets extremely poor in proteins, blood urea ceases to monitor the state of the patients. Patients have been observed to die with hemorrhage, restlessness, acidosis and hyperkalemia within a few days with rather low urea nitrogen values (100—120 mg-%). The main advantage of this type of treatment is the possibility to restitute to normal life and sometimes even to work some bedridden critically ill patients with very inadequate renal functions.

Finally, I wish to discuss the problem of the excretion and the dosage of drugs in patients with renal failure. Drugs mainly excreted by the kidneys may accumulate in patients with renal failure and cause symptoms of overdosage. This applies particularly to drugs which are used in the treatment of infections of the urinary tract by virtue of their high concentrations in urine. There are only few and scattered data on the doses of drugs useful in patients with renal failure. It appears particularly important to have data on antibiotics which must often be given to severly ill patients with restricted renal function. REUBI [62, 63] has provided such data for rolitetracycline (PMT, Reverin). He investigated the renal excretion of this antibiotic at different levels of glomerular filtration rate measured by the clearance of thiosulfate. The renal clearance of rolitetracycline (C_{PMT}) reached 65.8% of the clearance of thiosulfate (C_T) due to protein binding. The effect of the drug in the organism depends on the blood concentration. A stable value is usually reached two hours after an intravenous injection; the fall in plasma concentration after this time depends on the renal as well as the extra-renal excretion and degradation. The fall may be represented by a straight line when the logarithms of plasma concentration are plotted against time. From this straight line one may calculate the half life time (t/2) as well as the coefficient of elimination k which equals 0.693/t/2. REUBI found that k for rolitetracycline is linearily correlated to C_T. The elimination thus is good at higher values of GFR, but slow at low values of GFR. The y-axis-intercept at $C_T = O$ is positive and equal to the coefficient of elimination observed in patients with anuria or in nephrectomized subjects. In normal subjects 78% of injected rolitetracycline are excreted by the renal route, while 22% are eliminated extrarenally. These data allow us to adapt the doses of rolitetracycline to the state of the renal function in any given subject. In subjects with normal kidney functions, single doses of 275 mg induce a concentration of approximately 4 μg/ml after 2 hours which after 24 hours fall to approximately 0.5 μg/ml, and, with a subsequent injection, rise again to the original therapeutic values. If t/2 is increased from 8 to 24 hours, as observed with a decrease of GFR to 10 to 20 ml/min, adequate blood concentrations may be maintained with the same dose given once in 3 days. In patients with anuria, with t/2-values of approximately 40 hours, it is recommended to give the same dose once in four days.

Though there are no comparable precise data clinically useful data on other antibiotics have been published [40, 41].

References

1. ALLISON, J. B.: J. Amer. med. Ass. **164**, 283—289 (1957).

2. AVIOLI, L. V., and E. SLATOPOLSKY: The absorption and metabolism of vitamin D in chronic renal failure. J. clin. Invest. **46**, 1032 (1967).

3. Berlyne, G. M., A. B. Shaw, and S. Nilwarangkur: Dietary treatment of chronic. renal failure. Experiences with a modified Giovanetti diet. Nephron 2, 129—147 (1965).
4. Blaufox, M. D., A. E. Birbari, R. B. Hickler, and Merrill Jr.: Peripheral plasma renin activity in renal-homotransplant recepients. New Engl. J. Med. 275, 1165—1168 (1966).
5. Blumberg, A., R. M. Hegstrom, W. B. Nelp, and B. H. Scribner: Extracellular volume in patients with chronic renal disease treated for hypertension by sodium restriction. Lancet 1967 II, 69—73.
6. Bonar, J. R., B. B. Johnson, K. Hatton, C. Deraps, and H. G. Langford: Salvage of far advanced malignant hypertension. Abstract. Clin. Res. 12, 248—252 (1964).
7. Brown, J. J., D. L. Davies, A. F. Lever, and J. I. S. Robertson: Plasma renin concentration in human hypertension. Brit. med. J. 1966 I, 505—508.
8. Cerletty, J. M., and N. H. Engbring: Azotemia and glucose intolerance. Ann. intern. Med. 66, 1097—1108 (1966).
9. Cohen, B. O.: Abnormal carbohydrate metabolism in renal disease. Blood glucose unresponsiveness to hypoglycemia, epinephrine and glucagon. Ann. intern. Med. 57, 204—210 (1962).
10. Comty, C., H. Rottka, and S. Shaldon: Blood pressure control in patients with endstage renal failure treated by intermittent hemodialysis. EDTA Proceedings 1, 209—305 (1964).
11. Cummings, N. B., and S. M. Zottu: Glucose and pyruvate metabolism in liver slices of chronic uremic rats. Amer. J. Physiol. 198, 1079—1084 (1960).
12. Curtis, F. K., R. C. Davidson, and J. P. Pendras: Metabolic bone disease and chronic dialysis. Abstract Internat. Congr. Nephrol. 1966, p. 176.
13. Dalla Rosa, C., G. Gallanti, G. Ancona, E. Bruschi, and P. Confortini: Proceedings EDTA Conference 3, 107—115 (1966).
14. Deane, N., W. Desir, and T. Omeda: The production and extrarenal metabolism of urea in patients with chronic renal failure treated with diet and dialysis. Proc. E.D.T.A. conference 4, 244—249 (1967).
15. Dent, C. E., C. M. Harper, and G. R. Philpot: Treatment of renal glomerular osteodystrophy. Quart. J. Med. 30, 1—7 (1961).
16. Dustan, H. P., and I. M. Page: Some factors in renal and renoprival hypertension. J. Lab. clin. Med. 64, 948—951 (1964).
17. Fankhauser, S., et J. P. Felber: Les perturbations du métabolisme des hydrates de carbone dans l'azotémie chronique. Journées Annuelles de Diabétologie de L'Hôtel-Dieu 1966, p. 92.
18. Forsyth, B. T., M. E. Shipman, and L. C. Plough: J. clin. Invest. 34, 1653—1659 (1955).
19. Funck-Brentano, J. L., P. Chaumont, D. Perrin, J. Zingraff et J. Vantelon: Traitement de l'urémie chronique par hémodialyses répétés. Actualités néphrol. Hôp. Necker 1965, 43—47.
20. Giordano, C.: Use of exogenous and endogenous urea for protein synthesis in normal and uraemic subjects. J. Lab. clin. Med. 62, 231 (1963).
21. — R. Esposito, N. G. de Santo, and C. de Pascale: Dietary treatment in acute and chronic renal failure. Abstracts Intern. Congr. Nephrol., p. 50 (1966).
22. Giovanetti, S., and Q. Maggiore: A low-nitrogen diet with proteins of high biological value for severe chronic uraemia. Lancet 1964 I, 1000—1003.
23. Goldberg, B.: Lancet 1957 I, 74.
24. Goodman, A. D., J. Lemann, E. C. Lemon, and A. S. Relman: Production, excretion and net balance of fixed acid in patients with renal acidosis. J. clin. Invest. 44, 495—506 (1965).
25. Haas, E., and H. Goldblatt: Biochem. Z. 338, 164—178 (1964).
26. Hammerström, S., and P. Bechgaard: Amer. J. Med. 8, 53 (1950).
27. Hampers, C. L., J. J. Skillman, J. H. Lyons, J. E. Olsen, and J. M. Merrill: A hemadynamic evaluation of bilateral nephroctomy and hemodialysis in hypertensive man. Circulation 35, 272—288 (1967).
28. — J. S. Soeldner, P. B. Dvak, and J. P. Merrill: Effect of chronic renal failure and hemodialysis on carbohydrate metabolism. J. clin. Invest. 45, 1719—1731 (1966).

29. HEGSTROM, R. M., J. S. MURRAY, J. P. PENDRAS, J. M. BURNELL, and B. H. SCRIBNER: Hemodialysis in the treatment of chronic uremia. Trans. Amer. Soc. Artif. Int. Organs **7**, 136—141 (1961).

30. HERDMAN, R. C., A. F. MICHAEL, R. L. VERNIER, W. D. KELLY, and R. A. GOOD: Renal function and phosphorus excretion after human renal homotransplantation. Lancet **1966 I**, 121—125.

31. HILDEN, T.: Diskussionsbemerkungen in: Die Spätwirkungen der medikamentösen Hochdrucksbehandlung auf die Nierenfunktion bei Patienten mit essentieller Hypertension. In: Essentielle Hypertonie. Ein internationales Symposium, p. 373. Berlin-Göttingen-Heidelberg: Springer 1960.

32. HODLER, J.: Personal communication.

33. HOOBLER, S. W.: Hypertensive disease. Diagnosis and treatment, p. B. New York: Hoeber 1959.

34. HOOD, B., M. AURELL, T. FALKHEDEN, and S. BJÖRK: Essential hypertension, an international Symposium, p. 307. Berlin-Göttingen-Heidelberg: Springer 1960.

35. HUME, D. M., H. M. LEE, G. M. WILLIAMS, H. J. O. WHITE, J. FERRÉ, J. S. WOLF, G. R. PROUT JR., M. SLAPAK, J. O'BRIEN, S. J. KILPATRICK, H. M. KAUFFMAN JR., and R. J. KLEVELAND: Comparative results of cadaver and related donor renal homografts in man, and immunologic implications of the outcome of second and paired transplants. Ann. Surg. **164**, 352—357 (1966).

36. HUTCHINGS, R. H., R. M. HEGSTROM, and B. H. SCRIBNER: Glucose intolerance in patients on long-term intermittent dialysis. Ann. intern. Med. **65**, 275—285 (1966).

37. KEITH, N. M., H. P. WAGNER, and N. W. BARKER: Amer. J. Med. Sci. **197**, 332—338 (1939).

38. KINKAID-SMITH, P., J. MCMICHAEL, and E. A. MURPHY: The clinical course and pathology of hypertension with papilledema (malignant hypertension). Quart. J. Med. **27**, 117—125 (1958).

39. KOLFF, W. J., S. NAKAMATO, E. F. POUTASSE, R. A. STRAFFON, and J. E. FIGUEROA: Effect of bilateral nephrectomy and kidney transplantation on hypertension in man. Circulation **30**, Suppl. II, 23—28 (1964).

40. KUNIN, C. M.: Problems of drug therapy in renal failure. A guide to use of antibiotics in patients with renal disease. Ann. intern. Med. **67**, 151—158 (1967).

41. — S. B. REES, J. P. MERRILL, and M. FINLAND: Persistence of antibiotics in blood of patients with acute renal failure. J. clin. Invest. **38**, 1487—1491 (1959).

42. LEMANN, J., J. R. LITZOW, and E. J. LEMON: The effects of chronic acid loads in normal man: further evidence for the participation of bone mineral in the defense against chronic metabolic acidosis. J. clin. Invest. **45**, 1608—1614 (1966).

43. LIEBER, S. C., and A. LEFÈVRE: Ammonia as a source of gastric hypoacidity in patients with uremia. J. clin. Invest. **38**, 1271—1275 (1959).

44. LITZOW, J. R., J. LEMANN, and E. J. LEMON: The effect of treatment of acidosis on calcium balance in patients with chronic azotemic renal disease. J. clin. Invest. **46**, 280—286 (1967).

45. MCDONALD, S. J., E. M. CLARKSON, and N. E. DE WARDENER: The effects of a large intake of calcium citrate in normal subjects and patients with chronic renal failure. Clin. Sci. **26**, 27—39 (1964).

46. MCDONALD, L., and B. GOLDBERG: Lancet **1957 I**, 77.

47. MCINTOSH, D. A., E. W. PETERSON, and J. J. MCPHAUL: Anatomy of parathyroid function after renal homotransplantation. Ann. intern. Med. **65**, 900—907 (1966).

48. MERRILL, J. P., and E. SCHUPAK: Mechanisms of hypertension in renoprival man. Canad. med. Ass. J. **90**, 328—335 (1964).

49. MONASTERIO, G., S. GIOVANETTI e Q. MAGGIORE: La dieta nelle nefropatie. Boll. Soc. med.-chir. Pisa, Suppl. **4**, 1 (1963).

50. MOYER, J. H., C. HEIDER, K. PEVEY, and R. V. FORD: The vascular status of a heterogeneous group of patients with hypertension with particular emphasis on renal function. Amer. J. Med. **24**, 164—171 (1958).

51. — The effect of treatment of the vascular deterioration associated with hypertension with particular emphasis on renal function. Amer. J. Med. **24**, 177—185 (1958).

52. Muirhead, E. E., E. Booth, B. Brooks, M. Kosincki, E. G. Daniels, and J. W. Hinman: Renomedullary antihypertensive principle in renal hypertension. J. Lab. clin. Med. **64**, 989—996 (1964).
53. — B. Brooks, M. Kosincki, E. G. Daniels, and J. W. Hinman: Renomedullary antihypertensive principle in renal hypertension. J. Lab. clin. Med. **67**, 778—783 (1966).
54. Myers, V. C., and C. V. Bailey: The Lewis and Benedict method for the estimation of blood sugar with some observations obtained in disease. J. biol. Chem. **24**, 147—153 (1916).
55. Onesti, G., J. Cangiano, C. Swartz, O. Ramirez, and A. N. Brest: Blood pressure regulation in renoprival man. Intern. Congr. of nephrology Washington 1966, Abstract p. 251.
56. Palmer, R. S., D. Loofbourow, and C. R. Doering: New Engl. J. Med. **239**, 990 (1948).
57. Pellegrino, E. D., and R. M. Biltz: The composition of human bone in uremia. Medicine (Baltimore) **44**, 397—405 (1965).
58. Pendras, J. P., and R. V. Erickson: Hemodialysis — a successfull therapy for chronic uremia. Ann. intern. Med. **64**, 293—311 (1966).
59. Perkoff, G. T., C. L. Thomas, J. D. Newton, J. C. Sellman, and F. H. Tyler: Mechanism of impaired glucose tolerance in uremia and experimental hyperazotemia. Diabetes **7**, 375—377 (1958).
60. Rasmussen, H., H. de Luca, C. Arnaud, C. Hawker, and von M. Stedingk: The relationship between vitamin D and parathyroid hormone. J. clin. Invest. **42**, 1940—1974 (1963).
61. Reubi, F.: Die Spätwirkungen der medikamentösen Hochdrucksbehandlung auf die Nierenfunktion bei Patienten mit essentieller Hypertension. In: Essentielle Hypertonie. Ein internationales Symposium, p. 343. Berlin-Göttingen-Heidelberg: Springer 1960.
62. — Blutspiegel, Ausscheidung und Dosierung von N-Pyrrolidino-methyl-tetracyclin (PMT, Reverin) bei Nierenkranken. Klin. Wschr. **45**, 133—140 (1967).
63. —, u. C. Münger: Renale und extra-renale Ausscheidung von Pyrrolidino-methyl-tetracyclin (Reverin) bei Patienten mit normaler und eingeschränkter Nierenfunktion. Z. Klin. Pharmakol. **1**, 8—18 (1967).
64. Scholz, A.: Investigations on distribution and turnover-rate of ^{14}C-urea and tridiated water in renal failure. Proc. 4th Congr. E.D.T.A. **4**, 240—248 (1967).
65. Schottstaedt, M. F., and M. Sokolow: Natural history and course of malignant hypertension with papilledema. Amer. Heart J. **45**, 331—335 (1953).
66. Schroeder, H. A.: Hypertensive vascular disease. Therapy with modern drugs and its limits. J. chron. Dis. **1**, 497—499 (1955).
67. —, and H. M. Perry Jr.: Essential hypertension. An Internat. Symposium, p. 307. Berlin-Göttingen-Heidelberg: Springer 1960.
68. Scribner, B. H.: Proc. 3rd EDTA Conference **3**, 32 (1966).
69. Shaw, A. B., F. J. Bazzard, E. M. Booth, S. Nilwaragkur, and G. M. Berlyne: The treatment of chronic renal failure by a modified Giovanetti diet. Quart. J. Med. **35**, 237—241 (1965).
70. Shibagaki, M., W. J. Wolff, E. Haas, and H. Goldblatt: Concentration of renin in kidneys of patients with renal hypertension. Lancet **1965 I**, 1247—1248.
71. Smirk, F. H.: Prognosis in retinal grade I and II patients. In: Antihypertensive therapy. An International Symposium, p. 355. Berlin-Heidelberg-New York: Springer 1966.
72. Smithwick, R. H., and J. E. Thompson: J. Amer. med. Ass. **152**, 1501—1507 (1953).
73. Stanbury, S. W.: The treatment of renal osteodystrophy. Editorial Ann. intern. Med. **65**, 1133—1138 (1966).
74. —, and G. A. Lumb: Parathyroid function in chronic renal failure. Quart. J. Med. **35**, I (1966).
75. — —, and W. F. Nicholson: Elective subtotal parathyroidectomy for renal hyperparathyroidism. Lancet **1960 I**, 793—799.

76. Tchobroutsky, G. C., G. die P'Hurtet, G. Rosselin, R. Assan et M. Dévot: Étude de la glycorégulation dans l'insuffisance rénale chronique. Diabetologia **1**, 101—103 (1965).
77. Teuscher, A., S. Fankhauser u. F. R. Küffer: Untersuchungen zum Kohlehydratstoffwechsel bei Niereninsuffizienz. Klin. Wschr. **41**, 715—721 (1963).
78. Toussaint, Ch., M. Cremer, A. Heuse, P. Vereerstraeten, J. van Gertruyden, J. I. Cuykens et A. Vernivry: L'hypertension artérielle maligne incontrôlable, indication à la nephrectomie bilatérale dans le mal de Bright an stade ultime. EDTA Proceedings **3**, 65—69 (1966).
79. Westervelt, F. B., Jr., and G. E. Schreiner: The carbohydrate intolerance of uremic patients. Ann. intern. Med. **57**, 266—268 (1962).
80. Wilson, R. E., D. S. Bernstein, D. E. Murray, and F. D. Moore: Effects of parathyroidectomy and kidney transplantation in renal osteodystrophy. Amer. J. Surg. **110**, 384—389 (1965).
81. Wood, J. W., and W. B. Blythe: Management of malignant hypertension complicated by renal insufficiency. New Engl. J. Med. **277**, 57—61 (1967).

Discussion

Fritz:

You mentioned the possibility that secondary hyperparathyroidism in renal failure may evolve into "autonomous" hyperparathyroidism. Which arguments prove the transformation of an initially secondary hyperparathyroidism into the primary type in renal failure? Hypercalcemia is rare in chronic renal failure. It, therefore, appears quite possible that hyperparathyroidism of the primary type, in renal failure, is not a sequel to secondary hyperparathyroidism, but either a disease entity independent of the renal disease, or even responsible for the renal disease if the latter is a nephrocalcinosis leading to renal failure. This interpretation agrees with the fact that adenomatous changes are regularly observed in parathyroids which became autonomous in the course of renal failure.

Blumberg:

In the majority of patients with chronic renal failure subjected to parathyroidectomy hyperplasia of all glands (and not adenoma as you mentioned) was found [1,5]. This is of particular interest in patients who after successful renal homotransplantation continued to demonstrate signs of hyperparathyroidism necessitating parathyroidectomy [2—4]. In my opinion this finding can only be explained by the assumption that the parathyroid glands continued their hypersecretion in an autonomous fashion after the initial stimulus had been removed.

References

1. Felts, J. H., J. E. Whitey, D. D. Anderson, H. M. Caprentier, and H. H. Bradshaw: Medical and surgical treatment of azotemic osteodystrophy. Ann. intern. Med. **62**, 1272—1279 (1965).
2. Herdmann, R. C., A. F. Michael, R. L. Vernier, W. D. Kelly, and R. A. Good: Renal function and phosphorus excretion after human renal homotransplantation. Lancet **1966 I**, 121—123.
3. McIntosh, D. A., E. W. Peterson, and J. J. McPhaul: Autonomy of parathyroid function after renal homotransplantation. Ann. intern. Med. **65**, 900—907 (1966).
4. McPhaul, J. J., D. A. McIntosh, W. S. Hammond, and O. K. Park: Autonomous secondary (renal) parathyroid hyperplasia. New Engl. J. Med. **271**, 1342—1345 (1964).
5. Stanbury, S. W., G. A. Lumb, and W. F. Nicholson: Elective subtotal parathyroidectomy for renal hyperparathyroidism. Lancet **1960 I**, 793—795.

1.5.2. Contribution to the Dietetic Management of Chronic Renal Failure*

R. KLUTHE[1]

With 2 Figures

Good results obtained by GIOVANNETTI and MAGGIORE (1964) with a low nitrogen diet with proteins of high biological value in cases of advanced renal failure induced other clinicians to adapt this diet to the eating habits of other countries. The GIOVANNETTI diet was thus adapted to English eating habits by BERLYNE et al. (1965) — to Polish eating habits by POLEC (1966) — to French eating habits by SUC et al. (1966) — and to German eating habits by ourselves.

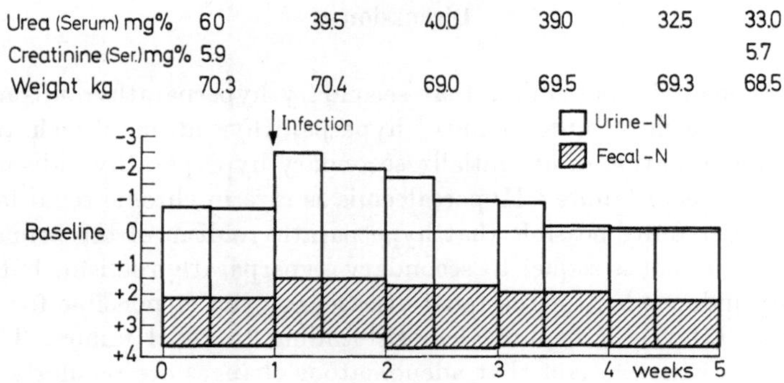

Fig. 1. Nitrogen balance in a patient with advanced chronic renal failure in the course of a pyelonephritis, given the potatoe-egg-diet. (Presentation according to REIFFENSTEIN, ALBRIGHT and WELLS, 1945). Equilibration after 4 weeks

The latter adaption is an almost purely vegetarian diet (KLUTHE and QUIRIN, 1966; KLUTHE et al., 1967), which proved satisfactory in the treatment of more than 60 patients with advanced chronic renal failure. The most important ingredients of our diet are potatoe and egg protein (in a fixed proportion, about 60/40 after KOFRANYI and JEKAT, 1964). We therefore called it potatoe-egg-diet. It contains: 1. a potatoe-egg mixture (ratio potatoe protein/egg protein about 60/40 ording to KOFRANYI and JEKAT, 1964). — 2. Low protein bread. — 3. Low protein noodles. — 4. Special vegetable pastes. — 5. Low protein vegetable and fruit. — 6. Carbohydrates and fats rich in unsaturated fatty acids. — An example of a nitrogen balance and the clinical course of a patient given the potatoe-egg-diet are shown in Figs. 1 and 2.

Successful management appears to depend on the following properties of the diet: 1. A high calory content (only 1/3 of the calories in the form of fat). — 2. A satisfactory spectrum of amino acids allowing equilibration of N-balance

* Supported by the Deutsche Forschungsgemeinschaft.

[1] Medizinische Poliklinik der Universität Freiburg i. Br., West Germany.

by 0.375 g/kg weight/day. — 3. Low osmotic residue (estimated in healthy persons) 360—380 mOsm/day (a pure carbohydrate diet of 2000 Cal. has an osmotic residue of ~ 300 mOsm/day (SARGENT and JOHNSON, 1956). — 4. Low acid residue: net acid excretion 15 mEq/day (normal food: about 70—80 mEq/day). — 5. Normal potassium content. — 6. Digestibility. — 7. May be prepared in the patient's home according to easy recipes (KLUTHE and QUIRIN, 1967).

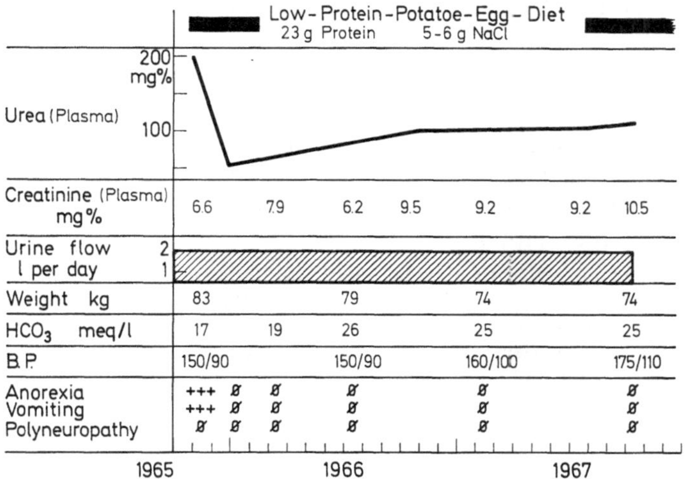

Fig. 2. Clinical course of a patient with an advanced chronic glomerulonephritis who was fully able to work under the low protein potatoe-egg-diet

References

BERLYNE, G. M., A. B. SHAW, and S. NILWARANGKUR: Dietary treatment of chronic renal failure. Experiences with a modified diet. Nephron **2**, 129—147 (1965).

GIOVANNETTI, S., and Q. MAGGIORE: Low protein diet in uremia . Lancet **1964 I**, 1000—1003.

KLUTHE, R.: Probleme des Eiweißstoffwechsels bei chronischer Niereninsuffizienz. In: Peritonealdialyse. Ed.: F. SCHELER, p. 28—36. München-Berlin-Wien: Urban & Schwarzenberg 1967.

—, u. H. QUIRIN: Experimentelle Untersuchungen zur eiweißarmen Diät bei chronischen Nierenerkrankungen. In: Aktuelle Probleme der Klinischen Naphrologie. Ed.: D. P. MERTZ u. R. KLUTHE, p. 142—144. Stuttgart: Georg Thieme 1966.

— — Diätbuch für Nierenkranke. Stuttgart: Georg Thieme 1967.

— — D. OECHSLEN u. A. WENIG: Kartoffel-Ei-Diät bei fortgeschrittener Niereninsuffizienz. Med. Klin. **62**, 1020—1022 (1967).

KOFRANYI, E., u. F. JEKAT: Die Wertigkeit gemischter Proteine. Hoppe-Seylers Z. physiol. Chem. **335**, 174—179 (1964).

POLEC, R.: Dieta ziemniaczana w leczeniu przewleklej niewydolnosci nerek. Pol. Arch. Med. wewnet. **5**, 647—665 (1966).

REIFENSTEIN, E. C., F. ALBRIGHT, and S. L. WELLS: The accumulation, interpretation of data pertaining to metabolic balances, notably those of calcium, phosphorous and nitrogen. J. clin. Endocr. **5**, 367—395 (1945).

SARGENT II, F., and R. E. JOHNSON: The effects of diet on renal function in healthy men. Amer. J. clin. Nutr. **4**, 466—481 (1956).

SUC, J. M., M. RUMEAU, TON-THAT HUNG, J. CONTE, P. MERIEL et J. BERNARD-GRIFFITHS: Régimes pauvres en proteines, completés en acides aminés essentiels dans le traitment au long cours de l'insuffisance ren. chron. grave. Proceedings of the Euro. Dialysis and Transplantant Ass. Vol. III (1966), p. 81—89.

1.5.3. Clinical Experience with the Combined Treatment of Chronic Renal Failure with Peritoneal Dialysis and a Strict Low-Protein "Potatoe-Egg-Diet"*

H. QUIRIN, V. HEINZE, A. TOURKANTONIS and R. KLUTHE[1]

With 4 Figures

Patients with far-advanced chronic renal-failure can be successfully treated over long periods of time by intermittent peritoneal dialysis and our modification of the Giovannetti-diet, the so-called low-protein "potatoe-egg-diet" (QUIRIN and KLUTHE, 1966; KLUTHE and QUIRIN, 1967).

Fig. 1 shows an example:

This 42-year-old patient with amyloidosis of the kidneys due to chronic osteomyelitis was admitted as an emergency-case in a uremic state. After 4 peritoneal dialyses the uremic symptoms disappeared. We then started the combined peritoneal-dialysis/diet-therapy which was continued on an outpatient basis, for 8 months. His urine-flow amounts to 400 ml per day, the daily nitrogen-excretion in urine to 0.7 g. With one weekly peritoneal dialysis the serum urea averaged 133 mg-% before dialysis, 83 mg-% after dialysis. The corresponding values of the serum creatinine were 14.2 and 10.5 mg-%. The patient feels well and performs minor household tasks.

In many cases it cannot be decided immediately, if a chronic patient in chronic renal failure is suitable for chronic extracorporeal dialysis. In other cases, patients cannot be included early enough into an extracorporeal chronic treatment-program for technical reasons. In this emergency the combined peritoneal-dialysis/diet-therapy may afford temporary relief (Fig. 2).

A 24-year-old chronic uremic patient was treated a few weeks by diet. When the urine-flow fell to 500/ml per day, she was treated by intermittent peritoneal-dialysis and the low-protein "potatoe-egg-diet" for 3 months, before she could finally be admitted to the chronic hemodialysis program. The daily nitrogen-excretion of the patient amounted to 0.8 g.

In some cases of acute uremic exacerbations of chronic nephritis the uremic symptoms can be eliminated by a few peritoneal dialyses followed by dietary treatment. Fig. 3 shows such a case.

After an initial peritoneal dialysis the 27-year-old patient with chronic pyelonephritis was successfully treated with the low-protein "potatoe-egg-diet" for 6 months. She is now able to take care of her household and children without assistance. Her serum urea hardly exceeds 100 mg-%, the serum creatinine averages 11 mg-%. The plasma standard bicarbonate, under the influence of alcalinizing drugs rose to 16 meq/l and, within the following 2 months, it reached the normal value of 25 meq/l under dietetic treatment. This increase may be due to the low-protein content of the diet.

Finally we measured the increase in serum urea during the interval between peritoneal dialyses under different dietetic conditions (Fig. 4). 102 observations were made in patients, receiving the low protein "potatoe-egg-diet" with a

* Supported by the Deutsche Forschungsgemeinschaft.

[1] Medizinische Poliklinik der Universität Freiburg i. Br., West Germany.

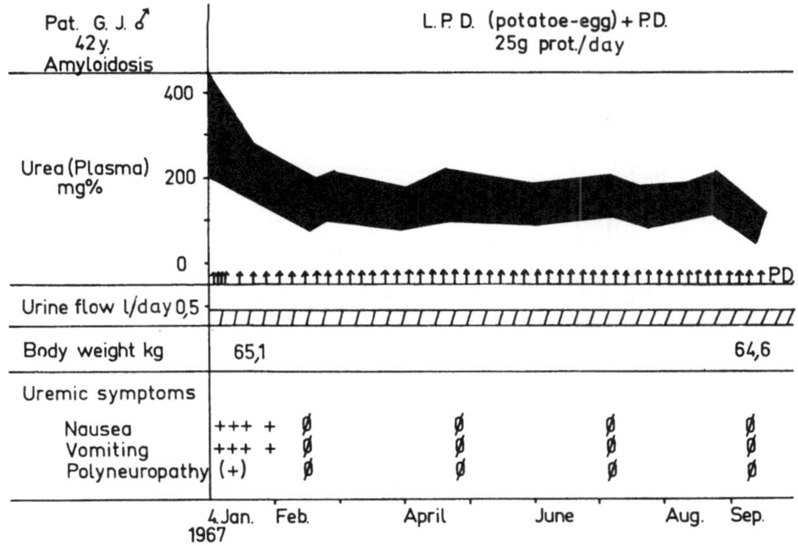

Fig. 1. Progress of a 42-year-old uremic patient with amyloidosis of the kidneys, treated now for eight months with combined low protein "potatoe-egg-diet" and one weekly peritoneal dialysis. Abbreviations: *L.P.D.* low protein "potatoe-egg-diet"; *P.D.* peritoneal dialysis; S_{Cr} serum creatinine; S_U serum urea

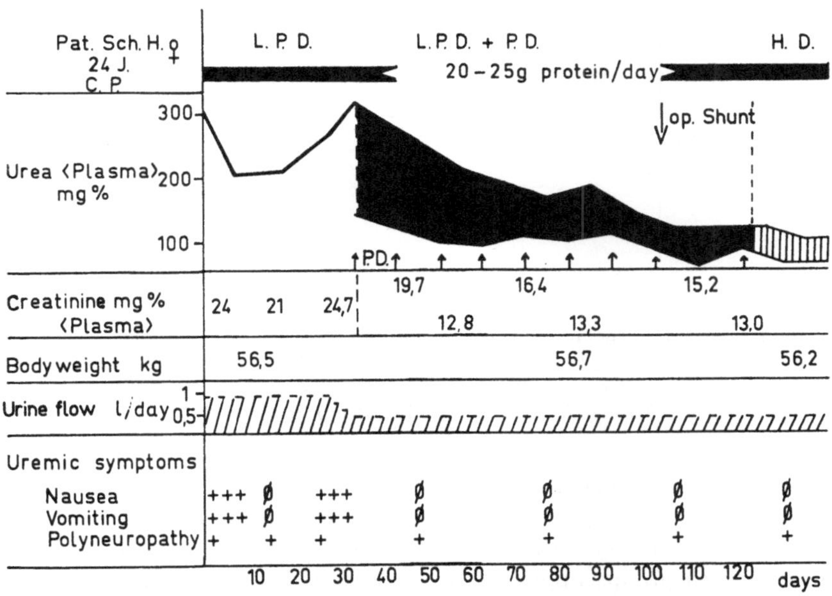

Fig. 2. "Potatoe-egg-diet" combined with peritoneal dialysis as interim therapy before chronic hemodialysis, in a case with uremia in the course of chronic pyelonephritis. Abbreviations: *L.P.D.* low protein diet; *P.D.* peritoneal dialysis; *H.D.* haemodialysis

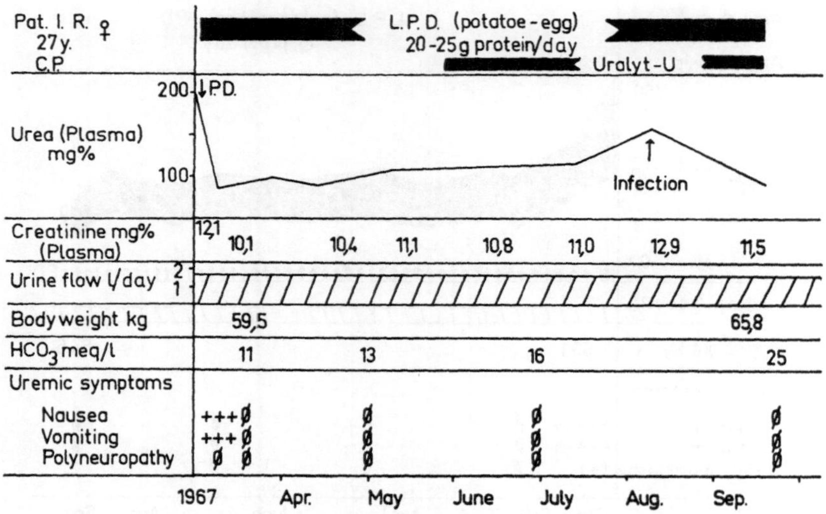

Fig. 3. Progress of a 27-year-old female patient with chronic renal failure due to chronic pyelonephritis. By means of one peritoneal dialysis the uremic symptoms were improved. During the following six months the patient was treated only with a low protein "potatoe-egg-diet". Abbreviations: *L.P.D.* low protein potatoe-egg-diet; *P.D.* peritoneal dialysis

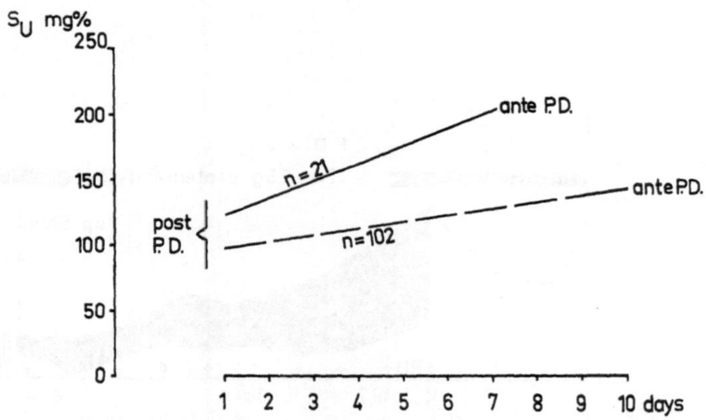

Fig. 4. Serum urea during the intervals between two sessions of peritoneal dialysis in patients given the "potatoe-egg-diet" (dotted line) or the usual 40 g protein-containing-diet (drawn line). The average increase per day of the group given the "potatoe-egg-diet" amounted to 7.7 mg-%, that in the other group to 14 mg-%

protein content between 20 and 25 g, and 21 observations with a diet containing 40 g protein. In both groups, the average urine excretion amounted to 500 ml/per day. No patient was hypercatabolic. The daily increase of serum creatinine averaged in both groups approx. 0.6 mg-% per day. Under the low-protein "potatoe-egg-diet" the daily increase of serum-urea was half of that of the group given 40 g of protein. We, thus, could extend the interval between our sessions of peritoneal dialysis up to 10 days, as compared to 7 days with a 40 g protein-containing-diet. The post- and predialytic serum-urea levels of both groups also different clearly. They averaged 98 to 147 mg-% under the "potatoe-egg-diet", 124 to 205 mg-% with 40g of protein per day. The difference was statistically significant ($p < 0.01$).

References

1. Giovannetti, S., and Q. Maggiore: Low protein diet in uremia. Lancet **1964I**, 1000—1003.
2. Heinze, V.: In: H. Sarre, Nierenkrankheiten, S. 443—452. Stuttgart: Georg Thieme 1967.
3. Kluthe, R., H. Quirin, D. Oechslen, and A. Wenig: Kartoffel-Ei-Diät bei fortgeschrittener Niereninsuffizienz. Med. Klin. **62**, 1020—1023 (1967).
4. Quirin, H., and R. Kluthe: Experimental contribution to the dietetic managment of chronic uremia in patient. VII. Int. Congr. of Nutrition Hamburg 1966, vol 5, p. 230—235. Braunschweig: Friedrich Vieweg & Sohn GmbH 1967.

1.5.4. The Pathology of Uremia

H. U. Zollinger[1]

With 12 Figures

The description of the morphological picture of uremia is more difficult than it appears at a first glance. Uremia is characterized by a host of renal disturbances other than the decreased ability to excrete nitrogenous waste products; these other disturbances influence the morphological picture. Thus, a decrease of renal blood flow induces hypertension which, in turn, causes morphological changes in the circulatory organs. Distal tubular damage induces acidosis and secondary hyperparathyroidism. These changes do not quantitatively depend on the blood urea concentrations. Finally, I wish to mention the consequences of a lack of erythropoietin which is presumably of tubular origin. I shall, therefore, discuss not only the "purely uremic" changes, i.e. those changes which are due to an increased concentration of urea in body fluids and which could be described in a few sentences, but shall try to describe the tissue changes often observed in uremia, which may or may not be related to retention of urea. Retention of urea and other substances usually excreted by normal kidneys is doubtlessly the main primary change in uremia. As a morphologist, I shall, however, abstain from discussing the properties and the effects of such substances.

I first wish to comment, briefly, on the diagnosis of uremia at autopsy. The currently used Nessler reaction on the gastric mucosa is unreliable, because it demonstrates only the presence of ammonia. NPN determinations in post-mortal blood are unreliable for similar reasons.

In contrast, measurements of NPN in cardiac muscle may be useful within 72 hours after death [13]: normal values may reach 220 mg-% while values above 300 mg-% are characteristic for uremia. On the other hand, the demonstration of crystals of triple phosphate in pharyngeal mucus, as described by Wegelin [22] and Riva [17], did not prove useful in our hands.

As shown in Fig. 1, the presence of increased amounts of urea in the brain, the lungs or the intestine may be demonstrated by the formation of dixanthyl urea crystals after application of xanthydrol. As a diagnostic method the procedure is, unfortunately, time-consuming, and its results depend on the purity of the xanthydrol solution used. Experienced pathologists very rarely refer to these methods for reaching a diagnosis of uremia, because other organ changes, i. e. the urinous odor of the tissues and morphological changes of the kidneys, usually allow a reliable diagnosis. Lesions at the so-called vicarious sites of excretion of nitrogenous metabolites normally excreted by the kidneys, i.e., the epicardium, the gastro-intestinal mucosa, the lungs and the pleura, are quite characteristic in uremic states, but may sometimes occur in other circumstances.

[1] Pathologisches Institut der Universität Basel, Switzerland.

The best known change of this type in the heart is uremic pericarditis which, however, usually does not occur in uremia due to acute renal failure. It also occurs only in a fraction of cases of chronic uremia: in 20% according to RIVA [17], in 50% according to SELDIN et al. [19]. We found uremic pericarditis in 60% of autopsies done on uremic patients; this figure comprizes cases with a slight opalescence of the surface of the heart, or hyperemia of the pericardium. In typical cases of uremic pericarditis, the pericardium contains an exsudative liquid rich in fibrin which is precipitated in strands resembling sand strands. The

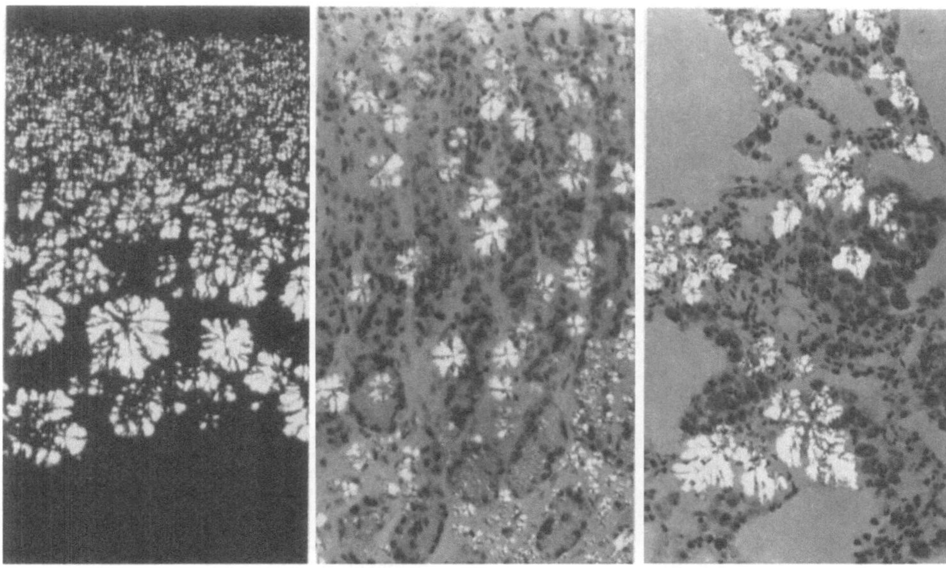

a b c

Fig. 1a—c. Xanthydrol reaction in uremia. a) Cerebral cortex. b) Stomach. c) Lungs. Enlargement 120 times

fibrinous precipitates often contain a brown pigment derived from the residues of hemorrhages. In spite of the presence of a small number of polynuclear leucocytes the fibrin precipitates do not undergo liquefaction (Fig. 2). The apparent absence of fibrinolytic processes in uremia will also retain our attention when discussing the aspect of the lungs. In one third of the cases of uremic pericarditis, pericardial liquid is serous, in one fifth of the cases it contains much blood. Uremic pericarditis may be a cause of death by pericardial tamponade [4]. Neither calcification nor scar-formation were observed in the pericardial exsudate of patients whose lives had been prolonged by hemodialysis.

It is more difficult to describe the myocardial changes. We called them uremic myocardosis (ZOLLINGER [23]). Microscopically the myocardium appears opalescent and pale. Its colour is a brownish yellow (color of "feuille morte"). The changes are due to two sequences of events. On the one hand, hyperkalemia is responsible for the occurrence of numerous very small necrotic areas without any inflammatory reaction (MEISTER) [16] ("micronecrosis"). On the other hand, hypertrophy of the myocardium, as a consequence of renal hypertension, is responsible for the paleness of the tissue. This paleness has been ascribed to inadequate oxygenation by the increased thickness of intercapillary layers. This does not, however, appear to be the only explanation. Many investigations demonstrate an inadequate utilization of energy-rich phosphates and of oxygen

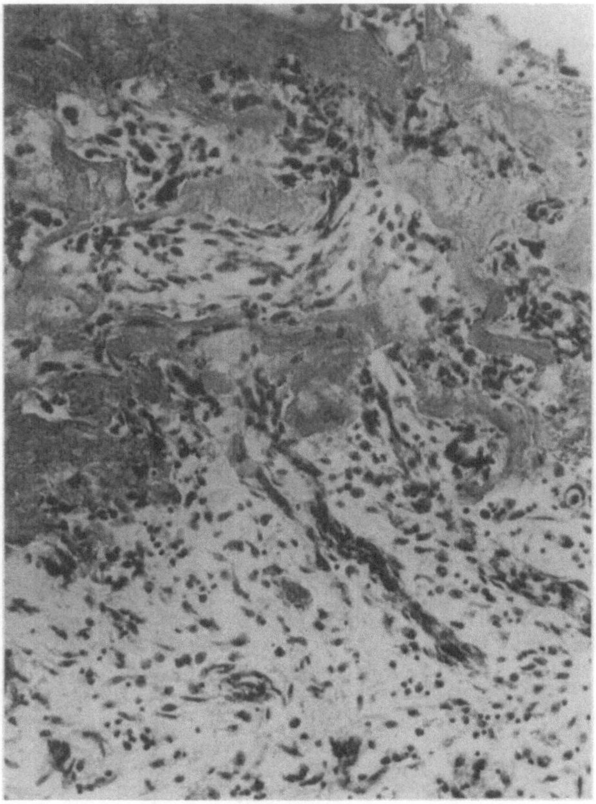

Fig. 2. Typical subacute pericarditis in chronic uremia. The epicardial side is the lower margin of the picture, while the pericardial space would be situated above the upper margin. Plump fibrin deposits without fibrinolysis by leucocytes. Capillaries proliferating into the fibrin. Some lymphocytic and histiocytic infiltrations. HE. Enlargement 150 times

(FLECKENSTEIN) [9], primarily due to a disturbance of calcium transports. The morphological sequelae to this disturbance of calcium transport are breaks and other changes of the sarco-plasmatic reticulum of the cardiac muscle fibers.

With light microscopy, the typical picture of myocardosis consists in minimal degenerative changes in the cardiac muscle fibers and pronounced interstitial edema between the fibers, particularly within the septa, where adventitial cells are also mobilized (Fig. 3). If life is prolonged by hemodialysis, these primary changes may evolve into diffuse interstitial sclerosis. True interstitial myocarditis is often found in patients dying in uremia, but is presumably due to simultaneous infections rather than to the retention of nitrogenous metabolites

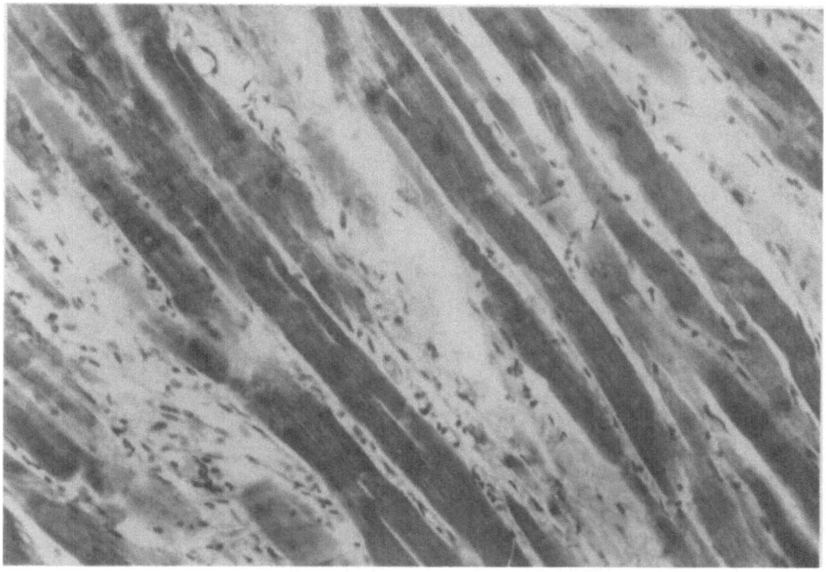

Fig. 3. Uremic myocardosis. Edema of the interstitial tissues. The adventitial cells of the capillaries are easily recognized. HE. Enlargement 170 times

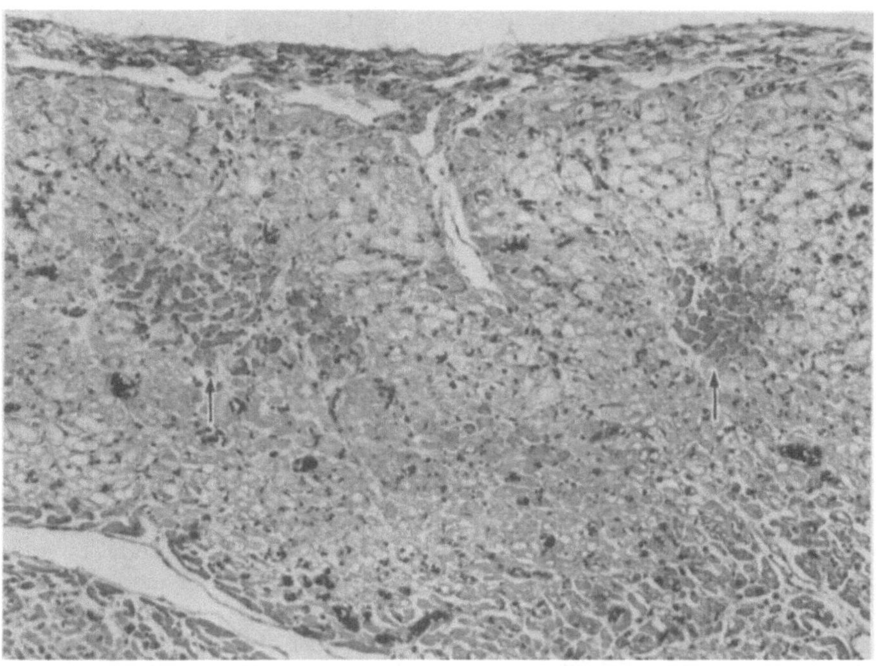

Fig. 4. "Fleckmyokard" in a uremic patient with malignant nephrosclerosis. The endocardium is seen at the upper margin of the section. Two necrotic foci surrounded by fibres containing vacuoles which presumably represent glycogen deposition. HE. Enlargement 90 times

(RIVA) [17]. One is struck by the rarity of the propagation of pericarditis to the myocardium which should result in inflammatory changes in the outer layers of the heart muscle (ALLEN) [1].

Cuts through the myocardium sometimes reveal lenticular or smaller yellowish opalescent spots, which produce the picture of a "Fleckmyokard". Microscopically, they are points of anoxic necrosis or fat deposition (Fig. 4) due to necrotic changes in the corresponding arterioles. These changes are not related to uremia as such, but to renal hypertension.

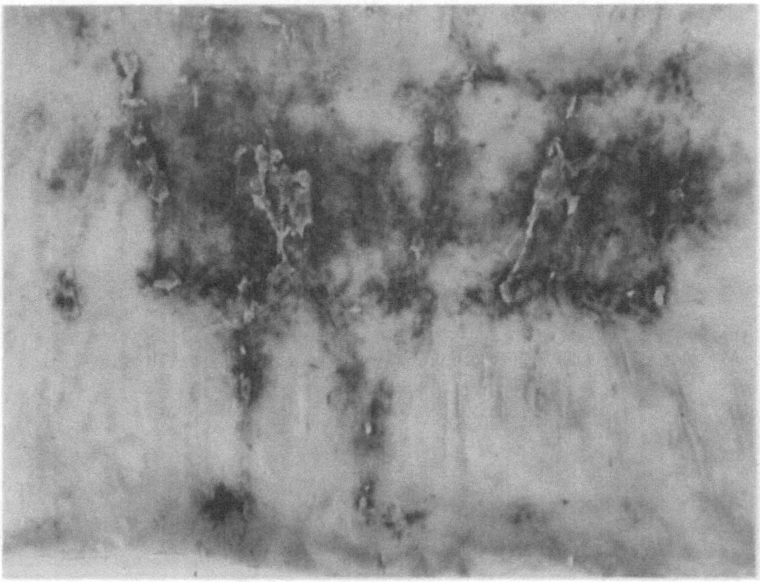

Fig. 5. Uremic colitis with extensive mucosal hemorrhages and small ulcers. The ulcers are covered with fibrin

A characteristic finding in uremia is gastro-enteritis which can only be reliably identified if autopsy is done immediately after death. The gastric mucosa is slightly red, clearly thickened and covered by viscous transparent mucus. The intestinal mucosa is mainly hyperemic and often shows small ulcerations (Fig. 5). Which are assumed to be due to bacterial liberation of ammonia from urea (RIVA [17]; SELDIN et al. [19]). We find these changes in approximately 80% of all autopsies on uremic subjects, while pseudomembranous or necrotizing colitis, which formerly was considered as a typical lesion in uremia, occurs very rarely. Since mercury intoxications were frequent in autopsy material in earlier days, this error may be due to a confusion between effects of mercury and of uremia. The microscopic picture of uremic gastroenteritis is not very characteristic. The only striking feature is the small number of polynuclear leucocytes, particularly around the small intestinal ulcerations (Fig. 6). The histological appearance suggests failure of the leucocyte defense mechanism. The submucosal layer is usually edematous. Increased secretion of mucus from the gastric mucosa is also seen in the microscopic preparations (Fig. 7).

Deep ulcers, as sometimes seen in the intestine in malignant hypertension, may be due to arteriolonecrosis. We recently observed, in the intestine of a 21 year old girl, confluent ulcerations which resulted in the clinical picture of intestinal infarction and necessitated surgical resection. Microscopically, ar-

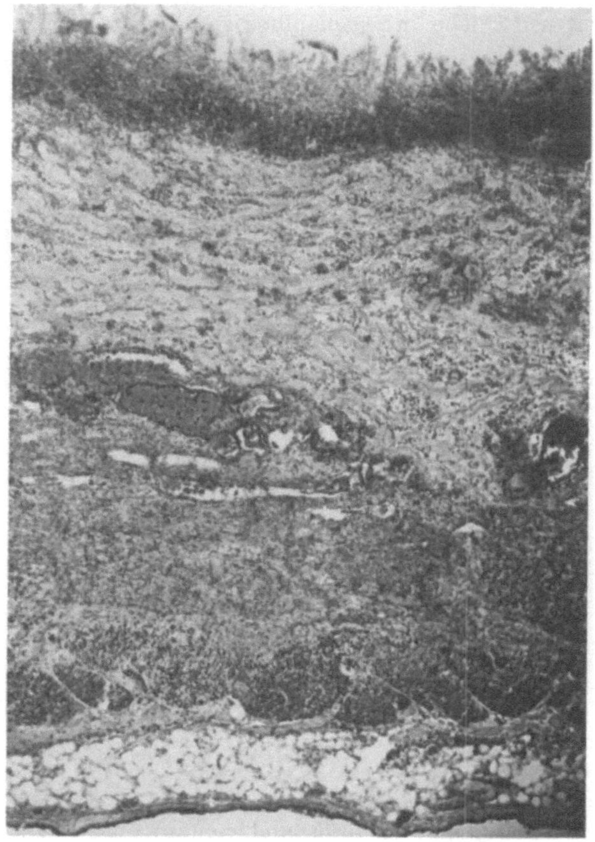

Fig. 6. Uremic enteritis. The mucosa is necrotic and partially desquamated. Large inflammatory infiltrations of the mucosal layers which extend into the muscular layer. HE. Enlargement 15 times

teriolonecrosis could be demonstrated in the diseased parts of the intestine (Fig. 8), while the only change observed in the big vessels was hypertrophy of the muscular coat due to hypertension. Thus, intestinal disturbances, observed in renal failure with hypertension, may be due to vascular damage rather than to retention of urea.

Pulmonary changes, as observed in approximately two thirds of all cases of uremia (HOPPS and WISSLER [12]), may result from many single lesions and are difficult to evaluate. The lungs are usually enlarged, heavy and show a spleen-like consistency, particularly the hilus, where the color is usually a dark bluish red. Ordinary hypostatic changes, on the other hand, occur in the peripheral lower parts of the lungs, rather than in the perihilar region. Fibrinous or fibrinoserous pleuritis, in our experience, occurs extremely rarely, and only in cases with secondary pneumonia. This statment contrasts with RIVA's [17] observation of pleuritis in 9.3% of the cases, and the data of HOPPS and WISSLER [12], who found it in 20% of uremic patients.

Microscopic examination discloses different types of changes which occur with variable intensity. The most characteristic change, in our view, is the occurrence of bulb-or mushroom-shaped precipitates of fibrin in single alveoles or groups of alveoles (Fig. 9). SCHNEITER's careful investigations [18] show that

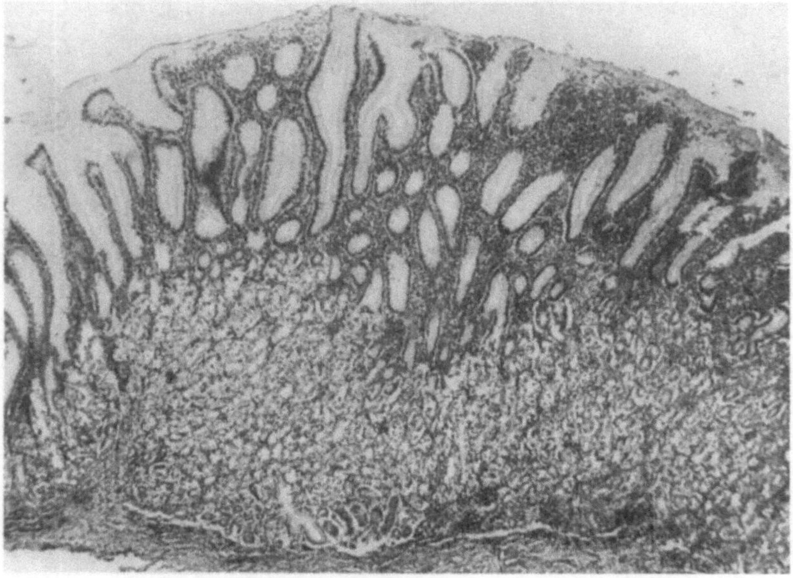

Fig. 7. Uremic gastritis with increased secretion of mucus and dense inflammatory infiltration of the stroma. HE. Enlargement 22 times

the fibrin layers are very poor in cells and contain only a few desquamated alveolar cells easily recognized by their PAS-positivity. Schneiter thought that these precipitates contained "fibrinoid". We think, however, that they contain in fact, fibrin as shown by their reactions with different dyes. As in uremic pericarditis the fibrin precipitates never undergo fibrinolysis in spite of the presence of polynuclear leucocytes. The fibrin precipitated in the pulmonary tissue is progressively "organized". The final result is the picture of relapsing "carnified" pneumonia (Fig. 10). Fibrin deposition appears to occur repeatedly at variable intervals. On the other hand, the deposition of fibrin stimulates an inflammatory reaction which, in the lungs, produces mainly lympho-plasmo-histiocytic focal pneumonia (Fig. 10). This type of focal pneumonia, together with the deposition of fibrin, is responsible for the typical "butterfly" X-ray picture with pronounced perihilar condensations.

The second type of changes of the lungs are hemorrhages similar to those occurring in the pericardium. A frequent trend to hemorrhage in uremia is a clinically well-known fact. Microscopically we did not succeed in detecting any

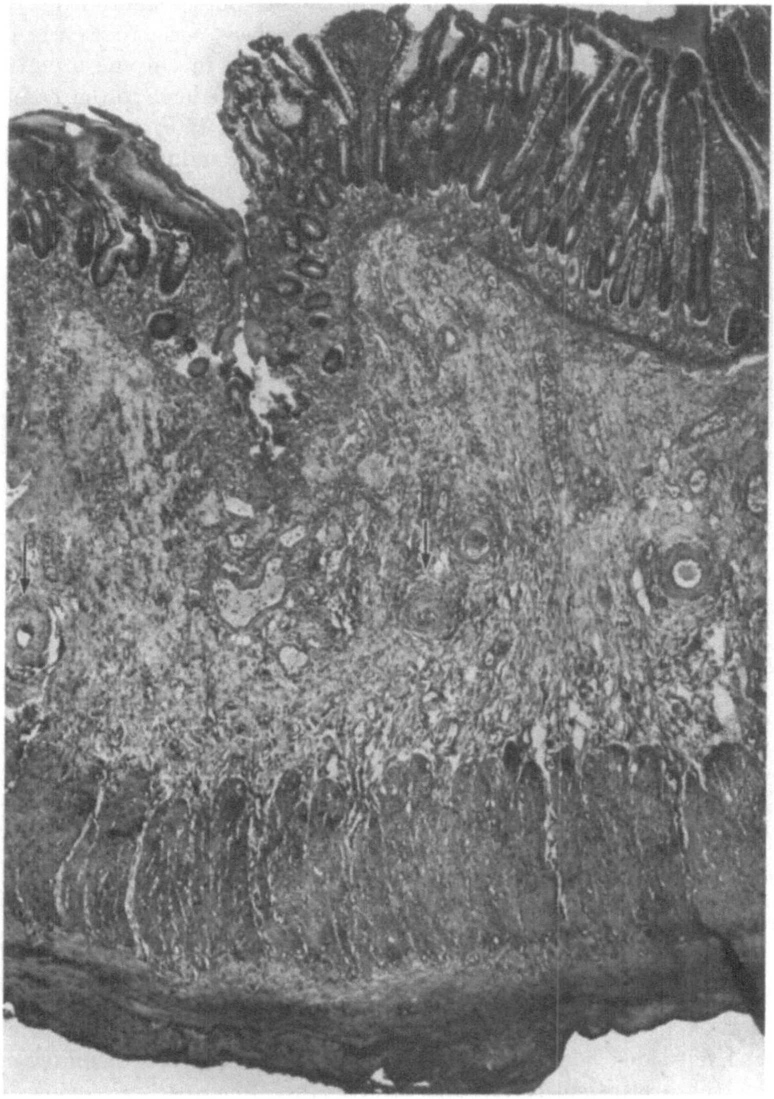

Fig. 8. Incipient ulceration of the jejunum, in uremia due to malignant nephroscleroses. Severe hypertensive changes in small arteries. Fibrinous deposits on the serosa are due to an earlier perforation at an other site. HE. Enlargement 12 times

lesions of small vessels which could be responsible for the fibrin exsudation or the tendency to hemorrhage. The pulmonary hemorrhages, thus, differ from those seen in cases of the Goodpasture syndrome, where we often find fibrinoid vascular necrosis (Zollinger and Hegglin [25]). We think that the bleeding in uremia is due to some functional disturbance of the bone marrow. Hemosiderin-containing alveolar phagocytes are often observed in the lungs of uremic patients. They occur probably in small hemorrhagic areas (Fig. 11).

A third type of pulmonary change in uremia is pulmonary edema due to left-sided heart failure, as a consequence of myocardosis, pericarditis and hypertension. Left heart failure is a frequent cause of death in chronic uremia with hypertension. Morphologically, cardiogenic pulmonary edema often cannot be distinguished from the so-called toxic edema of uremia. If the patient recovers from heart failure, absorption of pulmonary edema may induce the formation of hyaline membranes (Fig. 11), resembling those frequently seen in radiation

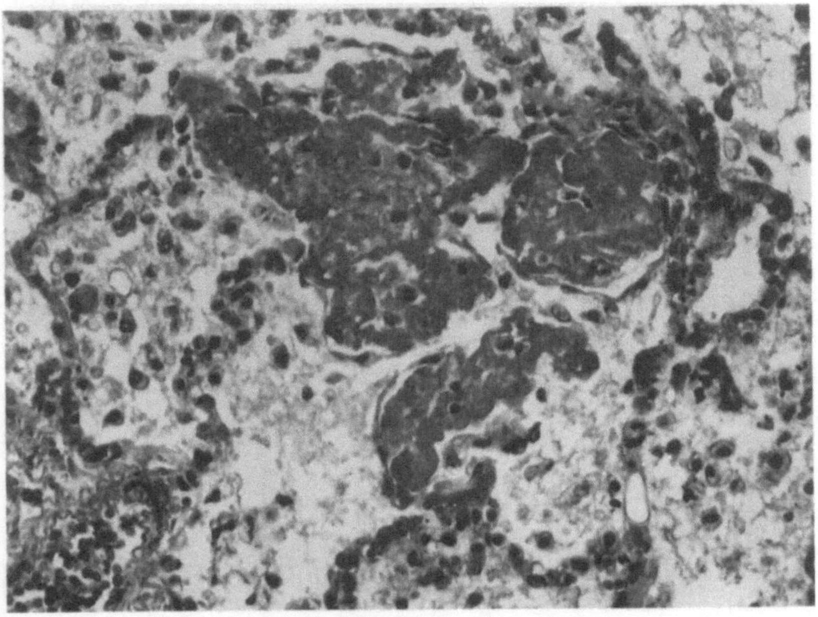

Fig. 9. Pneumonia in a uremic patient. Plump fibrinous deposits in the al veolar spaces Absence of leucocytes. Many phagocytic cells surround the fibrinous areas. HE. Enlargement 300 times

damage to the lungs or in asphyctic newborns or infants. As opposed to radiation damage or anoxia, uremia has not been demonstrated to cause capillary lesions. Long lasting left-sided heart failure and pulmonary stasis induce induration of the lungs which are primarily red and later change to brown as a consequence of the transformation of hemoglobin into hemosiderin. In many cases, the final composite picture comprises brown induration of the lungs (Fig. 10), acute agonal edema of the lungs, hyaline membranes, fibrin deposits in pulmonary tissue and interstitial inflammatory processes. Many pathologists call this state "uremic pneumonia". We prefer the term "pneumonia in a uremic patient", since the morphological appearance lacks specific features.

Inflammatory changes of the upper respiratory tract, oral cavity, pharynx, larynx and the esophagus, presumably due to the excretion of nitrogenous metabolites, are very frequent and will not be further discussed. Parotitis (parotitis marantica) appears to be much more frequent than generally assumed. At autopsy, the parotis is not often investigated. We found suppurative parotitis in 16 out of 20 cases of chronic uremia. It is unknown, to what degree this change may be due to retention of urea. Dryness of the oral mucosa in the course of the uremic coma, when the patient breathes through an open mouth, may contribute to this complication which is also facilitated by the lack of defense against infections in uremic subjects (HAMBURGER et al. [10]).

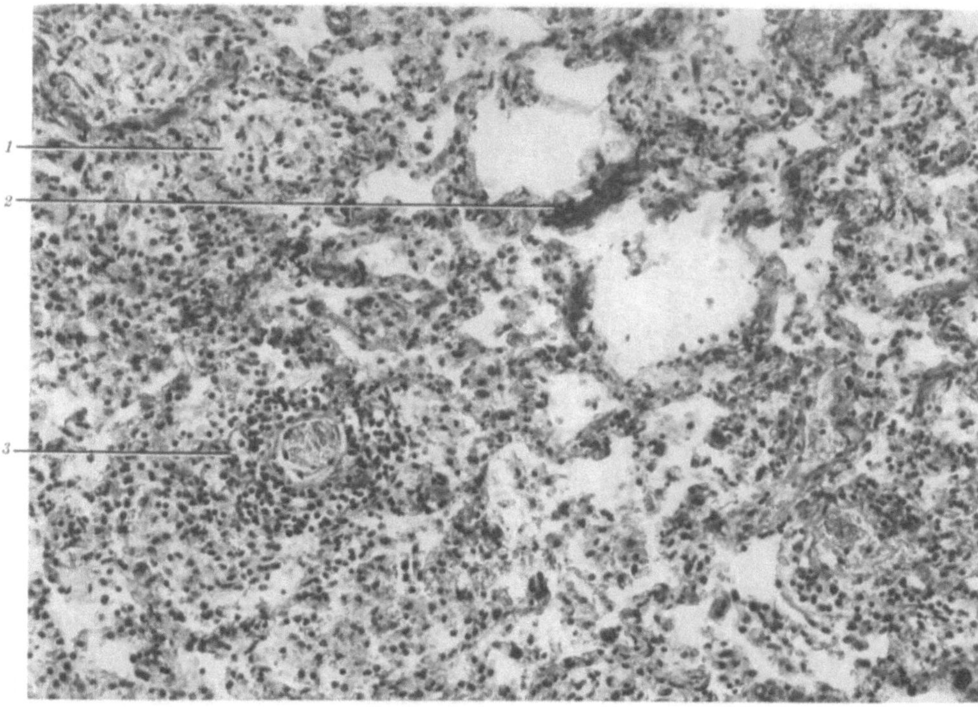

Fig. 10. Picture of the lung in uremia. Pneumonia with focal carnification (*1*), dark collagen fibers in the septa (*2*), atelectasis due to a pleural exsudate, perivascular-interstitial pneumonia (*3*). VAN GIESON. Enlargement 100 times

An enlargement of the pancreatic acini is a frequent, though not specific change in uremia (Fig. 12). The epithelial cells are often destroyed, which results in a non-suppurative interstitial inflammation. BAGGENSTOSS [3], who first described this change found it in 40% of his uremic subjects, but also in many other diseases of the stomach or the intestine. The change is thought to be due to a lack of secretin which increases the viscosity of the pancreatic secretion, as often observed in patients with diarrhea or vomiting. The pancreatic changes are not correlated with any known functional disturbance.

The absence of characteristic morphological changes in the brain of uremic subjects contrasts with the specificity of the clinical picture of uremic coma. Cerebral edema is generally observed and may be partly due to an accumulation of urea, but may as well be induced by heart failure, or occur partly as a consequence of the frequent nephrotic syndrome. Furthermore, cerebral vascular spasms occur and play an important role in patients with serious grades of

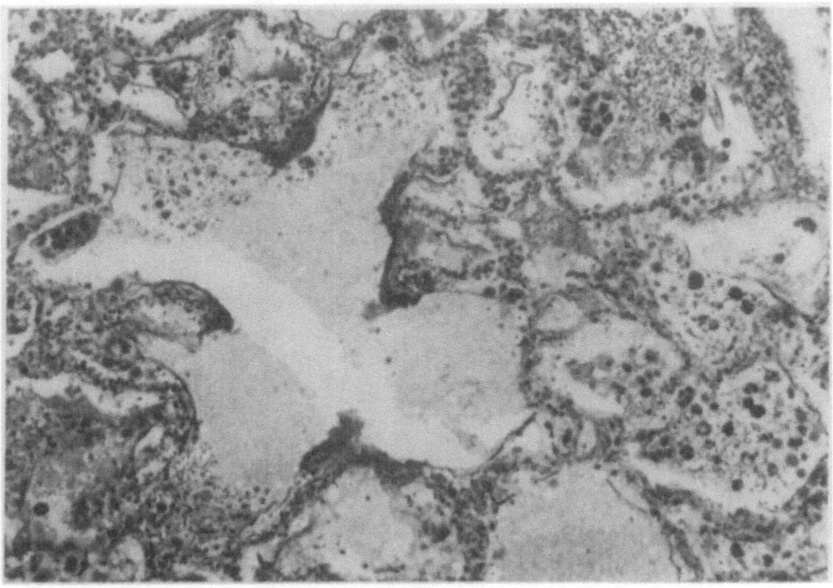

Fig. 11. Lungs in uremic patient: severe edema. In the middle of the picture formation of a hyaline membrane (dark layer in the alveole). Other alveoles contain large numbers of dark hemosiderin containing phagocytic cells as a consequence of chronic stasis and repeated small hemorrhages. Little inflammatory interstitial infiltration. HE. Enlargement 200 times

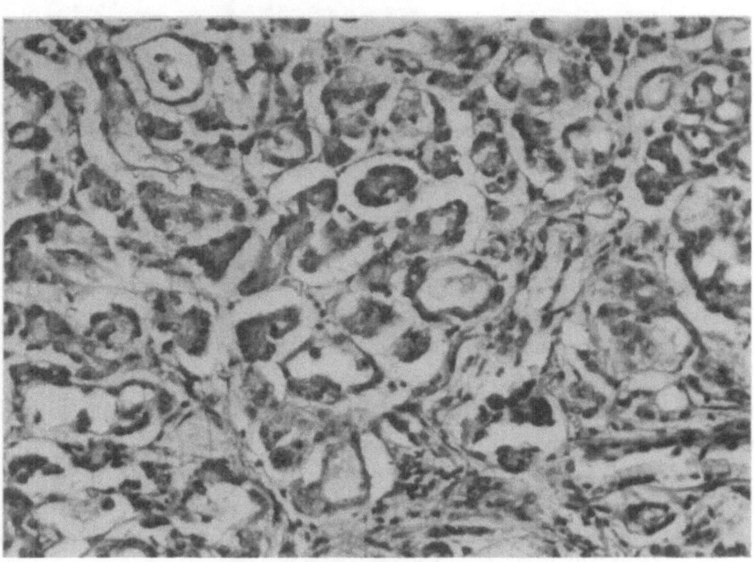

Fig. 12. Pancreas of a uremic patient. Enlargement of the acini, edema of the interstitium. HE. Enlargement 300 times

hypertension as shown experimentally by BYROM [7]. Eclampsia-like fits in uremic patients are due to vascular spasms rather than to the retention of urea. There is, thus, no morphological substrate of uremic coma. The changes described by BODECHTEL and ERBSLÖH [5] are vague and non-specific. Slight grades of meningitis, as observed by other pathologists, did not occur in our material.

At autopsy the bone marrow of the uremic subject appears pale; blood-forming marrow is largely replaced by yellow marrow in the metaphyses of long bones. Microscopic examination discloses a depression of red blood cell formation and a smaller inhibition of leucocyte formation (ANDRY [2]). The number of medullary plasma cells may be increased; this increase is not due to uremia, but depends on the type of the primary disease of the kidney. It does not occur in primarily vascular renal diseases. The inhibition of red blood cell formation is now usually ascribed to diminished secretion of renal erythropoietin in the diseased kidneys. The incorporation of radioactive iron into red blood cell precursors is depressed in uremia. Many authors think, however, that a hemolytic and a toxic component contribute to the anemia. Hemolysis may be responsible for the usually moderate hemosiderosis of the spleen. The life-span of red blood cells is usually decreased in uremia, while the number of reticulocytes is increased in spite of the inhibition of medullary red blood cell formation (SHAW and SCHOLER [20]). The mechanism of the inhibition of white blood cell formation is unknown. Leucopenia plays an important role in the pathogenesis of uremia. It may contribute to the absence of fibrinolysis which may, however, be partly due to a peripheral inhibition of the activation of leucocytes (MCLEOD [15]). The frequency of infections in uremia may also be related to the leucopenia (BULL [6]). As a consequence of such infections, there may be a destruction of tissue which, in turn, imposes a further burden on the excretory capacity of the kidneys, and, thus, induces a circulus vitiosus. Finally, it has been shown that antigen-antibody reactions are depressed in uremic patients, which may facilitate the "taking" of transplants. The depression of antigen-antibody reaction is not due to decreased antibody formation, but may be related to leucopenia or to functional incompetence of the leucocytes (KROE and VAZQUEZ [14]).

The hemorrhagic diathesis of uremia has been ascribed by CASTALI et al. [8] to damage to the platelets due to a change in the composition of the blood. These authors assumed that the damage results in a decrease in platelet aggregation and stickiness. Other investigators (HEINTZ [11]; HAMBURGER et al. [10]) ascribe the proneness to hemorrhage to arteriolar or capillary damage. The lack of morphological evidence for such vascular damage does not exclude its existence. Electron microscopic studies on this subject have not been published to my knowledge.

There are no characteristic uremic changes of the spleen. One sometimes sees hemosiderosis as the consequence of hemolysis and, in patients with malignant hypertension, necrotic areas due to arteriolonecrosis. There are no specific changes in the lymph nodes.

Some clinicians think that a hepatic disturbance contributes to the mechanism of the uremic coma. There are no known specific liver changes in uremia. The liver often contains a brown pigment which may be derived from hemolyzed red blood cells. Investigations of the last years demonstrated that this brown pigment occurs nearly exclusively in cases of chronic pyelonephritis or chronic interstitial nephritis observed after prolonged and heavy abuse of phenacetin. Experimentally, this type of pigmentation of the liver has been reproduced, and the pigment was identified as a lipofuscin (STUDER et al. [21]).

An analogous pigmentation of the skin also occurs after chronic abuse of phenacetin. It is believed that the skin and the liver pigments are identical. A frequent skin change is an atrophy of the epidermal layer, which is called "uremide" by clinicians and is presumably due to the accumulation of nitrogenous metabolites.

There are no known renal changes secondary to uremia. — Renal osteopathy and hypertrophy of the parathyroids are not true uremic changes, since they are also observed in partial renal failure with normal NPN values.

While the morphological appearance of uremia appears simple at first sight, a detailed analysis of the changes in different tissues results in a fairly complicated picture. While the sum of these lesions is highly characteristic for uremia, the single lesions are non-specific. Like a painting, which results from the quantitative and topographic distribution of simple basic colors, the characteristic disease entity observed in the human body is the sum of a specific distribution of non-specific changes. A better understanding of the picture of uremia and its pathogenetic mechanisms will probably be reached in the near future, since each of the different functional disturbances which occur in uremia may be eliminated by therapeutic measures, as e.g. hemodialysis, antihypertensive drugs, control of the concentration of electrolytes in body fluids, etc.

References

1. ALLEN, A. C.: The kidney, Ist ed. New York: Grune & Stratton 1951.
2. ANDRY, E.: Besondere Formen von Knochenmarkschädigung bei Urämie. Inaug.-Diss. 1951.
3. BAGGENSTOSS, A. H.: The pancreas in uremia: a histopathologic study. Amer. J. Path. **24**, 1003—1112 (1948).
4. BEAUDRY, C., S. NAKAMOTO, and W. J. KOLFF: Uremia pericarditis and cardiac tamponade in chronic renal failure. Ann. intern. Med. **64**, 990—995 (1956).
5. BODECHTEL, G., u. F. ERBSLOH: Die Veränderungen des Zentralnervensystems bei Nierenkrankheiten. In: HENKE-LUBARSCH, Handbuch der speziellen Pathologie, Bd. 13/II, S. 1392—1427. Berlin-Göttingen-Heidelberg: Springer 1958.
6. BULL, G. M.: The uremias. Lancet **1955 I**, 777—779.
7. BYROM, F. B.: The pathogenesis of the hypertensive encephalopathy and its relation to the malignant phase of hypertension. Lancet **1954 II**, 201—204.
8. CASTALI, P.: The bleeding disorder of uremia. A qualitative platelet defect. Lancet **1966 II**, 66—68.
9. FLECKENSTEIN, A.: Stoffwechselprobleme bei der Myocardinsuffizienz. 51. Verh. Dtsch. Ges. Path. 1967, 15—29.
10. HAMBURGER, J., G. RICHET, J. GROSNIER et J.-L. FUNCK-BRENTANO: L'insuffisance rénale. In: C. E. ALKEN et al., Handbuch der Urologie, Bd. IV. Berlin-Göttingen-Heidelberg: Springer 1962.
11. HEINTZ, R.: Nierenfiebel. Stuttgart: Georg Thieme 1964.
12. HOPPS, H. C., and R. W. WISSLER: Uremic pneumonitis. Amer. J. Path. **31**, 261—273 (1955).
13. KÖHLER, M.: Zur Bedeutung des Reststickstoff- und Harnstoffgehaltes im Herzmuskel für die Urämiediagnostik an der Leiche. Frankfurt. Z. Path. **74**, 465—473 (1965).

14. Kroe, D. J., and J. J. Vazquez: Hypersensitivity reactions in experimental uremia. Amer. J. Path. **50**, 401—419 (1967).
15. MacLeod, M., A. L. Stalker, and D. Ogston: Fibrinolytic activity of lung tissue in renal failure. Lancet **1962 I**, 191—193.
16. Meister, H.: Über Mineralanalysen an Leichenherzen bei Urämie. Virchows Arch. Path. Anat. **338**, 16—20 (1964).
17. Riva, G.: Die Diagnose der Urämie an der Leiche. Helv. med. Acta **10**, Suppl. XII (1943).
18. Schneiter, R.: Pneumonies urémiques aiguë et chronique. Ann. anat. Path. **6**, 59—98 (1961).
19. Seldin, D. W., N. W. Carter, and F. C. Rector: Consequences of renal failure and their management. In: M. B. Strauss and L. G. Welt, Diseases of the kidney, p. 173—217. Boston: Little, Brown & Comp. 1963.
20. Shaw, A. B., and M. C. Scholes: Reticulocytosis in renal failure. Lancet **1967 I**, 799—802.
21. Studer, A., u. K. Schärer: Langfristige Phenacetinbelastung am Hund mit Berücksichtigung der Leber- und Nierenpigmentierung. Schweiz. med. Wschr. **95**, 933—941 (1965).
22. Wegelin, C.: Zur mikroskopischen Diagnose der Urämie. Schweiz. med. Wschr. **71**, 1517—1522 (1941).
23. Zollinger, H. U.: Die Dysorosen. Schweiz. med. Wschr. **75**. 777—779 (1945).
24. — Niere und ableitende Harnorgane. In: W. Doerr u. E. Uehlinger, Lehrbuch der speziellen pathologischen Anatomie, Bd. III. Berlin-Heidelberg-New York: Springer 1966.
25. —, u. R. Hegglin: Die idiopathische Lungenhämosiderose als pulmonale Form der Purpura Schönlein-Henoch. Schweiz. med. Wschr. **88**, 439—442 (1958).

Discussion

Rotter:

At what level of liver-pigmentation, may a pathologist recognize previous abuse of phenacetin?

Pinggera:

Did you ever find calcium-oxalate deposits in tissues other than the kidney of patients with chronic uremia?

Cottier:

Does the proliferation of endothelial cells in small arteries, which you observe in uremic patients, ressemble the one seen by Imhof et al. (Essential Hypertension. Internat. Symposium, ed. K. D. Bock, and P. Cottier, p. 381, Berlin-Göttingen-Heidelberg: Springer 1960) in the kidneys of patients with malignant hypertension successfully treated with hypotensive drugs over a long period of time?

Scheitlin:

Severe hypercalcemia up to 15 mg per 100 ml was observed, in our department, in a patient with chronic glomerulonephritis after successful renal transplantation. The parathyroids were surgically explored and a large adenoma was removed. Since that time the blood calcium values of the patient are normal. The hyperparathyroidism, in this case, could be due to subsequent autonomy after an initial stage of secondary hyperparathyroidism in uremia.

1.5.5. Functional Patterns in Chronic Renal Failure*

A. HEIDLAND, K. KLÜTSCH, T. TAKUMA and E. SCHEITZA[1]

With 2 Figures

In 22 patients undergoing chronic dialysis, the renal excretory capacity was studied by determination of inulin-, PAH-, urea-, sodium-, and potassium-clearances (C_{In}, C_{PAH}, C_{Urea}, C_{Na}, C_K) as well as fractional excretion of water, sodium and potassium $\left(\frac{V}{GFR} \times 100, \frac{C_{Na}}{C_{In}} \times 100, \frac{C_K}{C_{In}} \times 100\right)$. The following results were obtained:

C_{In} (ml/min)	C_{PAH} (ml/min)	"F.F." (%)	C_{Urea} (ml/min)	$\frac{C_{Urea}}{C_{In}}$	Diuresis (ml/min)
m 3.32	7.88	51.0	3.40	0.99	1.30
σ 1.26	4.81	18.8	1.27	0.20	0.54
ε 0.17	0.67	2.6	0.21	0.03	0.07

Inulin $\frac{U}{P}$	$\frac{V}{GFR} \times 100$ (%)	C_{Na} (ml/min)	$\frac{C_{Na}}{C_{In}} \times 100$ (%)	C_K (ml/min)	$\frac{C_K}{C_{In}} \times 100$ (%)
m 2.86	40.5	0.85	26,9	5.33	170.1
σ 1.20	13.5	0.39	12.0	2.75	78.1
ε 0.16	1.8	0.05	1.6	0.37	10.6

Fractional elimination of water increased up to 74%, of sodium up to 64% and that of potassium up to 375%. There was an inverse relationship between $\frac{V}{GFR} \times 100$ and C_{In} (r = —0.299) and a positive correlation with plasma potassium (r = —0.499), but not with plasma urea concentration.

An exponential function could be observed between inulin U/P ratio and fractional water and sodium elimination (Fig. 1).

Decreased reabsorption of fluid results partially from osmotic diuresis [1, 2], which is induced by a combination of glomerular hypertrophy [18] and increased plasma concentrations of urea and some anions and cations. The relationship between hyperpotassemia and fractional diuresis, also observed by SIEBERTH, may be due to the above mentioned phenomena. In patients with an increased extracellular fluid volume the hypothetical natriuretic hormone [6, 7, 11, 14, 15], and an altered geometry of proximal convoluted tubule [4, 19] has to be discussed.

* Mit Unterstützung der Deutschen Forschungsgemeinschaft.

[1] Medizinische Universitätsklinik Würzburg, West Germany.

Finally, one must also consider the diuretic effect of parathormone [8] in patients with secondary hyperparathyroidism.

Maximal potassium secretion could be due to increased sodium — potassium exchange in the distal tubule [5], an elevated potassium concentration in peritubular capillaries [16] and a hyperaldosteronism, induced by hyperkalemia [13].

As in acute renal failure produced experimentally by aristolochic acid intoxication [17], in our patients the urea clearance increased to the level of inulin clearance. The $\frac{C_{Urea}}{C_{In}}$ ratio was 0.99 ± 0.20 with highest values in patients with an inulin U/P ratio below two. An increased $\frac{C_{Urea}}{C_{In}}$ ratio above one in patients with acute renal failure has been observed by others [20, 23].

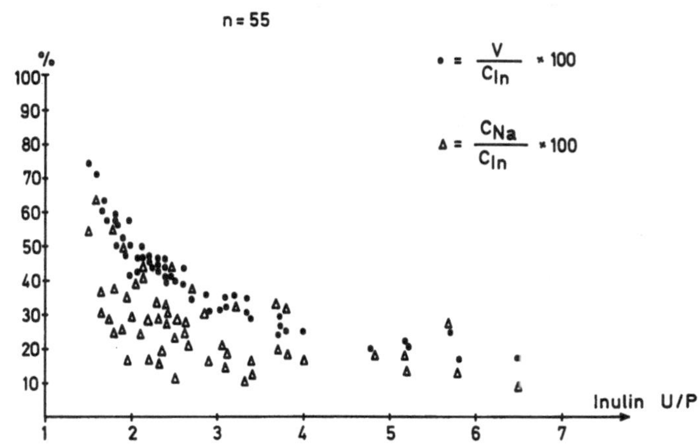

Fig. 1. Relationship between inulin U/P ratio and fractional elimination of water and sodium $\left(\frac{V}{C_{In}} \times 100, \frac{C_{Na}}{C_{In}} \times 100\right)$ in 55 studies on 22 patients with chronic renal failure

In order to study whether an additional inhibition of fluid reabsorption might reveal a masked secretion of urea, 10 patients received 1 g furosemide i.v. In spite of an increase of urine flow from 1.43 to 3.50 ml/min ($p < 0.0005$) with a decrease of the inulin U/P ratio from 2.64 to 1.54 ($p < 0.01$), the increase of C_{Urea} from 3.34 to 4.83 ml/min ($p < 0.05$) was similar to that of C_{In} from 3.36 to 5.17 ml/min ($p < 0.025$).

In the frog, administration of arginine results in an remarkable increase of renal urea production [21]. We, however, found no change in $\frac{C_{Urea}}{C_{In}}$ ratio in 3 uremic patients who were given 120 mmol arginine. According to in vitro studies of Brodsky and Huang [3] the mammalian kidney should be able to synthesize urea.

Relationship between uremic intoxication and renal function.

Seldin [22], Hoeffler, Wigger and Scheeler [10] discussed the possibility that the end stage of renal failure might be impaired additionally by the retention of uremic metabolic products. In order to gain information on this point, renal function

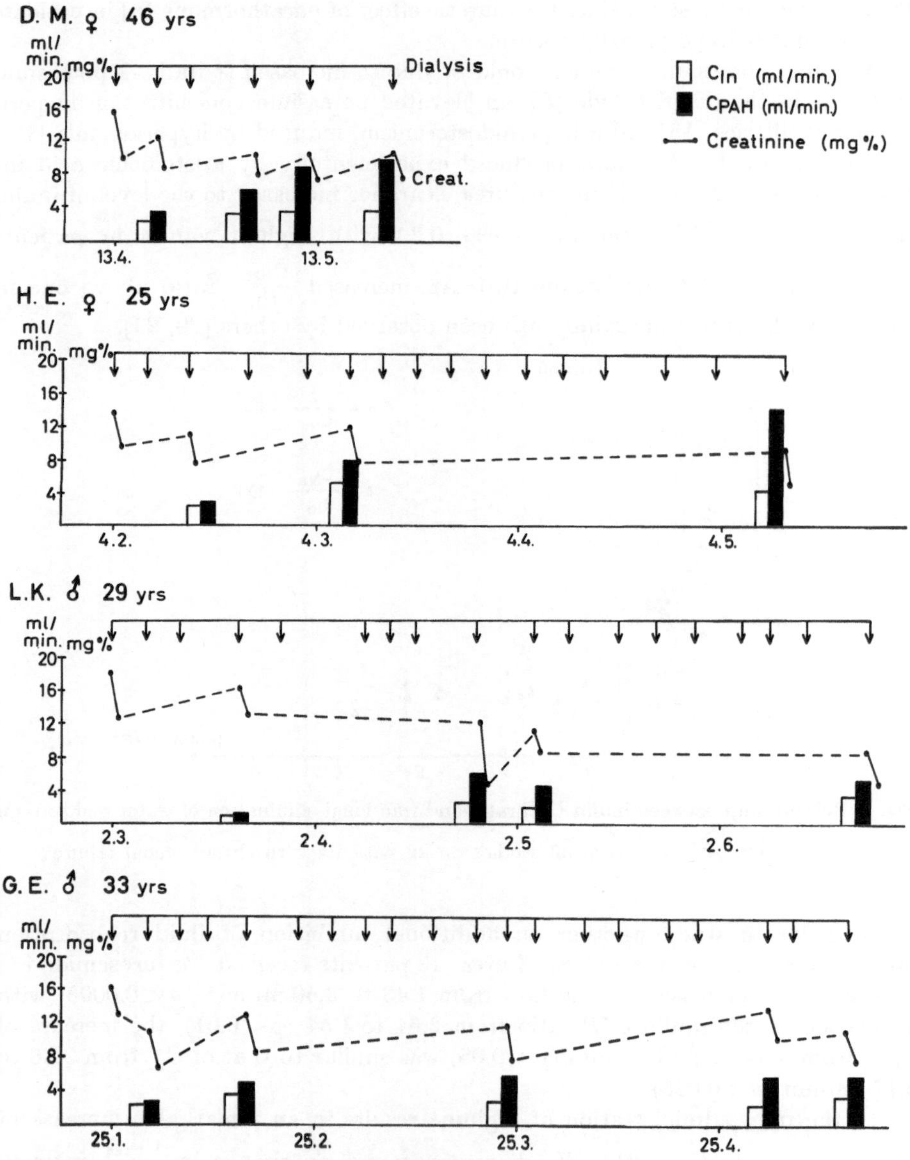

Fig. 2. Plasma creatinine, inulin- and PAH-clearances in 4 patients with stable chronic glomerulonephritis during prolonged dialytic therapy. All patients demonstrated an improvement of kidney functions. The first patient has not needed any dialysis for 4 months

was studied in 10 patients with stable chronic glomerulonephritis during uremic intoxication and after prolonged therapy by dialysis. In 4 patients, initial urea and creatinine concentrations were 249 ± 35 mg-% and 14.3 ± 2.8 mg-% respectively. They did not show any signs of heart failure, pericarditis or bacterial infection. Dialysis-induced loss of uremic symptoms was associated with some improvement in renal function. There was an increase of C_{In} from 2.0 ± 0.28 to 3.57 ± 0.4 ml/min, of C_{PAH} from 2.5 ± 0.30 to 9.08 ± 4.38 ml/min and of urine-flow from 0.65 ± 0.21 to 1.56 ± 0.40 ml/min fall. The plasma urea and creatinine concentration fell to 176 ± 87 mg-% and 8.1 ± 3.3 mg-%, respectively (Fig. 2).

The other 6 patients demonstrated stability or progressive deterioration of residual function, due to underlying disease.

The functional study reveals that uremic intoxication may impair the function of residual nephrons. The findings are in agreement with in vitro studies of HEINTZ and RENNER [9], who observed a diminished PAH uptake of kidney slices in the presence of uremic plasma.

Summary

In 22 patients from a chronic dialysis program, with an inulin clearance of 3.3 ml/min, the fractional elimination of water averaged 40.5% (maximal 74%), of sodium 26.9% (maximal 64%) and that of potassium 170% (maximal 375%). The urea clearance was equal to glomerular filtration rate. The administration of diuretics or arginine did not alter the $\frac{C_{Urea}}{C_{In}}$ ratio.

4 uremic patients with stable chronic glomerulonephritis, without any signs of immunologic activity, infection or heart failure, demonstrated after prolonged dialysis, with loss of uremic symptoms, a progressive increase in urine flow, inulin- and PAH-clearances. These findings may have been due to the elimination of toxic substances during dialysis.

References

1. BRICKER, N. S., J. DORHOUT MEES, S. KLAHR, B. ORLOWSKI, R. E. RIESELBACH, and L. E. TODD: The rate limiting and adaptive events in the tubular and glomerular functions of the chronically diseased kidney. Proc. II. Intern. Congr. Nephrology, pg. 39—47. Excerpta Medica Foundation 1964.
2. — S. KLAHR, and R. E. RIESELBACH: The functional adaptation of the diseased kidney. J. clin. Invest. **43**, 1915—1921 (1964).
3. BRODSKY, W. A., and K. C. HUANG: Biosynthesis of urea in kidney tissue without exogenous substrate. J. clin. Invest. **40**, 1026 (1961).
4. BRUNNER, F. P., F. C. RECTOR, and D. W. SELDIN: Mechanism of glomerulotubular balance. J. clin. Invest. **45**, 590—610 (1966).
5. DAVIDSON, D. G., N. G. LEVINSKY, and R. W. BERLINER: Maintenance of potassium excretion despite reduction of glomerular filtration during sodium diuresis. J. clin. Invest. **37**, 548—555 (1958).
6. DE WARDENER, H. E., I. H. MILLS, W. F. CHAPMAN, and C. J. HAYL: Studies on the efferent mechanism of sodium diuresis which follows the administration of intravenous saline in the dog. Clin. Sci. **21**, 249—258 (1961).
7. DIRKS, J. H., W. J. CIRKSENA, and R. W. BERLINER: The effect of saline infusion on sodium reabsorption by the proximal tubule of the dog. J. clin. Invest. **44**, 1160—1170 (1965).
8. GEKLE, G., D. ROSTOCK u. G. KURTH: Mikropunktionsuntersuchungen über den Einfluß von Parathormon auf die Flüssigkeitsresorption im proximalen Konvolut der Rattenniere. V. Symp. d. Ges. f. Nephrologie, Lausanne 1967.
9. HEINTZ, R., u. D. RENNER: In: Aktuelle Probleme der klinischen Nephrologie. Zellstoffwechselstörungen bei Urämie, hrsg. von MERTZ u. KLUTHE. Stuttgart: Georg Thieme 1967.

10. Höffler, D., W. Wigger u. F. Scheler: Befristete Hämodialyse bei chronischen Nierenerkrankungen. In: Melsunger Med. Pharmaz. Mitt. 1965.
11. Johnston, C. L., and J. O. Davis: Evidence from cross circulation studies for a humoral mechanism in the natriuresis of saline loading. Proc. Soc. exp. Biol. (N.Y.) **121**, 1058—1063 (1966).
12. Kleeman, C. R., R. Okun, and R. J. Heller: The renal regulation of sodium and potassium in patients with chronic renal failure and the effect of diuretics on the excretion of these ions. Proc. N.Y. Acad. Sci. 1966.
13. Laragh, J. H., and H. C. Stoerk: A study of the mechanism of secretion of the sodium retaining hormone (aldosterone). J. clin. Invest. **36**, 383—392 (1957).
14. Levinsky, N. G.: Non-aldosterone influences on renal sodium transport. Proc. N.Y. Acad. Sci. 1966.
15. Lichardus, B., and J. W. Pearce: Evidence for a humoral natriuretic factor released by blood volume expansion. Nature (Lond.) **209**, 407—409 (1966).
16. Orloff, J., and D. G. Davidson: The mechanism of potassium excretion in the chicken. J. clin. Invest. **38**, 21—31 (1959).
17. Peters, G., and P. R. Hedwall: Aristolochic acid intoxication. A new type of impairment of urinary concentrating ability. Arch. int. Pharmacodyn. **145**, **334—355** (1963).
18. Platt, R.: Structural and functional adaptations in renal failure. Brit. med. J. **1952** I, 1372.
19. Rector, C. F., J. C. Sellman, M. Martinez-Maldonado, and D. W. Seldin: The mechanism of suppression of proximal tubular reabsorption by saline infusions. J. clin. Invest. **46**, 47—56 (1967).
20. Schirmeister, J., H. Willmann u. H. W. Lotzen: In: Aktuelle Probleme der klinischen Nephrologie, hrsg. von Mertz u. Kluthe, S. 67. Stuttgart: Georg Thieme 1967.
21. Schmidt-Nielsen, B., and C. R. Shrauger: Handling of urea and related compounds by the renal tubules of the frog. Amer. J. Physiol. **205**, 483—488 (1963).
22. Seldin, D. W., N. W. Carter, and F. C. Rector: Consequences of renal failure and their management. Diseases of the kidney, ed. by M. B. Strauss and L. G. Welt. Boston: Little Brown & Co. 1963.
23. Wetzels, E., u. W. Herms: Untersuchungen über die tubuläre Funktion in Bezug auf Electrolyte und Harnstoff beim akuten Nierenversagen. In: Normale und pathologische Funktionen des Nierentubulus, hrsg. von Ullrich und Hierholzer, S. 361—365. Bern: Huber 1965.

Discussion

Sarre:

Could you please state the plasma urea and creatinine concentrations at the beginning and at the end of the treatment period in your four cases?

Wiederholt:

Could the fall of C_{Inulin} below the value of C_{urea} mean that the tubular walls become permeable to inulin?

Gessler:

Were some of your observations made in cases of pyelonephritis? We observed an improvement in renal functions and an increase in urine flow, which sometimes even allowed us to discontinue regular hemodialysis in some patients with pyelonephritis, but never in patients with glomerulonephritis.

Brunner:

How did the blood pressure evolve in the four patients in whom C_{In} and C_{PAH} improved after intermittent hemodialysis?

HEIDLAND to SARRE: During the first clearance studies the average plasma concentration of urea was 249 mg-% and of creatinine 14.3 mg-%. At the end of treatment there was a decrease to 176 mg-%, and 8.1 mg-% respectively. Much more impressive than the blood chemistry was the clinical improvement of all patients. To WIEDERHOLT: Considering the molecular weights it appears difficult to imagine that the back-diffusion of inulin could be greater than that of urea. One might conceive an incomplete filtration of inulin due to pathological changes in glomerular membranes, as discussed by SCHIRMEISTER. To GESSLER: We studied only patients with stable chronic glomerulonephritis and intentionally excluded cases with pyelonephritis, since these patients might show improvement as a consequence of antibiotic therapy. To BRUNNER: There was no significant change in arterial blood pressure during the period of observation. The mean values were 157/85 mm Hg, and 150/90 mm Hg respectively.

1.5.6. Immunologic Findings in Chronic Glomerulonephritis *

H. E. SCHÄFER and ANNELORE SCHÄFER [1]

With 3 Figures

Currently the immunopathogenesis of acute glomerulonephritis with its varied course is generally accepted. Numerous experimental and clinical investigations support immunologic mechanisms. Nevertheless many questions in regard to the immunopathogenesis are still unanswered. We do not know the specific

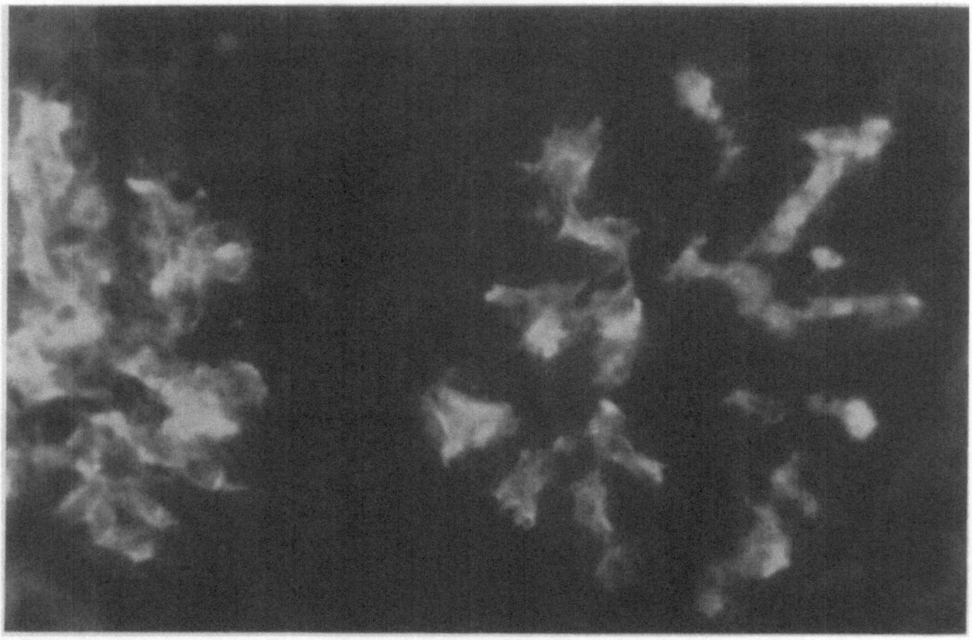

Fig. 1. Renal biopsy: chronic glomerulonephritis. Glomeruli stained with fluorescein-conjugated anti-human-gamma-globulin. Typical fluorescence localized in the mesangium and the axial regions of the glomeruli. A similar picture is obtained by staining the tissue with fluorescein-conjugated anti-human-complement and its fractions. (Cryostat section 3 μ, orig. magn. $\times$ 250)

initiating antigen and we cannot classify the corresponding antibody. Furthermore, the mode of localization of the antigen-antibody-complement complex on the glomerular basement membrane is unknown. This, in addition, puts emphasis on the divergent results with reference to the presence of streptococcal M-protein in the glomeruli [13, 14, 8, 5, 6].

* Supported by Deutsche Forschungsgemeinschaft.

[1] Medizinische Universitätsklinik Würzburg, West Germany.

The purpose of the present investigation was to study the localization and the persistence of fixed immune-complexes in chronic glomerulonephritis. Kidney tissue obtained by biopsy or antopsy from 96 patients, in different stages of the disease, was examined. Furthermore the immune deposits were examined after immunosuppressive therapy (ACTH, cortisone, cytostatic drugs) and chronic intermittent hemodialysis.

The immune complexes in the glomeruli, in acute post-streptococcal glomerulonephritis, appeared as granular continuous fluorescent lines of variable intensity

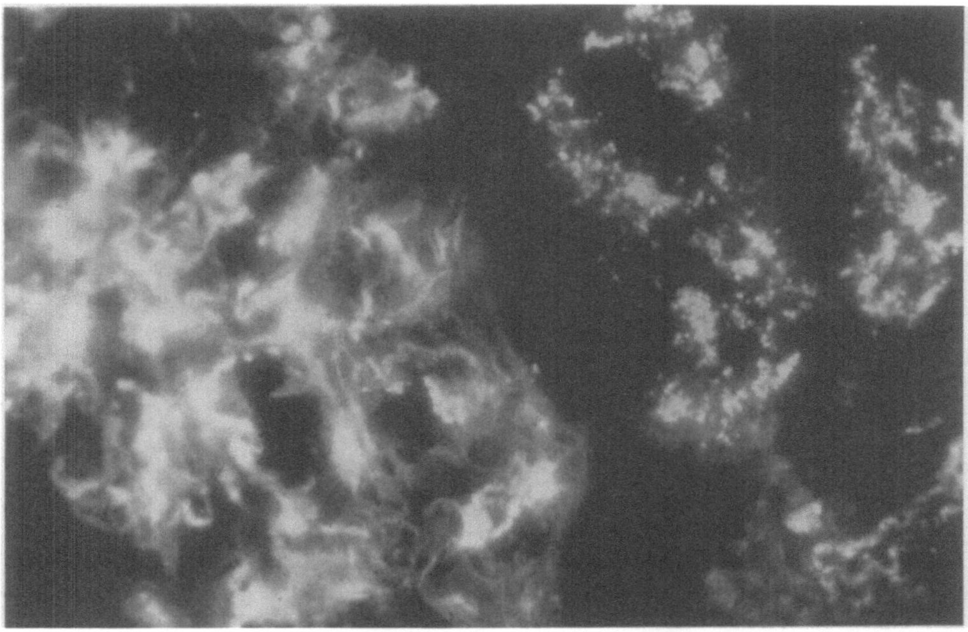

Fig. 2. Renal biopsy: chronic hypocomplementemic glomerulonephritis with nephrotic syndrome. Visualization of the fixed immune-complexes by fluorescein-conjugated anti-human-complement. Deposits in the basement membrane, mesangium, and the proximal tubules. Same reactions by staining with anti-beta$_{1C}$-globulin and anti-human globulin. (Cryostat section 3 μ, orig. magn. × 250)

on the glomerular basement-membrane. We demonstrated the presence of these immune-complexes either by electron microscopy or by means of fluorescein-conjugated anti-human gamma globulin. The gamma globulin represents an immune globulin because various complement fractions are found in the same region [4, 1, 12, 5, 6, 11, 3, 15, 9]. After clinical recovery (normalization of blood pressure, normal urinanalysis as well as clearance values), renal biopsies demonstrated the disappearance of the previously detectable immune-complexes. Lange et al. [5, 6] had already referred to these immunologic findings.

In other cases these immune complexes persisted. At present the causes of the persistence are unknown. In such cases, the immune-complexes were always found in morphologically damaged glomeruli. Rotter [10] and Lapp [7] recently re-classified the stages of the disease from a pathohistological and electron-microscopic viewpoint. According to our immunological studies the course of progression of glomerulonephritis seemed to be correlated to the localization and expansion of these immune complexes. The degree of expansion ranged from minute focal markings in the glomerular tufts, to wide irregular extensions of the entire capillary wall. Cases with clinically progressive disease showed immune deposits in the axial region of the glomeruli and demonstrable throughout the mesangium. The latter localization is considered to be typical for the chronically progressive course of the disease [5]. Fig. 1 shows this localization of immuno-

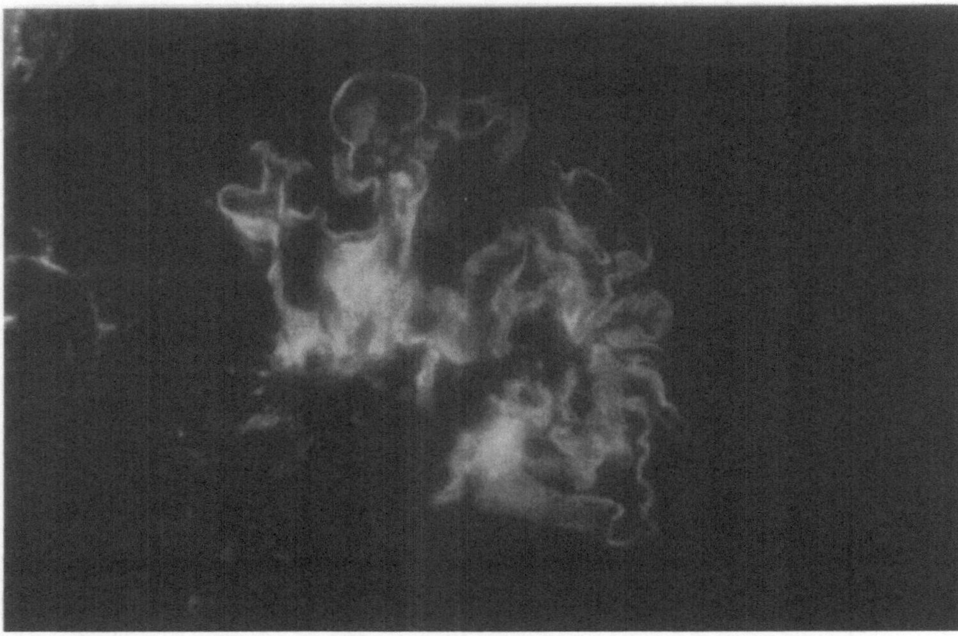

Fig. 3. Autopsy-tissue: chronic progressive glomerulonephritis, 14 weeks after the beginning of immunosuppression. No change of the immune deposits by staining with fluorescein-conjugated anti human gamma globulin. Same findings by staining for complement. Pathohistologically: progressive glomerulonephritis. (Cryostat section 3 μ, orig. magn. × 250)

globulins. In the same regions complement may be demonstrated. The glomerular immune-reactions sometimes were so extensive, that immune-complexes penetrated the glomerular basement membrane and were reabsorbed in the tubules (Fig. 2). In these cases complement depletion was always found in the serum [12]. Following WEST et al. [16] we call this form "hypocomplementemic chronic glomerulonephritis" in contrast to the more frequent normocomplementemic form.

The localization and persistence of the immune complexes of chronic glomerulonephritis leads to the problem of possible influences of cortisone and cytostatic drugs. In no patient with glomerulonephritis associated with the nephrotic syndrome [2], who received ACTH or prednisone could we detect an elimination or dissolution of the immune complexes. The duration of therapy had no influence. The antigen-antibody-complement complexes in these patients were quite similar to those usually observed in patients with chronic glomerulonephritis. It is, however, difficult to determine gradual differences in intensity of fluoresence. Fig. 3 shows the persistence of the immune-reactions 14 weeks after the beginning of therapy.

High blood urea concentrations observed in spite of prolonged extracorporeal hemodialysis in oligo-anuric patients did not influence the immune complexes of the glomeruli. In addition to hyalinization of the glomeruli, typical immune complexes always appeared in partially functional nephrons. Particularily the mesangium was always affected. Furthermore, in this stage continued expansion in site of the immune-reaction is still possible. In 4 out of 6 cases of this type, additional immune complexes were localized in the arterioles and smaller arteries. The stage of malignant hypertension in chronic glomerulonephritis was always initiated by this extension of the immune-reaction [12].

Summary

In chronic glomerulonephritis the primary glomerular immunoreaction persists to a variable extent. Its persistence in the axial regions of the glomeruli (proliferated mesangium) is typical. Immunecomplexes in the tubules primarily originate from glomerular depositions, which are found particularily in hypocomplementemic chronic glomerulonephritis with the nephrotic syndrome. In chronic progressive glomerulonephritis the immune-complexes are neither eliminated nor influenced by ACTH, cortisone, immunosuppressive therapy or chronic intermittent hemodialysis.

References

1. Dixon, E. J.: The pathogenesis of immunologically induced nephritis. Proc. III. Congr. Nephrol. Washington 1966, vol. II, p. 97. Basel: Karger 1967.
2. Ellis, A.: Natural history of Bright's disease. Lancet **1942 I**, 34—72.
3. Heymann, W.: Experimental analogues of human nephropathy. Proc. III. Congr. Nephrol., Washington 1966, vol. II, p. 164. Basel: Karger 1967.
4. Klein, P., u. P. M. Burkholer: Ein Verfahren zur fluoreszenzoptischen Darstellung der Komplementbindung und seine Anwendung zur histoimmunologischen Untersuchung der experimentellen Nierenanaphylaxie. Dtsch. med. Wschr. **84**, 2001 (1961)
5. Lange, K., G. Treser, J. Sagel, A. Ty, and E. Wasserman: Routine immunohistology in renal diseases. Ann. intern. Med. **64**, 25 (1966).
6. — — A. Ty, and E. Wasserman: The histologic and immunologic features of acute, subacute and chronic glomerulonephritis. Trans. Amer. Ass. Phycns **128**, 117 (1965).
7. Lapp, H.: Elektronenmikroskopische Befunde bei Glomerulonephritis. Verh. dtsch. Ges. Path. **49**, 80 (1965).
8. Miller, F.: Renal localization and persistence of type 12 streptococcal M-protein. Proc. Soc. exp. Biol. (N.Y.) **108**, 539 (1961).
9. Pfeiffer, E. F., and K. Federlin: Experimental chronic glomerulonephritis. Proc. III. Congr. Nephrol., Washington 1966, vol. II, p. 113. Basel: Karger 1967.
10. Rotter, W.: Pathologische Anatomie der Glomerulonephritis. Verh. dtsch. Ges. Path. **49**, 67 (1965).
11. Schäfer, H. E.: Untersuchungen über die Bedeutung des Serumkomplementes bei experimenteller und humaner Glomerulonephritis. Z. klin. Med. **158**, 221 (1964).
12. —, u. A. Schäfer: Aspekte zur Immunpathogenese der malignen Hypertonie. Med. Welt **1965**, 1144.

13. Seegal, B. C., K. C. Hsu, E. Fiaschi e G. Andres: La tecnica degli anticorpi fluorescenti applicata allo studio della patogenesi della nefrite umana. Rass. Fisiopat. clin. ter. **31**, 1 (1959).
14. — G. A. Andres, K. C. Hsu, and J. B. Zabriskie: Studies on the pathogenesis of acute and progressive glomerulonephritis in man by immunofluorescein and immunoferritin techniques. Fed. Proc. **24**, 100 (1965).
15. Thoenes, W.: Feinstrukturen des normalen und des funktionsgestörten Nephron. Verh. dtsch. Ges. Path. **49**, 14 (1965).
16. West, C. D., A. J. McAdams, J. M. McConville, N. C. Davis, and N. H. Holland: Hypocomplementemic and normocomplementemic persistent (chronic) glomerulonephritis, clinical and pathologic characteristics. J. Pediat. **67**, 1089 (1965).

Discussion

Sarre:

Did you also demonstrate the presence of streptococcal antigens in the glomeruli? Such antigens have been demonstrated by Miss Seegal (B. C. Seegal, G. Andress, K. Msu, J. Zabriskie: Fed. Proc. **24**, 100 (1965)]. Precipitation of gamma globulin and complement in the glomerulus is sometimes assumed to be a non-specific effect which may also occur with other types of inflammation. Were such precipitates found in aminonucleoside nephrosis, which is a toxic type of experimental nephropathy?

Pinggera:

What were the doses of the immuno-suppressive drugs? Did the patients improve clinically under immunosuppressive treatment?

Bohle:

Did you observe deposits in cases of acute or chronic membranous glomerulonephritis? Were they located within the glomerulus?

I know of at least one case of chronic proliferative glomerulonephritis which progressed under immunosuppressive treatment.

Schäfer to Sarre: The humoral action of the streptococcal M-protein is an important factor in the pathogenesis of early glomerulonephritis. The demonstration of the presence of these M-proteins in the glomouli particularly by fluorescent microscopy is difficult. These streptococcal proteins may not be responsible for the progression of the disease.

The insudation of gamma-globulin and other protein-fractions must be excluded, before one is entitled to speak about specific fluorescence. Our methods have previously been described in detail (Z. klin. Med. **158**, 221, 1964). They consist of "negative stainings" with non-specific fluorescein-conjugated proteins, examination at different pH values and at different urea concentrations. Therefore, the fluorescence seen may be considered as specific. We have not carried out immunological studies in aminonucleoside nephrosis.

To Pinggera: During the Imuran (1—200 mg/die) and additional prednisone therapy the white cell count ranged from 2—4,000/mm^3. The gamma globulin determined by electrophoresis was suppressed to 60% of its initial value. Penicillin was also given. Under immunosuppressive therapy we did not see any recovery nor tendency toward improvement of chronic glomerulonephritis.

I might also stress again the importance of the extension of the immune-complexes to the arterioles and smaller arteries, which produces malignant hypertension (SCHÄFER et al.: Med. Welt 1965, p. 1144).

To BOHLE: Immune deposits in the basement membrane of the glomeruli are demonstrable, by fluorescence microscopy, in acute and chronic membranous glomerulonephritis. Furthermore, electron microscopic studies show, that they are mostly localized subepithelially. The persistence of the immune complexes and the pathohistological progression of the chronic glomerulonephritis during therapeutic immunosuppression demonstrated by Dr. BOHLE leaves in doubt the local effect of such treatments in chronic glomerulonephritis. The issue probably depends on the onset of treatment.

1.5.7. The Retention of Urea, Uric Acid and Creatinine in Renal Failure and their Relations to Protein Changes in Blood and Cerebrospinal Fluid. Quantitative Immunochemical Findings

A. GOTTESLEBEN, A. PRILL, E. QUELLHORST, E. VOLLES and F. SCHELER [1]

With 4 Figures

Neurological complications in kidney diseases were mentioned already in 1839 by ADDISON and in 1873 by CHARCOT. But only recently, after the introduction of dialysis and the consequent longer survival of patients, have the often severe central and peripheral involvement of the nervous system been seen more frequently [2, 10, 12, 13, 15, 17].

We were interested in the following problem; how does the retention of nitrogen o ntaining metabolic end products in the blood affect their level in the CSF?

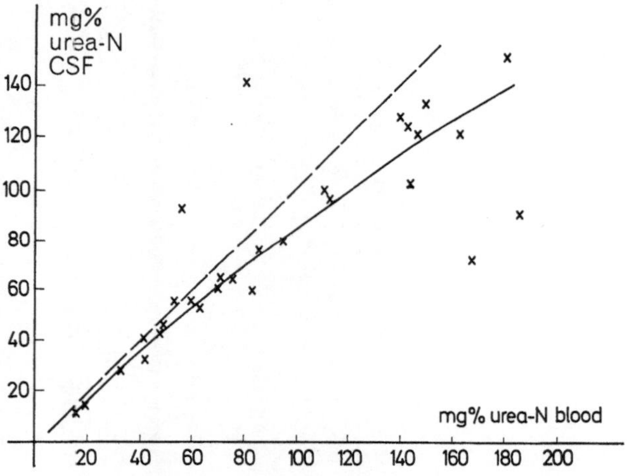

Fig. 1. The relation of urea nitrogen in serum and CSF in patients with renal failure.

Continuing our previous investigations [14] we investigated the question of whether the level of urea, creatinine etc. may be related to disturbances in central nervous function.

Blood and CSF (lumbar puncture) were obtained simultaneously. Both fluids were analyzed for urea, creatinine and, in several cases, uric acid. — Fig. 1 shows a comparison of *urea nitrogen* values. In blood we observed urea nitrogen levels between 15 and 185 mg-%, in CSF between 11 and 150 mg-%. We found that the value of CSF urea nitrogen was about 85% that of the serum. The only exceptions were 2 patients, in whom the examinations were done immediately

[1] Neurologische und Medizinische Universitätskliniken, Göttingen.

after dialysis. Our findings agree with studies in animals [5, 6, 7, 9]. — Fig. 2 represents the results of *creatinine* determinations. The ratio of creatinine in CSF to creatinine in serum at slightly elevated serum levels varied from 0.5 to 0.8, but at higher blood levels fell to about 0.3. Similar results were obtained to animal experiments [7]. — Tests for *uric acid* were performed only in a few cases, so that definite conclusions cannot be made. The value for uric acid in CSF did not appear to depend on the serum level and varied between 2 and 5 mg-%.

The changes of urea nitrogen and creatinine levels were not usually correlated to the severity of neurological symptoms. Therefore, we carried out quanti-

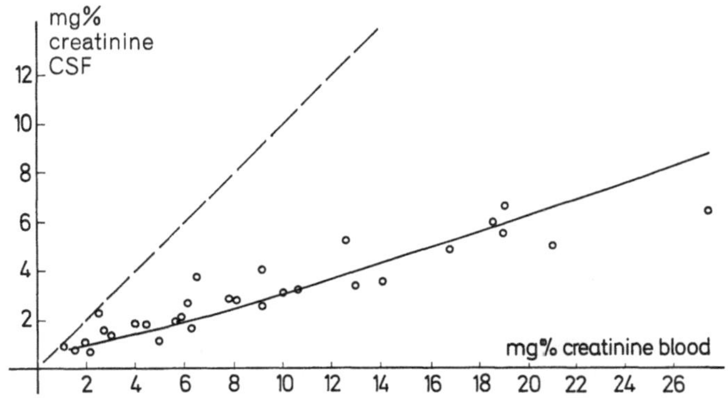

Fig. 2. The relation of creatinine in serum and CSF in patients with renal failure.

tative tests for some protein fractions in serum and CSF. We used the method of quantitative immunodiffusion [11, 16] which we adjusted for CSF [8].

We measured IgG-, IgA-, Igm-globulin, haptoglobin, alpha-1-glycoprotein and alpha-2-macroglobulin. In the serum the average value was 1,147 mg-%, which is slightly lower than the average in the serum of healthy men, but still within the "normal" range between 800 and 1,800 mg-%. Values for IgA (226 mg-%), Igm (140 mg-%) and alpha-2-macroglobulin (253 mg-%) did not differ from mean values of normal serum. In contrast, haptoglobin with 316 mg-% (normal range between 10 and 220 mg-%) and alpha-1-glycoprotein with 227 mg-% were significantly increased.

The findings in CSF were different. The mean value of IgG was 2.72 mg-%, which is slightly higher than the normal range with our method. IgA (0,34 mg-%) and haptoglobin (0.48 mg-%) were found in the normal range. Igm, which does not occur in CSF of healthy persons, was found in 9 patients. There were striking increases of occur in alpha-1-glycoprotein to a mean concentration of 1.17 mg-%, while the normal range is from 0 to 0.747 mg-%. In Fig. 3 alpha-1-glycoprotein, which shows the most pronounced pathological changes in CSF, is related to the values of blood urea nitrogen.

As stated above, there was only a very loose correlation between the changes in CSF urea-N or creatinine and the neurological symptoms. In order to find out whether there was a relation between the protein changes in the CSF and the severity of neurological symptoms, we divided the patients into 5 groups of different and progressive severity. Criteria of classification were: 1. the findings of the neurological examination; 2. findings in the EEG with special consideration of preconvulsive states; 3. the level of conciousness.

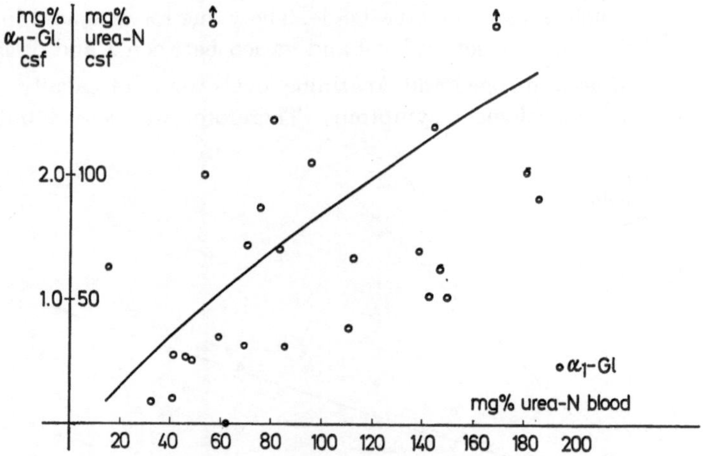

Fig. 3. Relations between urea nitrogen and alpha-1-glycoprotein in CSF.

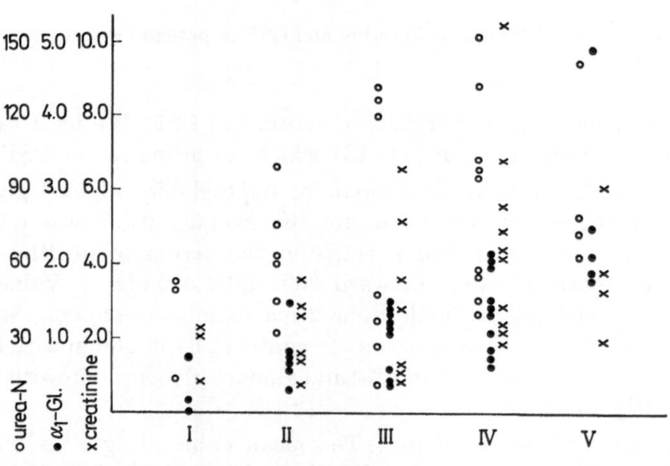

Fig. 4. Relations between the amount of urea nitrogen, alpha-1-glycoprotein and creatinine and the severity of the neurological symptoms in patients with renal failure.

Fig. 4 shows the values for alpha-1-glycoprotein in the five groups. Alpha-1-glycoprotein showed the most significant changes in the cerebrospinal fluid. The corresponding values of urea nitrogen and creatinine are also shown. Values for urea nitrogen and creatinine values were widely spread. The average value for urea nitrogen rose from 40 to 80 mg-%, those for creatinine from 1.7 to 4.5 mg-%. There was no further increase of levels from group 4 to 5. Alpha-1-glycoprotein, however, showed a steady increase from 0.25 to 2.5 mg-%, i.e. by 10 times. —

Also two other protein fractions appeared to be correlated to the clinical symptoms: they were the alpha-2-macroglobulins and gamma macroglobulins.

How could the protein changes in the CSF be explained? The following possibilities may be suggested. Proteins of the blood may enter into the CSF and appear there in a lower total concentration with the same distribution as in serum. The simultaneous increase of alpha-1-glycoprotein in both body fluids might support this hypothesis. On the other hand, the ratio of alpha-1-glycoprotein serum/CSF in the individual patients fluctuated widely and there was an evident discrepancy between the levels of haptoglobins in both body fluids. — Secondly one may hypothesize, that in the course of kidney disease the so called blood-CSF barrier may "break down" with an increased permeability for proteins. This assumption is supported by the appearance of Igm and the increased alpha-2-macro globulin, which presumably, according to investigations in inflammatory, neoplastic and vascular diseases of the central nervous system [8, 18], are indicators for a damaged function of the blood-CSF barrier. Several other findings [2, 3, 4, 19] suggest a third possibility, which is a production of proteins in the central nervous system itself.

References

1. Asbury, A. K., M. Victor, and R. D. Adams: Uremic polyneuropathy. Trans. Amer. neurol. Ass. **87**, 100—103 (1962).

2. Bauer, H.: Zur Frage der Identität der Liquorproteine mit den Eiweißkörpern des Blutserums. I. Besonderheiten der Liquorproteine hinsichtlich der Vorfraktion der Gamma-Globuline und der proteingebundenen Lipide. Dtsch. Z. Nervenheilk. **175**, 354—377 (1956).

3. — II. Die proteingebundenen Kohlehydrate des Liquors. Dtsch. Z. Nervenheilk. **175**, 488—510 (1957).

4. — III. Die Mucoproteine des Liquors. Dtsch. Z. Nervenheilk. **176**, 126—142 (1957).

5. Bradbury, M. W. B., and R. V. Coxon: The penetration of urea into the central nervous system at high blood levels. J. Physiol. (Lond.) **163**, 423—435 (1962).

6. — J. Stubbs, I. E. Hughes, and P. Parker: The distribution of potassium, sodium, chloride and urea between lumbar cerebrospinal fluid and blood serum in human subjects. Clin. Sci. **25**, 97—105 (1963).

7. —, and H. Davson: The transport of urea, creatinine and certain monosaccharides between blood and fluid perfusing the cerebral ventricular system of rabbits. J. Physiol. (Lond.) **170**, 195—211 (1964).

8. Gottesleben, A., and H. J. Bauer: Quantitative Immunochemistry of cerebrospinal fluid proteins in inflammatory diseases of the nervous system. Germ. med. Mth. **12**, 331—334 (1967).

9. Kleeman, C. R., H. Davson, and E. Levin: Urea transport in the central nervous system. Amer. J. Physiol. **203**, 739—749 (1962).

10. Locke, S., J. P. Merril, and H. R. Tyler: Neurologic complications of acute uremia. Arch. intern. Med. **108**, 519—531 (1961).

11. Mancini, G., A. D. Carbonara, and J. F. Heremans: Immunochemical quantitation of antigens by single radial immunodiffusion. Immunochemistry **2**, 235 (1965).

12. Prill, A.: Neurologische Komplikationen unter Peritonealdialyse. In: Peritonealdialyse. Ed. by F. Scheler. München: Urban & Schwarzenberg 1967.

13. — E. Quellhorst, and F. Scheler: Epilepsy, clinical and electroencephalographical findings among patients with renal insufficiency. In: The physiopathogenesis of the epilepsies. Ed. by H. Gastaut et al. Springfield, USA: Ch. C. Thomas 1968 (in press).

14. Prill, A.: E. Volles, E. Quellhorst, A. Gottesleben u. F. Scheler: Beobachtungen über akute nephrogene Elektrolyt- und Wasserhaushaltsstörungen in ihren Auswirkungen auf das zentrale Nervensystem. In: Kienle: Hydrodynamik, Säure-Basen- und Elektrolythaushalt im Liquor und Nervensystem. Stuttgart: Thieme 1967.
15. Riecker, G.: Encephalopathie als Folge von Elektrolytstörungen (unter besonderer Berücksichtigung der Niereninsuffizienz). Verh. Dtsch. Ges. Inn. Med. 1966, S. 125—141. München: Bergmann 1967.
16. Schwick, G., u. K. Störiko: Ergebnisse der quantitativen immunologischen Bestimmung von Human-Plasma-Proteinen. Proc. 10th Congr. Europ. Soc. Haemat. Strasbourg 1965, 1 (1967).
17. Tenckhoff, H. A., u. B. H. Scribner: Langzeiterfolge und Komplikationen der Dialysebehandlung. Verh. Dtsch. Ges. Inn. Med., S. 645—648. München: Bergmann 1967.
18. Ursing, B., S. J. Dencker, and B. Swahn: Protein pattern of cerebrospinal fluid in meningitis and meningoencephalitis. Acta med. scand. **171**, 715 (1962).
19. Warecka, K., and H. Bauer: Studies on "brain-specific" proteins in aqueous extracts of brain tissue. J. Neurochem. **14**, 783—787 (1967).

1.5.8. Studies on Blood Acetoacetate, Pyruvate, Lactate, α-Oxoglutarate and Citrate in Chronic Renal Failure

L. Campanacci, G. F. Guarnieri, N. Siliprandi and E. Fiaschi [1]

With 3 Figures

A great deal of emphasis has been placed in the past on the accumulation of phosphate and sulphate anions in the blood, as well as on the failure of the tubules to remove H^+ in the acidosis due to renal failure [5, 10]. In contrast, very little attention has been paid to other blood anions — e.g. acetoacetate and lactate — which can accumulate and produce acidosis.

The present paper deals with the measurement of blood acetoacetate and lactate in chronic uremia.

Table

	Plasma acetoacetate (mM/l)	Plasma citrate (mM/l)	Blood α-oxoglutarate (mM/l)
Chronic uremic patients mean ± S.D.	0,2160 ± 0,0140 (No. = 35)	0,1123 ± 0,0057 (No. = 35)	0,011014 ± 0,003840 (No. = 27)
Normal controls mean ± S.D.	0,0838 ± 0,0043 (No. = 20)	0,1690 ± 0,0053 (No. = 17)	0,013128 ± 0,003000 (No. = 15)
P (t test)	< 0,001	< 0,001	∼0,05
	Blood lactate (mM/l)	**Blood pyruvate (mM/l)**	**Lactate/pyruvate ratio**
Chronic uremic patients mean ± S.D.	1,3540 ± 0,0744 (No. = 15)	0,1002 ± 0,0049 (No. = 15)	13,52 ± 1,32 (No. = 15)
Normal controls mean ± S.D.	1,1249 ± 0,0091 (No. = 14)	0,0968 ± 0,0036 (No. = 19)	10,18 ± 0,95 (No. = 14)
P (t test)	> 0,05	> 0,5	> 0,05

No. = number of cases.

Plasma acetoacetate and citrate were determined in 9 women and 26 men, aged 20—55; 13 had chronic pyelonephrytis, 21 chronic glomerulonephrytis and 1 hypertensive nephropathy.

Blood α-oxoglutarate was determined in 13 women and 14 men, aged 20—55; 12 had chronic pyelonephrytis, 12 chronic glomerulonephrytis, 2 hypertensive nephropathy and 1 renal amyloidosis.

Lactate and pyruvate were determined in 3 women and 12 men, aged 19—57; 5 had chronic pyelonephrytis and 10 chronic glomerulonephritis.

---

[1] Institutes of Medical Pathology and of Biological Chemistry, University of Padua, Padua, Italy.

Pyruvate, α-oxoglutarate and citrate were also studied as they are metabolites closely related to lactate and acetoacetate.

These results have been compared with the plasma acetoacetate, citrate and pyruvate levels in normal adults after the intravenous administration of glycine. It is in fact known that in idiopathic hyperglycinemia there is often a temporary increase in ketonemia [8]. On the other hand an increase of the blood glycine level has been demonstrated in the chronic uremic patients by SALISBURY et al. [17].

The results of the investigations could be of some value in the interpretation of the findings in uremic patients.

Materials and Methods

All metabolites were determined in patients maintained on a normocaloric, normolipidic, high carbohydrate, low-protein (18—40 g proteins daily) diet, used routinely in the treatment of chronic uremia. None of the patients suffered from obvious liver damage, diabetes, or any of the diseases that can affect the blood pyruvate level [2].

The blood was withdrawn without stasis after a 10 hour period of fasting.

Acetoacetate was measured in plasma and urine by a modification [7] of the Walker-Allred method [18, 1]. The KRAUS' method was used for plasma citrate [13]. Pyruvate [6], lactate [12] and α-oxoglutarate [3] were measured enzymatically.

Glycine (150 mg/kg body weight) was injected intravenously after 10 hours of fasting. In these experiments, healthy adult subjects of both sexes without any clinical or functional symptom or sign of kidney and/or liver disease were chosen. Venous blood was withdrawn at intervals after the injection and plasma acetoacetate, pyruvate and citrate were estimated. The method used for the measurement of blood acetoacetate seems to be sufficiently specific; particularly glycine [18] and its metabolites cysteine and reduced glutathione [1], do not interfere with it. Moreover, glyoxilic acid was also carefully checked.

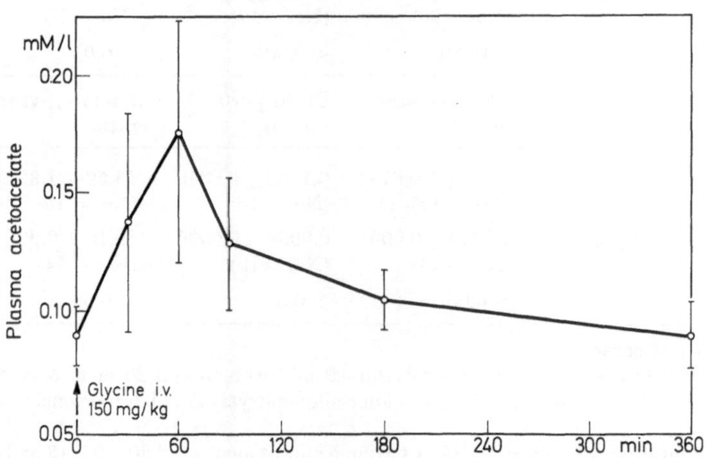

Analysis of variance

Source	Sum of squares	D.f.	Variance	F	P
Between groups	0.062045	5	0.012409	5.19	< 0.01
Within groups	0.143449	60	0.002391		

Fig. 1. Plasma acetoacetate in normal subjects after i.v. injection of 150 mg/kg of glycine.

Results

The table shows that in uremic patients plasma acetoacetate is significantly increased in comparison with normal subjects, whereas plasma citrate and blood α-oxoglutarate are decreased.

Blood pyruvate and lactate do not show any significant change.

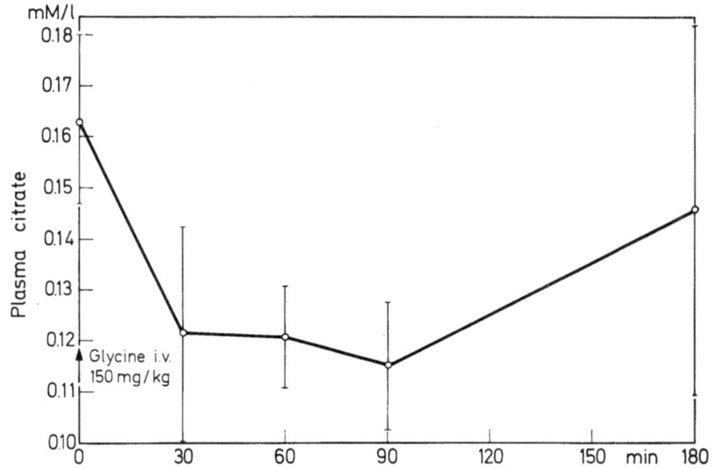

Analysis of variance

Source	Sum of squares	D.f.	Variance	F	P
Between groups	0.011733	4	0.002933	5.29	< 0.01
Within groups	0.016771	30	0.000559		

Fig. 2. Plasma citrate in normal subjects after i. v. injection of 150 mg/kg of glycine.

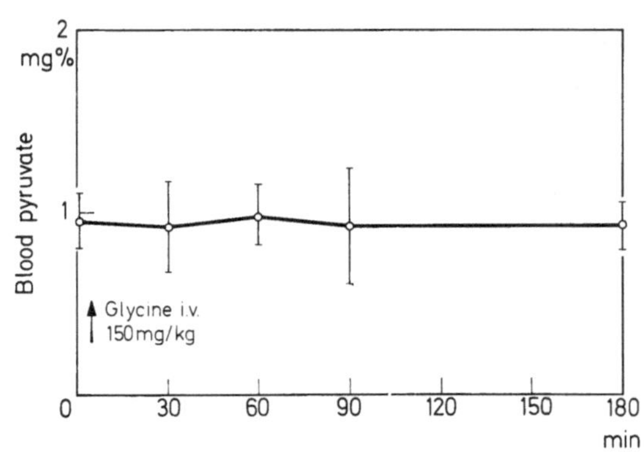

Analysis of variance

Source	Sum of squares	D.f.	Variance	F	P
Between groups	0.01	4	0.025		> 0.05
Within groups	0.68	20	0.034	0.073	(n.s.)

Fig. 3. Blood pyruvate in normal subjects after i. v. injection of 150 mg/kg of glycine.

The glycine load in normal adults produced a progressive increase in the plasma acetoacetate (Fig. 1). In contrast, the plasma citrate decreased (Fig. 2). In both cases, the results obtained were statistically significant ($P < 0.01$). The blood pyruvate level did not show any significant change ($P > 0.05$) (Fig. 3).

Discussion and Conclusions

The first question arising from the results obtained is whether impaired renal function in uremic patients could account for the plasma acetoacetate increase. Since the urinary excretion of acetoacetate in many uremic patients with varying degrees of kidney damage was the same as in normal adults [11], such a relationship can be excluded. Moreover, failure of renal function and the consequent decrease of citrate clearance [15] should also result in an increased plasma citrate level.

Since blood lactate and pyruvate levels are normal, it seems likely that there is no increased glycolysis in uremic patients that could lead to an accumulation of AcCoA and, in consequence, to ketosis.

It follows that some other metabolic disorder, in which both acetoacetate, α-oxoglutarate and citrate are involved, could very probably explain the above results. It is well known that the tissue levels of NH_4^+ and the blood level of amino compounds such as aminoacids [17], some of which can transaminate [14], are increased in the uremic patient. One might infer that this excess of ammonium ions and of amino compounds could lead to an increase in the transamination reactions with oxaloacetate and α-oxoglutarate [9, 16,19]. The speed of the citric acid cycle could be consequently slowed down, with the result that incompletely oxidized AcCoA could form acetoacetate instead [11].

This hypothesis could also explain the decrease in the plasma citrate level, since a lack of some citric acid cycle intermediates may result in a lack of oxaloacetate with which AcCoA forms citrate.

The results obtained after a glycine load confirm this hypothesis. The blood pyruvate, which could arise from glycine and produce acetoacetate, does not show any alteration.

The ketonemia might in part contribute to the much more severe acidosis found in chronic uremic patients.

Summary

Plasma acetoacetate, α-oxoglutarate, lactate, pyruvate and citrate levels were measured in patients suffering from chronic uremia. The results showed an increase of acetoacetate and a decrease of citrate and α-oxoglutarate in comparison with the values obtained from normal subjects. On the other hand, no significant alterations were observed in either blood pyruvate and lactate in the same uremic patients.

A defective excretory function, per se, cannot account for the increased plasma acetoacetate level. However, it may be suggested that this metabolic disorder could be produced through an accumulation of ammonium ions and amino compounds, such as aminoacids, which undergo massive transamination resulting in the subtraction of some key citric acid cycle intermediates necessary for the optimal utilization of AcCoA.

This hypothesis seems to be substantiated by the results obtained following the intravenous injection of glycine in normal subjects. Under these circumstances, a marked increase of acetoacetate and a decrease of citrate was observed in the plasma.

References

1. ALLRED, J. B.: Analyt. Biochem. **11**, 138 (1965).
2. AMATUZIO, D. S., and S. NESBITT:. J. clin. Invest. **29**, 1486 (1950).
3. BERGMEYER, H. U., and E. BERNT: In: H. U. BERGMEYER, Methods of enzymatic analysis, p. 324. New York and London: Academic Press 1965.
4. BITTAR, E. E.: Cell pH, cap. 11, Butterworth, London 1964.
5. BRIGGS, A. P.: Exp. Med. Surg. **5**, 128 (1947).
6. BÜCHER, T., quoted by B. HESS, Klin. Wschr. **33**, 540 (1955).
7. CAMPANACCI, L., G. F. GUARNIERI, B. PICCINELLI e A. D'ALBERTON: Boll. Soc. ital. Biol. sper. **42**, 1730 (1966).
8. CHILDS, B., W. L. NYHAN, M. BORDEN, L. BARD, and R. E. COOKE: J. Pediat. **27**, 522 (1961).
9. CLARK, G. M., and B. EISEMAN: New Engl. J. Med. **259**, 178 (1958).
10. FALBRIARD, A.: Schweiz. med. Wschr. **94**, 75 (1964).
11. FIASCHI, E., N. SILIPRANDI, L. CAMPANACCI, and G. F. GUARNIERI: Minerva nefrol. **14**, 44 (1967).
12. FIELD, M.: J. B. BLOCK, and D. P. RALL: Amer. J. Med. **40**, 528 (1966).
13. KRAUS, P.: Clin. chim. Acta **12**, 462 (1965).
14. MEISTER, A.: Biochemistry of the amino acids, vol. I, p. 354. New York: Acad. Press 1965.
15. NORDMANN, J., and R. NORDMANN: Clin. Chem. **3**, 462 (1957).
16. RECKNAGEL, R. O., and V. R. POTTER: J. biol. Chem. **191**, 263 (1951).
17. SALISBURY, P. F., M. S. DUNN, and E. A. MURPHY: J. clin. Invest. **36**, 1227 (1957).
18. WALKER, P. G.: Biochem. J. **58**, 699 (1954).
19. WILLIAMSON, D. H., P. LUND, and H. A. KREBS: Biochem. J. **103**, 514 (1967).

1.5.9. Plasma Phenols in Renal Failure and their Elimination through the Artificial Kidney

H. E. KELLER, H. J. KRAMER, G. A. JUTZLER, D. DOENECKE, G. TRAUT and D. MÜTING[1]

With 3 Figures

The early investigations of BECHER, LITZNER and DOENECKE [1, 2, 3] concerning the relationship of phenolic compounds to uremic symptoms has induced many further studies [8, 10, 12, 20, for a review see 18].

Recent in-vitro-experiments support the assumption, that phenolic compounds in certain concentrations may inhibit different enzyme systems [8, 9, 19]. The biochemical role of phenols in the disturbed metabolic pathways in uremia, therefore, deserves some studies.

The present investigation was carried out in order to determine the plasma concentrations of free and conjugated phenolic compounds in renal failure and their relationship to the concentration of creatinine in plasma, and to study the kinetic aspects of the elimination of phenolic compounds through the artificial kidney us compared to those for creatinine.

Clinical experiments were made with the artificial kidney, primarily with reference to the toxicity of phenols in uremia. Toxic factors responsible for the symptoms of uremia, should have been removed at adequate values by the artificial kidney [6, 7, 14, 15].

Methods

The free and conjugated phenolic substances, initially separated by ether extraction [13], were quantitatively determined using the method of E. G. SCHMIDT [17].

The "free phenol" fraction contained the free volatile phenols and the free aromatic hydroxyacids. The conjugated phenolic substances appeared in the "conjugated phenol" fraction. The data we obtained, using this method, were calculated in equivalent concentrations of p-hydroxyphenylacetic-acid.

Normal plasma values were:

free phenols	100—300 μg/100 ml
conjugated phenols	200—600 μg/100 ml

The simultaneous determinations of serum creatinine were made using JAFFÉ'S method.

Results

In a group of 16 patients suffering either from compensated or non-compensated renal failure, the plasma levels of the free phenols ranged from 100 to 1750 μg/

[1] Dialyse-Abteilung der I. Medizinischen Univ-Klinik der Universität des Saarlandes, Homburg/Saar, West Germany.

100 ml. The conjugated phenolic compounds reached levels of 800 to 4,800 μg/100 ml. The values of the simultaneous creatinine concentrations ranged from 1.4 to 20 mg/100 ml.

Fig. 1 shows the relationship of the plasma concentrations of the free and conjugated phenolic compounds to that of creatinine. The positive correlation coefficients are statistically highly significant. The ratio between the free and

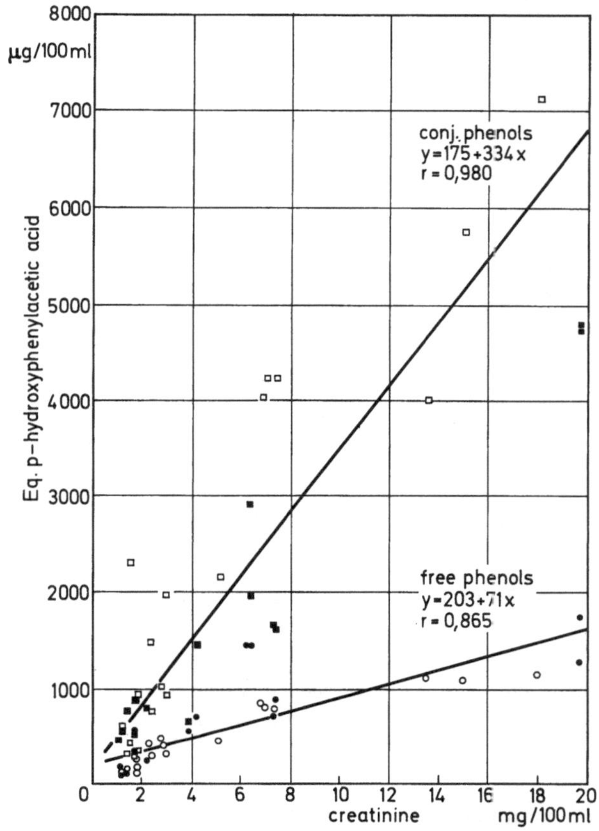

Fig. 1. The relationship of the plasma concentrations of the free and conjugated phenols to that of creatinine. ● Free phenols, authors' values; ○ free phenols, values of E. G. Schmidt; ■ conjugated phenols, authors' values; □ conjugated phenols, values of E. G. Schmidt

Table. *Mean values of plasma concentrations of the free and conjugated phenols and of creatinine before and after 6-hour hemodialyses. (Travenol standard artificial kidney, twin coil 145)*

	6-hrs-Hemodialysis		
	Pre	After	%
Free phenols (μg/100 ml)	1,030	620	~60
Conjugated phenols (μg/100 ml)	2,800	2,100	~75
Creatinine (mg/100 ml)	13.5	8.5	~63

the conjugated phenols ranged from 1:2 to 1:4. This finding supports the conclusion that conjugation of phenols is generally not disturbed in uremia [17].

A total of 20 hemodialysis treatments of 7 patients suffering from chronic renal failure was studied. The table shows the mean values of free and conjugated phenols and creatinine before and after hemodialysis of 6 hours duration. The values fell resp. to 75 and 60 percent of the initial concentrations, the ratio between free and conjugated phenols remaining nearly constant.

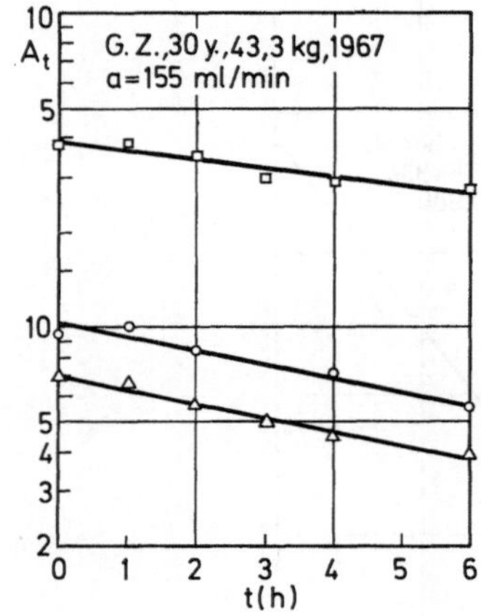

Fig. 2

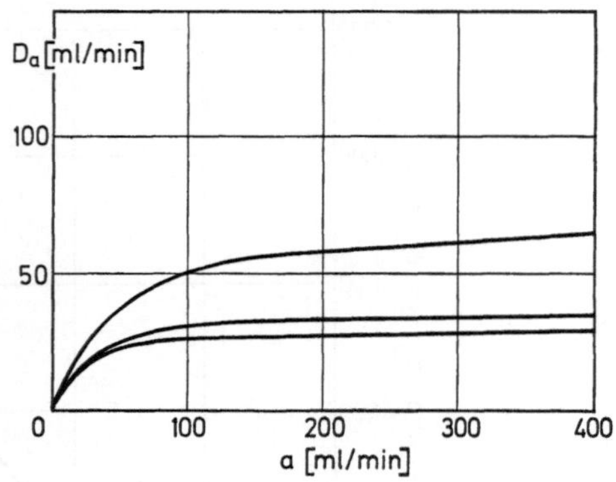

Fig. 3

Fig. 2. The above semilogarithmic graph illustrates the decline of plasma concentrations of creatinine, free and conjugated phenols during a 6-hour hemodialysis. (Travenol standard-artificial kidney, twin coil 145). □ Conjugated phenols [μg/100 ml]: $\ln A_t = 8.280-0.062\,t$; ○ free phenols [μg/100 ml]: $\ln A_t = 6.927-0.095\,t$; △ creatinine [mg/100 ml]: $\ln A_t = 1.651-0.104\,t$

Fig. 3. The relationship of the in vivo dialysance (D) of creatinine and the free and conjugated phenols to the blood flow rate (a). P permeability (cm/min); S surface area (cm²) $PS_{\text{creatinine}} = D_{a\to\infty} = 72$ [ml/min]; $PS_{\text{free phenols}} = D_{a\to\infty} = 37$ [ml/min]; $PS_{\text{conj. phenols}} = D_{a\to\infty} = 31$ [ml/min]

Fig. 2 shows an example of a course of treatment by the artificial kidney. As expected the decline of serum concentrations of the free and conjugated phenols and that of creatinine followed an exponential function. The concentrations of these substances in the dialysate and the ultrafiltrate were negligible.

Referring to the simplified formula of MACEY and WOLF [11], dialysance is defined as follows:

$$D = -\frac{\frac{d(bA)}{dt}}{A-U} \tag{1}$$

If A, the plasma concentration of a substance is much higher than U, the urinary, concentration, and if the concentrations in the dialysate and the ultrafiltrate are negligible, integration yields the simplified Eq. (2):

$$\ln A_t = \ln A_o - \frac{D_a}{b_o} \cdot t. \tag{2}$$

The slope of the regression line (Fig. 2) is given by the quotient of dialysance (D_a) at a given flow rate (a) and the virtual dialysable volume (b_o).

In order to obtain values of clinical significance, the dialysance was determined in vivo in regard to standards set by FRITZ [4]. The relationship between the dialysance of phenols and creatinine and the different flow rates is shown in Fig. 3. At flow rates greater than 100—150 ml/min, dialysance of phenols is essentialy determined by permeation through the dialyser membrane ($D_{max} = P \cdot S$) (Fig. 3). The dialysance of phenols is approximately one-half that of creatinine (Fig. 3).

Abbreviations:

A = plasma concentration (µg/100 ml, resp. mg/100 ml)
a = blood flow rate at the entrance to the dialyser tubing
a_i = blood flow rate at the end of the dialyser tubing including effects of filtration (ml/min)
b_o = virtual dialysable volume in the filtration-free case
b = virtual dialysable volume with uniform dispersion of a substance including the effects of filtration (ml)
D = dialysance (ml/min)
t = time (min)

Summary

1. In the compensated and decompensated retention of renal failure, the retention of free and conjugated phenols is an approximately linear function of that of creatinine. The relationship of the concentrations of free phenols to that of conjugated phenols supportis the conclusion that conjugation of phenolic compounds is not disturbed in uremia.

2. During dialysis, the plasma concentrations of the free and conjugated phenols fell, following, as expected, an exponential function of time, similar to that observed for creatinine and other dialysable substances. The in vivo dialysance of the phenols was calculated to be approximately one-half that of creatinine.

Through these results do not allow any direct conclusion about the toxicity of phenolic compounds in uremia, their retention in renal failure and their fairly easy removal by dialysis, support a possible role in the pathogenesis of uremia. Further investigations are needed in order to determine the role of single phenolic compounds in renal failure, their kinetics in dialysis and their inhibitory effects on enzyme systems.

Inhibitory effects of aromatic hydroxyacids, in vitro, on certain cerebral enzymes were demonstrated by HICKS et al. [9]. Furthermore, the breakdown of certain free aromatic hydroxyacids as possible uremic blood constituents depends on "energy-rich" compounds. Thus, the synthesis of coenzyme-A-compounds (HEINTZ and RENNER) may be disturbed in uremia.

References

1. BECHER, E.: Studien über die Pathogenese der echten Uraemie, insbesondere über die Bedeutung der retinierten Phenole und anderer Darmfäulnisprodukte. Zbl. inn. Med. **46**, 369—383 (1925).
2. — F. DOENECKE u. ST. LITZNER: Quantitative Studien über die Fraktion der aromatischen Oxysäuren im Blut bei Krankheiten. Z. klin. Med. **104**, 29—43 (1926).
3. — ST. LITZNER u. W. TÄGLICH: Der Phenolgehalt des Blutes unter normalen und pathologischen Verhältnissen. Z. klin. Med. **104**, 182—194 (1926).
4. FRITZ, K. W.: Hämodialyse. Stuttgart: Georg Thieme 1966.
5. HARTNETT, J. C.: Possible role of free phenols in renal uremia. Proc. Soc. exp. Biol. (N.Y.) **69**, 177—179 (1948).
6. HEINTZ, R., u. D. RENNER: Uraemie. Neue Ergebnisse der Ätiologie und Pathogenese. Med. Welt **31**, 1803—1807 (1967).
7. HENKIN, R., P. BYATT, and M. MAXWELL: Evidence for the presence of a dialysable toxic factor in the sera of uremic subjects. Clin. Res. **9**, 202 (1961).
8. HICKS, J. M., D. S. YOUNG, and I. B. P. WOOTTON: Abnormal blood constituents in acute renal failure. Clin. chim. Acta **7**, 623—633 (1962).
9. — — — The effect of uremic blood constituents on certain cerebral enzymes. Clin. chim. Acta **9**, 228—235 (1964).
10. KRAMER, B., H. SELIGSON, H. BALDRUSH, and D. SELIGSON: The isolation of several aromatic acids from the hemodialysis fluid of uremic patients. Clin. chim. Acta **11**, 363—371 (1965).
11. MACEY, R. J., and A. V. WOLF: Kinetics of ultrafiltration hemodialysis. Bull. Math. Biophys. **22**, 217—226 (1960).
12. MÜTING, D.: Studies on the pathogenesis of uremia. Clin. chim. Acta **12**, 551—554 (1965).
13. — Persönliche Mitteilung.
14. NIETH, H.: Pathophysiologie und Klinik des Coma uraemicum. Mels. Med. Mitt. **37**, 162—170 (1963).
15. SARRE, H.: Nierenkrankheiten, 3. Aufl. Stuttgart: Georg Thieme 1967.
16. SCHMIDT, E. G.: Urinary phenols. IV. The simultaneous determination of phenol and p-cresol in urine. J. biol. Chem. **179**, 211—215 (1949).
17. — N. F. MCELVAIN, and J. J. BOWEN: Plasma amino acids and ether-soluble phenols in uremia. Amer. J. clin. Path. **20**, 253—261 (1950).
18. SCHREINER, G., and J. MAHER: Uremia: Biochemisty pathogenesis and treatment. Springfield, Ill.: Ch. C. Thomas 1961.
19. WEDDING, R. T., C. HANSCH, and T. R. FUKUTO: Inhibition of malate dehydrogenase by phenols and the influence of ring substituents on their inhibitory effectivness. Arch. Biochem. **121**, 9—21 (1967).
20. YOUNG, D. S., and J. D. P. WOOTTON: The retention of amines as a factor in ureaemic toxaemia. Clin. chim. Acta **9**, 503—505 (1964).
21. WOOTTON, J. D. P.: Retention of aromatic compounds in acute renal failure. The Scientific Basis of Medicine. Ann. Rev. 235—248 (1963).

1.5.10. The Effect of Blood Reinfusion and of THAM on Experimental Hypovolemic Acidosis*

K. Klütsch, A. Heidland, L. Griebel and F. Günther[1]

Hemorrhagic shock induces metabolic acidosis [2—4]. While normovolemic respiratory acidosis does not affect renal the resistance or diuresis, even when vascular pH decreases to 7.1 [1], normovolemic metabolic acidosis results in a reduction in renal blood flow and in cessation of diuresis at a pH of 7.25 [4].

In the present investigation acid-base-balance and renal functions were studied in untreated experimental hemorrhagic hypotension, as well as after volume substitution and the infusion of alkaline solutions.

Table 1. *Group I (n = 6)*

	Arterial pH	pCO_2 (mm Hg)	Base excess (mEq/l)	Mean a. p. (mm Hg)	Blood volume (ml/kg b. w.)	C_{In} (ml/min)
Control value	7.337 ±0.018	43.9 ±12.3	−3.6 ±4.7	110.0 ±23.0	99.2 ±15.4	106.8 ±28.0
2 hours hemorrhage	7.264 ±0.129	30.6 ±15.4	−12.6 ±5.8	40.0 ±0	62.6 ±12.6	4.3 ±5.3
4 hours hemorrhage	7.231 ±0.075	45 ±2.0	−8.7 ±5.2	40.0 ±0	61.2 ±13.7	3.33 ±1.6
Blood	7.214 ±0.125	46.8 ±15.7	−8.5 ±6.5	106.7 ±13.3	100.6 ±19.1	73.17 ±18.8
THAM	7.352 ±0.081	44.7 ±13.6	−1.6 ±5.8	108 ±10.3	102.4 ±18.4	91.6 ±29.9

	C_{PAH} (ml/min)	C_{osm} (ml/min)	Urine flow (ml/min)	Na-excretion (μEq/min)	K-excretion (μEq/min)
Control value	392.2 ± 126	2.62 ± 0.83	0.96 ± 0.32	203.4 ± 110	54.0 ± 18.5
2 hours hemorrhage	5.7 ± 5.4	0.05 ± 0.17	0.16 ± 0.09	24.2 ± 13.7	3.2 ± 4.4
4 hours hemorrhage	5.9 ± 1.8	0.0 ± 0.0	0.15 ± 0.15	7.5 ± 4.5	2.5 ± 0.7
Blood	332.2 ± 158	4.12 ± 0.69	2.67 ± 1.11	323.4 ± 116	143.8 ± 70.5
THAM	363.6 ± 138,5	5.98 ± 1.73	4.63 ± 2.0	286 ± 210	188 ± 74

* Supported by Deutsche Forschungsgemeinschaft.
1 Medizinische Universitätsklinik Würzburg, West Germany.

Method

15 female mongrel dogs (body weight 24.7 ± 4.3 kg) were anesthetized with sodium pentobarbital and urethane. Arterial blood pH, pCO_2, base excess, mean arterial pressure, plasma volume (I^{131}-albumin), the renal clearance of inulin and PAH, urine flow, plasma and urine osmolarity, sodium- and potassium concentrations in plasma and in urine were measured.

After obtaining base values, the mean arterial pressure was lowered, within 15 minutes, by arterial bleeding and maintained at the level obtained by further withdrawal of blood and/or reinfusion for a time of 2 to 4 hours. During hypotension all measurements were repeated. Thereafter, 11 dogs received the volume of blood withdrawn previously, as ADC-blood. After the reinfusion of blood, 6 dogs (group I) were given THAM (trishydroxymethylaminomethane) intravenously as a 0.3 M solution, the amount infused being calculated (in ml) as the product of negative base excess and body weight. The remaining 4 dogs received a comparable amount of 0.9% NaCl-solution (group II). In group III (4 dogs) THAM and ADC-blood were infused simultaneously.

Measurements were repeated for periods up to 11 days after single experiments.

Table 2. *Group II* ($n = 5$)

	Arterial pH	pCO_2 (mm Hg)	Base excess (mEq/l)	pm (mm Hg)	Blood volume (ml/kg KG)	C_{In} (ml/min)
Control value	7.304 ± 0.059	31.9 ± 5.4	−11.0 ± 2.7	138 ± 12.4	102 ± 10.4	111.0 ± 14.6
2 hours hemorrhage	7.225 ± 0.09	18.6 ± 5.8	−18.5 ± 3.9	40 ± 0	62.2 ± 9.1	1.6 ± 2
4 hours hemorrhage	7.240 ± 0.11	19.7 ± 4.5	−15.7 ± 3.7	40 ± 0	58.1 ± 7.6	2.5 ± 3.5
Blood ($n = 4$)	7.207 ± 0.12	23.2 ± 9.0	−16.6 ± 4.3	114 ± 26.9	94.1 ± 8.0	60.22 ± 31.1
NaCl	7.210 ± 0.14	21.0 ± 7.0	−14.8 ± 4.1	110 ± 25.5	95.2 ± 7.8	73.0 ± 23.6

	C_{PAH} (ml/min)	C_{osm} (ml/min)	Urine flow (ml/min)	Na excretion (μEq/min)	K excretion (μEq/min)
Control value	321.6 ± 100.5	1.94 ± 0.71	1.35 ± 0.57	225.7 ± 120.5	67.8 ± 32.7
2 hours hemorrhage	4.95 ± 4.8	0.01	0.21 ± 0.02	3.5 ± 6.9	7.5 ± 1.5
4 hours hemorrhage	3.1 ± 0.4	0 ± 0	0.21 ± 0.01	2.07 ± 4.1	0 ± 0
Blood ($n = 4$)	209.2 ± 108.9	3.31 ± 1.76	3.85 ± 2.99	300.8 ± 113.0	204 ± 182
NaCl	200.6 ± 99.6	4.21 ± 2.88	3.55 ± 2.66	315 ± 339.3	137.6 ± 50.1

Results

Presumely as a result of barbiturate anaesthesia, the initial mean arterial pH had decreased to 7.31 ± 0.043, base excess to-6.9 ± 4.4 mEq/l and pCO_2 to 38.1 ± 9.1 mm Hg.

Lowering of mean arterial pressure to 40 mm Hg required the removal of 1294 ± 209.7 ml of blood, approximately 52% of the initial blood volume or 5.2% of body weight. After 2 hours of hypotension, the arterial pH had decreased in all three groups to 7.23—7.29, pCO_2 to 30.6—18.6 mm Hg, negative base excess had increased to −10.0 to −18.5 mEq/l. The inulin-clearance in all groups was lowered to 1—4%, the PAH-clearance to 0.9—1.5% of the control values. Urine flow, osmolar clearance, sodium and potassium excretion fell proportionally. After four hours of hypotension, group I exhibited a further drop of arterial pH to 7.24 ± 0.075, whereas the pH in group II had increased slightly to 7.24 ± 0.11.

During reinfusion of the ADC-blood, one dog died. In the remaining experiments of groups I and II, mean arterial blood pressure and blood volume increased approximately to control values, arterial pH, however, decreased further to 7.21 ± 0.125 in group I and 7.21 ± 0.120 in group II respectively.

The inulin- and PAH-clearances reached 69.5 and 85% of the control values in group I and 54.3 and 65.2% in group II. The subsequent administration of

Table 3. *Group III* ($n = 4$)

	Arterial pH	pCO_2 (mm Hg)	Base excess (mEq/l)	Mean a. p. (mm Hg)	Blood volume (ml/kg KG)	C_{In} (ml/min)
Control value	7.293 ± 0.063	39.7 ± 7.7	− 6.9 ± 1.6	112 ± 18.5	104.8 ± 11.5	93.2 ± 14.5
1 hour hemorrhage	7.283 ± 0.097	31.2 ± 7.8	− 10.0 ± 1.9	40 ± 0	77.2 ± 17.7	0.72 ± 0.9
2 hours hemorrhage	7.268 ± 0.106	22.8 ± 10.3	− 15.2 ± 4.1	40 ± 0	72.0 ± 13.1	0.0 ± 0
Blood + THAM	7.403 0.020	37.9 ± 4.9	+ 0.5 ± 3.1	110 ± 8.2	100.3 ± 12.6	85.34 ± 26.0

	C_{PAH} (ml/min)	C_{osm} (ml/min)	Urine flow (ml/min)	Na excretion (μEq/min)	K excretion (μEq/min)
Control value	267.6 ± 55.6	1.23 ± 0.01	0.9 ± 0.5	109.3 ± 38.0	52.5 ± 28.2
1 hour hemorrhage	2.43 ± 3.0	0.0 ± 0	0.4 ± 0.1	22.4 ± 18.2	0.7 ± 0.02
2 hours hemorrhage	0.0 ± 0	0.0 ± 0	0.2 ± 0.1	13.0 ± 10.7	0.1 ± 0.2
Blood + THAM	243.3 ± 65.4	4.98 ± 0.96	6.5 ± 2.4	301.8 ± 173	150.6 ± 28.0

THAM resulted, in group I, in an almost complete correction of the metabolic acidosis. Concommitantly, the inulin clearance increased further to 86% and the PAH-clearance to 93% of the control values. This increase was associated with a rise of urine flow to 4.63 ± 2.0 and of osmolar clearance to 5.98 ± 1.73 ml/min. In group II, which had obtained a comparable amount of 0.9% NaCl-solution, the metabolic acidosis and the depression of renal functions remained unaffected. Group III, which had received blood and THAM simultaneously showed a complete normalization of the acid base balance and a return of inulin- and PAH-clearance to 92 and 91% of the control values respectively (average values with standard deviations: Tables 1, 2, 3).

Control studies in the animals, which had received THAM revealed in 4 experiments lasting up to 10 days almost normal mean arterial pressure- and volume conditions. The inulin- and PAH clearances remained within normal limits. In contrast, 4 out of 5 dogs, which had received only ADC-blood, died within 24 hours. In the fifth dog, inulin- and PAH-clearance had decreased to 10 and 12% of the control values after 24 hours. There was still a partially compensated metabolic acidosis with a pH of 7.3, a pCO_2 of 25 mm Hg and a negative base excess of -10.5 mEq/l.

References

1. Emanuel, D. A., M. Fleischmann, and F. J. Haddy: Effect of pH change upon renal vascular resistance and urine flow. Circulat. Res. **5**, 607—611 (1957).
2. Lauson, H. D., S. E. Bradley, and A. Cournanand: The renal circulation in shock. J. clin. Invest. **23**, 381 (1944).
3. Selkurt, E. E.: Nierendurchblutung und renale Clearances bei Blutverlust und im hämorrhagischen Schock. In: Schock, Pathogenese und Therapie, S. 162—168. Berlin-Göttingen-Heidelberg: Springer 1962.
4. Zimmermann, W. E.: In: Genese und Therapie des hämorrhagischen Schocks, S. 115—127. Stuttgart: Georg Thieme 1966.

1.5.11. Isolated Renal Polyarteriitis

W. Friedrich, A. Lackenschweiger, W. Weissel and E. Zimmermann[1]

With 1 Figure

The case-history of a 36 year old woman in chronic progressive renal failure is presented. After 14 months of conventional conservative treatment with relatively high doses of anabolic hormones she had to undergo chronic hemodialysis, twice weekly, by means of a twin-coil kidney. A shunt-infection necessitated large doses of penicillin. The patient died 9 months later (Fig. 1). Post mortem studies revealed the unusal finding of polyarteriitis of arcuate and interlobular

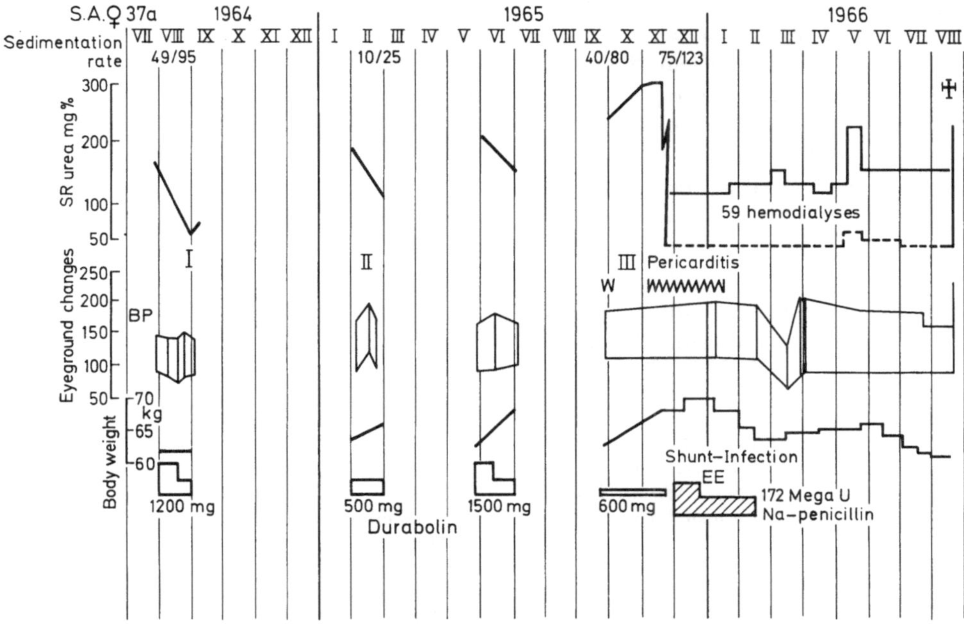

Fig. 1

arteries in both kidneys, complicating a preexisting chronic glomerulonephritis. No other organ showed similar arterial lesions.

The interpretation of the picture as a locally complicating polyarteriitis was based on the following anatomo-pathological arguments:

1. Complete or incomplete infarction — as typical for the Kussmaul-Maier disease — were totally lacking in our case. The only possible explanation for this

[1] Department of Pathology and 3d Medical Department, Wilhelminenspital, Vienna, Austria.

fact is that the renal tissue was already scarred before the onset of polyarteriitis.

2. Several other renal arteries showed intimal fibrosis, as observed in for long-dialysed chronic glomerulonephritis ("adaptive intima fibrosis [9]").

The present case has some clinical importance. Polyarteriitis is a very rare cause of renal failure [8]. Though detection by biopsy is hardly to be expected [2], histologic diagnosis by either biopsy or in a removed kidney could be mistaken as proof for generalized arterial disease. This conclusion does not appear to be compelling, so that the exclusion of such patients from a chronic dialysis or transplantation-program would not be justified.

The etiology of polyarteriitis (panarteriitis or periarteriitis nodosa) in its localized form is as obscure as that of the generalized disease. The allergic-hyperergic character of the tissue reactions (in our case) directs attention towards "traumatic dialysis" in view of the large volumes of preserved blood given to the patient, or towards possible drug reactions. We dispose of two thoroughly investigated comparable cases, who died after 6 and 9 months, respectively, of similar dialysis treatment. None of them showed arterial vascular changes in their kidneys or other organs. The case reported is the only one of these three cases which was treated with high doses of anabolic hormones and very large doses of penicillin. There is no reference in the literature to arterial lesions from anabolic steroids, whereas periarteriitis nodosa after penicillin is frequently mentioned [1, 3, 4, 5 and 6]. Nephrotoxicity of penicillin, though only in the form of interstitial nephritis without arterial lesions, has been demonstrated in animal experiments [7].

The observation of allergic-hyperergic arteriitis in a previously diseased organ should stimulate experimental investigations.

References

1. ADELSON, J.: Periarteritis nodosa in infancy. J. Pediat. **39**, 346—349 (1951).
2. BANGE, F., K. W. FRITZ, and W. DINTER: Akutes Nierenversagen durch Periarteriitis nodosa. Münch. med. Wschr. **107**, 375—379 (1965).
3. BERNE, R. N.: An unusual sensitivity reaction to penicillin. Report of a case with autopsy finding. New Engl. J. Med. **242**, 814—816 (1950).
4. KIPKIE, G. F., and D. S. JOHNSON: Possible pathogenic mechanism responsible for human periarteritis nodosa as suggested of two instances of this disease in association with glomerulonephritis. Arch. Path. **51**, 387—391 (1951).
5. MCCOMBES, R. P.: Drug allergies. Case report of unusual sequelae in three patients. Bull. New Engl. J. med. Cent. **13**, 39—42 (1951).
6. PICKERING, G. W.: Cit. after F. REUBI, Nierenkrankheiten, S. 656. Bern u. Stuttgart: Hans Huber 1960.
7. POLSTER, A.: Über die Wirkung von Penicillin auf die Nieren von Mensch und Tier. Dtsch. med. Wschr. **91**, 1646—1650 (1966).
8. SCHUBERT, G. E., u. H. KÖBERLE: Über die Häufigkeit des pathologisch-anatomischen Bildes der Schockniere und anderen Nierenerkrankungen im unausgewählten Obduktionsgut. Dtsch. med. Wschr. **91**, 147—150 (1966).
9. ZOLLINGER, H. U.: In: Probleme der renovasculären Hypertonie. Arzneimittel-Forsch. 8, 1065—1073 (1967).

2. Toxic Disturbances of Renal Functions

2.1. General Toxicology

2.1.1. Morphological Aspects of the Acute Toxic Nephropathies

F. Gloor[1]

With 14 Figures

The prevalence and importance of the toxic nephropathies has increased considerably in the course of the last few years. This increase has created therapeutic problems in practical medicine, since the number of drugs and chemicals used in industry and agriculture, which influence human bodily functions, increases steadily. On the other hand, experimental toxic nephropathies may be good models for studying functional and structural changes of diseased glomeruli and tubules.

We define toxic nephropathy as a type of renal damage due to a nephrotoxin. A nephrotoxin is a synthetic or a natural chemical which enters the body by inhalation, ingestion, absorption or injection and damages renal tubular or glomerular cells, either by its own action or after having undergone some metabolic transformation. In order to be considered as a true nephrotoxin, a chemical must have the following properties:

1. its ingestion by man should regularly, or at least frequently, induce renal damage;

2. the type and the localization of the renal damage should be similar in all individuals exposed to the same nephrotoxin;

3. renal damage, as seen in man, should be reproducible in animal experiments;

4. the grade of structural and functional damage should be proportional to the dose of the substance given.

Renal damage occurring as a consequence of sensitization of the body to various substances, therefore, is not considered as nephrotoxic nephropathy in the present context. Renal damage caused by an increase in the blood concentration of physiologically occurring substances as in hypercalcemia, hypokalemia, hyperuricemia, hyperoxalemia, or after infusing large amounts of concentrated glucose solutions, are equally outside of the scope of the present review.

Most nephrotoxins are also toxic to other tissues. Their prevalent action on the kidneys is due to the large fraction of the cardiac output running through these organs and to the high concentrations which such toxic substances may reach in tubular fluid. It is, therefore, not astonishing that a large number of drugs are known to be nephrotoxins; as shown in table 1 they belong to widely differing chemical groups.

[1] Pathologisches Institut der Universität Basel, Switzerland.

Table 1. *Nephrotoxines*

Metals: Arsenic, Bismuth, Cadmium, *Chromium, Gold,* Iron, *Lead, Mercury* (organic and inorganic), Silver, Thallium, *Uranium*
Organic Solvents: Carbon tetrachloride, Chloroform, Dinitrophenol, Methanol, Tetrachloroethylene, Trichloroethylene, Tetrachloromethane
Glycols: Ethylene glycol (glycol diacetate), Propylene glycol, *Diethylene glycol,* Dipropylene glycole (Dioxane)
Antibiotics: Amphotericin B, Bacitracin, Colistin, Kanamycin, *Neomycin,* Novobiocin, Polymyxins, Tetracyclines (Degradation Products), Vanomycin, *Viomycin*
Sulfonamides: Sulfonamides of low solubility (crystallization)
X-Ray Contrast Media: Contrast agents in high concentration
Various Therapeutics: Halogenated Quinolines and Quinaldines, Cyclophosphamide (Endoxan), Hexadimethrinbromide, Phenacetin, Quinine, Salicylate, Trimethadione
Miscellaneous Agents: Calcium-EDTA (Versene), *Chlorate,* Deuterium, Glycerol, Maleic acid, Mushrooms, Oxalic acid, Phosphate, D,L-Serine, Snake Venoms, Tannic acid, *Tartrate*

In man the most important nephrotoxic agents are inorganic or organic compounds of mercury, carbon tetrachloride and related solvents, glycols, and, more recently antibiotics, cystostatics and radiocontrast agents [3, 13, 27, 29, 51, 52, 67]. As known from animal experiments, different species of mammals differ largely in their sensitivity to various nephrotoxins. It is, therefore, extremely difficult to extrapolate from the results of animal experiments to human disease [9, 25, 31, 40].

Only in acute intoxications are the clinical and the morphological picture primarily determined by the nephrotoxic agent, while in chronic intoxications, many additional influences modify the picture. For this reason we shall discuss only the morphologic appearance of toxic nephropathies induced by one single exposition to a nephrotoxic agent.

The macroscopic picture of toxic nephropathies does not differ much with different toxic agents. Both kidneys are enlarged, their surfaces are smooth. On section the cortex is enlarged and moist, its color is a pale yellow. The medullary cones appear reddened. The kidney-weight is increased (Fig. 1).

The microscopic picture also is very similar with different nephrotoxins. The first change, usually observed with light microscopy, is a swelling of tubular cells with a decrease in optical density of the cytoplasm, due to an increased water content of the cells (Fig. 2). On the swollen cell body appear rings of constriction which tend to severe the apical cell parts. With heavier damage, the apical cell membrane ruptures and the content of the cell flows out into the tubular lumen. While cytolysis by hyperhydration is the more frequent form of cell destruction, one sometimes also sees a type of cell necrosis initiated by cellular dehydration. In this type of damage, the epithelial cells contract, their cytoplasm becomes more eosinophilic, while their nuclei become pycnotic. The picture is that of "necrosis by coagulation". The necrotic epithelial cells, finally, separate from the basal membrane and fall into the tubular lumen (Fig. 3).

Both types of epithelial necrosis may occur simultaneously in one kidney; neither is specific for a given type of nephrotoxin. Proximal convoluted tubular cells tend to undergo necrosis by overhydration, while cells in the pars recta of the proximal tubules and of the distal convoluted tubules tend to undergo necrosis by dehydration.

With nephrotoxins inducing glomerular proteinuria, the tubular cells contain translucent droplets which denote protein storage. Cell damage usually depresses, within a short time, the cellular storage capacity for protein as well as for vital dyes. The tubular basement membrane usually remains intact, even after an

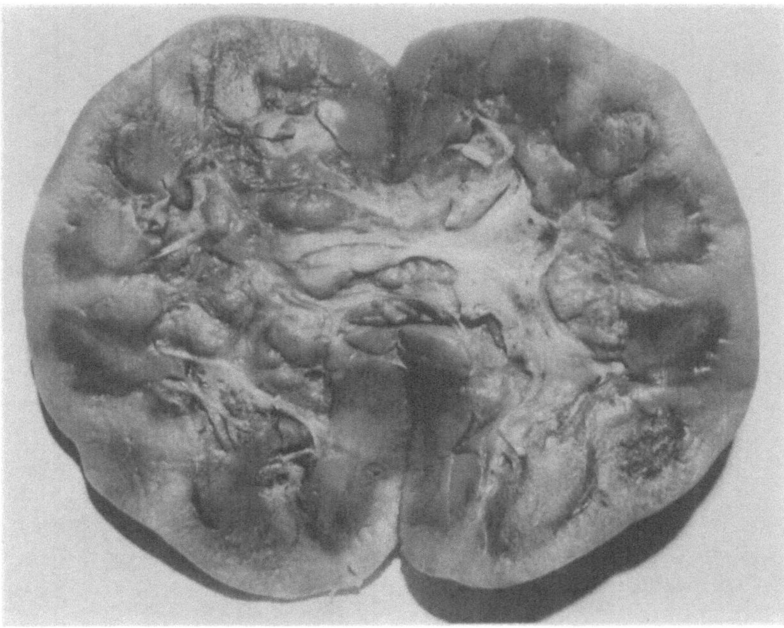

Fig. 1. Human mercuric chloride nephropathy. ♀ aged 20 y., death twelve days after ingestion of approximately 2 gm of mercuric chloride. Weight of both kidneys: 590 gm

extensive necrosis of epithelial cells, as shown by Oliver et al. [43] using the microdissection technique. After epithelial destruction, the basement membrane remains as the only layer which separates the tubular lumens from the capillaries (Fig. 4). 2 to 3 days after acute toxic damage, the tubular epithelial layer begins to be regenerated. Mitoses appear in epithelial cells close to the necrotic zone (Fig. 14). If the intoxicated subject survives for more than 3 to 4 days with acute tubular necrosis, there occurs a more or less pronounced interstitial edema together with a lympho-plasmocytic infiltration of the interstitial space (Fig. 5). At this stage, necrotic desquamated epithelial cells are no longer visible in cortical tubules, since they usually have been carried away by the tubular fluid. They sometimes are caught in the thin parts of Henle's loops. Necrotic epithelial cells tend to become calcified not earlier than 4 days after acute damage. Such calcification is characteristic for intoxication with mercuric chloride (Fig. 5), but is also found after intoxications with chloroform [25] or hexadimethrin-bromide (Polybrene) [35].

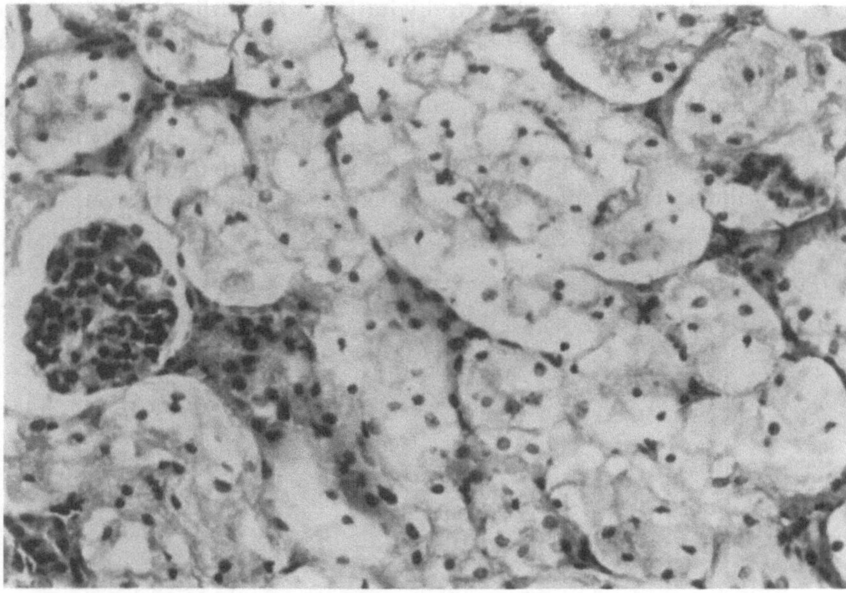

Fig. 2. Tartrate nephropathy. Rat. Renal cortex. Six hours after i.p. injection of 2.5 mg/kg of sodium-potassium-tartrate at pH 7.2. Marked swelling of proximal tubular epithelial cells by fluid retention. (× 350)

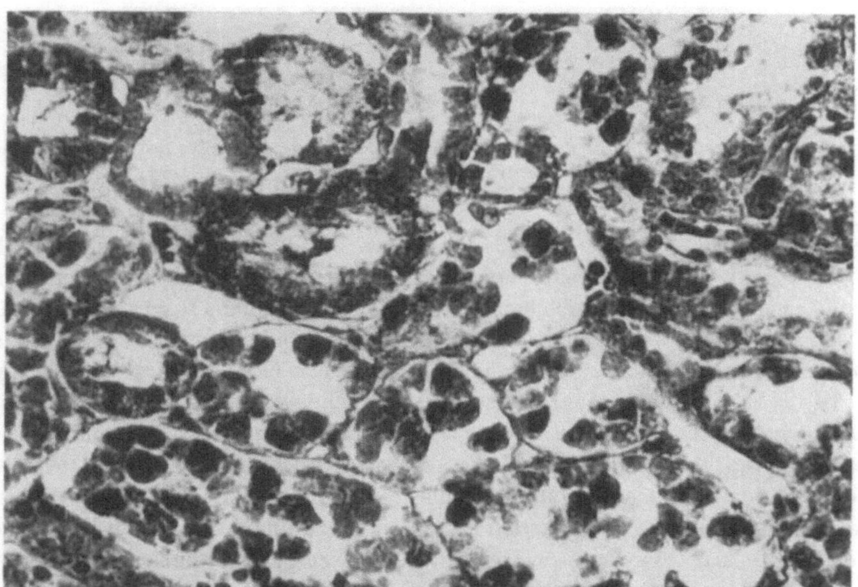

Fig. 3. Sublimate nephropathy. Rat. Renal cortex. Twenty hours after i.p. injection of 1 mg/kg mercuric chloride. Coagulation necrosis of epithelial cells of the pars recta of proximal tubules. Epithelium detached from the intact basement membrane. (× 400)

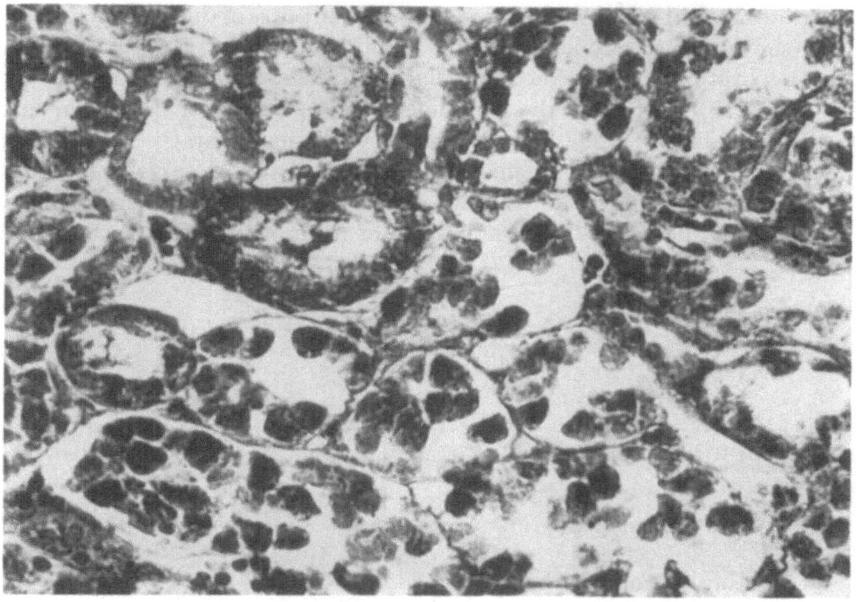

Fig. 4. Nephropathy caused by hexadimethrine bromide. Rat. Outer medulla. Twenty-four hours after i.v. injection of 32 mg/kg hexadimethrine bromide. Necrosis of epithelial cells in Henle's loops. Intact tubular basement membranes. (× 400)

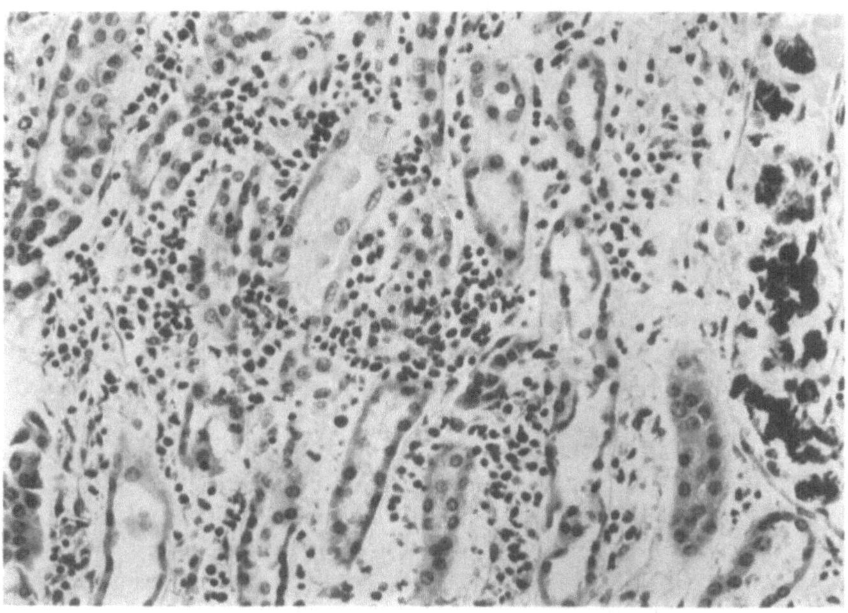

Fig. 5. Human mercuric chloride nephropathy. ♀, 20 y. Twelve days after ingestion of approximately 2 gm of mercuric chloride. Edema and interstitial infiltration at the medullary-cortical border. Dystrophic calcification of tubular epithelia. (× 225)

Nephrotoxins differ mainly by damaging different sites of the nephrons. SUZUKI [59] has shown, in experiments on the cellular deposition of vital dyes, that different nephrotoxins act on the nephrons at different levels. These results were confirmed and completed by the experiments of OLIVER et al. [43] who introduced the microdissection method. Different localizations characteristic for different nephrotoxins can only be demonstrated with shmall doses of nephrotoxin and by examining the kidneys within the first minutes or hours after administration of the toxic substance. With high doses of nephrotoxins the whole nephron

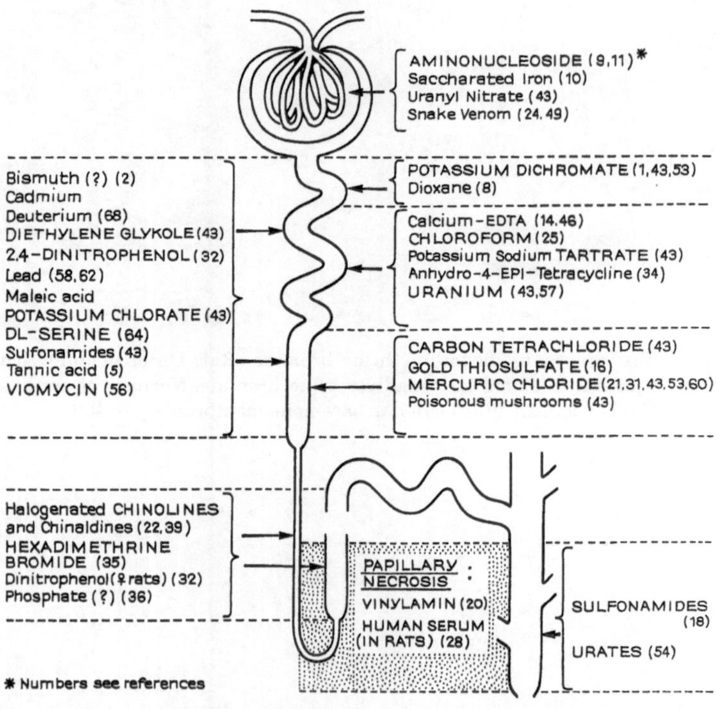

Fig. 6. Localization of nephrotoxic damage in various forms of poisoning

is usually damaged. Furthermore, high doses of nephrotoxins tend to cause circulatory disturbances which further modify the microscopic picture [50]. Finally, there are species differences in the localization of epithelial necrosis at different tubular levels (Fig. 6).

The best method for localizing nephrotoxic effects is micro-dissection. In the usual microscopic slices identification of different parts of the tubules is difficult under pathological conditions [43, 54, 67]. Identification of tubular segments is facilitated, in our experience, by the use of enzyme histochemistry. We used the method developed by MEIER and SIMON [38]: a kidney of an experimental animal and a control kidney are simultaneously frozen on the freezing table and the cryostat-sections obtained from both kidney are incubated simultaneously. It, thus, becomes possible to compare the enzyme activities in the experimental and control animals (Fig. 7). Damage to the rat kidney by tartrate causes a complete loss of non-specific α-naphthyl-esterase activity in the proximal convolutions, while the enzyme activity does not disappear from the lower parts of the proximal tubules (Fig. 7)[2]. In contrast, in animals intoxicated with mercuric chloride, the enzyme activity disappears from the lower half of the proximal tubule, while it remains unchanged in the outer cortical zone (Fig. 8). Damage to the thick part of the ascending limb of Henle's loop may be demonstrated by a decrease in the activity of succinic dehydrogenase or of lactic dehydrogenase which are

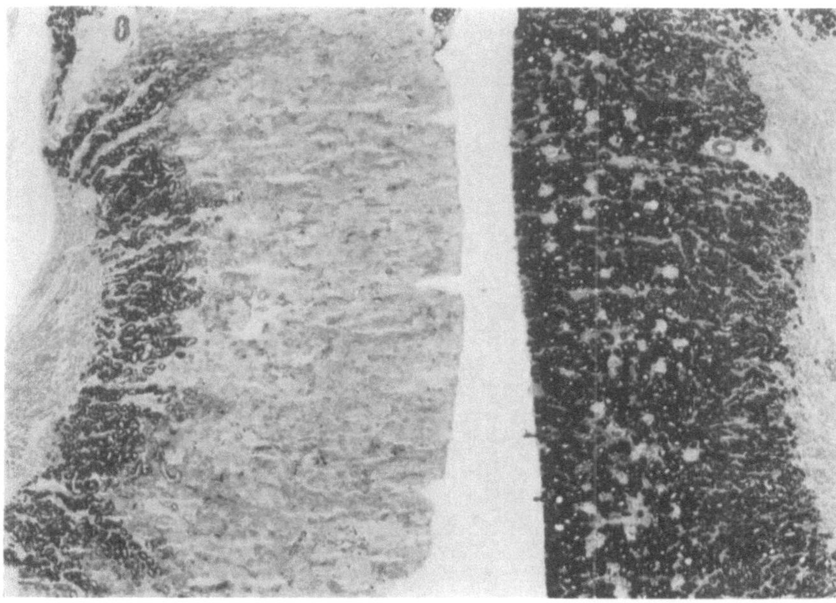

Fig. 7. Tartrate nephropathy. Rat. Renal cortex. Six hours after 2.5 mg/kg sodium-potassium-tartrate i.p. Non-specific alpha-naphthyl-esterase according to GÖSSNER (see 39). Incubation time: 4 min. Loss of enzyme activity in the outer cortex. Right side: control kidney incubated simultaneously

both normally present in high concentrations in this part of the nephron. Intoxication with hexadimethrine bromide considerably depresses the succinic dehydrogenase activity in the thick parts of the ascending limbs. The activity is only very slightly depressed in the pars recta of the proximal tubule and remains unchanged in the proximal convolutions (Fig. 9).

The causes of the different topographical distribution of tubular damage with different nephrotoxins are still largely unknown. The absence of visible damage to the glomeruli, which are the first renal structures to be reached by the toxic substances, is surprising. ZOLLINGER [67] stated that light microscopy often demonstrates a discrete non-specific glomerulo-nephrosis. Electron microscopy, however, shows only very slight changes of glomerular capillaries in the early stages of most types of toxic damage to the kidney, at a time when necrotic changes of tubular cells are already fairly prevalent [5, 8, 22, 26, 65]. The selective

2. The histochemical methods are described in the legends.

attack of nephrotoxins on proximal tubular cells may be due to the fact that these cells are the first highly differentiated cells of the nephron which are reached by the nephrotoxins in adequate concentrations. This applies particularly to nephrotoxins which are filtered through the glomeruli and are then concentrated, either in tubular fluid or in the tubular cells, as a consequence of water and salt reabsorption. Even nephrotoxins bound to serum proteins and, therefore, escaping glomerular filtration, may reach renal cells by peritubular

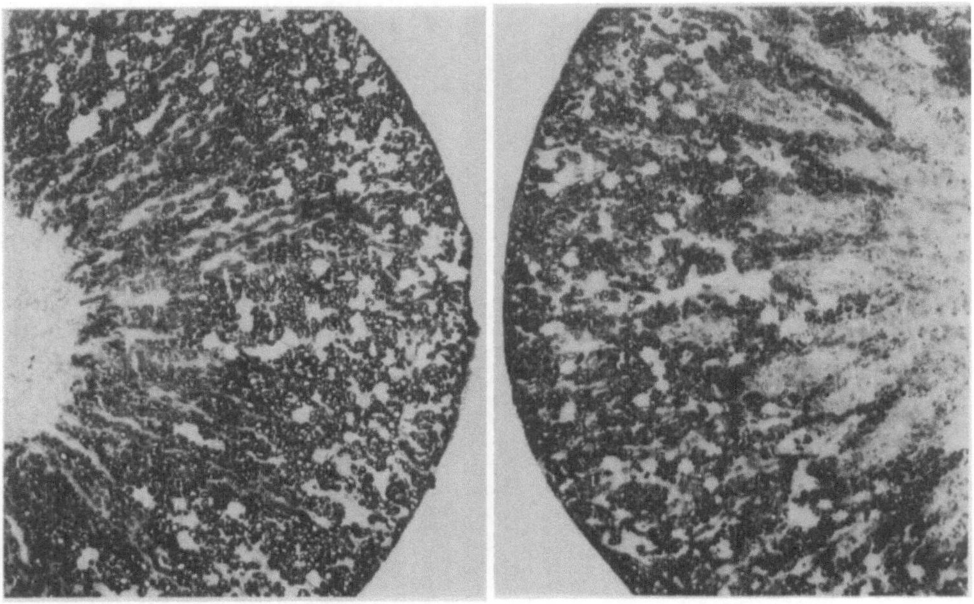

Fig. 8. Sublimate nephropathy. Rat. Renal cortex. Twenty-four hours after 1.0 mg/kg mercuric chloride i.p. Reaction for non-specific alpha-naphthyl-esterase. Decrease of enzyme activity in the inner cortex with normal activity in the outer cortex. Right side: control kidney incubated simultaneously-

capillaries in higher concentrations than cells of other tissues. It is, however, not clear why some nephrotoxins attack preferably the upper half, and others preferably the lower half, of the proximal tubules. The point of attack of a nephrotoxin within the proximal tubule may depend on its molecular weight, since Gerard and Cordier [19] showed that the site of reabsorption of proteins depends on molecular weight: low molecular weight proteins are reabsorped in the upper proximal convolutions, while the site of reabsorption descends down to the pars recta as a function of increasing molecular weight. Simonds and Heplar [53] conclude that the site of damage in intoxications with metal salts depends on the atomic weight of the metal: with increasing atomic weight the site of damage tends to be displaced towards the pars recta.

Damage to the thick part of the ascending limb of Henle‘s loop, may be due to a low grade of nephrotoxicity of the offending substance. In this case the concentration in proximal tubular fluid may not rise sufficiently to induce damage to the epithelial cells, while the abstraction of water from tubular fluid in the

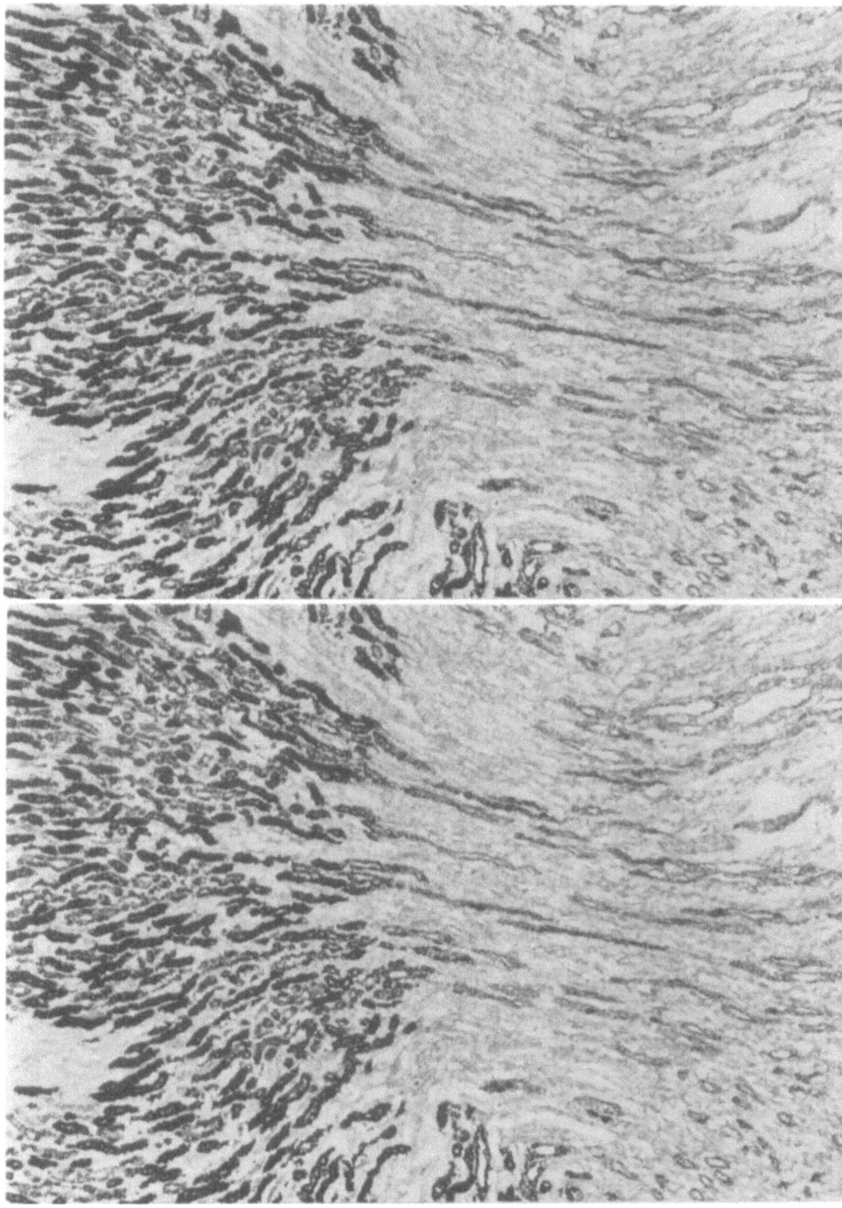

Fig. 9. Nephropathy due to hexadimethrine bromide. Rat. Outer medulla. 48 hours after 16 mg/kg hexadimethrine bromide i.v. Demonstration of lactic dehydrogenase according to HESS et al. (see 39). Incubation for 20 min. Extensive loss of enzyme activities in epithelial cells of Henle's loops. Left side: control kidney incubated simultaneously

hairpin-countercurrent system of Henle's loop may raise the concentration to toxic levels in the early distal tubules. Preferential damage to the thick part of the ascending limb may be due to the high degree of differentiation of the cells at this site, which have a complicated ultrastructure and high enzyme activities. The less differentiated thin part of Henle's loop and the equally less differentiated collecting ducts are apparently less sensitive. The hypothesis that urinary concentration occurring in Henle's loop is responsible for nephrotoxic damage to medullary early distal tubules is supported by observations by MEIER-RUGE [40]. He showed that halogenated quinoline derivatives induce distal tubular damage only in animals capable of elaborating a highly concentrated urine. The most severe grades of damage were found in desert rats, while the damage was less severe in ordinary white rats or in golden hamsters. In the cat, the dog and in man the quinoline derivatives do not damage the kidneys.

As stated above, the morphologic appearance of tubular damage as revealed by light microscopy is usually similar for different nephrotoxins. The hope that there might be specific *ultrastructural changes* in renal damage induced by different nephrotoxins has not yet been fulfilled. Electron microscopic studies on early changes in tubular epithelial cells under the influence of different nephrotoxins yielded quite similar pictures [5, 7, 8, 16, 22, 26, 30, 37, 41, 57, 58, 62, 65, 66, 68]. Though the site of damage differs with different nephrotoxins, the type and pattern of ultrastructural changes remain the same. The main changes are related to disturbances in the transport of fluid through the tubular cells (Table 2). Such disturbances first cause the appearance of an increased number of vesicles in the apical pole of the cell. Within the first hours after an intoxication, these vesicles are transformed into smaller or larger vacuoles, which first remain limited to the apical part of the cytoplasm, but later reach the basal part. At this time the cytoplasm is diluted by fluid and the whole cell swells. In the apical part of the cell, the vacuoles blister and extend into the tubular lumen (Fig. 10).

Table 2. *Renal tubular fine structure during reaction to various nephrotoxins*

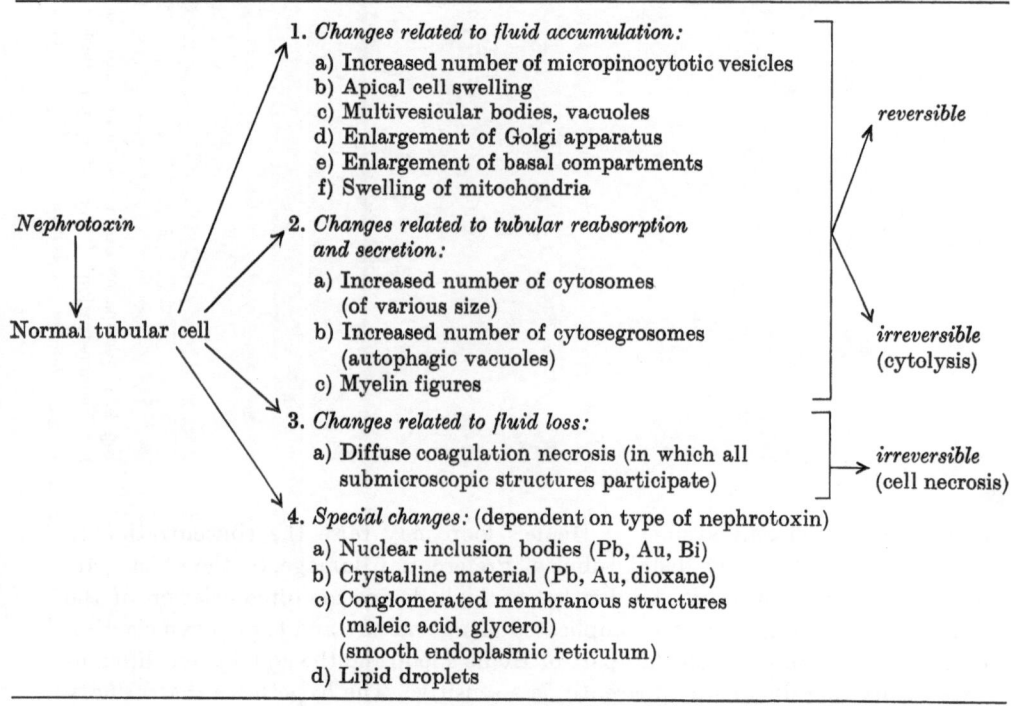

Nephrotoxin ↓ Normal tubular cell →	1. *Changes related to fluid accumulation:* a) Increased number of micropinocytotic vesicles b) Apical cell swelling c) Multivesicular bodies, vacuoles d) Enlargement of Golgi apparatus e) Enlargement of basal compartments f) Swelling of mitochondria 2. *Changes related to tubular reabsorption and secretion:* a) Increased number of cytosomes (of various size) b) Increased number of cytosegrosomes (autophagic vacuoles) c) Myelin figures	(1. and 2.) → *reversible* / → *irreversible* (cytolysis)
	3. *Changes related to fluid loss:* a) Diffuse coagulation necrosis (in which all submicroscopic structures participate)	→ *irreversible* (cell necrosis)
	4. *Special changes:* (dependent on type of nephrotoxin) a) Nuclear inclusion bodies (Pb, Au, Bi) b) Crystalline material (Pb, Au, dioxane) c) Conglomerated membranous structures (maleic acid, glycerol) (smooth endoplasmic reticulum) d) Lipid droplets	

With increasing cellular swelling the apical cell membrane is torn; a fraction of the cytoplasm flows into the tubular lumen (Fig. 11). The basement membrane of the tubule remains intact. Even after destruction of an epithelial cell, fragments of the cell-base remain attached to the basement membrane. Rarely, one sees an enlargement of basal compartments. The brush-border is well preserved in the first hours after intoxication, but soon begins to become sparse. In early stages of intoxication the mitochondria show an either increased or decreased density, while the outer and inner membranes are intact. The Golgi-complex is often enlarged, while the endoplasmic reticulum is unchanged. In later stages the mitochondria may swell more markedly and the cristae may be destroyed. Besides these changes, which are characteristic consequences of cellular overhydration and which induce necrosis by cytolysis, there is usually an increase in the number of electron dense small bodies of various size and shape ("cytosomes"). The cytosomes are mainly found in the apical parts of the cells. Besides, one also finds cytosegrosomes, i.e. inclusion bodies containing cell organells (Fig. 12). Cytosomes and cytosegrosomes usually occur simultaneously with cell swelling. Cell necrosis as a consequence of cellular dehydration is observed more rarely. In this type of damage, the density of the cytoplasm as well as of cell organells increases, while the nuclei become pycnotic [65]. In electron microscopic studies, the differences in sensitivity of different cells to toxic damage appear still more impressive than in light microscopic studies. In one section through a tubule, cells with marked hydropic changes or undergoing cytolysis may be seen next to completely intact cells (Fig. 13). Factors which may be responsible for the different sensitivity may be an alternating activity of different cells [61] or the co-existence of cells of different ages within the epithelial layer [48].

Electron microscopic and histochemical studies contribute to the understanding of the mechanism of toxic damage to the kidney and of cell destruction, though this mechanism is still largely unknown. The major primary morphological change is an edematous swelling of the cell, which is explained as a consequence of failure of cellular energy production needed for the functioning of pumps responsible for maintaining the normal ionic composition of the cellular fluid [6]. A deficient energy production by the mitochondria may depress the activity of the pumps, while their efficacy may simultaneously be limited by changes in permeability of the cell membrane. At the same time, catabolic hydrolysis of cellular proteins causes an accumulation of osmotically active material within the cell [61]. An increased number of cytosomes and cytosegrosomes denotes a disturbance of reabsorption and excretion by tubular epithelial cells [12. 23].

The intra-cellular site of action of most nephrotoxins is still unknown. Mercury and other heavy metals are thought to block sulfhydryl groups of cellular proteins [17, 47]. 2,4-dinitrophenol inhibits adenosin-triphosphatase of cell membranes and mitochondria [32].

The possiblity has been raised that some other nephrotoxins may exert a primary effect on terminal blood vessels and induce tubular necrosis as a consequence of primary ischemia. An argument in favor of this hypothesis is the similarity of the electron microscopic picture of ischemic and toxic tubular damage [48]. In ischemic tubular damage swelling of the cells is also prevalent. As opposed to nephrotoxic changes, ischemic changes are usually accompanied

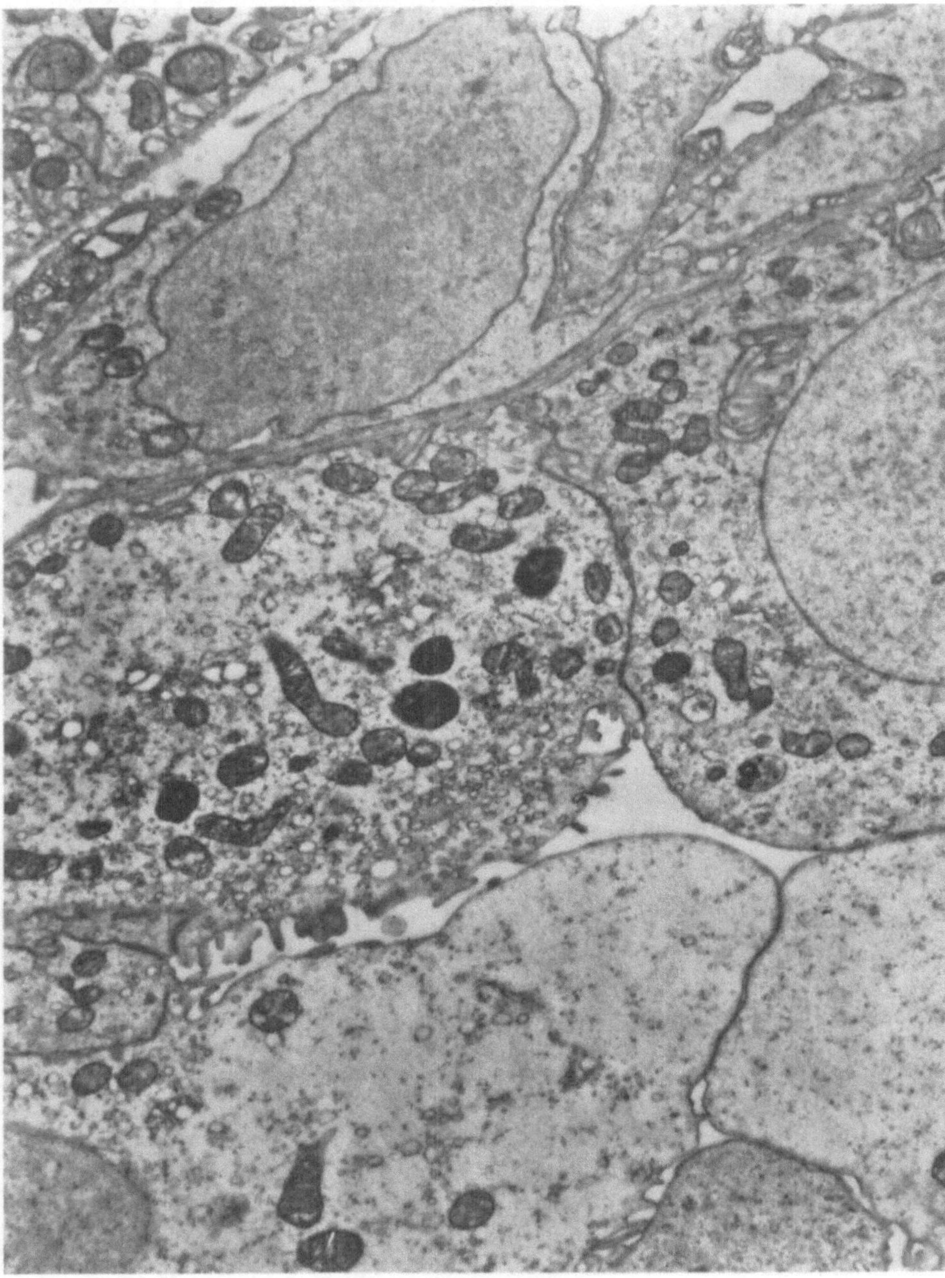

Fig. 10. Nephropathy due to halogenated quinaldine. Rat. 48 hours after 200 mg/kg of 5,7-dichloro-8-hydroxyquinaldine. Thick part of ascending limb of Henle's loop. Apical vesicles with narrowing of the lumen. Increased vesiculation. (× 18,000)

by more pronounced mitochondrial alterations while there is no increase in the number of cytosomes [61]. As opposed to toxic nephropathy, ischemic nephropathy rarely proceeds to epithelial necrosis [4, 61, 63]. However many nephrotoxins are known to cause focal ischemia when injected in large doses [43, 50].

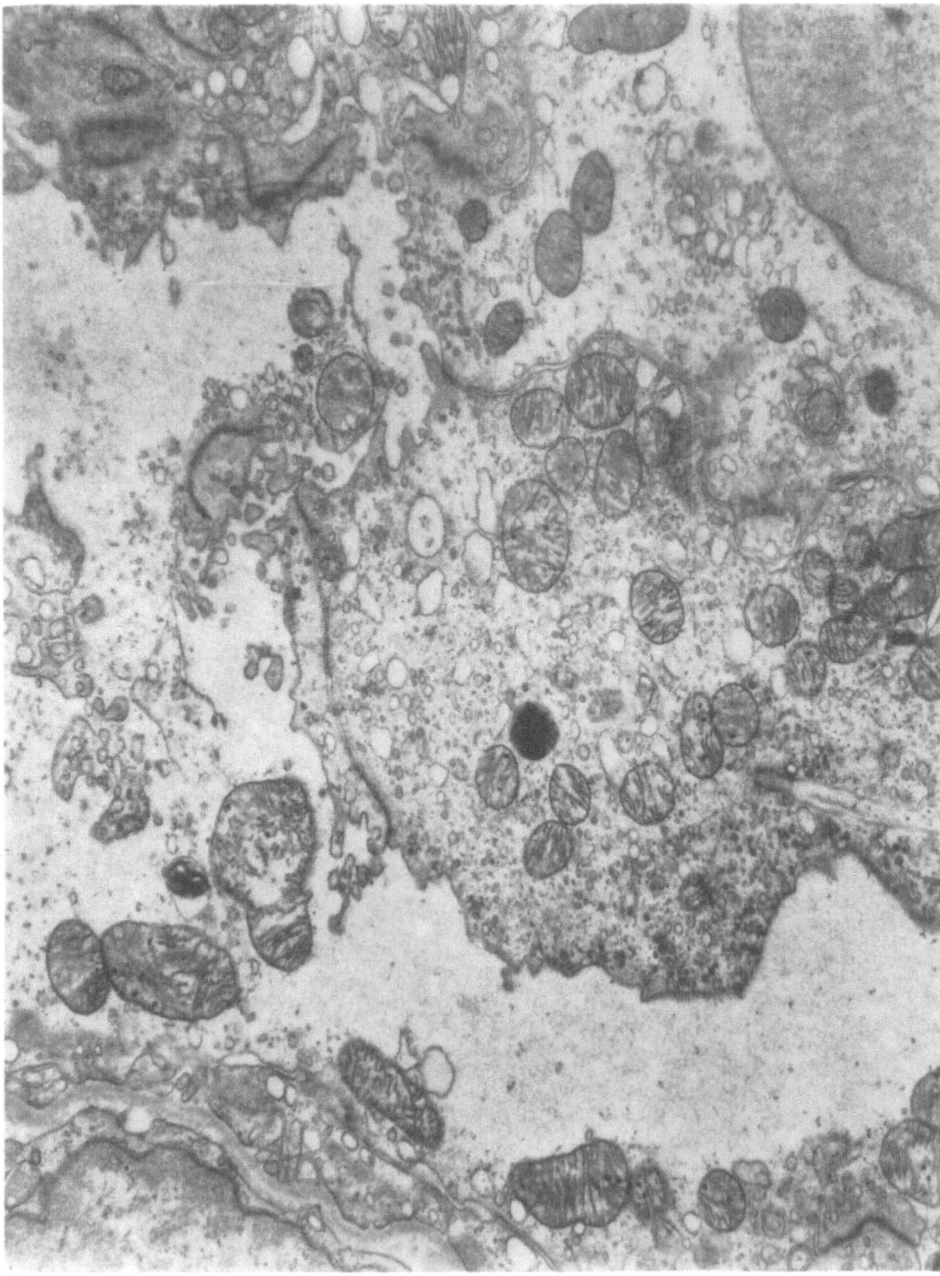

Fig. 11. Nephropathy due to halogenated quinaldine. Rat. 7 days after daily oral administration of 200 mg/kg of 5,7-dichloro-8-hydroxyquinaldine. Thick part of ascending limb of Henle's loop. Cytolysis with rupture of the apical cell membrane and emptying of cell contents into the tubular lumen. Mitochondria well preserved. (× 16,000)

The focal ischemia after large doses of the nephrotoxins appears to represent an unrelated second type of damage, rather than a mechanism of nephrotoxic action. Most nephrotoxins are believed to interfere directly with cellular metabolism.

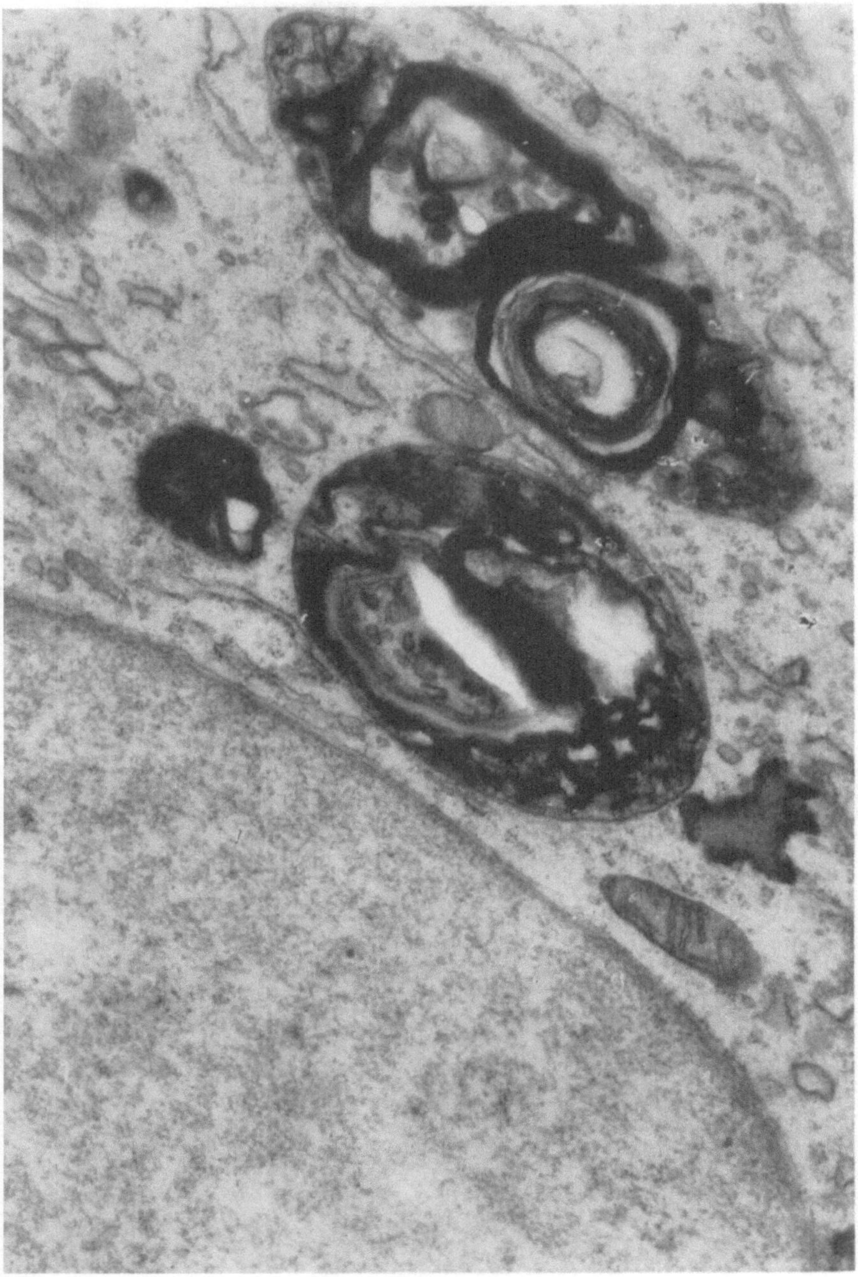

Fig. 12. Nephropathy due to halogenated quinaldine. Rat. 20 days after daily oral administration of 200 mg/kg of 5,7-dichloro-8-hydroxyquinaldine. Epithelial cells from the thick part of the ascending limb of Henle's loop. Cytosegrosomes and "myelin figures". (× 34,000)

Histoautoradiographic studies by Noltenius et al. [42] using H^3-thymidine showed that regeneration, after mercuric chloride nephropathy, begins after a latent period of approximately 72 hours. Regeneration reaches its highest rate on the 5th to 7th day; it is practically complete by the 10th day. Cells are

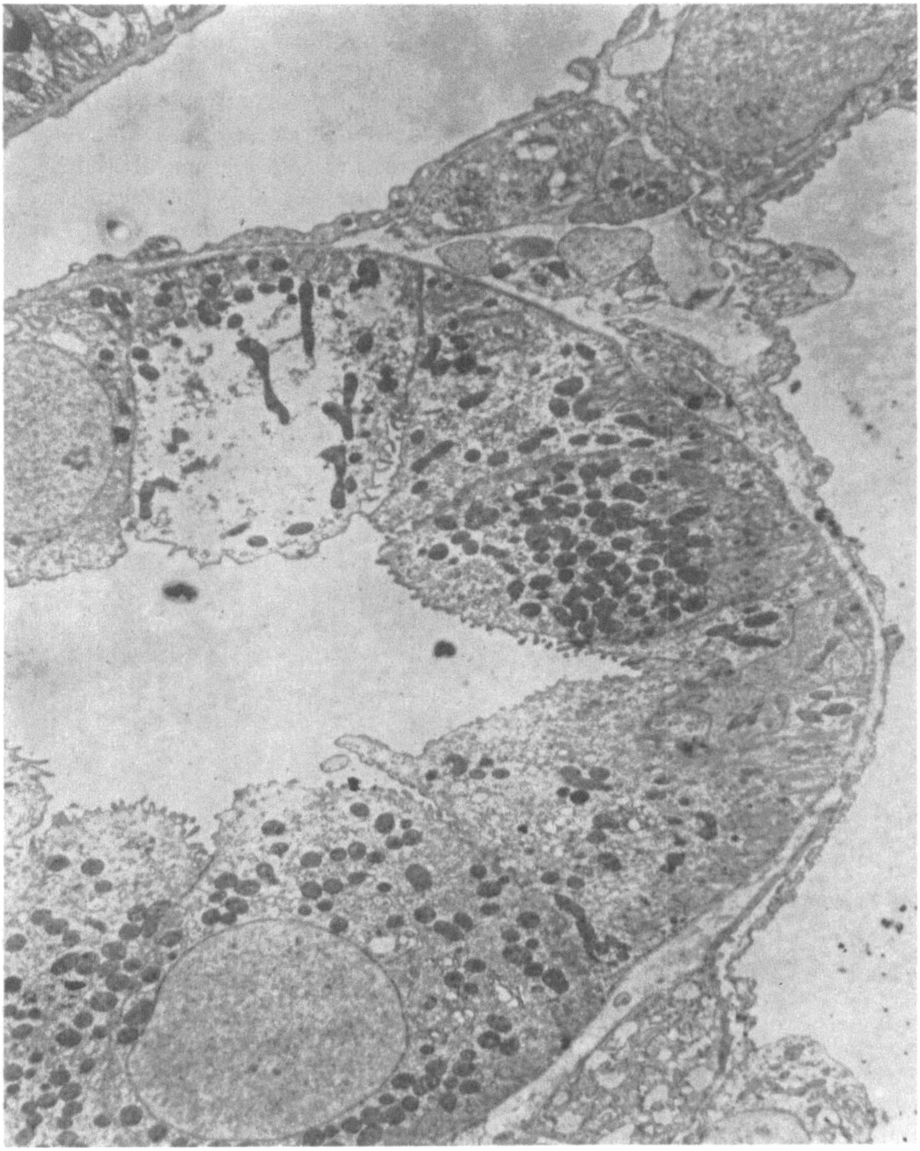

Fig. 13. Nephropathy due to halogenated quinaldine. Rat. Treatment as in fig. 10. Thick part of ascending limb of Henle's loop: difference in sensitivity of neighboring cells. Hydropic next to intact cells. (× 8,600)

regenerated by the surviving cells at the margins of the necrotic zone. On the 2nd and 3rd days after damage, many mitoses can be seen in these regions. The new epithelial cells first appear flat (Fig. 14). A continuous layer of cells covering the whole luminal surface of the tubule is found after 5 to 7 days. The new epithelial cells at first lack histochemically detectable enzyme activity. Acid phosphatase and non-specific esterase activities first appear on the 3rd day. Succinic dehydrogenase, lactic dehydrogenase and NAD-cytochrome-C-reductase can first be demonstrated on the 7th day. The last enzymatic activity to reappear is alcaline phosphatase in the brush border [1, 32]. The ability of tubular epithelial cells to store vital dyes and proteins is a particularly sensitive indicator of the functional competence of tubular cells: it recovers its original efficacy 15 to 20 days after damage [33, 55]. The ultrastructural changes in regenerating epithelial cells reflect the progressive maturation found in the histochemical studies. Newly formed epithelial cells have a swollen nucleus and a cytoplasm of low

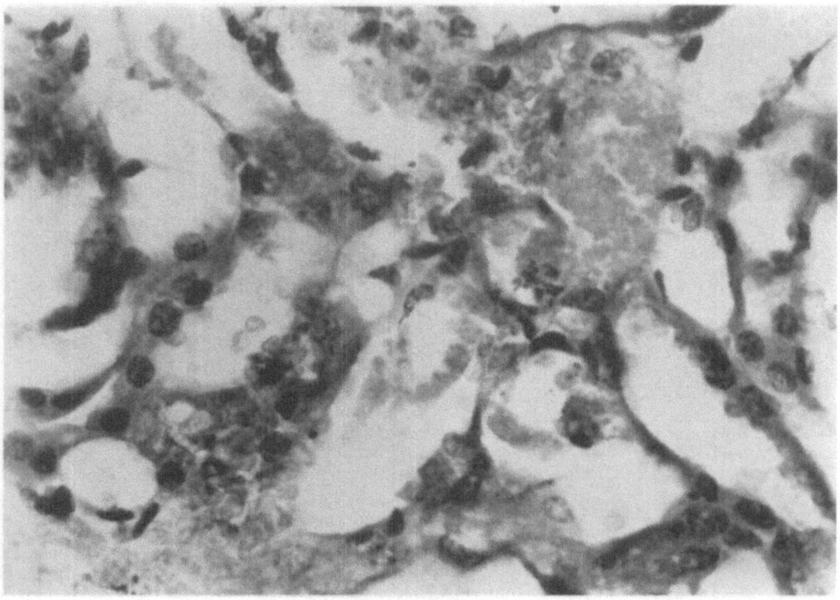

Fig. 14. Nephropathy due to hexadimethrin-bromide. Rat. Outer medulla. 72 hours after 32 mg/kg 5,7-dichloro-8-hydroxyquinaldine i. v. Regenerative mitotic activity in the vicinity of a necrotic focus. (× 600)

density containing many small vesicles. The mitochondria at first are small, sparse and distributed evenly over the whole cytoplasm. The brush border appears disorganized. With increasing maturation the mitochondria increase in size and become grouped in the basal cell compartments. The brush border regains its usual shape [26, 44]. During maturation the newly formed epithelia are insensitive to toxins and ischemia [45, 55]. The continuity of the nephron during regeneration is preserved by the survival of the basement membranes which are seldom ruptured in toxic nephropathies. According to Oliver et al. [43] this fact constitutes the main difference between toxic and ischemic nephropathies. Ischemic nephropathy induced tubulorhexis with rupture of the basement membrane. Epithelial regeneration begins as rapidly as in toxic nephropathies but does not re-establish the continuity of the tubule. These morphologic findings are in agreement with the clinical observation that functional revovery in toxic nephropathies is better than in ischemic nephropathies [27].

Summary

Light microscopic, electron microscopic and histochemical findings in acute toxic nephropathies are discussed. Nephrotoxins are substances which, in animal experiments, cause reproducible and dose-dependent renal damage. Though belonging to many different chemical classes, different nephrotoxins usually induce strikingly similar histological changes. The main changes are necrosis of tubular epithelia. Different nephrotoxins differ in the site of the main tubular damage. Most nephrotoxins act on the proximal tubules. No specific changes characteristic for a given nephrotoxic substance could, until now, be demonstrated by electron microscopy or histochemistry. The electron microscopic picture is characterized by hydropic cell swelling, presumably due to disturbances of the liquid transport through the cell membrane and by metabolic disturbances resulting in an increased number of cytosomes. These changes are independent of the type of nephrotoxin responsible for the damage. The pathogenetic mechanisms of these changes and the morphological features of cellular regeneration are discussed.

References

1. Baines, A. D.: Cell renewal following dichromate induced renal tubular necrosis. An enzyme histochemical study. Amer. J. Path. **47**, 851—876 (1965).
2. Beaver, D. L., and R. E. Burr: Electron microscopy of bismuth inclusions. Amer. J. Path. **42**, 609—618 (1963).
3. Bluemle, L. W., C. D. Webster, and R. J. Elkinton: Acute tubular necrosis. Arch. intern. Med. **104**, 180—186 (1959).
4. Bohle, A.: Pathologische Anatomie des akuten Nierenversagens. Verh. dtsch. Ges. Path. **49**, 56—66 (1965).
5. Boler, R. K., J. S. Broom, and R. B. Arhelger: Ultrastructural renal alterations following tannic acid administration to rabbits. Amer. J. Path. **49**, 15—32 (1966).
6. Burck, H. C.: Die Zellschwellung als Folge des passiven Wasserwechsels. Ionenbilanzstudien an inkubierten Leberschnitten. Virchows Arch. path. Anat. **336**, 326—341 (1963).
7. Caesar, R.: Die Bedeutung der Lysosomen für die formale Genese der Viomycin-Nephrose. Verh. dtsch. Ges. Path. **49**, 157—161 (1965).
8. David, H.: Elektronenmikroskopische Befunde bei der dioxanbedingten Nephrose der Rattenniere. Beitr. path. Anat. **130**, 187—212 (1964).
9. Dubach, U. C.: Aminonucleosid-Nephrose. Fortschr. Arzneimittel-Forsch. **7**, 341—463 (1964).
10. Ellis, J. T.: Glomerular lesions and the nephrotic syndrome in rabbits given sacchareted iron dioxide intravenously, with special reference to the part played by intracapillary precipitates in the pathogenesis of the lesions. J. exp. Med. **103**, 207—210 (1956).
11. Ericsson, J. L. E., and G. A. Andres: Electron microscopic studies on the development of the glomerular lesions in aminonucleoside nephrosis. Amer. J. Path. **39**, 643—663 (1961).
12. — B. F. Trump, and J. Weibel: Electron microscopic studies of the proximal tubule of the rat kidney. Lab. Invest. **14**, 1341—1365 (1965).
13. Fink, H. E., W. J. Roenigk, and G. P. Wilson: An experimental investigation of the nephrotoxic effects of oral cholecystographic agents. Amer. J. med. Sci. **247**, 201—215 (1964).
14. Foreman, H., C. Finnegan, and C. C. Lushbangh: Nephrotoxic hazard from uncontrolled edethamil calcium-disodium therapy. J. Amer. med. Ass. **160**, 1042—1046 (1956).
15. Foster, C. L., and E. Cameron: Observations on the histological effects of subletal doses of cadmium chloride in the rabbit. II. The effect on the kidney cortex. J. Anat. (Lond.) **97**, 281—288 (1963).

16. Ganote, C. E., D. L. Beaver, and H. L. Moses: Renal gold inclusions. Arch. Path. **81**, 431—438 (1966).
17. Gayer, J., u. R. Partowi: Ein Beitrag zur Pathogenese der Sublimatnephrose. Z. ges. exp. Med. **135**, 419—430 (1962).
18. Geiser, W.: Experimentell erzeugte chronisch-interstitielle Nephritis. Virchows Arch. path. Anat. **330**, 463—482 (1957).
19. Gérard, P., et R. Cordier: Sur l'interprétation des altérations morphologiques caractéristiques observées dans le rein au cours de la néphrose lipidique. Arch. int. Méd. exp. 8, 225—235 (1933).
20. Gloor, F., et M. Jenny: Nécrose papillaire et néphrite interstitielle chronique (Étude expérimentale). Helv. med. Acta **27**, 218—227 (1960).
21. Harber, M. H., and R. B. Jennings: Renal response of the rat to mercury. Arch. Path. **79**, 218—222 (1965).
22. Hodel, C., F. Gloor u. W. Meier-Ruge: Elektronenmikroskopische und histochemische Befunde bei primären Alterationen am distalen Nierentubulus. Verh. dtsch. Ges. Path. **49**, 162—167 (1965).
23. Hruban, Z., B. Spargo, H. Swift, R. W. Wissler, and R. G. Kleinfeld: Focal cytoplasmic degradation. Amer. J. Path. **42**, 657—684 (1963).
24. Huth, F., u. E. McClure: Morphologische Veränderungen der Nieren von Kaninchen nach Injektion von Schlangengift (Bothrops jararaca). Frankfurt. Z. Path. **74**, 91—108 (1964).
25. Jacobsen, L., E. K. Anderson, and J. V. Thorberg: Accidental chloroform nephrosis in mice. Acta path. microbiol. scand. **61**, 503—513 (1964).
26. Kemmer, Ch., K. D. Kunze u. W. R. Herrmann: Das elektronenmikroskopische Bild der Rattenniere nach oraler Applikation von 2,4-Dinitrophenol (DNP). Frankfurt. Z. Path, **77**, 83—97 (1967).
27. Kiley, J. E., S. R. Powers, and R. T. Beebe: Acute renal failure. New Engl. J. Med. **262**, 481—486 (1960).
28. Klavins, J. V., P. L. Patrick, and D. J. Kroe: Experimental renal papillary necrosis. Fed. Proc. **22**, 549—550 (1963).
29. Kleeman, C. R., and M. H. Maxwell: The nephrotoxicity of antibiotics. In: Biology of pyelonephritis. Boston: Little, Brown & Co. 1960.
30. Klein, H. J., E. Steinbach u. N. Schümmelfeder: Ultrastrukturelle und histochemische Untersuchungen zur Entstehung der Viomycin-Nephrose. Frankfurt. Z. Path. **75**, 432—445 (1966).
31. Kriz, W.: Histophysiologische Untersuchung an der Rattenniere bei Sublimatvergiftung. Z. Zellforsch. **57**, 914—952 (1962).
32. Kunze, K. D., u. W. R. Herrmann: Histologische und fermenthistochemische Befunde an der Rattenniere nach oraler Belastung mit 2,4-Dinitrophenol. Frankfurt. Z. Path. **76**, 213—226 (1967).
33. Lapp, H., u. K. Schafé: Morphologische, histochemische und Speicherungs-Untersuchungen über den Verlauf der Sublimatnephrose bei der Ratte. Beitr. path. Anat. **123**, 77—100 (1960).
34. Lowe, B. M., D. Obst, and E. Tapp: Renal damage caused by anhydro-4-epi-tetracycline. Arch. Path. **81**, 362—364 (1965).
35. Lutterbeck, P., F. Gloor, W. Meier-Ruge, and E. C. Yasargil: Localization of renal dysfunction following polybrene medication. J. cardiovasc. Surg. (Torino) 8, 515—519 (1967).
36. MacFarlane, D.: Zit. nach K. O. Rother, Experimentelle Nierenkrankheiten. In: Handbuch der experimentellen Pharmakologie, Bd. XVI/4. Berlin-Heidelberg-New York: Springer 1965.
37. Martines, G.: Ultrastructural findings of rat kidney treated with carbon tetrachloride. Riv. Pat. Clin. **6**, 171 (1965).
38. Meier, W., u. H. Simon: Über eine Möglichkeit zur halbquantitativen Auswertung histochemischer Fermentnachweise und anderer histochemischer Reaktionen. Acta histochem. (Jena) 8, 1—8 (1959).

39. MEIER-RUGE, W.: Untersuchungen über primäre Alterationen am distalen Nierentubulus der Ratte mit Störung des Haarnadelgegenstromsystems. Virchows Arch. path. Anat. **337**, 470—482 (1964).
40. — Der Aussagewert des experimentellen pathologischen Nierenbefundes für die Pathologie der menschlichen Niere. Path. Microbiol. **30**, 266—282 (1967).
41. MÖLBERT, E., D. KUHN u. F. BÜCHNER: Elektronenmikroskopische Untersuchungen am Tubulusepithel der Niere sublimatvergifteter Ratten. Beitr. path. Anat. **129**, 222—246 (1963/64).
42. NOLTENIUS, H., H. SCHELLHAS u. W. OEHLERT: Histoautoradiographische Untersuchungen mit 3H-Thymidin der Tubulusregeneration nach akuter Sublimatvergiftung von Ratten. Beitr. path. Anat. **129**, 90—117 (1963/64).
43. OLIVER, J., M. MACDOWELL, and A. TRACY: The pathogenesis of acute renal failure associated with traumatic and toxic injury. J. clin. Invest. **30**, 1305—1440 (1951).
44. PORTE, A., Y. CUSSAC, P. STOEBNER et J. P. ZAHND: Sur la formation et l'ultrastructure des "cellules de régéneration" dans les tubes rénaux de souris intoxiquées par le nitrate d'uranyle. C. R. Soc. Biol. (Paris) **157**, 2079—2081 (1963).
45. REBER, K.: Blockierung der Speicherfunktion der Niere als Schutz bei Sublimatvergiftung. Schweiz. Z. Path. **16**, 755—771 (1953).
46. REUBER, M. D.: Accentuation of Ca edetate nephrosis by cortisone. Arch. Path. **76**, 382—386 (1963).
47. RODIN, A. E., and C. N. CROWSON: Mercury nephrotoxicity in the rat. II. Investigation of the intracellular site of mercury nephrotoxicity by correlated serial tissue histologic and histoenzymatic studies. Amer. J. Path. **41**, 485—495 (1962).
48. ROTTER, W., H. LAPP u. H. ZIMMERMANN: Pathogenese und morphologisches Substrat des „akuten Nierenversagens" und seine Erholungszeit. Dtsch. med. Wschr. **87**, 669—677 (1962).
49. SAKAGUCHI, H., and S. KAWAMURA: Electron microscopic observations of the mesangiolysis. The toxic effects of the "Habu snake" venom on the renal glomerulus. Keiô J. Med. **12**, 99—106 (1963).
50. SCHLEGEL, J. U., and J. B. MOSES: A method for visualization of kidney blood vessels applied to studies of the crush syndrome. Proc. Soc. exp. Biol. (N.Y.) **74**, 832—837 (1950).
51. SCHREINER, G. E.: Nephrotoxicity and diagnostic agents. J. Amer. med. Ass. **196**, 413—415 (1966).
52. —, and J. F. MAHER: Toxic nephropathy. Amer. J. Med. **38**, 409—432 (1965).
53. SIMONDS, J. P., and O. E. HEPLER: Experimental nephropathies I. A method of producing controlled selective injury of renal units by means of chemical agents. Arch. Path. **39**, 103—108 (1945).
54. SMITH, J. F., and YIN CHEN LEE: Experimental uric acid nephritis in the rabbit. J. exp. Med. **105**, 615—621 (1957).
55. STAEMMLER, M.: Die akuten Nephrosen. IV. Tubuläre Schädigung und Wiederherstellung. Virchows Arch. path. Anat. **330**, 139—155 (1957).
56. —, u. B. KARKHOFF: Die akuten Nephrosen. II. Nierenschäden durch Antibiotika. Virchows Arch. path. Anat. **328**, 481—502 (1956).
57. STONE, S. R., S. A. BENCOSME, H. LATTA, and S. C. MADDEN: Renal tubular fine structure. Studied during reaction to acute uranium injury. Arch. Path. **71**, 160—174 (1961).
58. SUN, C. N., R. A. GOYER, M. MELLIES, and M. W. YIN: The renal tubule in experimental lead intoxication. Arch. Path. **82**, 156—163 (1966).
59. SUZUKI, T.: Zur Morphologie der Nierensekretion unter pathologischen Bedingungen. Jena: Fischer 1912.
60. TAYLOR, N. S.: Histochemical studies of nephrotoxicity with sublethal doses of mercury in rats. Amer. J. Path. **46**, 1—22 (1965).
61. THOENES, W.: Mikromorphologie des Nephron nach temporärer Ischämie. Zwangslose Abhandlung aus dem Gebiet der normalen und pathologischen Anatomie, H. 15. Stuttgart: Georg Thieme 1964.

62. Totovíc, V.: Elektronenmikroskopische Untersuchungen an dem Tubulusapparat der Niere bei experimenteller chronischer Bleivergiftung der Ratte. Virchows Arch. path. Anat. **339**, 151—167 (1965).
63. — Elektronenmikroskopische Untersuchungen über das Verhalten der Hauptstückepithelien beim experimentellen Niereninfarkt der Ratte. Virchows Arch. path. Anat. **340**, 251—269 (1966).
64. Wachstein, M.: Nephrotoxic action of DL-serine in the rat. I. Localization of the renal damage, the phosphatase activity and the influence of age, sex, time and dose. Arch. Path. **43**, 503—514 (1947).
65. —, and M. Besen: Electron microscopy of renal coagulative necrosis due to DL-serine, with special reference to mitochondrial pyknosis. Amer. J. Path. **44**, 383—400 (1964).
66. Worthen, H. G.: Renal toxicity of maleic acid in the rat. Enzymatic and morphologic observations. Lab. Invest. **12**, 791—801 (1963).
67. Zollinger, H. U.: Niere und ableitende Harnwege. W. Doerr u. E. Uehlinger, Spezielle pathologische Anatomie, Bd. 3, S. 198. Berlin-Heidelberg-New York: Springer 1966.
68. Zunker, H. O. H., and D. G. McKay: Ultrastructural alterations in deuterium intoxication. Arch. Path. **82**, 18—26 (1966).

Discussion

Gessler:

In experiments on mercuric chloride intoxication, which we did a few years ago together with M. Steinhausen (Physiologisches Institut der Universität, Heidelberg), we regularly found a decrease in GFR and a prolonged tubular passage-time of lissamine-green. If the macula densa is not destroyed by the intoxication, it could possibly be responsible for the observed decrease in GFR. Do you find morphological changes in the region of the macula densa in mercurial nephropathy?

Gloor:

In our experiments with 1.0 mg/kg mercuric chloride i.p., in the rat, we did not find any morphological changes of the macula densa. The macula densa was not investigated by histochemical methods in these experiments.

2.1.2. Experimental Studies of Acute Renal Failure*

D. E. OKEN[1]

With 4 Figures

Despite marked variability in the etiologic circumstance and the histologic appearance of kidneys with acute renal failure, the end functional results appear to be quite comparable from case to case. Theories commonly suggested as the cause of renal insufficiency include tubular obstruction with casts, tubular obstruction by interstitial edema causing external compression of tubules, and passive back flow of filtrate through "holes" in the tubular epithelium. Some authors have postulated a vascular origin for the observed abnormalities. Because of the oliguria seen with acute renal failure, classical physiologic techniques have failed to distinguish between the possible mechanisms responsible for renal impairment. We, therefore, decided to study this problem utilizing renal micropuncture techniques in an attempt to find out more about the mechanisms involved.

Two models of experimental acute renal failure have been studied in our laboratory to date: the first, mercury poisoning, and more recently, glycerol induced hemoglobinuric acute renal failure in the rat. Interestingly, the mechanisms operative in these widely different models were found to be qualitatively similar, and I shall restrict my talk to the hemoglobinuria model which is more similar to acute renal failure seen in man. Drs. MANUEL L. ARCE, DOUGLAS R. WILSON, GILBERT THIEL, and FRANKLIN D. MCDONALD participated in various portions of the work I shall report on today.

Acute renal failure was produced in rats by injecting 10 ml/kg body weight of 50% glycerol into the muscles of both hind limbs. Within two hours after the injection, the urine became burgundy wine color due to the presence of a high concentration of heme pigment. The animals were anesthetized with pentobarbital, and their blood pressure was continuously monitored by carotid manometry. The animals were subjected to micropuncture at intervals ranging from 30 minutes to 26 hours after glycerol was given. Hypotension typically did not occur after glycerol injection despite a marked diminution in plasma volume. The micropuncture methods used have been described in earlier papers [1, 2]. In short, proximal tubular hydrostatic pressure was measured by direct manometry. Glomerular filtration rate and fractional water absorption of individual nephrons were determined using C^{14} labelled inulin. The puncture site in the proximal tubules was determined by the intratubular injection of latex and subsequent microdissection of the nephron. Direct qualitative estimates of proximal tubule water absorption also were made without relying on the assumption of

* This work was supported by U.S.P.H.S. Grant AM 08695.

[1] Department of Medicine, Peter Bent Brigham Hospital and Harvard Medical School, Boston, Massachusetts.

tubular impermeability to inulin. In such experiments, a droplet of isosmolar NaCl solution was injected between oil drops, and its rate of absorption observed directly at 160× magnification. Most often, after the injection of glycerol, proximal tubular fluid flow rates were so slow that it was impossible to collect samples of adequate size for accurate measurement. In order to obtain some estimate of flow rate in such nephrons, a small drop of Sudan black stained mineral oil was injected into the tubules, and its rate of progress down the lumen was observed. Reasonable qualitative correlation was found between flow rate estimated in this manner and that measured by volume collection.

There was a very rapid change in the appearance of the kidney surface after glycerol injection. Despite normal blood pressure, the kidney surface became markedly pale, peritubular capillary circulation being markedly decreased. The tubule lumens became very small and the tubule epithelium appeared pale and granular. In fifteen to thirty minutes, hemoglobin stained fluid first appeared in the tubules. Within one to two hours all tubules contained hemoglobin stained fluid and tubule fluid flow rate was greatly reduced. Two to four hours after glycerol injection, approximately a third of the tubules had no visible lumen while the lumens of the remaining two-thirds of the tubules were variable in size, their tubule fluid was hemoglobin stained and tubule fluid flow rate was grossly but variably reduced. Eighteen to twenty-six hours after glycerol injection, islands of white granular tubules with no visible lumen were interspersed with tubules of variable sized lumens containing clear tubular fluid, and an occasional tubule containing dark hemoglobin stained casts. The severity of the renal lesions observed in animals deprived of water for 24 hours prior to glycerol injection was considerably greater than that of animals allowed free access to water. The BUN of dehydrated animals rose to a mean value of 222 mg-% 48 hours after glycerol injection in comparison with a rise to only 78 mg-% in nondehydrated rats. The highly significant difference in BUN values between dehydrated and nondehydrated animals occurred regardless of the fact that dehydrated animals were allowed free access to water immediately after glycerol injection and often reattained their predehydration weight.

In Fig. 1, is shown the estimated proximal tubule fluid flow rate determined qualitatively by the rate of progression of an oil droplet. As may be seen, proximal tubule fluid flow was somewhat diminished just by the process of dehydration under control conditions. After glycerol, flow was minimal or absent in the majority of tubules. A smaller percentage had grossly reduced flow while a few tubules had moderately reduced flow. Almost all tubules of dehydrated animals, shown in columns marked B, had insignificant volumes of flow. Eighteen to twenty-six hours after glycerol, tubules of both dehydrated and nondehydrated animals had grossly reduced flow, the dehydrated group still showing considerably worse function than that of their nondehydrated counterparts. As can be seen from this slide, very few of the nephrons within a kidney had sufficient function to permit quantitative measurement of glomerular filtration and tubule fluid flow rate. The quantitative values obtained in those very best nephrons are shown in Table 1. It may be seen that the process of dehydration alone caused a modest decrease in glomerular filtration rate and tubule fluid flow rate in the rat, as was detected by oil droplet injection.

Thirty minutes to four hours after glycerol injection, the GFR and tubule fluid fow rate of nondehydrated glycerol animals were even further reduced, this reduction persisting beyond eighteen to twenty-six hours after glycerol injection. It should be stressed again that these quantitative values were obtained only from those few most normal nephrons on the kidney surface. The kidneys of dehydrated rats were universally so severely abnormal that virtually no samples adequate

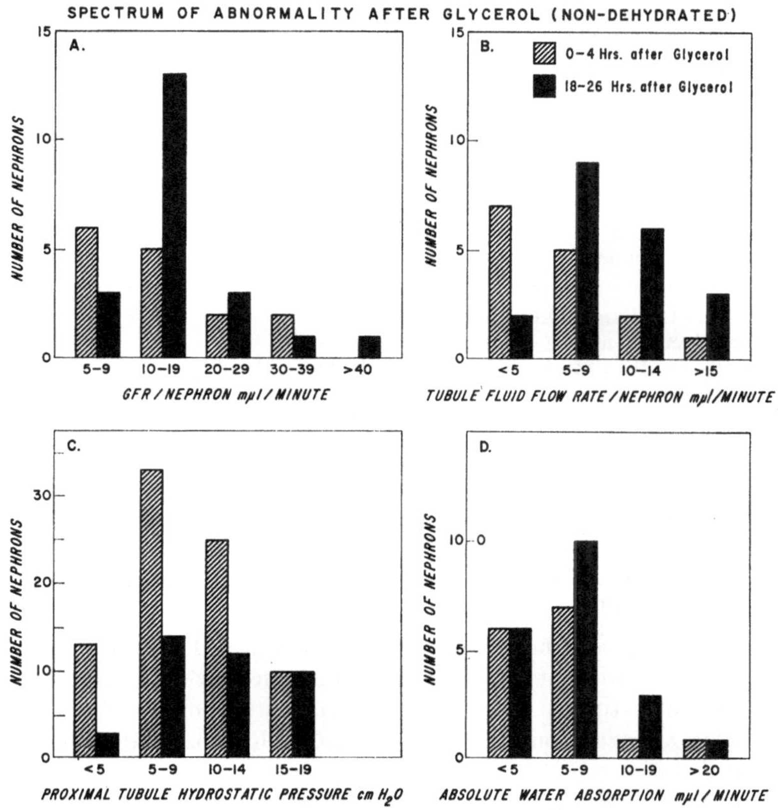

Fig. 1. Qualitative estimates of proximal tubule fluid flow rate in non-dehydrated (A) and dehydrated (B) rats

in size for quantitative assessment could be obtained at either four hours or in the later period, eighteen to twenty-six hours.

In order to determine whether this apparent decrease in glomerular filtration and tubule fluid flow rate was the result of leakage of tubule fluid content because of disrupted epithelium, fractional water absorption was measured in the proximal tubules. Although no difference in fractional water absorption could be observed in control hydrated rats, control dehydrated rats and rats studied four hours after glycerol, a distinct difference in water absorption was observed eighteen to twenty-six hours after glycerol injection, as is shown in Fig. 2. Fractional water absorption of the rats injected with glycerol eighteen to twenty-six hours earlier was distinctly lower with statistical significance at the 5%

Table 1. *Functional parameters of individual nephrons studied 0—4 hours and 18—26 hours after glycerol injection*

No. of tubules/No. of rats	Control		Glycerol, 0 to 4 hours glycerol, 18 to 26 hours	
	non-dehydrated (29/9)	dehydrated (17/8)	non-dehydrated (15/9)	non-dehydrated (20/8)
Tubular fluid flow rate (mμl per tubule per minute)	17.3 ± 1.2[b]	9.2 ± 0.8[c]	7.0 ± 1.4[c]	10.0 ± 0.9[c]
Glomerular filtration rate (mμl per tubule per minute)	38.8 ± 2.2	23.3 ± 1.9[c]	14.7 ± 2.3[c]	18.4 ± 2.5[c]
TF/P_{In}[a]	2.4 ± 0.2	2.7 ± 0.2	2.4 ± 0.2	1.8 ± 0.1[e]
Absolute water absorption (mμl per tubule per minute)	21.4 ± 1.7	14.1 ± 1.6[d]	9.1 ± 1.5[c]	8.4 ± 1.8[c]

[a] Tubular fluid to plasma inulin concentration ratio.
[b] All values given are mean ± standard error.
[c] Statistically less than nondehydrated control value, $p < 0.001$.
[d] Statistically less than nondehydrated control value, $p < 0.01$.
[e] Statistically less than nondehydrated control value, $p < 0.05$.

confidence level. Again, these values were derived from the least abnormal nephrons. When isosmolar fluid was injected into the more seriously abnormal nephrons and observed under the dissecting microscope, water absorption was found to be very severely diminished. There was, then, no evidence to support the "passive backflow" theory.

The role of tubular obstruction as a cause of diminished glomerular filtration was assessed by measurement of proximal tubule hydrostatic pressure. As shown in Fig. 3, proximal tubule hydrostatic pressure was considerably lower in glycerol injected animals than the 15.6 cm H_2O value observed in the control period. Accurate assessment of hydrostatic pressure could be made only in those best nephrons containing significant volumes of tubule fluid. Since fluid could be injected readily into tubules with collapsed lumina at pressures under 5 cm H_2O, it is apparent that tubular collapse was not the result of extrinsic compression. It is also apparent that tubular obstruction was not the prime cause of cessation of glomerular filtration since, under those circumstances, intratubular pressure should be supernormal rather than grossly subnormal.

The intact nephron hypothesis suggests that the urine obtained in acute renal failure is derived from normal nephrons, the remainder of nephrons being non-functional. As may be seen from Fig. 4, however, such is certainly not the case in this experimental model. Rather, a number of nephrons do have minimal or no function, but the remainder show a wide spectrum of abnormality in glomerular filtration rates, tubule fluid flow rates, proximal tubule hydrostatic pressures, and absolute water absorption. We have found that such measures as the prophylactic administration of mannitol and saline or plasma may have a distinct salutary effect upon renal function both by decreasing the number

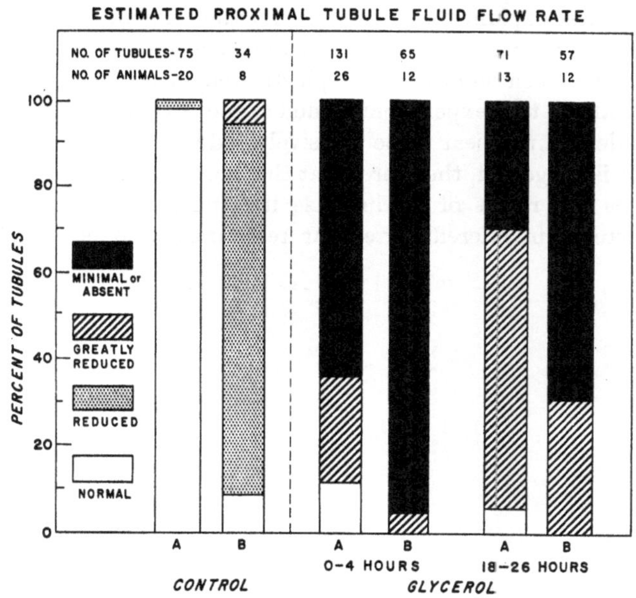

Fig. 2. Fractional water absorption in proximal tubules of dehydrated and non-dehydrated rats

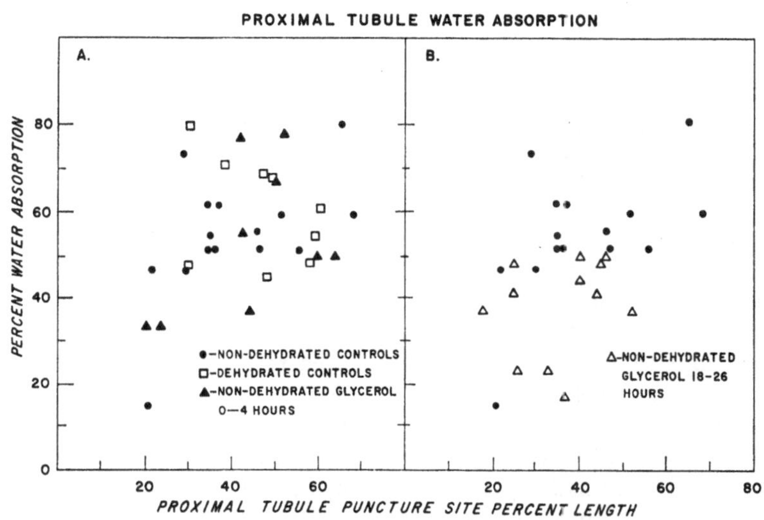

Fig. 3. Proximal tubule hydrostatic pressure

of nonfunctioning nephrons and by weighting the spectrum of function more towards normal.

We can now say that renal insufficiency in this experimental model of acute renal failure is the result of a primary diminution of glomerular filtration rate which is independent of obstruction and is not artifactual as the result of non-selective absorption of tubular contents. A glomerular vasomotor phenomenon would appear to best explain these findings. Further explanation must take into account the fact that renal blood flow in acute renal failure in man and experimental animals has been shown with sophisticated methodology to be from $^1/_3$ normal to normal. In this experimental model, too, capillary blood flow on the kidney surface does not appear to be massively reduced after the first few hours post-glycerol. It is suggested, therefore, that the marked diminution in glomerular filtration rate is the result of an increase in afferent arteriolar resistance, a comparable decrease in efferent arteriolar resistance perhaps permitting total

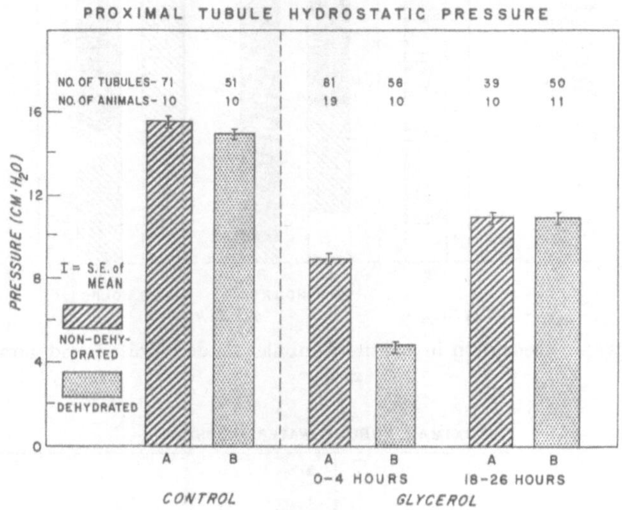

Fig. 4. The spectrum of abnormality in GFR proximal tubule fluid flow rate, proximal tubule fractional water absorption and absolute water absorption of individual nephrons of nondehydrated rats 18 hours after glycerol

resistance to remain within reasonable limits. In this way, intraglomerular pressure would be markedly reduced, and glomerular filtration greatly diminished despite adequate perfusion of the glomeruli themselves. The mechanism responsible for this vasomotor phenomenon remains unsettled.

In an attempt to elucidate mechanisms which might be operative as predisposing factors to the development of ARF, we looked again at the nondehydrated group. Although the mean BUN of these rats 48 hours after glycerol was 78 mg-%, approximately one-third of the total number of animals had BUN's lower than 30 mg-%, another third had BUN's between 30 and 80 mg-% and the remainder had BUN's greater than 80 mg-% with a mean BUN of 151 mg-%. Control values of blood hematocrit, plasma sodium and potassium concentration, plasma volume, body weight, water intake, urine volume, urine osmolality, urine sodium and potassium concentration, were compared in these three groups of nondehydrated animals. No differences could be found in those parameters to account for the different severity of renal insufficiency observed in the three groups. There was, however, a very slight, but statistically significant difference in urine pH, the least azotemic group having a urine pH of 6.7 prior to glycerol injection while the other two groups had a urine pH of 6.3. Aciduria has frequently been cited as a predisposing factor in the development of acute renal failure. It seems doubtful that the difference in urine pH itself was important, but perhaps reflected other differences in these animals. The acid-hematin theory suggests that aciduria promotes precipitation of hematin within the kidney, yet at the time of hemoglobinuria, during the first hour after glycerol, the urine pH of all three groups of rats was the same, pH 6.1. Furthermore, as may be seen in Table 2, manipulation of urinary pH before giving glycerol did not reveal any relationship between urine pH and the severity of renal insufficiency. There was little difference in the 48-hour BUN values of animals given ammonium chloride to achieve a urine pH of 5.4 before glycerol injection and that observed in acetazolamide treated rats that had a urine pH of 7.8. By contrast, methionine treated animals had a urine pH of 5.6, a value very similar to that of ammonium chloride treated animals, and yet they had the lowest BUN of the four groups studied. We were left with no adequate explanation for the variability in the degree of renal insufficiency observed among nondehydrated glycerol injected rats.

The question then was raised as to the manner in which dehydration exerts its predisposition to renal insufficiency in acute renal failure. It has been suggested previously that the effect of dehydration is mediated through the renal concentrating mechanism. According to this view, the striking increase in the incidence and severity of acute renal failure associated with dehydration has been thought to be mediated by increased absorption of toxic products, by increased levels of circulating antidiuretic hormone, or by changes in urine flow rate and urine concentration leading to intratubular cast formation. We tested these postulates by repeating the studies described above in rats with congenital hypothalamic diabetes insipidus [5]. These animals, kindly supplied by Dr. HEINZ VALTIN, drink a volume of water approximating their body weight each day. Nonetheless, because of their large obligatory urine volume, they are effectively dehydrated as manifest by a serum osmolality higher than normal and a plasma volume intermediate between that found in normal nondehydrated rats and normal rats deprived of water for 24 hours. The mean individual nephron GFR of diabetes insipidus rats in the control period, furthermore, was not significantly different from that of the dehydrated normal rats but was significantly less than that of normal nondehydrated rats. Although the mean urine volume fell to approximately 15% of the control value after glycerol injection, these animals were still polyuric with a urine volume of 25 ml/24 hours. Despite polyuria,

Table 2. *Effect of changes in urine pH on subsequent azotemia 48 hours after glycerol injection*

	Urine pH		48 hr. BUN
	before glycerol	after glycerol	mg-%
NH_4Cl ($N = 27$)	5.4 ± 0.02 (S.E.)	5.9 ± 0.1 (S.E.)	143 ± 15 (S.E.)
Methionine (n = 14)	5.6 ± 0.04	6.1 ± 0.1	34 ± 5
$NaHCO_3$ (N = 14)	8.0 ± 0.02	6.2 ± 0.1	74 ± 13
Acetazolamide (N = 16)	7.8 ± 0.05	6.4 ± 0.2	123 ± 19

their BUN rose to 152 mg-% 48 hours after glycerol. At micropuncture, both the degree of abnormality of the kidneys judged by eye and the proportion of nephrons with severe impairment of glomerular filtration and tubule fluid flow rate, were intermediate between that of dehydrated and nondehydrated rats without diabetes insipidus, a finding consistent with the degree of BUN elevation. Even in the presence of marked polyuria, severe abnormality of renal function again correlated with the degree of dehydration. It is difficult to invoke any aspect of the concentrating mechanism as a cause of the severe nephropathy manifest by these animals. Presumably, then, the effect of dehydration is mediated by other means.

It is well established that dehydration is a potent stimulus for the production of renin. Increasing evidence suggests, moreover, that the renin-angiotensin-system may have important effects within the kidney itself. SCHNERMANN and THURAU have provided evidence that acute volume depletion produced by hemorrhagic hypotension in the rat results in an increased sodium concentration in fluid obtained by micropuncture from the early distal tubules. Other experiments by these workers indicate that an increase in sodium concentration in the region of the macula densa decreases glomerular filtration in the same nephron, presumably by afferent arteriolar constriction, and that this effect is dependent on the concentration of renin in the kidney. Whether such a mechanism is operative in acute renal failure is not yet known, but it is entirely possible that renin release, regardless of cause, may have a profound effect on glomerular filtration rate. To study this further, 1% saline was substituted for drinking water of a series of rats for more than two months. The single nephron GFR, proximal tubule pressure, and fractional water absorption values of saline loaded rats in the control period was no different from that of their counterparts drinking tap water. Forty-eight hours after glycerol injection, however, the mean BUN of the saline loaded rats was only 16 mg-% compared with the 78 mg-% value found in their water-drinking counterparts. It is of some interest that the renal ischemia and tubular collapse seen in water-drinking rats in the first four hours after glycerol was duplicated in the saline-drinking animals. After the first four hours post-glycerol, however, almost all surface tubules were full of clear fluid, and the kidney continued to have greatly better function thereafter. Individual nephron GFR returned to more than 75% of normal within twelve hours. It appears, therefore, that although saline loading does not prevent the initial ischemic phase with cessation of glomerular filtration and tubular collapse resulting from glycerol injection, it does abolish continued functional impairment. Chronic saline loading of rats seems to uncover separate phases in the development of glycerol induced acute renal failure. Whatever mechanism is responsible for this protection either is not operative during the first four hours after glycerol, or is overwhelmed by another mechanism which is not abolished by chronic saline loading.

In summary, the oliguria and renal insufficiency of glycerol induced hemoglobinuric acute renal failure in the rat are the result of a primary decrease in glomerular filtration rate. The abnormality in glomerular filtration rate is not due to tubular obstruction with casts or compression by edema. There is no evidence to support the contention that increased absorption of a normal volume of filtrate is responsible for the renal insufficiency observed. Differences in the degree of renal insufficiency observed are attributable in part to the degree of abnormality of the best functioning nephrons, but are more importantly related to the proportion of nephrons with minimal or absent filtration. There is no evidence to support the "intact nephron" hypothesis that nephrons function either normally or not at all in this experimental model of acute renal failure. Rather, a spectrum of abnormality in the nephron population is found routinely. Although dehydration predisposes to the development of severe renal insufficiency, its effect does not appear to be related either to antidiuretic hormone or to any feature of the renal concentrating process.

The abnormality in glomerular function may be the result of two or more mechanisms affecting afferent arteriolar tone. Since glomerular function soon returns towards normal in rats whose kidneys are renin depleted due to chronic saline loading, it is suggested that the renin-angiotensin-axis may play an important role in the perpetuation of renal functional abnormalities caused by glycerol injection and its resultant myohemoglobinuria.

References

1. Flanigan, W. J., and D. E. Oken: Renal micropuncture study of the development of anuria in the rat with mercury-induced acute renal failure. J. clin. Invest. **44**, 449—451 (1965).
2. Oken, D. E., M. L. Arce, and D. R. Wilson: Glycerol-induced hemoglobinuric acute renal failure in the rat. I. Micropuncture study of the development of oliguria. J. clin. Invest. **45**, 724—735 (1966).
3. Thiel, G., D. R. Wilson, M. L. Arce, and D. E. Oken: Glycerol induced hemoglobinuric acute renal failure in the rat. II. The experimental model, predisposing factors, and pathophysiologic features. Nephron **4**, 276—297 (1967).
4. Wilson, D. R., G. Thiel, M. L. Arce, and D. E. Oken: Glycerol induced hemoglobinuric acute renal failure in the rat. III. Micropuncture study of the effects of Mannitol and isotonic saline on individual nephron function. Nephron **4**, 337—355 (1962).
5. Wilson, D. R., G. Thiel, M. L. Arce, and D. E. Oken: The role of the concentration mechanism in the development of acute renal failure: Micropuncture studies using diabetes insipidus rats. Nephron (in press).

Discussion

Campanacci:

A few years ago we studied, by renal biopsy and functional tests, the kidneys of patients suffering from hemoglobinuric favism. In agreement with Dr. Oken's findings we saw an irregular patchy distribution of tubular lesions. Functionally, there was a slight decrease of tubular activity as measured by Tm_{PAH}. The renal lesion and the impairment of Tm_{PAH} improved rapidly in the days following the hemoglobinuric crisis and had disappeared 20 to 30 days later.

How do you explain the mechanism of the hemoglobinuria produced by glycerol? Could the type of renal impairment be similar to that observed in hemoglobinuric favism?

Steinhausen:

Your observations on the fate of hemoglobin cylinders in the renal cortex of rats agree with results of investigations on the golden hamster's papilla [6].

We demonstrated, microcinematographically, that chromoprotein cylinders are usually washed out from the collecting ducts at normal arterial blood pressure and with an adequate rate of urine flow [7].

6. Steinhausen, M.: Pflügers Arch. ges. Physiol. **279**, 195—213 (1964).
7. — In: Aktuelle Probleme der Nephrologie. Berlin-Heidelberg-New York: Springer 1966.

Truniger:

Would you care to comment on recent studies indicating tubular obstruction [8], or total reabsorption of filtrate [9] as the cause of oliguria?

8. Bank, N., B. F. Mutz, and H. S. Aynedjian: The role of leakage of tubular fluid in anuria due to mercury poisoning. J. clin. Invest. **46**, 695—704 (1967).
9. Jaenike, J. R.: The renal lesion associated with hemoglobinemia: A study of the pathogenesis of the excretory defect in the rat. J. clin. Invest. **46**, 378—387 (1967).

Gessler:

In rats intoxicated with hematin we found a considerable depression of GFR. Anuria was due to two different mechanisms, i.e. complete suppression of glomerular filtration and complete reabsorption of the reduced amount of filtrate still produced. The localization of the tubular toxic effect could depend on GFR.

It, thus, appears probable that acute renal failure is due to the simultaneous occurrence of tubular damage and depression of GFR.

2.2. Special Toxicology

2.2.1. The Effect of Actinomycin D on Transepithelial Sodium Transport

M. WIEDERHOLT and K. HIERHOLZER[1]

With 5 Figures

Actinomycin, an antibiotic, which has been isolated from streptomyces [21] and which has been synthesized recently [1], is used in clinical medicine because of its cytostatic action. In this paper we shall discuss its use as an inhibitor of sodium transport, or more specifically: the action of actinomycin D as inhibitor of steroid dependent transport of sodium in isolated membranes and in the mammalian kidney.

This inhibitory action is due to a dose dependent, more or less specific inhibition of the DNA-dependent synthesis of RNA, which is the consequence of the binding of actinomycin D to DNA [16, for reference see also: 7, 14, and 17]. Accordingly, the effects of a large number of hormones, which are thought to exert their effects via a stimulation of the synthesis of RNA, as demonstrated first by KARLSON for ecdysone [10, 11], are blocked by actinomycin D [8, 18]. This interaction between antibiotic and DNA as well as hormones and DNA has been the starting point of the present experiments.

The first experiments, in which a direct effect of actinomycin D on transepithelial transport of sodium was be established, were conducted by EDELMAN et al. [4]. In these and subsequent experiments [3, 5, 19], it was demonstrated that in the isolated toad bladder aldosterone stimulation of sodium transport is completely blocked by the antibiotic. In a bathing medium with a concentration of 5 μg/ml, basal sodium transport in steroid depleted toad bladders was not affected[2], furthermore, normal sensitivity of the membrane preparation to vasopressin was maintained indicating a specific inhibition of the effect of aldosterone by actinomycin D. This inhibitory effect can be demonstrated in vitro when the antibiotic is administered before [3, 4, 5, 19] or after [19] aldosterone to the bathing medium. Comparable results have also been obtained in toad bladder and ventral toad skin by CRABBÉ and DE WEER [3], who observed an inhibition of the effect of d-aldosterone by administration of actinomycin D not only in vitro but also in vivo. The results obtained in isolated membranes are in keeping with the hypothesis that aldosterone affects sodium transport by induction of protein synthesis, a concept which has been explored further by EDELMAN et. al. [4] and PORTER et al. [15].

WILLIAMSON [22] has postulated that a similar sequence of events takes place in the mammalian kidney. In adrenalectomized rats, substituted

---

[1] Physiologisches Institut, Freie Universität, West-Berlin.

[2] In higher concentrations [5], actinomycin D apparently also depresses the basal transport activity of this membrane.

with d-aldosterone, he observed an augmentation of renal sodium excretion. The antinatriuretic effect of aldosterone was eliminated when actinomycin D (in a dose of 0.4 mg/kg b.w.) was administered simultaneously with or before aldosterone. However, when actinomycin D was given after the injection of the steroid hormone, no significant effect of sodium excretion could be detected [12]. Since these results are in contrast to the data obtained in vitro, as shown above, and since the measurement of electrolyte excretion in the urine does not permit

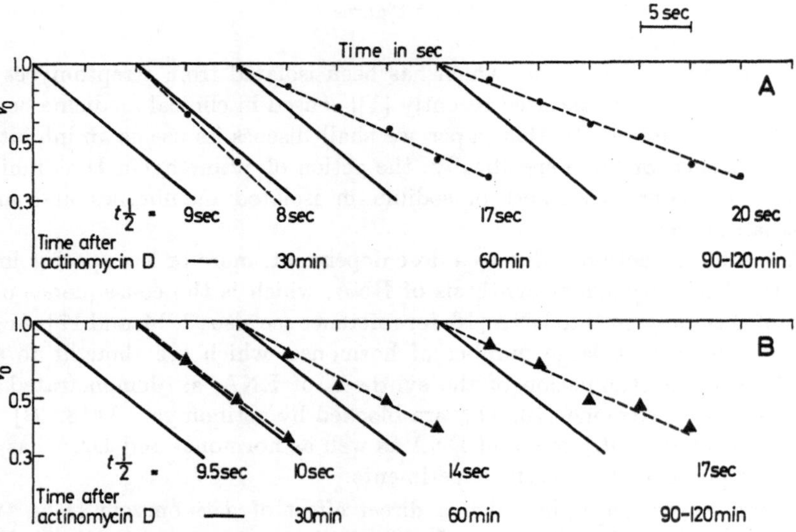

Fig. 1. *Effect of actinomycin D (2 μg/kg b.w. intravenously) on fluid reabsorption in the proximal convolution.* Split oil droplet method [6]. V/V_0 = volume of isotonic NaCl droplets at different times (on abscissa) divided by volume of droplets at time zero. *Upper part (A):* single experiment in a control rat with intact adrenals before (heavy line) and after (dotted line) actinomycin D. *Lower part (B):* adrenalectomized rat with aldosterone substitution (7.5 μgms d-aldosterone/100 gms b.w. for 3 days prior to the experiment) before and after actinomycin D. Data from [reference 23]

an analysis of site and action of actinomycin D we have attempted to evaluate the influence of aldosterone and actinomycin D on sodium reabsorption in the rat kidney. Micropuncture methods have been applied to proximal and distal surface tubules.

First, the rate of disappearance of saline injected into the tubular lumen was measured using the split oil droplet method of GERTZ [6]. Fig. 1 demonstrates proximal data obtained in one control rat (A) and in one adrenalectomized rat substituted with aldosterone (B). In both animals the half time of proximal fluid reabsorption was within the normal range of 8—10 sec [6, 9]. 30 minutes after intravenous injection of actinomycin D the results were essentially similar, but 60 minutes after the administration of the antibiotic the local transport capacity of the proximal tubular epithelium was reduced in both rats, as indicated by a smaller slope of the reabsorption line. A maximum inhibition of local sodium and fluid reabsorption was observed 30 to 60 minutes later, the $t\,^1/_2$ values being 20 sec and 17 sec respectively [24].

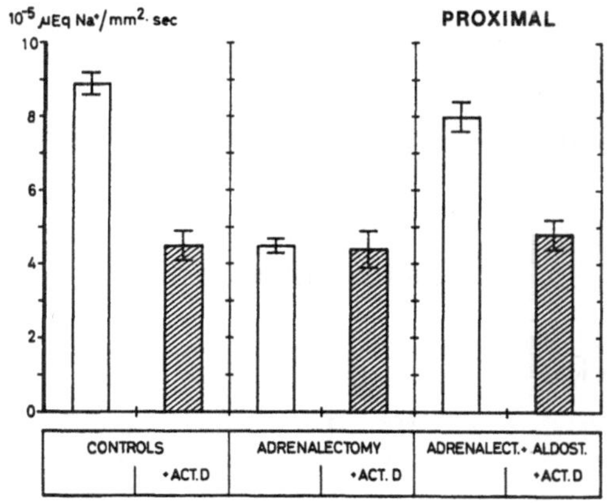

Fig. 2. *Effect of actinomycin D on transtubular net sodium transport in the proximal convolution.* Each column is a mean value (± S.E.) of 30—60 measurements (split oil droplet method) in 3 rats. Data from [ref. 23]. The difference between the first two columns (= intact rats without and with actinomycin D) and between the last two columns (= adrenalectomized and aldosterone-treated rats without and with actinomycin D) is significant ($P<0.001$)

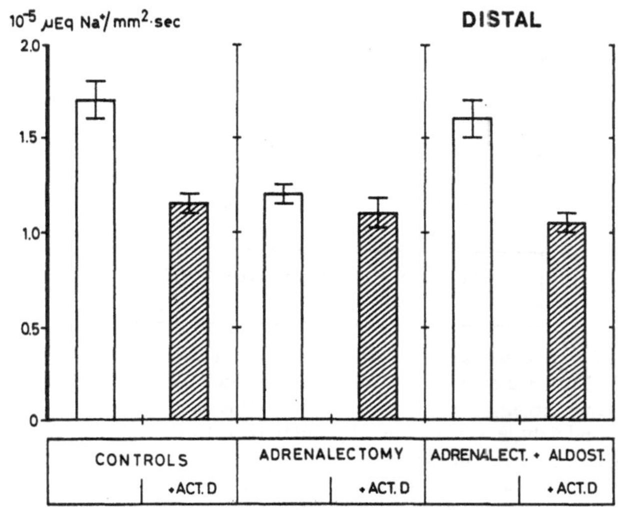

Fig. 3. *Effect of actinomycin D on transtubular net sodium transport in the distal convolution.* Compare to Fig. 2

Fig. 2 shows the rates of transtubular net sodium reabsorption as calculated from split droplet measurements in proximal convolutions. As seen in the first 2 columns (control rats[3]) and in the last 2 columns (adrenalectomized rats substituted with d-aldosterone), actinomycin D, 60 to 120 minutes after intravenous administration, reduces local sodium transport capacity by approximately 50%: from 8.6 ± 0.2 (S.E.) to $4.5 \pm 0.4 \times 10^{-5}$ μEq/mm² × sec in control rats and from

[3] Actinomycin D reduces endogenous aldosterone production in control rats by approx. 40% 30 min after administration [2].

7.8 ± 0.6 to $4.8 \pm 0.4 \times 10^{-5}$ μEq/mm² × sec in aldosterone-treated adrenalectomized rats.

The second pair of columns indicates that actinomycin D in the dose used (i.e. 2 mg/kg b.w.) did not depress basal, aldosterone-independent, sodium reabsorption.

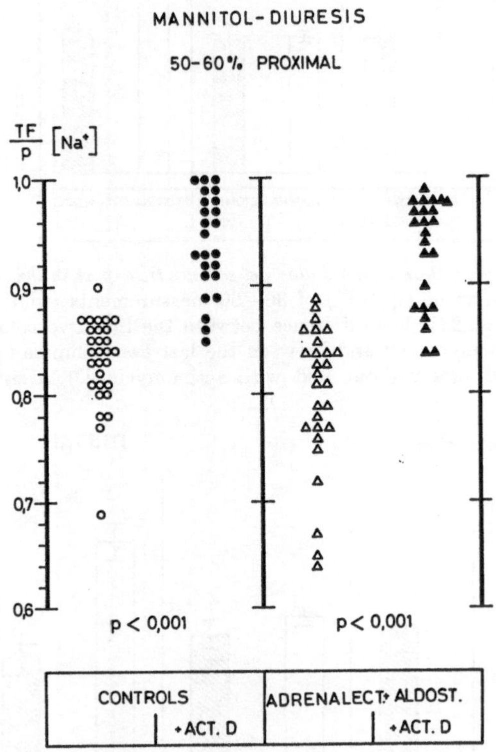

Fig. 4. *Free flow micropuncture experiments in osmotic diuresis (5 ml 20% mannitol in 0.9% NaCl/60 min i.v.).* Data from 16 rats. Only the last loop of the proximal convolution, as identified by lissamin green, has been punctured (this corresponds to 50—60% of total length of the proximal tubule as confirmed by microdissections of latex casts). Determination of Na concentrations (*TF* = tubular fluid, *P* = plasma) by micro-flamephotometry [13]. Samples were taken 60—90 min after the onset of the infusion of mannitol. Actinomycin D was injected 30 min prior to mannitol

Essentially, similar data (on a lower absolute level) were obtained in distal convolutions as shown in Fig. 3. Again, base line transport capacity was unaffected, but steroid-dependent activity was reduced to base level by actinomycin D.

Thus, in contrast to the experience of WILLIAMSON [22], and in agreement with the findings obtained in isolated membranes, steroid-dependent sodium transport in the rat kidney is inhibited also when actinomycin D is given after administration of exogenous aldosterone, or when actinomycin D is administered to control rats with intact adrenals. It should be emphasized here, that in the course of the micropuncture experiments which continued over a 2 hour-period following injection of actinomycin, the arterial blood pressure (105—125 mm Hg), the clearance of inulin (0.94 ± 0.06 ml/min·100 gms) and proximal transit time (10.0 ± 0.4 sec) remained virtually unchanged in control rats. This holds, also, for the two groups of adrenalectomized animals. Therefore, a direct effect of actinomycin D on the tubular epithelium has to be postulated. However, up to the present time we have not succeeded in interfering with tubular sodium reabsorption by intratubular infusion of the antibiotic.

An alternative method of characterization of renal sodium transport consists in the measurement of the transtubular concentration difference of sodium which can be established in osmotic diuresis by the tubular epithelium. Data

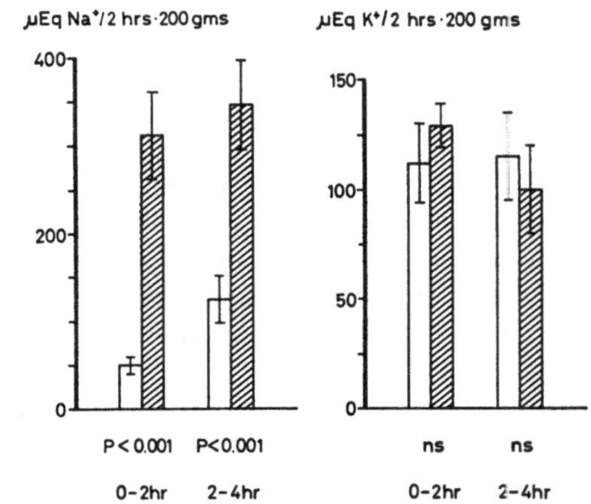

Fig. 5. *$U_{Na} \times V$ and $U_K \times V$ of unanethetized control rats.* First, the animals were kept in metabolic cages without actinomycin D and electrolyte excretion was measured during a 4 hour period following intraperitoneal injection of 2 ml isotonic NaCl/100 gms b.w. (white columns). Two days later, the experiment was repeated with actinomycin D. The drug was injected i.p. 1 hour before the administration of saline (shadowed columns). Each column represents the mean ($\pm$ S.E.) of data obtained in 8 rats. *ns* = no significance

from experiments performed in proximal convolutions in strong mannitol diuresis are shown in Fig. 4. On the left side, as shown, the sodium TF/P-concentration ratios in the terminal segment: they increased from 0.83 ± 0.01 (in control rats) to 0.94 ± 0.01 after actinomycin. This corresponds to an increase of the mean intraluminal sodium concentration from 115 to 132 mEq/l. Plasma sodium concentration was not affected significantly by the antibiotic. As seen on the right side of Fig. 4, data obtained from adrenalectomized and aldosterone treated rats (7.5 µg/100 gms b.w. and 24 hours for 3 days) are scattered within the control range, the mean TF/P-sodium value being 0.80 ± 0.01. Again actinomycin D reduces active sodium reabsorption as shown by an increase of sodium-TF/P to 0.93 ± 0.01. This latter value is similar to results obtained earlier by Stolte et al. (unpublished results) in adrenalectomized rats without hormone substitution.

The results obtained with two different and independent micropuncture methods lead us to the conclusion that in the rat kidney actinomycin D at the dose and during the time period of action tested here, inhibits specifically the aldosterone-dependent sodium reabsorption by interfering with the active transport system. Thus, the extent of inhibition of sodium reabsorption equals that induced by bilateral adrenalectomy. The steroid-independent fraction of sodium reabsorption is unaffected by the antibiotic. The similarity of proximal and distal data supports our previous conclusion that in the proximal as in the distal convolution a fraction of active sodium transport is under the influence of mineralocorticosteroids. One is therefore tempted (though not entitled) to assume a single mechanism of action of aldosterone on sodium transport in biological membranes. Whether the mode of action includes a change in sodium permeability of the passive diffusion barrier or whether the active transport step is directly affected cannot be decided at present (for references see 19).

There remains one observation to be discussed. In the face of the intimate coupling of transtubular transport of sodium and potassium we expected an interference of actinomycin D not only with sodium reabsorption but also with potassium excretion. Surprisingly, and for reasons unknown at the present time, such an inhibition does not occur. WILLIAMSON[22] observed, in adrenalectomized rats, that the kaliuretic effect of aldosterone could not be blocked. In further experiments we have measured sodium and potassium excretion of control rats before and after administration of actinomycin D.

Fig. 5 demonstrates that, although actinomycin inhibited tubular sodium reabsorption, potassium excretion was quite unaffected.

References

1. BROCKMANN, H., and M. LACKNER: Totalsynthese von Actinomycin C_3. Naturwissenschaften **47**, 230—230 (1960).
2. BURROW, G. N., P. J. MULROW, and P. K. BONDY: Protein synthesis and aldosterone production. Endocrinology **79**, 955—963 (1966).
3. CRABBÉ, J., and P. DE WEER: Action of aldosterone on the bladder and skin of the toad. Nature (Lond.) **202**, 298—299 (1964).
4. EDELMAN, I. S., R. BOGOROCH, and G. A. PORTER: On the mechanism of action of aldosterone on sodium transport: the role of protein synthesis. Proc. nat. Acad. Sci. (Wash.) **50**, 1169—1177 (1963).
5. FANESTIL, D. D., and I. S. EDELMAN: On the mechanism of action of aldosterone on sodium transport: effects of inhibitors of RNA and protein synthesis. Fed. Proc. **25**, 912—916 (1966).
6. GERTZ, K. H.: Transtubuläre Natriumchloridflüsse und Permeabilität für Nichtelektrolyte im proximalen und distalen Konvolut der Rattenniere. Pflügers Arch. ges. Physiol. **276**, 336—356 (1963).
7. GOLDBERG, I. H.: Mode of action of antibiotics. II. Drugs affecting nucleic acid and protein synthesis. Amer. J. Med. **39**, 722—752 (1965).
8. HECHTER, O., and I. D. K. HALKERSTON: Effects of steroid hormones on gene regulation and cell metabolism. Ann. Rev. Physiol. **27**, 133—162 (1965).
9. HIERHOLZER, K., M. WIEDERHOLT u. H. STOLTE: Hemmung der Natriumresorption im proximalen und distalen Konvolut adrenalektomierter Ratten. Pflügers Arch. ges. Physiol. **291**, 43—62 (1966).
10. KARLSON, P.: Biochemische Wirkungsweise der Hormone. Dtsch. med. Wschr. **86**, 668—674 (1961).
11. — New concepts on the mode of action of hormones. Perspect. Biol. Med. **6**, 203—221 (1963).
12. LUDENS, J. H., J. B. HOOK, and H. E. WILLIAMSON: Lack of effect of actinomycin D on aldosterone induced antinatriuresis when administered after the hormone. Proc. Soc. exp. Biol. (N.Y.) **124**, 539—541 (1967).
13. MALNIC, G., R. M. KLOSE, and G. GIEBISCH: Micropuncture study of renal potassium excretion in the rat. Amer. J. Physiol. **206**, 674—686 (1964).

14. NEUBERT, D.: Beeinflussung des Nucleinsäure- und Proteinstoffwechsels durch Pharmaka. Internist (Berl.) **7**, 435—454 (1966).
15. PORTER, G. A., R. BOGOROCH, and I. S. EDELMAN: On the mechanism of action of aldosterone on sodium transport: the role of RNA synthesis. Proc. nat. Acad. Sci. (Wash.) **52**, 1326—1333 (1964).
16. REICH, E., E. M. FRANKLIN, A. J. SHATKIN, and E. L. TATUM: Effect of actinomycin D on cellular nucleic acid synthesis and virus production. Science **134**, 556 (1961).
17. — Biochemistry of actinomycins. Cancer Res. **23**, 1428—1441 (1963).
18. SAMUELS, L. D.: Actinomycin and its effects. Influence on an effector pathway for hormonal control. New Engl. J. Med. **271**, 1301—1308 (1964).
19. SHARP, G. W. G., and A. LEAF: Mechanism of action of aldosterone. Physiol. Rev. **46**, 593—633 (1966).
20. STOLTE, H., M. WIEDERHOLT, and K. HIERHOLZER: Unpublished results.
21. WAKSMAN, S., and H. B. WOODRUFF: Bacteriostatic and bactericidal substances produced by a soil actinomyces. Proc. Soc. exp. Biol. (N.Y.) **45**, 609—614 (1940).
22. WILLIAMSON, H. E.: Mechanism of the antinatriuretic action of aldosterone. Biochem. Pharmacol. **12**, 1449—1450 (1963).
23. WIEDERHOLT, M.: Mikropunktionsuntersuchungen am proximalen und distalen Konvolut der Rattenniere über den Einfluß von Actinomycin D auf den mineralocorticoidabhängigen Na-Transport. Pflügers Arch. ges. Physiol. **292**, 334—342 (1966).
24. — H. STOLTE, J. P. BRECHT u. K. HIERHOLZER: Mikropunktionsuntersuchungen über den Einfluß von Aldosteron, Cortison und Dexamethason auf die renale Natriumresorption adrenalektomierter Ratten. Pflügers Arch. ges. Physiol. **292**, 316—333 (1966).

2.2.2. Metabolic Tubular Failure Induced by Local Application of Potassium Cyanide to the Surface of the Rat Kidney

K. H. LANGER, W. THOENES and A. WARNING[1]

With 3 Figures

Most experimental investigations on tubular failure due to metabolic disturbances are carried out on ischemic kidneys. Since ischemia induces many changes other than suppressing aerobic metabolic functions, we tried to induce metabolic tubular failure [see 1, 2] by direct application of potassium cyanide to the surface of the living kidney. Changes in the tubules were observed by surface microscopy and by light and electron microscopy after tissue fixation in vivo.

Method

Male white rats (weight 180—250 gm) were prepared as for micropuncture experiments. Inactin (80 mg/kg) was used for anesthesia. The surface of the left kidney was covered by a layer of mineral oil (37° C). A solution of M/50 potassium cyanide (pH 7,4; Sörensen buffer solution, M/10; 300 mOsm) was dropped on a circumscribed area (5 mm) of the kidney surface for 20 minutes. The KCN solution was applied with the aid of an injection needle (gauge No. 20) the point of which was placed under the mineral oil layer near to the surface of the kidney. For control animals a similar isotonic solution without potassium cyanide was used.

In vivo fixation of tissue was accomplished by removing the mineral oil and rinsing the surface with a 1% OsO_4 solution for 3 minutes. The kidney was removed immediately and excised tissue wedges of subcapsular regions were fixed once more in 1% OsO_4 at 4° C for 1—2 hours. After dehydration the tissue wedges were embedded in Epon in such a manner that the surface of the kidney was cut first. Sections were stained with silver methenamine for light microscopy [6]. Tubular diameters were measured with a screw eyepiece-micrometer (Zeiss). Thin sections for electron microscopy were cut on a Porter-Blum-Microtome MT 1 and examined with a Siemens Elmiskop I.

Results and Discussion

The following observations were made by surface microscopy on the kidney in vivo: the KCN-treated tissue showed the bright red color of capillary blood. There was a progressive increase in tubular diameter. The passage time of lissamine-green, measured according to the method of STEINHAUSEN [9], changed as follows: in KCN-treated kidneys, the dye appeared in proximal tubules at 32 ± 3.1 sec (controls: 11 ± 0.3 sec), in distal tubules at 133 ± 19 sec (controls: 44 ± 1.4 sec). The dye finally disappeared from the distal tubules after more than 300 sec in KCN-treated areas (controls: 130 ± 4 sec). The collapse time of proximal tubules after clamping the renal artery was measured in 10 animals. In KCN-treated areas the collapse time was 160 ± 16.9 sec (controls 12 ± 1.4 sec). It is of special interest to note that in the KCN-treated kidneys, the surface

[1] Pathologisches Institut der Universität Würzburg, West Germany.

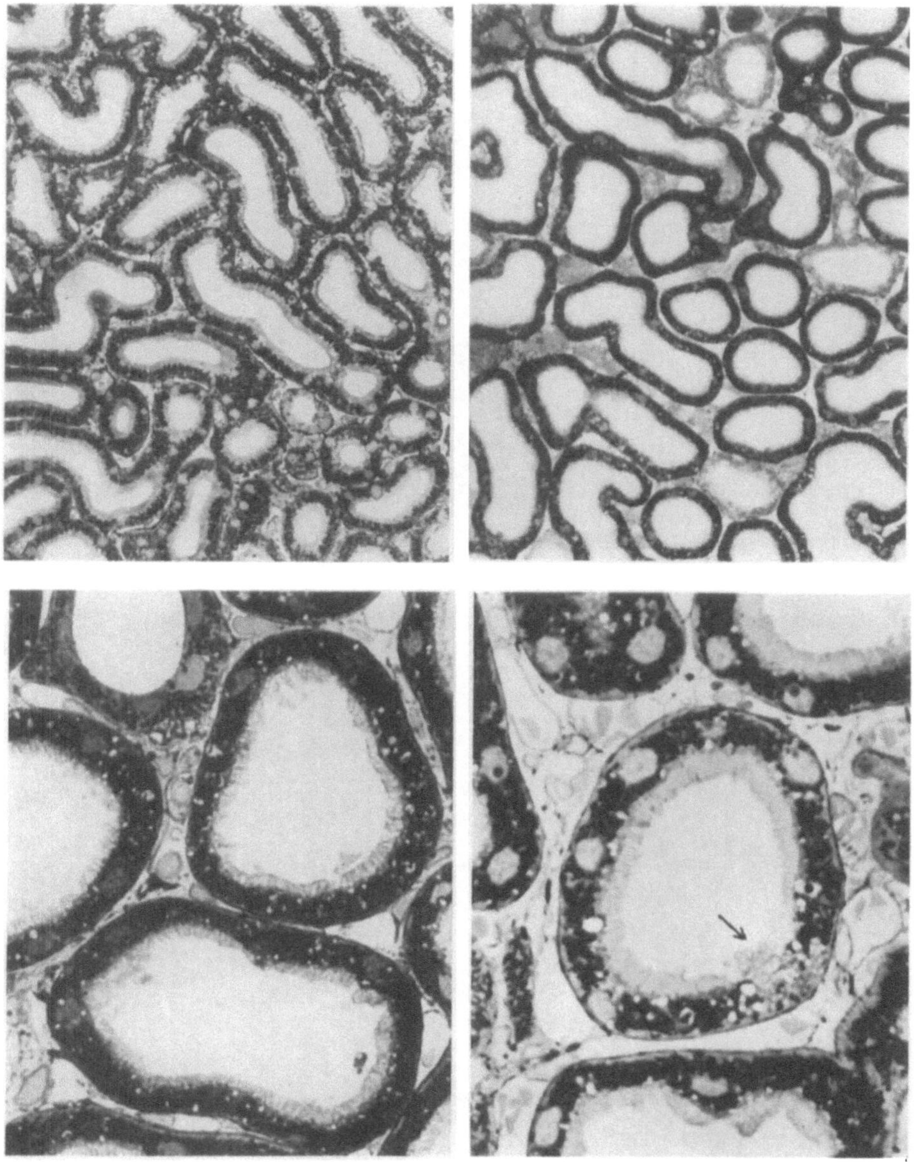

a b c d

Fig. 1a—d. Superficial renal cortical tissue of the rat kidney after 20 minutes of superfusion with a) control solution or b, c, d) 1/50 M KCN-solution. Intravital fixation, embedding in Epon, staining by silver methenamine. After KCN, diffuse dilatation of proximal and distal tubules. Excellent state of the tubular epithelial cells with a slightly altered brush border. One single incipient hydropic cellular necrosis (d). Magnification: a) and b) 185 times, c) 675 times, d) 800 times

areas which did not come into contact with KCN showed the same values of tubular diameter, lissamine-green passage time, and collapse time as did the control animals untreated with KCN.

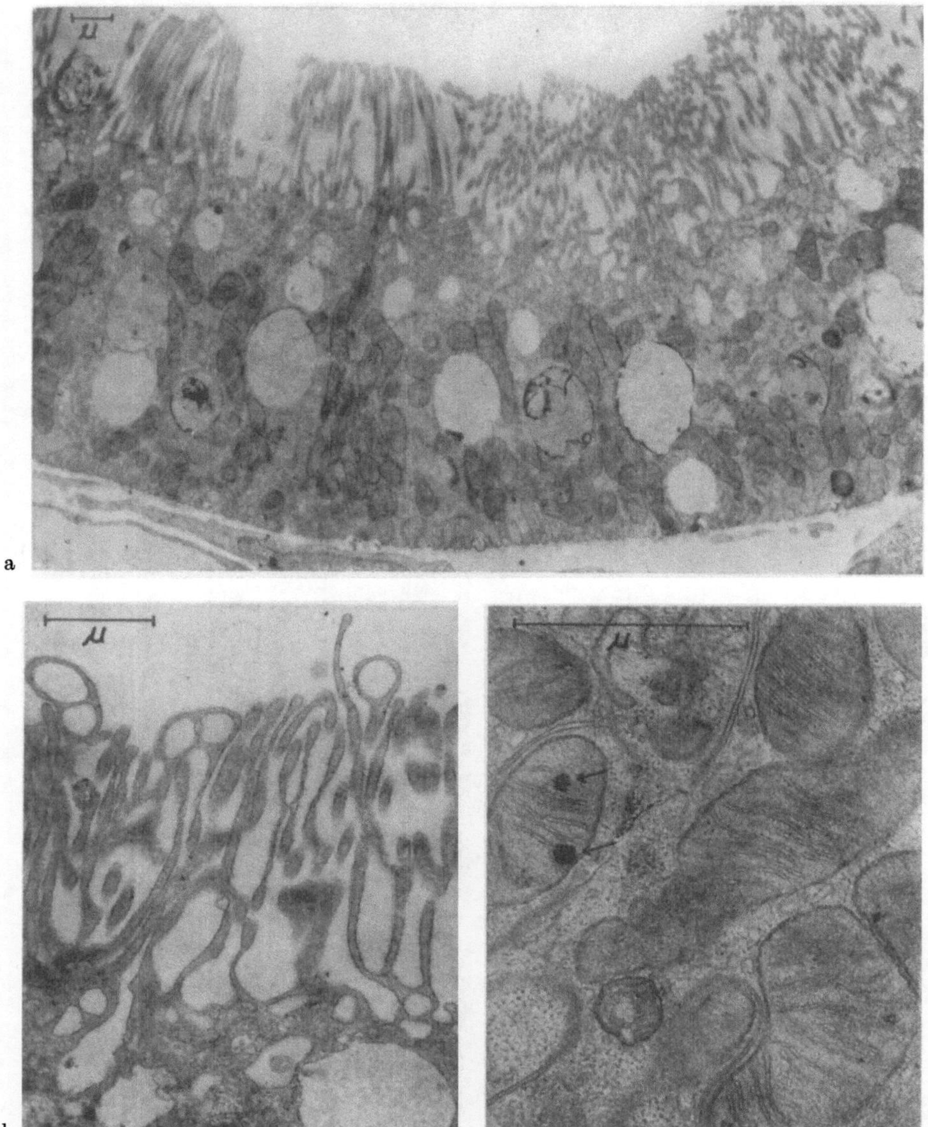

Fig. 2. a) Large field: section from proximal tubule near to the surface after superfusion with a KCN solution with lightening of the brush border, 4,400 times. b) Detail of changes in the brush-border: swelling of microvilli due to the formation of vacuoles, enlargement of intervillar spaces particularly at the base. Magnification 14,400 times. c) No hydropic changes of cytoplasm, no swelling of mitochondria. The matrix of a few mitochondria contains electron-dense material (see [14]). Magnification 31,000 times

Light microscopy revealed a dilatation of proximal and distal tubules. The mean diameter of proximal tubules in KCN-treated kidneys increased from $19 \pm 0.35\,\mu$ (controls) to $27 \pm 0.45\,\mu$ ($p < 0.0005$). If there was no change the in tubular length the intraluminal volume of proximal tubules, was thus, increased by 100% and that of distal tubules by 190%. The change in proximal epithelial surface was not statistically significant. The proximal epithelial surface in KCN-treated kidneys was $852 \pm 38\ \mu^2$, in control kidneys $800 \pm 12\ \mu^2$ ($p<0.15$).

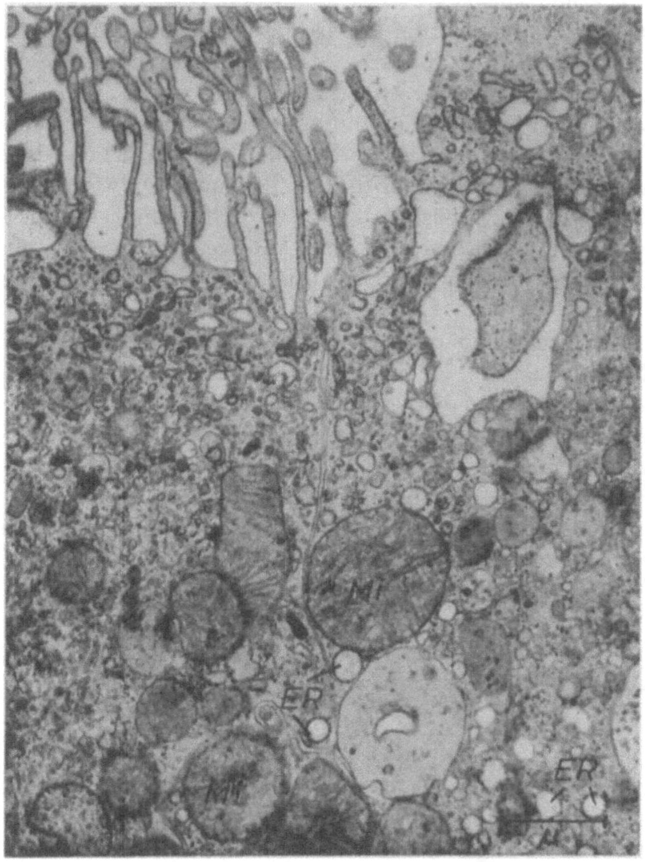

Fig. 3. Hydropic changes in two neighboring tubular cells (compare Fig. 1d) with mitochondrial swelling of the matrix type (*Mi*). Enlargement of the endoplasmatic reticulum. Magnification 12,000 times

The changes observed in the KCN-treated areas of the kidneys may well be considered as a consequence of an inhibition of oxidative metabolism. In this regard, tubular dilatation is interpreted as a consequence of an inhibition of fluid reabsorption (compare 3, 8, 15 a. o.). Since occlusion of normal proximal tubules after clamping the renal artery appears to be due to continued reabsorption of fluid [4, 5, 10, 11], the prolonged occlusion time in our experiments supports this interpretation. With a proximal intraluminal volume increased by 100%, one would expect doubling of the passage time. Since we actually found a three-fold increase, an additional depression of GFR, possibly due to an increased intratubular pressure, may have contributed to the delayed passage of the dye.

Microscopically, proximal as well as distal epithelial cells were very well preserved (Fig. 1b). Greater magnifications showed a slight irregular blanching of the brush borders, accompanied sometimes by partial or total disappearance of apical reabsorption vacuoles (Fig. 1c). Hydropic changes and cytolysis remained limited to a very few cells (Fig. 1d).

Like light microscopy, electron microscopy demonstrated only minor changes (Fig. 2a). The brush border appeared less tight than normally. The microvilli were elongated or thickened and sometimes stuck to each other. Some microvilli contained vacuoles (Fig. 2b). The mitochondria were not swollen, and there were no hydropic changes of the cytoplasm (Fig. 2c). These data agree with the lack of a significant increase of total cell volume. Only occasionally, we saw a few hydropic epithelial cells with swollen mitochondria (Fig. 3). Metabolic failure by cyanide intoxication thus may produce the type of change seen in ischemic kidneys [12]. The quantitative importance of these changes, however, is minimal.

Thus, in our experiment the reabsorptive failure of proximal tubular cells, after cyanide intoxication, is not accompanied by major cytomorphological changes. That this apparent discrepancy is not due to death of the cells is shown by the observation that cyanide-intoxicated cells still are capable of taking up ferritin after intratubular injection [14, method: 13]. However, the rate of uptake is slower than in normal kidneys. This may be an expression of the general rule that a disturbance of oxidative metabolism first depresses the functional and then the basal metabolism of tissues [7]. The occurence of structural changes may be limited to the stage in which the basal metabolism becomes disturbed. The present results indirectly support the opinion expressed by Bohle et al. [3] that the diffuse dilatation of proximal and distal tubules observed in acute renal failure of man is due to a disturbed reabsorption of fluid.

Summary

Under micropuncture conditions an isotonic 0.02 M KCN solution at pH 7.4 was superfused on a circumscribed area of the surface of one kidney of a living rat. KCN superfusion was followed by a marked dilatation of proximal and distal tubules, which was seen in the living animal. The diameter of the proximal lumens was found to be increased by 42%, and that of the distal lumens by 70%. The proximal passage time of lissamine-green was prolonged by 200%, while the occlusion-time of proximal tubules after clamping the renal artery reached more than 10 times its normal value. These changes are interpreted to express a disturbance of proximal sodium and fluid reabsorption due to an inhibition of oxidative metabolism. Only minor lesions were seen with light and electron microscopy. There were very slight changes in the structure of the brush border, but no mitochondrial swelling and only very sparse necrotic cells.

References

1. Bayliss, L. E., and E. Lundsgaard: The action of cyanide on the isolated mammalian kidney. J. Physiol. (Lond.) **74**, 279—293 (1932).

2. Becker, V.: Geweblich gebundener Sauerstoffmangel (histotoxisch bedingte Hypoxydosen). Klin. Wschr. **32**, 577—584 (1954).

3. BOHLE, A., CH. HERFARTH u. H.-J. KRECKE: Beitrag zur Morphologie der Niere beim akuten Nierenversagen. Klin. Wschr. **38**, 152—164 (1960).
4. HANSSEN, O. E.: Early post mortem renal changes studied in mice with one kidney exteriorized. Acta path. microbiol. scand. **49**, 280—296 (1960).
5. LEYSSAC, P. P.: Dependence of glomerular filtration rate on proximal tubular reabsorption of salt. Acta physiol. scand. **58**, 236—242 (1963).
6. MOVAT, H. Z.: Silver impregnation methods for electron microscopy. Amer. clin. Path. **35**, 528—537 (1961).
7. OPITZ, E.: Der Zellstoffwechsel in seiner Beziehung zur Zellstruktur. Verh. dtsch. Ges. Path. **33**, 18—20 (1949).
8. RANDERATH, E., u. A. BOHLE: Morphologische Grundlagen akuter extrarenal bedingter Nierenfunktionsstörungen. Verh. dtsch. Ges. inn. Med. **65**, 250—269 (1959).
9. STEINHAUSEN, M.: Eine Methode zur Differenzierung proximaler und distaler Tubuli der Nierenrinde von Ratten in vivo und ihre Anwendung zur Bestimmung tubulärer Strömungsgeschwindigkeit. Pflügers Arch. ges. Physiol. **277**, 23—35 (1963).
10. — J. JRAVANI, G. E. SCHUBERT u. R. TAUGNER: Auflichtmikroskopie und Histologie der Tubulusdimensionen bei verschiedenen Diuresezuständen. Virchows Arch. path. Anat. **336**, 503—527 (1963).
11. SWANN, H. G.: The functional distension of the kidney: a review. Tex. Rep. Biol. Med. **18**, 565—595 (1960).
12. THOENES, W.: Mikromorphologie des Nephron nach temporärer Ischämie. Zwangl. Abh Geb. norm. u. path. Anat., H. 15. Stuttgart: G. Thieme 1964.
13. — K. H. LANGER u. M. WIEDERHOLT: Resorption von Ferritin im proximalen Konvolut der Rattenniere. Klin. Wschr. **44**, 1379—1381 (1966).
14. — — u. A. WARNING: Funktionsmorphologische Studien zur energetischen Insuffizienz des Nierentubulus. Klin. Wschr. **46**, 696—708 (1968).
15. WALTHER, D.: Ein Beitrag zur Insuffizienz der proximalen Nierentubuli und zur Deutung der „Nephrohydrose". Münch. med. Wschr. **105**, 1370—1375 (1963).

Discussion

NOLTE:

We perfused rats' kidneys, through the renal artery for one minute with a Ringer solution containing 5×10^{-3} or 5×10^{-4} mol KCN, and fixed them intravitally by subsequent arterial infusion of glutaric acid. We did not find any dilatation of tubules nor any change in ultramicroscopic structure.

WIEDERHOLT:

Using GERTZ' split oil column method, we found that KCN intoxication inhibits proximal sodium reabsorption in the rat.

SCHOEPPE:

To what depth does cyanide, superfused on the surface of the living kidney, penetrate?

WALTHER:

Similar changes are found after temporary ischemia and after tourniquet shock. The passage times and the collapse times of the proximal tubules are increased, while the proximal and distal tubules are dilated. Simultaneously the intratubular pressures rise.

STEINHAUSEN:

Similar observations were made in the kidneys of animals treated subchronically with the metabolic inhibitor dinitrophenol. We observed a moderate dilatation of the proximal tubular lumina with considerably increased passage and collapse times.

THOENES:

The absence of tubular dilatation after intra-arterial injections of cyanide may be due to primary toxic lesions of the vascular system which depress GFR. Consequently, the intratubular pressure may become so low that an inhibition of fluid reabsorption does not induce tubular dilatation.

LANGER:

Microscopic studies on sections at a right angle to the surface show that the depth of penetration of KCN corresponds approximately to 2—3 layers of tubules.

2.2.3. Renal Lesions After the Intramuscular Injection of Glycerol in the Study of Acute Renal Failure*

H. C. Burck and F. Petruch[1]

With 3 Figures

Koslowski (1951), Finckh (1957) and Fajers (1959) commented for the first time on tubular necrosis, chromoprotein casts, and dilated tubular lumina after glycerol injections. While the possible nephrotoxic effect of hemoglobinemia remained controversial, speculation continued regarding the pathogenesis of these renal lesions. In previous investigations we studied the kidney of rabbits after clamping of the renal pedicle, using this as an experimental model of acute renal failure (Burck and Petruch, 1966—1967). In this paper we wish to describe our results after glycerol injection.

24 male rabbits, weighing 3 to 4.5 kg, received 13 ml per kg of body weight of a 25% aqueous glycerol solution during light anesthesia with Pernocton, equally distributed into both thighs. Groups of six were sacrificed after 1, 3, 4, and 10 days. 17 rabbits served as controls. After a blow on the head, all were exsanguinated, the blood was collected, and the kidneys quickly removed. The results were subjected to statistical evaluation.

Gross anatomy of the kidney showed a brownish surface with numerous reddish-brown spots. On section, it was possible to see a deep contrast between brown cortex and dark blue medulla, while the papillae remained grey with stripes of brown. These optical differences facilitated the preparation of cortex and medulla for O_2 measurements by the Warburg-apparatus. Because of edema, both kidneys were enlarged, sections were wet, and they were of brittle consistence. Microscopically, after one and three days, the kidneys exhibited dilated lumina regionally, or diffusely throughout the cortex and the outer zone (Fig. 1). The distal parts of the nephron contained chromoprotein casts, positive to benzidine. Bowman's space was distended, as in acute renal failure (Burck, 1967). Three days after glycerol injection, in addition to dilated tubular lumina, tubular necrosis and cellular water uptake was more prominent in the cortex, as well as in the outer medulla (Fig. 1). Ten days after glycerol injection, we noted focal areas of maximal tubular dilatation, much greater than noted previously in other experiments, with sharply demarcated boundaries to normal looking cortex (Fig. 1). Only after ten days was there an increased incidence of dystrophic calcification (Finckh, 1957) (Fig. 1d).

These morphologic lesions were associated with the following functional defects (Fig. 2). Increased serum creatinine and nonprotein-nitrogen (not shown in the graph) indicate that renal insufficiency starts the first day after glycerol injection, reaches its peak on the third day, and starts returning to normal from the fourth day on. Tissue electrolytes show a similar pattern. The cortex

---

* Supported by Deutsche Forschungsgemeinschaft.

[1] Medizinische Universitätsklinik Tübingen.

b

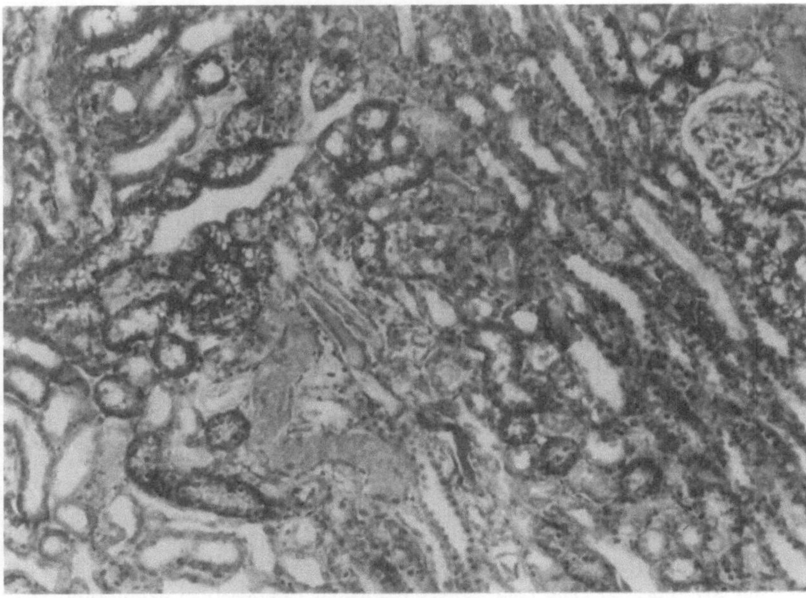

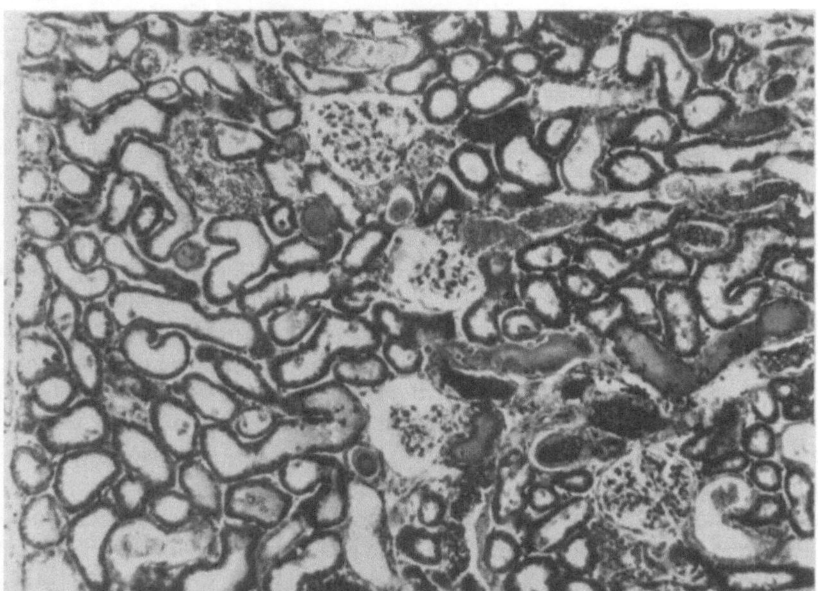

a

characteristically exhibits a dysionia (BURCK, 1963): potassium content was decreased and sodium increased. In contrast, the outer zone shows a loss of potassium as well as sodium (BURCK and PETRUCH, 1966). Because changes were insignificant, we give no figures for sodium, potassium, and chloride in urine and plasma, nor for osmolarity of serum and urine.

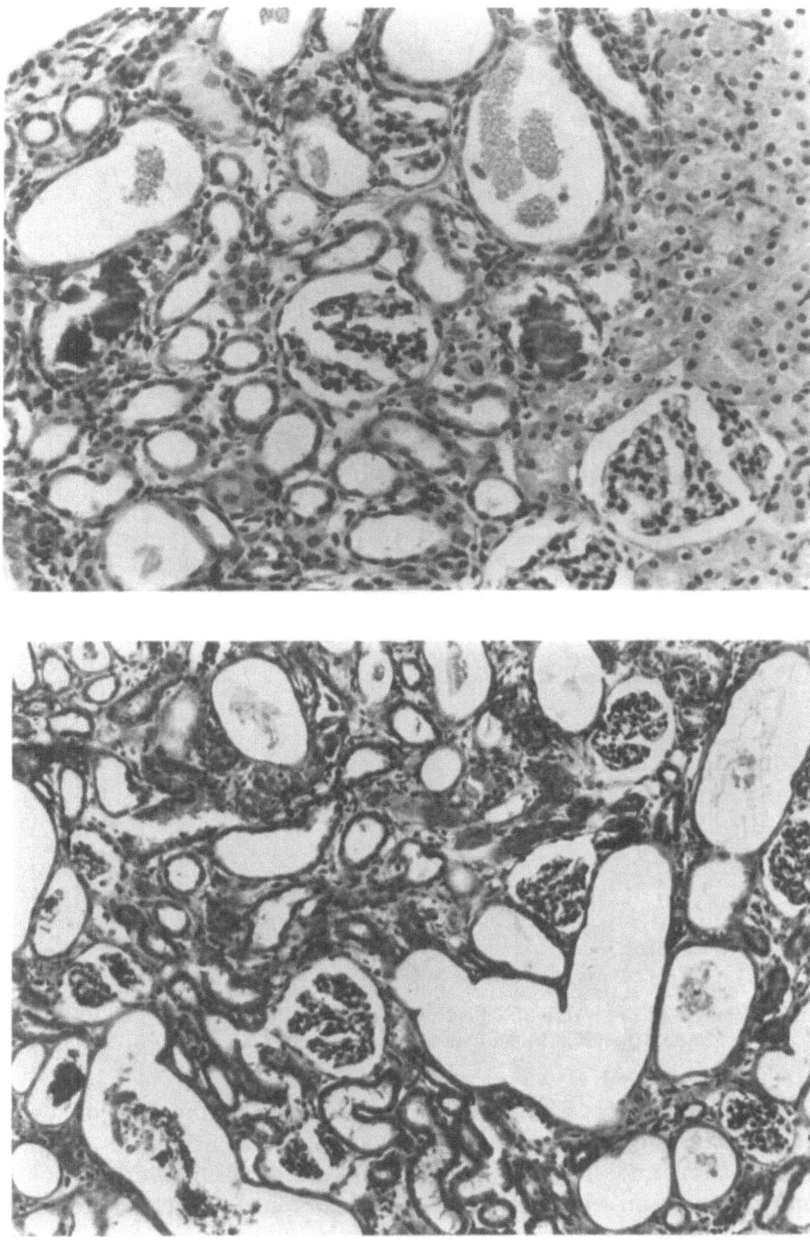

c d

Fig. 1a—d. Rabbit renal cortex after intramuscular injection of glycerol: widely patent tubular lumina, enlarged Bowman's spaces and chromoprotein casts after one day (a), necrosis in a few nephrons and cellular water uptake after three days (b), areas of maximally dilated tubular lumina with flattened epithelium, absent brush borders and basal stripes (c) and dystrophic calcification of some tubules; tubules with wide lumina beside normal nephrons ten days after injection (d) (×140, trichromic Masson-Goldner). Similar alterations of outer medulla could be demonstrated by slides

The oxygen consumption of the cortex and outer medulla was measured in different flasks, with a Na content of 150 mEq/l and of 350 mEq/l in Krebs medium III (1950) (for details see Burck and Petruch, 1967). In contrast to creatinine and tissue electrolytes, which improved after four days, cortical and outer medullary oxygen consumption was depressed even after ten days (Fig. 3).

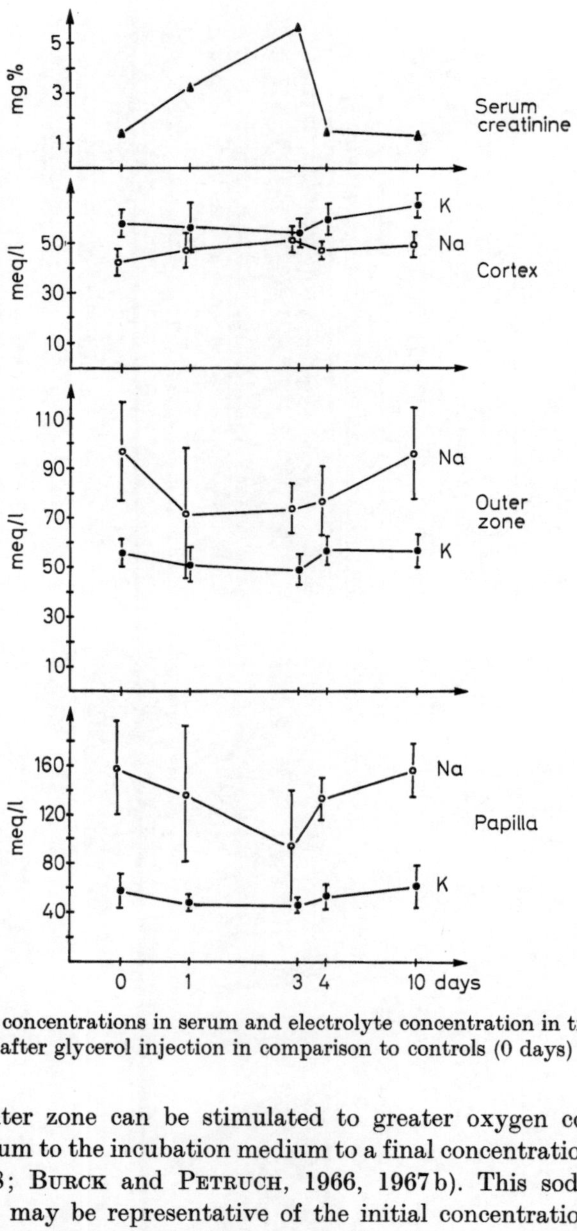

Fig. 2. Creatinine concentrations in serum and electrolyte concentration in tissue 1 to 10 days after glycerol injection in comparison to controls (0 days)

The normal outer zone can be stimulated to greater oxygen consumption by addition of sodium to the incubation medium to a final concentration of 350 mEq/l (Ullrich, 1958; Burck and Petruch, 1966, 1967b). This sodium-dependent increase, which may be representative of the initial concentration effect in the ascending part of the loop of Henle, is abolished at all stages after glycerol injection.

Discussion

Morphological and functional results of this study reflect renal lesions caused by intramuscular glycerol injections.

Fajers' (1959) hypothesis of tubular obstruction by chromoprotein casts is no longer attractive since Steinhausen succeeded in filming cast expulsion by

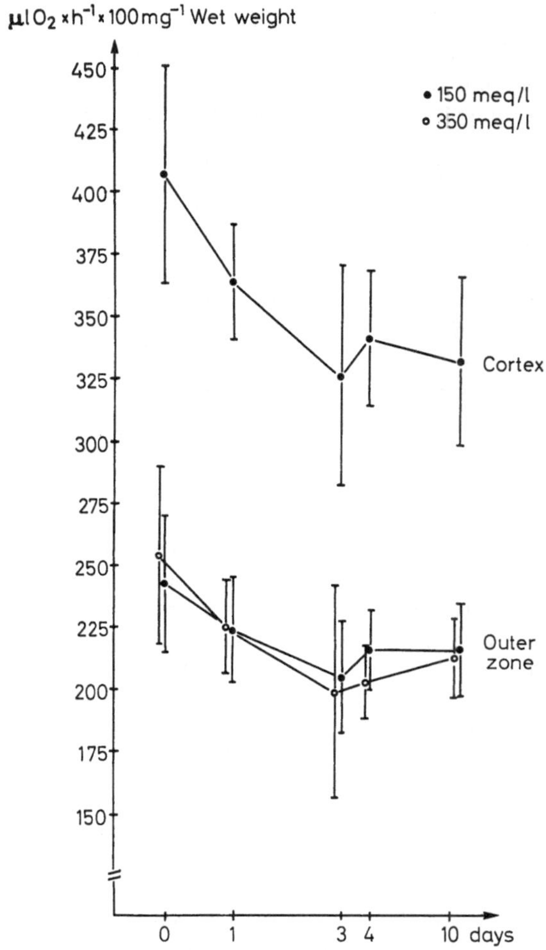

Fig. 3. Oxygen consumption of renal cortex and outer zone in comparison to controls (0 days): increase in oxygen consumption in a Krebs-solution containing 350 mEq/l sodium is abolished and O_2 drastically reduced in cortex as well as in medulla 1—10 days after glycerol application

papilla. Nevertheless, we are unable to give any other explanation for the pathogenesis of the lesions in those renal areas which show widely dilated tubular lumina ten days after glycerol injection, particularly when casts are still demonstrable in the medulla (Fig. 1c). It is possibly a quantitative problem. However, there is some doubt whether the entire disturbance can be explained in this way.

At first sight, one is tempted to blame a direct effect of intravascular myohemoglobin, because of the striking similarity of the histologic lesions after glycerol injection with the so-called human crush kidney (chromoprotein kidney of Zollinger, 1966). Although Finckh (1957) and Fajers (1959) noted a direct correlation between the degree of hemolysis and the amount of renal damage, experiments with intraperitoneal injection of glycerol, which caused renal lesions without hemolysis, are against this being due to merely a chromoprotein effect. This agrees with the conclusions of most workers, who deny any direct nephrotoxic effect of hemoglobin on the excretory function of the kidney (cf. Zollinger, 1966). However, Batolo (1964) and Jaenike (1966) showed that a great quantity of free hemoglobin in combination with dehydration could cause acute renal failure. In any case, a hemolytic or nephrotoxic effect of glycerol is unlikely, particularly since there is no evidence of hemolysis after adding glycerol to erythrocytes in vitro, nor any renal damage after giving glycerol intravenously (Cameron and Finckh, 1956; Finckh, 1959; Carrol et al., 1965). It thus seems impossible for us to comment on the importance of myolysis which we have observed in the areas of glycerol injection (slide). Since glycerol is effective only in concentrations over 10%, we consider dehydration, as a consequence of the osmotic effect of the glycerol, to be an important factor in the pathogenesis. This agrees with the conclusions of Koslowski (1962) and Carrol et al. (1965), who were the firsts to take hemodynamic factors into consideration. In previous experiments, we were able to show a similar reduction in oxygen consumption, a similar change in tissue electrolytes, and a similar loss of the sodium-dependent increase in oxygen consumption, as well as similar renal lesions after renal ischemia in rabbits, indistinguishable from the changes after glycerol injection (Burck and Petruch, 1966). Even though we are, as yet, unable to present a unified explanation, we believe that the "glycerol kidney" is remarkably similar to the kidney of human acute renal failure and, therefore, is likely to have a similar pathogenesis. It is thus possible that we may have an experimental model suitable for the study of acute renal failure and particularly suited to the investigation of the therapeutic problems associated with this disease.

Summary

Twenty-three male rabbits received intramuscular injections of a 25% glycerol solution (13 ml/kg body weight) and were then sacrificed one, three, four, and ten days thereafter and compared with 17 controls. Microscopic study of the enlarged, mottled, brownish-red kidneys showed areas of widely patent tubular lumina and a wide Bowman's space after one day, areas of necrosis and/or cellular water uptake after three days, diffuse and more marked cellular water increase after four days, with focal necrosis as well, and maximally dilated tubular lumina with flattened epithelium and calcification at the end of ten days. At every stage of investigation, there were more or less chromoprotein casts throughout the kidney, especially in the distal parts of the nephron. By means of the Warburg-apparatus, we measured a reduction in the oxygen consumption in the cortex and outer medulla, and abolition of the sodium-dependent stimulation of oxygen consumption in the outer zone. Tissue electrolytes showed the typical features of dysionia described earlier in ischemic renal disease. Three and four days after injection, creatinine and NPN were increased in the serum, while other serum parameters were unchanged. Numerous pathogenetic factors were discussed, with the conclusion that there exists a close relationship to human acute renal failure. It is felt that this experimental model is well suited to the further investigation of human acute renal failure, particularly with regard to therapy.

References

BATOLO, D., P. CALAPSO e C. INFERRERA: Richerche istochimiche ed ultrastrutturali sul rene da emoglobinuria sperimentale. Arch. De Vecchi Anat. pat. **43**, 419—434 (1964).

BURCK, H.-C.: Die Zellschwellung als Folge des passiven Wasserwechsels. Virchows Arch. path. Anat. **336**, 326—349 (1963).

— Zur Morphologie der Niere beim akuten Nierenversagen und beim akuten Tod. Klin. Wschr. **45**, 1208—1216 (1967).

—, u. F. PETRUCH: Struktur und Funktion der geschädigten Außenzone nach Ischämie als Beitrag zum akuten Nierenversagen. Arch. klin. Med. **212**, 313—326 (1966).

— — Tierexperimenteller Beitrag zur allgemeinen Pathologie des akuten Nierenversagens. Arch. klin. Med. **214**, 1—19 (1967a).

— — Natriumabhängige Atmungsänderungen der Nierenrinde, -außenzone und der Leber in vitro. Klin. Wschr. **45**, 1216—1219 (1967b).

CAMERON, G. R., and E. S. FINCKH: The production of an acute haemolytic crisis by the subcutaneous injection of glycerol. J. Path. Bact. **71**, 165—172 (1956).

CARROLL, R., K. KOVACS, and E. TAPP: The pathogenesis of glycerol-induced renal tubular necrosis. J. Path. Bact. **89**, 573—580 (1965).

FAJERS, C. M.: Experimental studies in hemoglobinuric nephrosis. II. The enhanced effect on the kidneys of glycerol-induced hemoglobinemia combined with unilateral nephrectomy. Acta path. microbiol. scand. **46**, 17—36 (1959).

— Experimental studies in hemoglobinuric nephrosis. III. The effect of acute hemolytic anemia (hemoglobinemia) combined with ten minutes' unilateral renal ischemia on the morphology and function of the rabbit's kidneys. Acta path. microbiol. scand. **44**, 177—196 (1959b).

FINCKH, E. S.: Experimental acute tubular nephrosis following subcutaneous injection of glycerol. J. Path. Bact. **73**, 69—85 (1957).

— The indirect action of subcutaneous injections of glycerol on the renal tubules in the rat. J. Path. Bact. **78**, 197—202 (1959).

— Glycerol-induced oliguria and reduced glomerular filtration in the rat. Brit. J. exp. Path. **16**, 119—124 (1965).

JAENIKE, J. R.: The renal lesion associated with hemoglobinemia. I. Its production and functional evolution in the rat. J. exp. Med. **123**, 523—535 (1966).

KREBS, H. A.: Body size and tissue respiration. Biochim. biophys. Acta (Amst.) **4**, 249—269 (1950).

KOSLOWSKI, L.: Experimentelle Untersuchungen zur Pathogenese und Morphologie des Crush-Syndroms. Zbl. allg. Path. path. Anat. **87**, 49—74 (1951).

— Die Pathogenese der akuten Niereninsuffizienz aus der Sicht des Chirurgen. In: Akutes Nierenversagen, S. 71—75. Stuttgart: Thieme 1962.

STEINHAUSEN, M.: Lissamingrün-Passagen in der Nierenpapille — Mesocricetus auratus (Muridae) Goldhamster. Film Nr. E 967. Institut für den wissenschaftlichen Film, Göttingen.

ULLRICH, K. J., u. G. PEHLING: Aktiver Natriumtransport und Sauerstoffverbrauch der äußeren Markzone der Niere. Pflügers Arch. ges. Physiol. **267**, 207—217 (1958).

ZOLLINGER, H. U.: Niere und ableitende Harnwege. In: Spezielle pathologische Anatomie, Bd. III. Hrsg. W. DOERR u. E. UEHLINGER. Berlin-Heidelberg-New York: Springer 1966.

We are indebted to Miss ULRIKE KRETSCHMANN for technical assistance.

Discussion

CAMPANACCI:

In order to obtain some information about the genesis of renal lesions during hemoglobinuric crises, we studied the oxidative phosphorylation in rat kidney sections, after injection of glycerol, after injection of hemoglobin or after injection of hemoglobin and bleeding of the animals.

A similar impairment of the enzymatic systems of the tubules and of the oxidative phosphorylation in the renal mitochondria was found during hemoglobinuria induced by glycerol, by hemoglobin injection or by hemoglobin injection in anemic animals. This observation appears to suggest that the renal lesions of hemoglobinuric nephropathy are caused by the hemoglobin load and not by renal anemia or hypoxia.

Gessler:

What changes of urine flow did you observe in your experiments?

Burck:

Urine flow was measured in a particular way: 24 hours after glycerol application we injected a 1% brillantsulfoflavine in 0.9% NaCl solution intravenously. This fluorescent dye is immediately excreted with the urine and thus traces of urine can be detected on a filter paper put underneath the cages. By this method we only once saw anuria. In all the other animals we had no evidence for complete anuria. Renal failure was indicated by the increase of creatinine and urea concentrations in serum.

2.2.4. Hypokalemia, Metabolic Alkalosis and Hypernatremia Induced by Treatment with high Doses of Sodium-Penicillin G

F. P. Brunner and P. G. Frick [1]

With 1 Figure

Intravenous penicillin had been considered as practically free of toxic side-effects until, a few years ago, central nervous system toxicity was observed mainly in patients with renal failure or cerebral disease [7]. We observed another dangerous side-effect of the drug in 3 patients who were given 100 million units per day of the sodium salt of penicillin-G for the treatment of subacute bacterial endocarditis.

This side-effect is a disturbance of electrolyte homeostasis. Table 1 shows the extreme values of plasma electrolytes which we observed in our first 3 patients (cases 1—3). All three had hypokalemia with potassium concentrations of 2.0 to 3.2 mEq/l and metabolic alkalosis with total CO_2 values from 30—42 mMol/l in venous plasma. Two of the three patients, furthermore, had hypernatremia which may be readily explained. In order to avoid overloading the circulation, the whole dose of 100 million U of penicillin was given in 1 liter of isotonic glucose solution without considering the fact that 100 million U of penicillin correspond to 170 mEq/l, i.e. 340 mOsm sodium + penicillin. When, as a consequence of increasing drowsiness and weakness induced by hypokalemia or by CNS toxicity of penicillin, the patients ceased to ingest fluid, the administration of 1 liter of water proved inadequate to compensate for urinary, cutaneous and pulmonary water losses, and to excrete the additional 340 mOsm of penicillin-sodium. Thus hypernatremia was the logical consequence of negative water balance.

Table 1. *Extreme values of serum-K, venous serum CO_2 content, arterial pH and serum-Na in 3 patients undergoing treatment with 100 million U of Na-penicillin G for subacute bacterial endocarditis*

Case	Serum-K mEq/l	Serum-CO_2 (ven.) mM/l	Art. pH	Serum-Na mEq/l
1	2.3	42	7.49	141
2	3.2	30	7.47	159
3	2.0	37	7.54	165

It appears more difficult to explain the mechanism of hypokalemia and alkalosis. The best known causes of the disturbances are inadequate ingestion of potassium as a consequence of anorexia, or, on the other hand, losses of potassium from the gastrointestinal tract by vomiting or by diarrhea, or through the kidneys due to hyperaldosteronism or diuretics. None of these factors explains

[1] Medizinische Universitätsklinik Zürich.

satisfactorily the disturbance observed in our patients. We therefore considered the possibility that penicillin itself could be responsible for the hypokalemia.

The excretion of penicillin occurs mainly through the kidneys. We, therefore, investigated the effect of penicillin on potassium excretion by measuring electrolyte excretion and serum electrolyte concentrations in 6 other patients who were treated by salt restriction and by 100 million U of penicillin per day (cases 4—9).

Fig. 1 shows the changes in serum potassium and total CO_2-content after 3—6 days of treatment. In 5 of these patients, all of whom had subacute bacterial

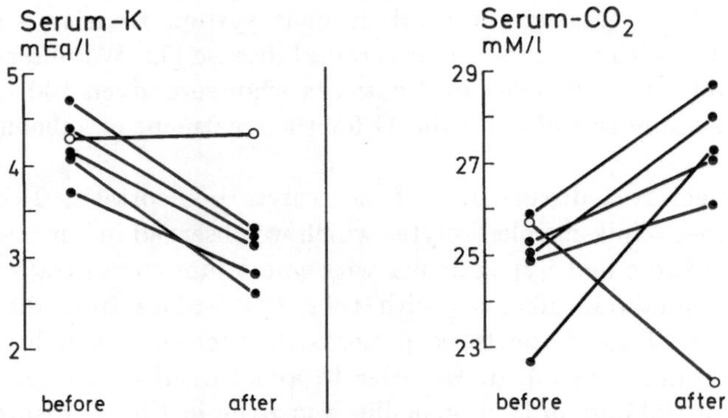

Fig. 1. Serum-K and arterial serum CO_2 content before and 3 to 6 days after treatment with 100 million U Na-penicillin G daily in 5 patients with subacute bacterial endocarditis (closed circles, case 4 to 8) and in one patient with coxitis (open circles, case 9)

endocarditis, we found hypokalemia and a tendency to metabolic alkalosis; the 6th patient (case 9) had no heart disease and did not incur any disturbance of electrolyte values.

Table 2 shows the serum potassium values and the urinary potassium excretion of our 6 patients. In the 5 patients (cases 4—8) with subacute bacterial endocarditis the urinary excretion of potassium was inappropriately high in relation to the low serum concentration [4]. Thus, it appears that high doses of sodium penicillin may induce dangerous renal losses of potassium.

Table 2. *Serum-K and urinary K excretion after 3 to 6 days of treatment with 100 million U Na-penicillin G daily (cases 4 to 8 suffering from SBE, case 9 from coxitis)*

Case	Serum-K mEq/l	Urinary K mEq/24 h
4	3.3	72
5	2.6	50
6	3.2	70
7	2.8	47 (?)
8	3.3	32 (?)
9	4.7	70

Potassium losses may be avoided by using the potassium salt of penicillin-G instead of the sodium salt. This could be shown in patient Nr. 8, in whom we were able to correct both the hypokalemia as well as the metabolic alkalosis by substituting 100 million U of potassium penicillin for sodium penicillin.

Since potassium-penicillin for medical use is practically not available in Switzerland or in Germany, high doses of sodium-penicillin should be given together with potassium-sparing diuretics as e.g. amiprazide (Amilorid), triamterene (Dyrenium) or spironolactone. In patient Nr. 7 we were able to rapidly correct the penicillin-induced hypokalemia by combined daily administration of 20 mg of amiprazide and 120 mEq of potassium citrate for 2 days. In spite of the use of an alkaline salt of potassium the alkalosis disappeared. Subsequently and with continued administration of 20 mg of amiprazide per day, serum potassium values remained normal in spite of continued treatment with 50 million U of sodium-penicillin G.

Discussion

The potassium-depleting effect of large doses of penicillin may be related to the physico-chemical properties of the antibiotic. Penicillin is a rather strong organic acid with a M.W. of 334 and a pK of approximately 2.8. It is, thus, a rather large molecule, which even with maximal urinary acidification is ionized in urine to more than 90%. The drug reaches the tubular fluid by glomerular filtration and active proximal tubular secretion. By its molecular size and its electric charge, it should then behave like a non-reabsorbed anion. The influence of such anions on distal tubular potassium movements in the secretory direction has been studied in micropuncture experiments by CLAPP et al. [1] as well as GIEBISCH et al. [3]. An increase in urinary potassium excretion induced by such an anion or by penicillin could be due to one or several of the following four mechanisms:

a) an increase in cation permeability of the luminal membrane of the tubular cells;

b) an increase in the potassium concentration within the tubular cells;

c) an increase in transtubular P.D. (intratubular electrical negativity);

d) an increase of sodium and fluid delivery to the distal tubule.

While nothing is known about a possible influence of penicillin or other anions on the cation permeability or the intracellular potassium concentration, it has been shown that non-reabsorbed anions as e.g. sulfate or bicarbonate increase the intratubular negativity and thereby facilitate the diffusion of potassium ions in the secretory direction, i.e. into the distal tubular fluid. At the same time, they interfere with sodium and water reabsorption from the proximal tubules and Henle's loops and increase the amount of fluid and sodium reaching the distal tubules.

The metabolic alkalosis induced by penicillin could be related to chloride loss similar to that observed after infusion of nitrate [2]. In our study the metabolic alkalosis was not as severe as the hypokalemia and could, furthermore, be readily corrected by administration of potassium. It appears, therefore, that it was mainly due to hypokalemia which is known to increase urinary acid excretion by stimulating renal production of ammonia [6] and to accelerate the proximal reabsorption of bicarbonate [5].

Urinary potassium losses induced by the action of penicillin as a non-reabsorbed anion do not, by themselves, determine the extent of potassium depletion in patients treated with high doses of sodium penicillin. Thus, one of our 6 patients did not show any electrolyte disturbance. Potassium depletion appeared to be facilitated by a low potassium intake as a consequence of anorexia and by incipient heart failure. In patients without heart failure, eating sufficient quantities of a normal or even a sodium restricted diet (case 9), 100 million U of sodium-penicillin G per day, in our experience, do not induce electrolyte disturbances.

Summary

Hypokalemia, metabolic alkalosis and hypernatremia were observed to occur in patients undergoing treatment with 100 million U Na-penicillin G daily for subacute bacterial endocarditis. The hypernatremia could be related to insufficient fluid administration in the face of an increased daily solute load represented by 340 mOsm Na-penicillin G. Hypokalemia as well as metabolic alkalosis appear to be explained by renal potassium losses due to penicillin, which acts as a non-reabsorbed anion and, thereby, promotes distal tubular potassium secretion. Potassium depletion may be prevented by using potassium-sparing diuretics or by substituting the potassium salt of penicillin G for the sodium salt.

References

1. Clapp, J. R., F. C. Rector Jr., and D. W. Seldin: Effect of unreabsorbed anions on proximal and distal transtubular potentials in the rat. Amer. J. Physiol. **202**, 781—786 (1962).
2. Gulyassy, P. F., C. van Ypersele de Strihou, and W. B. Schwartz: The mechanism of nitrate-induced alkalosis. The possible role of selective chloride depletion in acid-base regulation. J. clin. Invest. **41**, 1850—1862 (1962).
3. Malnic, G., R. M. Klose, and G. Giebisch: Micropuncture study of distal tubular potassium and sodium transport in the rat nephron. Amer. J. Physiol. **211**, 529—547 (1966).
4. Müller, A. F., E. L. Manning, and J. Hodler: Hypoaliaemie, Aldosteronausscheidung und primärer Hyperaldosteronismus. Schweiz. med. Wschr. **93**, 1265—1272 (1963).
5. Rector, F. C., Jr., H. A. Bloomer, and D. W. Seldin: Effect of potassium deficiency on the reabsorption of bicarbonate in the proximal tubule of the rat kidney. J. clin. Invest. **43**, 1976—1985 (1964).
6. Seldin, D. W., F. C. Rector, N. Carter, and J. Copenhaver: Nature of hypochloremic alkalosis induced by adrenal steroids. Amer. J. Med. **16**, 608 (1954) (Abstract).
7. Weinstein, L., P. I. Lerner, and W. H. Chew: Clinical and bacteriological studies on the effect of "massive" doses of penicillin G on infections caused by gram-negative bacilli. New Engl. J. Med. **271**, 525—533 (1964).

2.2.5. Clinical Observations on Drug-Induced Nephrotoxicity: DL-Penicillamine and Aristolochic Acid

K. G. THIELE and R. C. MUEHRCKE [1]

With 3 Figures

Renal disease occurred in three patients during treatment with DL-penicillamine and aristolochic acid. The clinical value of these observations is minimal, because DL-penicillamine is no longer commercially available and aristolochic acid was given in a much higher dose than is recommended today. Penicillamine (β,β-dimethylcysteine) is a degradation product of penicillin. It is an effective chelator of copper, mercury and lead and promotes the excretion of these metals in the urine. In 1956 WALSHE [17] first proposed the use of penicillamine in Wilson's disease.

We shall describe here a patient in whom a nephrotic syndrome developed during treatment with DL-penicillamine. A 32 year old house wife with Wilson's disease, first diagnosed in 1955, was treated in 1957 with DL-penicillamine with temporary improvement, but developed a severe dermatitis so that the drug had to be withdrawn. Since that time her neurological disease progressed steadily. In 1960 she was severely incapacitated and required assistance in eating, dressing and walking. Her speech was dysphonic and dysarthric. There was a coarse, static rest and intention tremor present in all extremities as well as in the head, associated with a moderate degree of rigidity. Urinalysis was normal. The total serum proteins were 6.9 g-%. She was placed on DL-penicillamine, 2 g/d. Under long-term treatment her illness improved remarkably. In July, 1962, she noted ankle edema and soon thereafter periorbital swelling in the morning. In September 1962 she was admitted to the hospital. She had a fine resting tremor of her hands. There was no evidence of a Kayser-Fleischer ring, but there was a 2+ leg edema. Urinalysis: pH of 6; 4+ protein; specific gravity of 1020; sugar negative. Microscopic examination revealed no red cells, occasional white cells, coarse granular and cellular casts and rare double refractile lipid bodies. Total serum protein was 5.0 g-%, albumin 2.2 g-% and γ-globulin 0.75 g-%, cholesterol 425 mg-%, creatinine 0.9 mg-%, endogenous creatinine clearance 71 ml/min, PSP excretion 35% in 15 minutes. In an ammonium chloride loading test the lowest urine pH was 5.3. A renal biopsy was unremarkable under light microscopy. On electron microscopy the width of the capillary basement membrane was normal. The capillary epithelial foot processes were fused in many areas.

Since the patient had shown such improvement on penicillamine, this was continued. Steroid therapy, 40 mg prednisone daily, was begun and she was put on a high protein diet. A week later the 24-hour urine proteins decreased

[1] Department of Medicine, West Suburban Hospital, Oak Park, and Research & Educational Hospital, University of Illinois, Chicago, Illinois, and I. Medizinische Abteilung des Allgemeinen Krankenhauses Barmbek, Hamburg.

from 11 g to 6 g. She lost weight and became edema-free. 11 months later her urine was protein-free: steroids were withdrawn. In 1964, during the 8th month of pregnancy, she had a left renal colic and passed two small stones. Stone-analysis: $CaHPO_4$ and $Mg(PO_4)_2$, no oxalate. A urogram post partum showed several areas of calcification in the papillae of both kidneys. The patient is now working as a secretary. She is on D-penicillamine, 1 g/d, and pyridoxine.

Several undesirable side effects of penicillamine have been encountered. The most serious reaction is the nephrotic syndrome. Until now seven cases have been reported [1, 3, 4, 6, 9, 16, 18]. STERNLIEB [16] first recognized that in all cases DL-penicillamine was the offending agent. This renal complication has never occurred during treatment with the D-isomer. There was a strikingly long interval between the onset of penicillamine therapy and the appearance of the nephrotic syndrome. It was about one year with a range of two months to two years. The renal toxicity of DL-penicillamine was reversible when administration of the drug was discontinued. A recurrence was noted after a dose of DL-penicillamine [1, 4] but not if the treatment was continued with D-penicillamine (RUBENSTEIN and BURKE, cit. by [16]). Our patient was changed to D-penicillamine during her hospital admission. We have no explanation to account for the nephrotoxicity of the racemic form. The L-form of penicillamine is known to be a potent antimetabolite to pyridoxine phosphate [7], but pyridoxine deficiency has never been associated with the nephrotic syndrome. AGNEW [2] described renal lesions in rats fed a pyridoxine-free diet. An immunologic mechanism could also cause this toxic effect; on the other hand similar allergic skin lesions are seen with D-penicillamine and with racemic penicillamin. Renal lesions were also described in untreated cases of Wilson's disease, but these were mainly tubular lesions [8, 15]. In one of 9 patients with chronic lead intoxication treated with D-penicillamine, a heavy proteinuria occurred after 4 months of treatment [5].

Another nephrotoxic drug is aristolochic acid (3,4-methylendioxy-8-methoxy-10-nitrophenanthren-carbonsäure-1) from Aristolochia clematis L., an officinal herb known since antiquity. Aristolochic acid causes renal damage in horses, rabbits and rats [10, 13, 14]. Nephrotoxic effects in man have not been described to our knowledge. There is renewed interest in this drug, since MÖSE [11, 12] discovered that aristolochic acid has a potent activating effect on the phagocytosis of leukocytes. In addition it has been tried in patients with cancer. During clinical investigations on aristolochic acid we observed acute oliguric renal failure in one patient, and a tremendous diuresis in another patient.

The first patient was a 53 year old woman with metastatic breast cancer. She had been treated with radioactive cobalt, 5-fluorouracil and bilateral oophorectomy and adrenalectomy. At the time of admission she was on cortisone acetate 100 mg/d, and Cushingoid features were present. Serum electrolytes were normal, BUN 24 mg-%. On May 6, 1962, she was started on aristolochic acid, 75 mg i.v. per day. After the third day she became oliguric, and aristolochic acid was discontinued (Fig. 1). Renal biopsy on the sixth day showed marked tubular necrosis (Fig. 2). She remained oliguric and, in spite of intensive therapy, died 25 days later.

The second patient, a 57 year old cachectic negro male, had a resection for rectal carcinoma 3 years before and now had severe pain over the lumbosacral

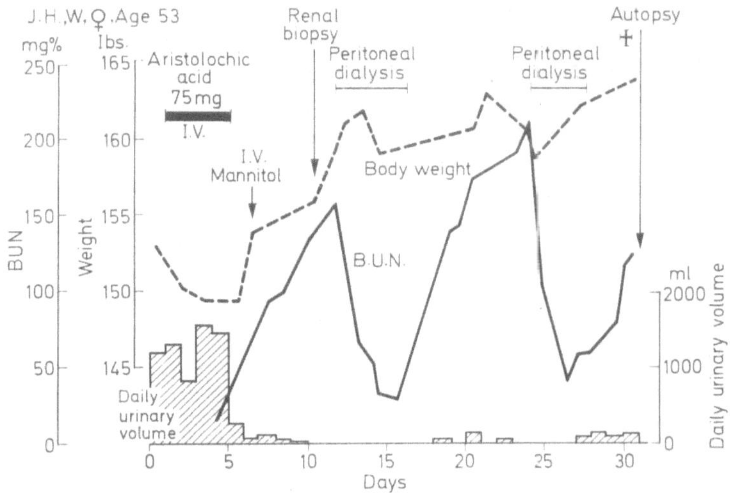

Fig. 1. Clinical findings in a patient with acute renal failure following aristolochic acid

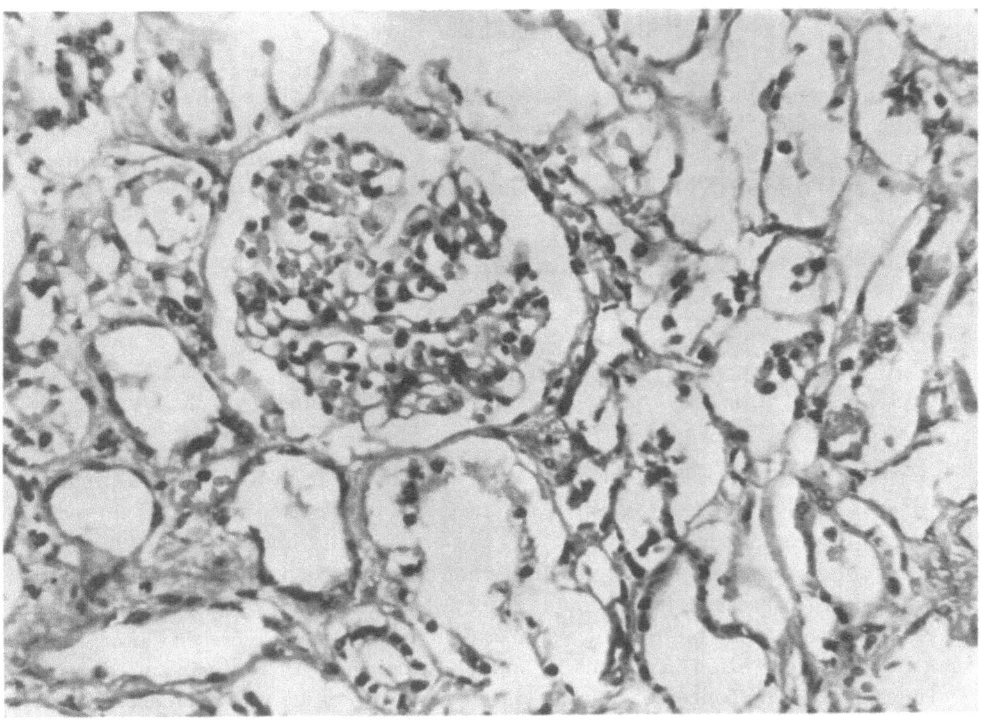

Fig. 2. Renal biopsy on the 6th day of acute renal failure following aristolochic acid

area due to a metastatic lesion. On March 13, 1962, the patient was given aristolochic acid in an intravenous drip starting with 4 mg/day. The total dose was 1069 mg, his last single dose.120 mg, on April 25, 1962. During this course an increasing urine-output was noted (Fig. 3). Aristolochic acid administration was stopped, but 7 days after the last dose his daily urine volume reached 18.5 L. The polyuria was not controlled by vasopressin or chlorothiazide. The patient was kept in water and electrolyte balance. He tolerated this fairlv well. Gradually, over a 3 week period, the diuresis subsided.

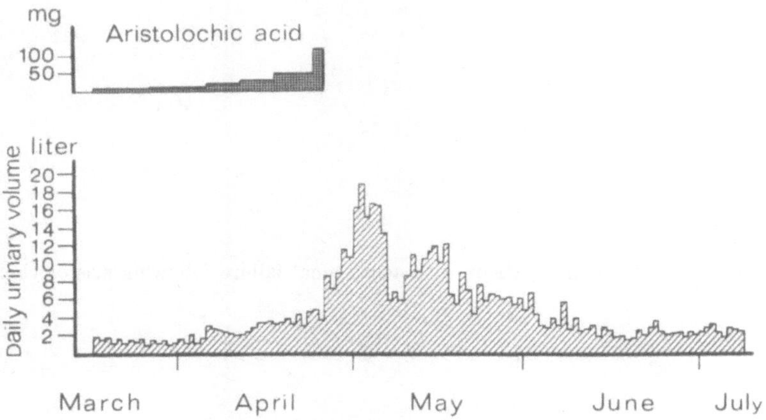

Fig. 3. Polyuria induced by aristolochic acid

The first renal biopsy on May 17 showed severe interstitial edema and degenerative changes in the tubuli. The second biopsy one month later revealed only focal interstitial fibrosis. During the entire time the serum values for creatinine, urea and uric acid were in the lower normal limit or below. We have measured the clearances for these substances only twice:

	5/15/1962	6/17/1962
Creatinine	69 ml/min	94 ml/min
Urea	24 ml/min	37 ml/min
Uric acid	58 ml/min	39 ml/min

Renal effects of aristolochic acid have previously been studied in animals. Pohl in 1892 [14] noted that in rabbits after 7 mg/kg AS a marked diuresis occurs. After a higher dose, 15 mg/kg, the animals die in acute renal failure. Méhes found later that this polyuria does not respond to ADH [10]. Peters and Hedwall [13] observed that a single injection of 30 mg/kg of aristolochic acid in rats induced renal failure with a decrease in GFR and increased urea and creatinine concentration in plasma as well as impairment of the urinary concentrating ability. The concentration of urea in papillary tissue was decreased, both when referred to (urea) plasma and to (urea) urine. The absolute values of the trans-collecting duct urea gradients rose with increasing urinary urea concentrations both in controls and in injected animals. The slope of the rise was steeper in rats injected with aristolochic acid. The data are interpreted to show that intoxication with aristolochic acid causes a decrease in the permeability of the walls of collecting ducts and possibly also of the proximal tubules to urea. Our clinical observations thus, have a counterpart in animal experiments. Whether aristolochic acid induces acute oliguric renal failure or renal diabetes insipidus may depend on the doses used.

References

1. Adams, D. A., R. Goldman, M. H. Maxwell, and H. Latta: Nephrotic syndrome associated with penicillamine therapy of Wilson's disease. Amer. J. Med. **36**, 330—336 (1964).
2. Agnew, L. R. C.: Renal lesions in pyridoxine-deficient rats. J. Path. Bact. **63**, 699—705 (1951).
3. Boudin, G., et B. Pépin: Accidente rénaux dans deux cas maladie de Wilson traités par la pénicillamine. Bull. Soc. méd. Hôp. Paris **116**, 833—842 (1965).
4. Fellers, F. X., and N. T. Shahide: Nephrotic syndrome induced by penicillamine therapy. Amer. J. Dis. Child. **98**, 699 (1959).
5. Goldberg, A., J. A. Smith, and A. C. Lockhead: Treatment of lead-poisoning with oral penicillamine. Brit. med. J. **1963 I**, 1270—1274.
6. Hirschman, S. Z., and K. J. Isselbacher: The nephrotic syndrome as a complication of penicillamine therapy for hepatolenticular degeneration (Wilson's disease). Ann. intern. Med. **62**, 1297—1300 (1965).
7. Jaffe, I. A., K. Altman, and P. Merryman: The antipyridoxine effect of penicillamine in man. J. clin. Invest. **43**, 1869—1873 (1964).
8. Kark, R. M.: Some aspects of nutrition and the kidney. Amer. J. Med. **25**, 698—707 (1958).
9. Karp, M., and M. Lurie: Nephrotic syndrome in the course of treatment of Wilson's disease with DL-penicillamine. Arch. Dis. Childh. **41**, 684—687 (1966).
10. Méhes, J., L. Desci, F. Varga u. S. Kovács: Selektive chemische Ausschaltung der Harnkanälchen I. Ordnung bei Kaninchen. Naunyn-Schmiedebergs Arch. exp. Path. Pharmakol. **234**, 548—565 (1958).
11. Möse, J. R.: Weitere Untersuchungen über die Wirkung der Aristolochia-Säure. Arzneimittel-Forsch. **16**, 118—122 (1966).
12. —, u. G. Lukas: Versuche über die Wirkungsweise von Aristolochia clematis L. Arzneimittel-Forsch. **11**, 33—36 (1961).
13. Peters, G., and P. R. Hedwall: Aristolochic acid intoxication: a new type of impairment of urinary concentrating ability. Arch. int. Pharmacodyn. **145**, 334—355 (1963).
14. Pohl, J.: Über das Aristolochin, einen giftigen Bestandtheil der Aristolochia-Arten. Naunyn-Schmiedebergs Arch. exp. Path. Pharmak. **29**, 282—302 (1892).
15. Reynolds, E. S., R. L. Tannen, and H. R. Tyler: The renal lesion in Wilson's disease. Amer. J. Med. **40**, 518—527 (1966).
16. Sternlieb, I.: Penicillamine and the nephrotic syndrome. J. Amer. med. Ass. **198**, 173—174 (1966).
17. Walshe, J. M.: Wilson's disease: New oral therapy. Lancet **1956 I**, 25—26.
18. Yonis, I. Z., and M. Karp: Chelating agents in Wilson's disease. Lancet **1963 II**, 689.

2.2.6. Reversible Fanconi Syndrome due to a Toxic Degradation Product of a Tetracycline*

J. Brodehl, K. Gellissen, W. Hagge and H. Schumacher [1]

With 4 Figures

The renal Fanconi syndrome (gluco-amino-phosphate diabetes) may be caused by various metabolic disturbances (cystinosis, galactosemia, Wilson's disease, etc.) or by exogenous intoxications (e.g. lead, uranium, maleic acid, dichromates, etc.). In 1963, reports appeared in the American literature [5, 7, 9, 15] describing toxic disturbances of proximal tubular function which were caused by degradation products of a tetracycline. We observed this type of intoxication in a girl, 3.5 years of age, and shall report on the evolution of the renal changes.

The girl, born 1963, had repeatedly had urinary tract infections since 1964. A relapse was treated from Feb. 27 to March 14, 1967 with chloramphenicol and a tetracycline containing proprietary drug marketed under the trade name of Tetra-citro. 4 days after finishing the treatment, proteinuria and glucosuria were noted by her physician, and the girl, therefore, was refered to the hospital.

On admission the girl did not appear to be acutely ill. She had, however, hyperchloremic acidosis (Fig. 1) with a serum chloride value of 116 mEq/l and a bicarbonate of 16.0 mEq/l. The serum phosphate concentration was 1.8 mg-%. The urine contained more than 0.5% of protein (Esbach), mainly albumin; there were no paraproteins [2]. The urine contained glucose at normal blood glucose levels. All findings reverted to normal within 30 days. Clearance studies were done on the days marked by "Cl" in Fig. 1; a final study was performed 4 months later.

The first clearance study was done 14 days after the end of tetracycline administration. The glomerular filtration rate (C_{In}) was decreased to 60 ml/min/1.73 m² and the C_{PAH} to 116 ml/min/1.73 m² (Fig. 2). The filtration fraction was, thus, considerably increased (0.51). One week later, C_{PAH} had increased and the filtration fraction had fallen to 0.23. 4 months later, both C_{In} and C_{PAH} were still slightly depressed. The renal clearance of potassium was first increased, and that of sodium decreased. Both became normal after 4 months.

The specific functions of the proximal tubules showed the following changes: the maximal tubular capacity for phosphate reabsorption (Tm_P) was first considerably depressed to 1 mg/min/1.73 m², and the ratio Tm_P/C_{In} was lowered to 15.0 µg/ml. 4 months later, phosphate reabsorption had almost completely recovered. The clearance of endogenous phosphate was not increased as a consequence of the depression of GFR. Maximal tubular reabsorption of glucose (Tm_G)

* Supported by Deutsche Forschungsgemeinschaft.

[1] Universitäts-Kinderklinik Bonn, West Germany.

[2] We gratefully acknowledge the help of Prof. Vorländer, Med. Univ.-Klinik Bonn, who carried out the urinary electrophoresis.

was measured only once, at a time when the renal glucosuria had already disappeared. The value of Tm_G/C_{In} at this time was normal (2.16 mg/ml).

The most conspicuous disturbances occurred in the reabsorption of amino acids. The clearances of amino acids were elevated (Fig. 3). In Fig. 3, black columns show the clearance rates of individual amino acids analyzed by column chromatography. White columns show the mean values of 12 healthy children. In our patient there was generalized hyperaminoaciduria similar to that described by

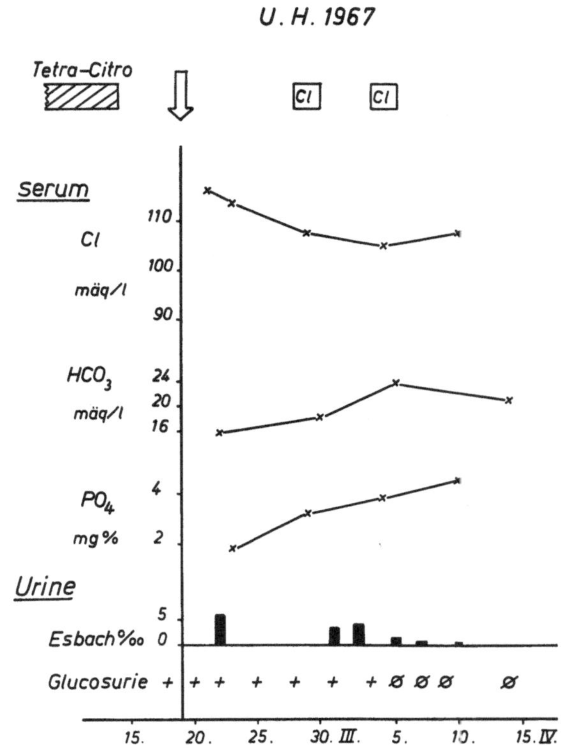

Fig. 1. Serum and urinary findings in a girl, 3.5 years old, with nephropathy due to degraded tetracycline

others [4, 10]. Of some amino acids less than 60% of the filtered loads were reabsorbed by the tubules.

Fig. 4 demonstrates the course of the hyperaminoaciduria. After 1 week amino acid clearances already had fallen to half of their initial values. After 4 months all the clearance rates had become normal.

The patient, thus, had a toxic Fanconi syndrome which was completely reversible, except for the still lowered values for C_{In} and C_{PAH} after 4 months, which may, however, have been low before the intoxication.

The etiological role of a degraded tetracycline could be proved by the demonstration of the presence of degradation products. The sugar coated pills contained a brownish powder, in which Prof. Roth (Dep. Pharmaceutics, University of

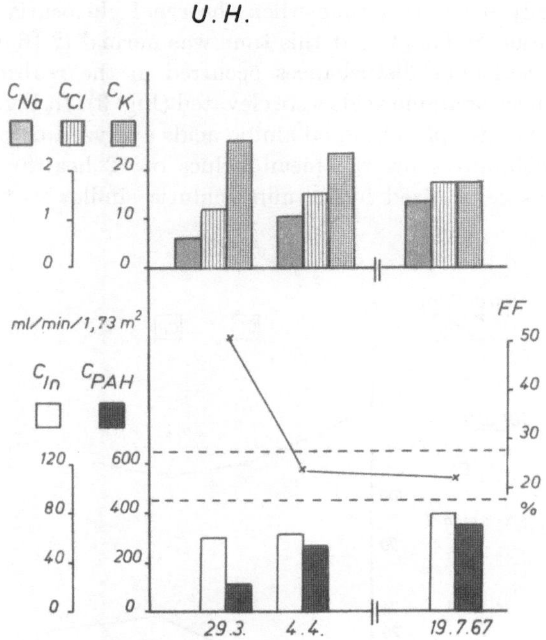

Fig. 2. Changes in glomerular filtration rate (C_{In}), renal plasma flow (C_{PAH}) and electrolyte clearance (C_{Na}, C_K, C_{Cl}) in the girl with nephropathy due to degraded tetracycline

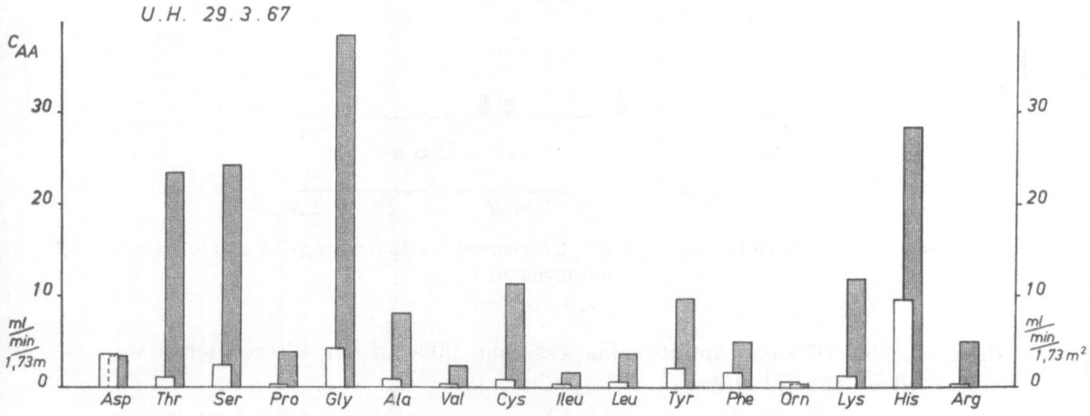

Fig. 3. Clearance rates of free amino acids in the girl with nephropathy due to degraded tetracycline (= black columns), compared to values of 12 normal children (= white columns)

Bonn) demonstrated the presence of 50% of anhydro-tetracycline by thin layer chromatography.

Among the degradation products of tetracycline (4-epi-tetracycline, anhydro-tetracycline, 4-epi-anhydro-tetracycline), the 4-epi-anhydro-tetracycline was shown to be the most nephrotoxic substance in animal experiments [1, 2, 6, 11].

The degradation of tetracycline is accelerated by humidity, high temperature and a low pH. The drug used in our case was tetracycline-citrate, a complex which is not used any more at the present time.

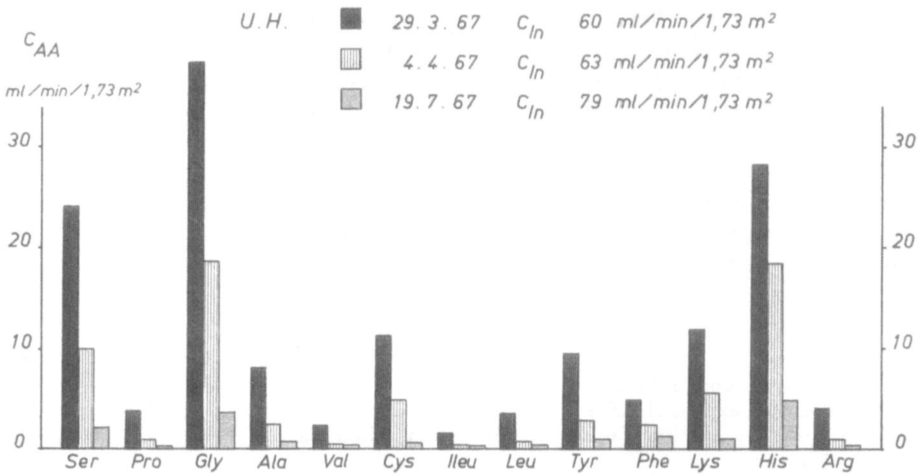

Fig. 4. Evolution of the clearance rates of free amino acids in the girl with Fanconi syndrome due to intoxication with degraded tetracycline

Table. *Symptoms of the nephropathy due to degradation products of tetracycline or tetracycline derivatives, summarized from 12 cases described in the literature* [4, 7,—9, 12, 16, 18]. *First figure in brackets = number of patients showing a given pathological sign; second figure in brackets = number of patients investigated for the presence of this particular sign*

Proteinuria	100%	(12/12)
Glucosuria	100%	(12/12)
Hyperaminoaciduria	100%	(11/11)
Phosphate diabetes	100%	(3/3)
Depressed GFR	100%	(3/3)
Hypophosphatemia	80%	(8/10)
Hypouricemia	80%	(4/5)
Hypokalemia	73%	(8/11)
Polyuria (or disturbed urinary concentration, dehydration)	70%	(7/10)
Acidosis	64%	(7/11)
Bence-Jones proteinuria	40%	(2/5)
Leukocyturia	33%	(3/9)
Azotemia	18%	(2/11)

Our observation resembles those of other observers (Table) [4, 7—9, 12, 16, 17—19]. Most often disturbances of proximal tubular functions were described leading to renal glucosuria, hyperaminoaciduria and depressed phosphate reabsorption. There also was proteinuria and a decreased GFR in all cases. In the majority of the patients a decrease of serum phosphates, uric acid and potassium also was described, as well as polyuria and sometimes very severe acidosis. Increased values of NPN were only found in 2 patients who had vomited and who were dehydrated. In a few other cases, a disturbance of renal acid secretion [18] or renal potassium conservation [8] were the most prominent features. Non-renal signs of the intoxication were severe neurologic disturbances which suggested the wrong diagnosis of a brain tumor.

It may be worthwhile mentioning that in one patient, nephrogenic diabetes insipidus without disturbances of proximal tubular functions was observed after demethyl-chloro-tetracycline [3]. Other disturbances due to ingestion of non-degraded tetracycline (increases of NPN in renal failure, liver damage or deposition of tetracycline in teeth or bone) cannot be discussed here [see 13, 14].

The treatment of tetracycline nephropathy is symptomatic, consisting of intravenous administration of fluid and electrolytes. Since all published cases recovered completely, the prognosis is good, which contrasts with the serious prognosis of Fanconi syndromes due to other causes.

References

1. BENITZ, K. F., and H. F. DIERMEIR: Renal toxicity of tetracycline degradation products. Proc. Soc. exp. Biol. (N.Y.) **115**, 930—935 (1964).
2. CAREY, B. W.: Abnormal urinary findings and achromycin V. Pediatrics **31**, 697—698 (1963).
3. CASTELL, D. O., and H. A. SPARKS: Nephrogenic diabetes insipidus due to demethylchlortetracycline hydrochloride. J. Amer. med. Ass. **193**, 237—239 (1965).
4. CLEVELAND, W. W., W. C. ADAMS, J. B. MANN, and W. L. NYHAN: Acquired Fanconi syndrome following degraded tetracycline. J. Pediat. **66**, 333—342 (1965).
5. EHRLICH, L. I., and H. S. STEIN: Abnormal urinary findings following administration of achromycin V. Pediatrics **31**, 339 (1963).
6. FELLERS, F. X., and R. LINDQUIST: Mechanism of induced nephropathy by old tetracycline. Fed. Proc. **23**, 573 (1964).
7. FRIMPTER, G. W., A. E. TIMPANELLI, W. J. EISENMENGER, H. J. STEIN, and L. I. EHRLICH: Reversible Fanconi syndrome caused by degraded tetracycline. J. Amer. med. Ass. **184**, 111—113 (1963).
8. FULOP, M., and A. DRAPKIN: Potassium-depletion syndrome secondary to nephropathy apparently caused by outdated tetracycline. New Engl. J. Med. **272**, 986—989 (1965).
9. GROSS, J. M.: Fanconi syndrome (adult type) developing secondary to ingestion of outdated tetracycline. Ann. intern. Med. **58**, 523—528 (1963).
10. HAGGE, W., u. J. BRODEHL: Die Veränderungen der Nierenfunktion bei der Cystinose. Teil II. Die Aminosäuren-Clearances. Ann. paediat. (Basel) **205**, 442—460 (1965).
11. LOWE, M. B., and E. TAPP: Renal damage caused by anhydro-4-epi-tetracycline. Arch. Path. **81**, 362—364 (1966).
12. MAVROMATIS, F.: Tatracycline nephropathy. J. Amer. med. Ass. **193**, 191—194 (1965).
13. MEYLER, L.: Side effects of drugs, 4th edit. Amsterdam-New York-London-Milan-Tokyo: Excerpta Medica Foundation 1964.
14. OLSON, C. A., and H. D. RILEY: Complications of tetracycline therapy. J. Pediat. **68**, 783—791 (1966).
15. ROSENTHAL, S., and P. ROTHMAN: Abnormal urinary findings and achromycin V. Pediatrics **31**, 697 (1963).
16. SULKOWSKI, S. R., and J. R. HASERICK: Simulated systemic lupus erythematosus from degraded tetracycline. J. Amer. med. Ass. **189**, 152—154 (1964).
17. THIELE, K. G., R. C. MUEHRKE u. H. BERNING: Nierenerkrankungen durch Medikamente. Dtsch. med. Wschr. **92**, 1632—1635 (1967).
18. WEGIENKA, L. C., and J. M. WELLER: Renal tubular acidosis caused by degraded tetracycline. Arch. intern. Med. **114**, 232—235 (1964).
19. ZIMMERMAN, M. J., and Z. L. WERTHER: Renal glycosuria, acidosis and dehydration following administration of outdated tetracycline. J. Mt Sinai Hosp. **31**, 38—42 (1964).

Discussion

KRUECK:

The metabolic acidosis observed in your case points to a disturbance of urinary acidification. Did you investigate this disturbance? Could you state the concentrations of ammonia, titratable acidity and bicarbonate and the pH of urine?

COTTIER:

At what rate did your patient excrete uric acid? We found, in a case of aquired Fanconi-syndrome, an increase of the clearance of uric acid which approached the clearance of inulin.

SCHUETTERLE:

How did you demonstrate Bence-Jones protein and how do you explain its presence?

BRODEHL: The metabolic acidosis of the Fanconi syndrome usually is due to inappropriate losses of bicarbonate in the urine. We did not measure the bicarbonate in our case. In the urines collected on March 26—29 the values for pH were 5.7 to 7.0, of titratable acidity 30.7 to 5.6 meq/l, and of ammonia 31 to 27.5 meq/l, in a urine volume of 465 to 520 ml/day. To COTTIER: Unfortunately, we did not determine the excretion of uric acid. To SCHUETTERLE: We did not demonstrate Bence-Jones proteinuria. This was done by some investigators mentioned before [7, 12]. These gave no further comment on the significance of this finding.

2.2.7. Absorption, Fate and Elimination of Phenacetin and N-Acetyl-p-Aminophenol in Renal Failure *

U. C. DUBACH[1]

Summary

In 13 patients with decreased glomerular filtration rate (24 h.–creatinine clearance 3—64 ml/min) of different etiology and in 3 persons with normal kidney function, unconjugated and total N-acetyl-p-aminophenol, the main metabolite of phenacetin, was determined in plasma and urine 1, 4, 8, 24 and 72 hours after ingestion of 1.5 gm of phenacetin in capsules, orally. The gastro-intestinal absorption of phenacetin in patients with renal failure was neither decreased nor delayed. Hepatic binding of the free metabolite was similar to the controls. However, the plasma concentrations of the unconjugated and the bound metabolite surpassed many times those of the controls and remained increased for days when kidney functions were markedly decreased. In 29 male and 34 female patients with or without renal failure due to various diseases a statistically significant correlation between the excretion of free and bound N-acetyl-p-aminophenol and the 24 h.–creatinine clearance was found after oral ingestion of 0.5 g in capsules (correlation coefficient $r = 0.454$ for males and $r = 0.547$ for females). No differences was found in the excretion patterns of patients with or without a regular intake of phenacetin containing analgesics. It is concluded that a decreased glomerular elimination of N-acetyl-p-aminophenol occurs with decreased kidney function.

---

* Supported by the World Health Organization in Geneva, F. Hoffmann-La Roche AG Basel, Farbenfabriken Bayer AG Wuppertal-Elberfeld and Burroughs Wellcome and Co. Inc. Tuckahoe, N.Y.; see: Klin. Wschr. **46,** 261 (1968).

[1] Medizinische Universitätspoliklinik Basel.

2.2.8. The Fanconi Syndrome in Hepatorenal Glycogen Storage Disease*

J. BRODEHL, K. GELLISSEN and W. HAGGE[1]

With 2 Figures

In 1949 FANCONI and BICKEL described a case with glycogen storage disease of the liver and renal gluco-amino-phosphate diabetes (Fanconi syndrome). This combination seems to be a very rare disorder since only a few reports appeared in the literature since then [2—6]. We had the opportunity to observe a boy with this syndrome during the last two years. At the age of 15 months he showed a moderate dystrophy, marked hepatomegaly and rachitic rosary. The glycogen content amounted to 9 g/100 g wet tissue (Prof. HERS, Louvain). The activities of the glycogenolytic enzymes were within the normal range. In clearance studies the boy showed the fully developed Fanconi syndrome (Table). The

Table. *Renal functions of a 15 months old boy with hepatorenal glycogen storage disease and Fanconi syndrome (renal glucose losing syndrome)*

Glomerular filtration rate	C_{In}	= 128 ml/min/1,73 m²
Effective renal plasma flow	C_{PAH}	= 434 ml/min/1,73 m²
Filtration fraction	FF	= 22,9%
Endogenous phosphate clearance	C_P	= 59 ml/min/1,73 m²
Percent tubular PO_4-reabsorption	TRP	= 54%
Maximal tubular PO_4-reabsorption[a]	Tm_P	= 2,4 mg/min/1,73 m²
Endogenous amino acid clearance[b]	C_{AA}	= 47,4 ml/min/1,73 m²
Percentage tubular amino acid reabsorption[b]	$\% T_{AA}$	= 63%
Renal glucose excretion[c]	UV_G	= 66,9 mg/min/1,73 m²
Tubular glucose reabsorption[c]	T_G	= 29,5 mg/min/1,73 m²
Glucose clearance[c]	C_G	= 89 ml/min/1,73 m²
Percent tubular glucose reabsorption[c]	$\% T_G$	= 30,5%

[a] Determined after beginning of vitamin D therapy.
[b] Mean value of 18 free amino acids.
[c] At blood glucose level of 75 mg-%.

hyperaminoaciduria was generalized and massive. The most remarkable changes, however, were observed in the renal glucose transport (Fig. 1). The ratio of the clearances of glucose and of inulin (C_G/C_{In}) remained constant at approximately 0.7 and did not change under glucose loads between 50 and 350 mg/min/1.73 m². Under treatment with vitamin D the rickets disappeared, the hyperaminoaciduria improved quite impressively, and the phosphate diabetes showed a marked improvement (Fig. 2). But the severe glucosuria did not change at all during the two years of observation and treatment.

* Supported by the Deutsche Forschungsgemeinschaft.

[1] Universitäts-Kinderklinik Bonn, West Germany.

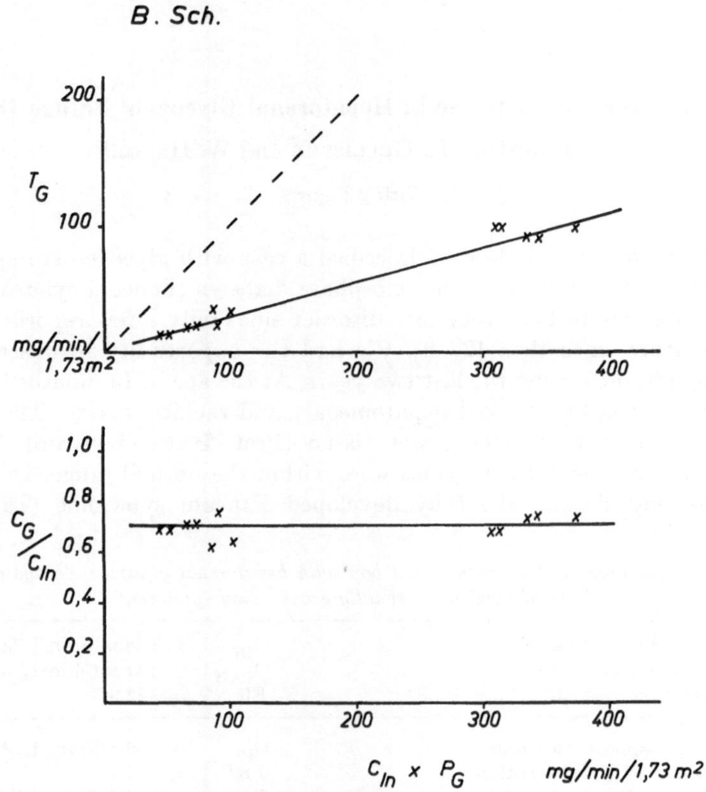

Fig. 1. The values of tubular glucose reabsorption (T_G, on the top part) and of the ratio C_G/C_{In} (below) under various glucose loads ($C_{In} \times P_G$) between 50 and 350 mg/min/1,73 m²

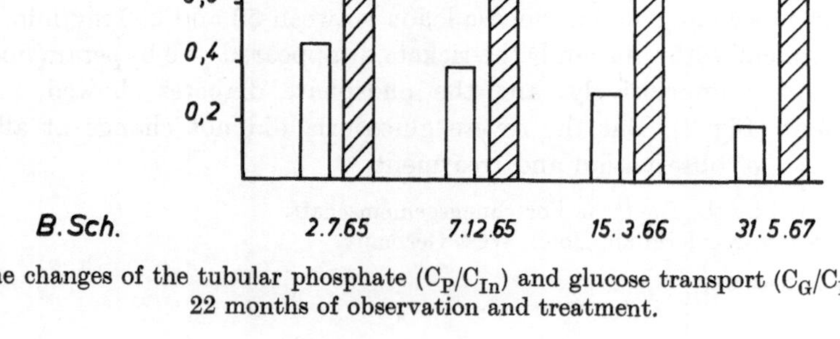

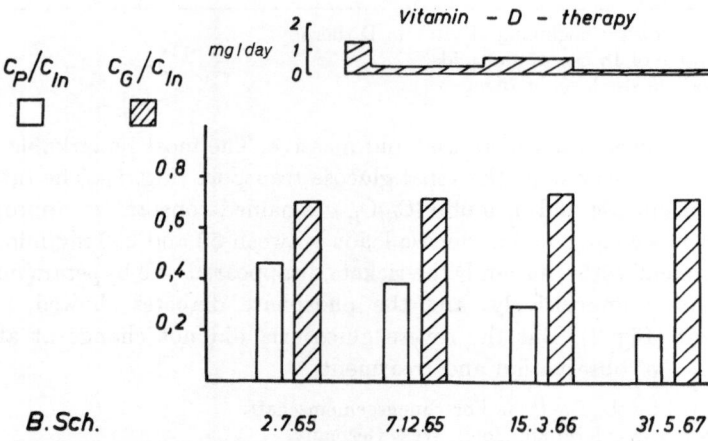

Fig. 2. The changes of the tubular phosphate (C_P/C_{In}) and glucose transport (C_G/C_{In}) during 22 months of observation and treatment.

The enzymatic defect of this type of glycogen storage disease is still unknown. It has been suggested by FELLERS et al. that the glycogen storage may be caused by a massively accelerated gluconeogenesis which is the consequence of the massive renal glucose loss. Assuming that this hypothesis is correct we must consider the renal glucosuria as the primary defect in these cases. Their inability to reabsorb glucose, indeed, is much more pronounced than in cases of benign renal glucosuria. This led FELLERS et al. to call this syndrome "pseudo-phlorizin-diabetes". Since phlorizin, however, does not produce hepatic glycogen storage, renal hyperaminoaciduria and phosphate diabetes in laboratory animals, we would suggest calling this syndrome "renal glucose losing syndrome" (= renales Glucose-Verlust-Syndrom).

References

1. FANCONI, G., u. H. BICKEL: Die chronische Aminoacidurie (Aminosäurendiabetes oder nephrotisch-glukosurischer Zwergwuchs) bei der Glykogenose und der Cystinkrankheit. Helv. paediat. Acta **4**, 359—396 (1949).
2. FELLERS, F. X., V. PIEDRAHITA, and E. M. GALAN: Pseudo-phlorizin diabetes. Ped. Res. **1**, 304 (1967).
3. KIRMSE, H., u. H. FRIEDRICH: Beitrag zur Glykogenose mit Aminoacidurie bei Geschwistern. Kinderärztl. Prax. **32**, 241— 250 (1964).
4. LAMPERT, F., u. H. MAYER: Glykogenose der Leber mit Galaktoseverwertungsstörung und schwerem Fanconi-Syndrom. Z. Kinderheilk. **98**, 133—145 (1967).
5. ODIEVRE, M.: Glycogénose hépato-rénale avec tubulopathie complex. Rev. int. Hépat. **16**, 1—70 (1966).
6. ROTTHAUWE, H. W., H. FICHSEL, H. W. HELDT, E. KIRSTEN, M. REIM, E. SCHMIDT, F. W. SCHMIDT u. W. WESEMANN: Glykogenose der Leber mit Aminoacidurie und Glucosurie. Klin. Wschr. **41**, 818—825 (1963).

2.2.9. Functional and Morphologic Investigation of the Effects of Subchronic Treatment with 2,4-Dinitrophenol on the Rat's Kidney *

G. M. Eisenbach, H. Cain and M. Steinhausen [1]

With 3 Figures

The experiments reported here are an attempt to reproduce the polyuric phase of acute renal failure in animal experiments and to investigate simultaneously tubular functions and tubular structure. 2,4-dinitrophenol (DNP) was chosen as a metabolic inhibitor [4], in order to induce metabolic failure of tubular cells, without interfering with the circulation of blood, lymph or tubular fluid by clamping the renal pedicle. Long-lasting tubular failure could only be obtained with a particular schedule of subchronic administration of DNP.

Male white rats of 300 g were treated for 3—4 days with 2 daily i.v. injections of 20 mg/kg of DNP and were then sacrificed by a blow on the neck. The kidneys were immediately fixed in formalin and Zenker's solution and were examined after suitable staining. The walls of the smaller arterial vessels and the afferent vessels contained occasional hydropic vacuoles. There were no necrotic smooth muscle cells. The epitheloid cells of the vasa afferentia and the smaller arterioles often appeared degranulated, when compared to those of normal control animals (Figs. 1 and 2). The granulations of epitheloid cells were very well stained in ultra-thin slices treated with silver. There were no major glomerular changes besides a slight increase in thickness of the epithelial cells. The proximal tubular lumina were enlarged and contained desquamated pieces of brush border, whole apical vesicles, as well as pycnotic or swollen epithelial nuclei. While the majority of the tubular epithelial cells showed hydropic changes with apical vesicles extending into the lumina, there were also always a few dehydrated cells as well as some instances of cytolysis and coagulation necrosis. The basal membranes were never torn; the intertubular areas were always narrow (Fig. 3).

When measured in metabolic cages, the urine volume was found to increase to 3.5 times its normal value 12 hours after the i.v. administration of DNP, and up to 2.5 times its normal value after i.p. administration. The polyuria lasted for approximately 5—7 days and subsided subsequently.

Microscopic investigations using incident light in living animals were done as follows: male white rats weighing 300 g were treated for 2 days with 2 daily i.p.injections of 20 mg/kg of DNP. They were then anesthetized with Inactin. The left kidney was prepared as usual for micropuncture experiments and was fixed in a plastic cup. The aorta above the ostium of the renal artery was freed from surrounding tissues, and the ureter of the prepared kidney was canulated. The blood pressure was recorded continuously from a polyethylene tube in the

* Supported by Deutsche Forschungsgemeinschaft.

[1] Pathologisches Institut am Städt. Katharinenhospital Stuttgart, Physiologisches Institut der Universität Heidelberg, Germany.

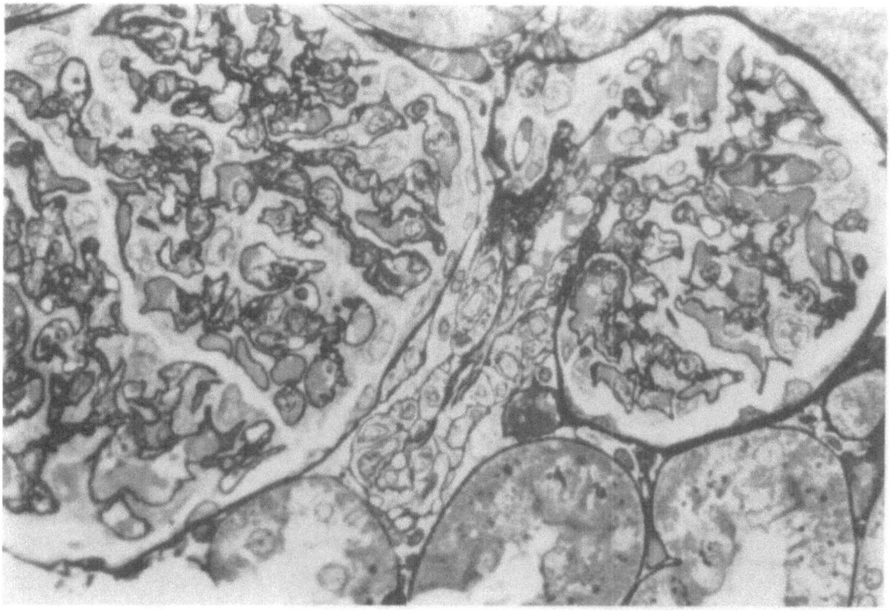

Fig. 1. 2,4-dinitrophenol. Two glomerula with their vasa afferentia. Degranulation of epitheloid cells. Ultrathin slice, silver impregnation according to Movat, enlargement approximately 750 times

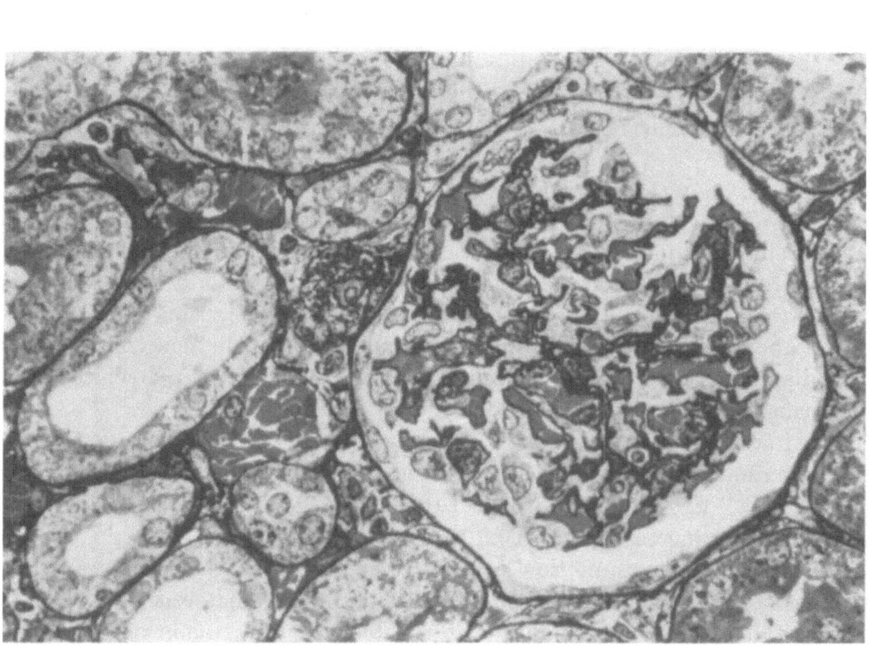

Fig. 2. Control. Glomerulum with vas afferens. Dense granulation of epitheloid cells. Ultrathin slice, silver impregnation according to Movat, enlargement approximately 750 times

carotid artery by Statham pressure transducer. Blood pressures in the DNP treated animals did not differ from normal control values. The renal surface was observed in incident light through an Ultropak optical system at a magnification of 65—100 times. Photographs of the renal surface were taken with a camera with an automatic film transporting device using an electronic flush apparatus (Ukatron UN-60, Zeiss). In the course of all observations, the renal surface and the open peritoneal cavity were continuously rinsed with mineral oil,

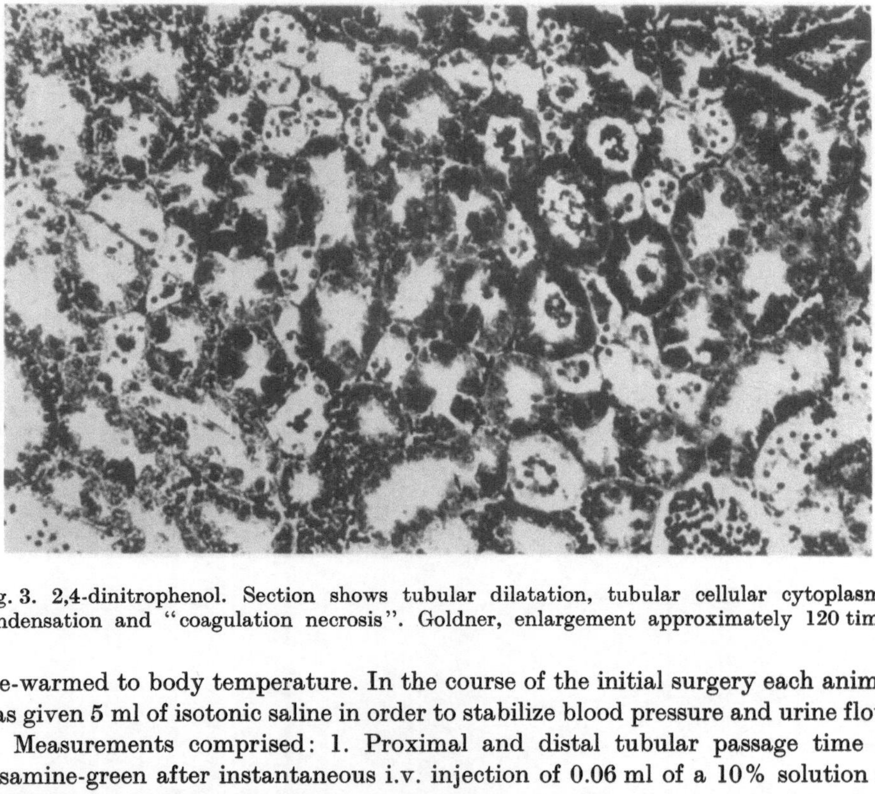

Fig. 3. 2,4-dinitrophenol. Section shows tubular dilatation, tubular cellular cytoplasmic condensation and "coagulation necrosis". Goldner, enlargement approximately 120 times

pre-warmed to body temperature. In the course of the initial surgery each animal was given 5 ml of isotonic saline in order to stabilize blood pressure and urine flow.

Measurements comprised: 1. Proximal and distal tubular passage time of lissamine-green after instantaneous i.v. injection of 0.06 ml of a 10% solution of lissamine-green [6]; 2. The "collapse time", i.e., the time elapsing after clamping the aorta above the renal artery until the proximal tubular lumens collapse [3, 5]; 3. The diameter of the proximal lumens between the 2 luminal white seams; 4. The urine flow from the investigated kidney.

Table 1 summarizes the results.

The proximal passage time was increased from 10.0 to 14.4 sec, i.e., by 44%. "Collapse time" was prolonged from 9.1 to 19.9 sec, i.e. by 118.2%. The proximal tubular diameter increased from 20.3 to 24.4 μ, i.e. by 20.5%.

Proximal tubular volume flow may be calculated from the proximal passage time of lissamine-green and from the proximal luminal diameter as $V = \pi \cdot r^2 \cdot L \cdot t^{-1}$ (r = proximal tubular luminal radius, L = tubular length, taken as one mm in the present calculations, and t = proximal passage time). The volume of tubular fluid reabsorbed from the proximal tubules per unit of time may be calculated using the same formula but taking t as the collapse time. Both types of calcula-

Table 1

	Proximal passage time [sec]	Distal passage time [sec]	Collapse time [sec]	Proximal tubular lumen diameter [μ]	Urine flow unanesthetized rats [μl/min]	anesthetized rats [μl/min]
2.4 DNP 2×20 mg/kg per day i.p.	14.4 ∓ 0.9 ($n=15$)	74.9 ∓ 8.4 ($n=13$)	19.9 ∓ 0.9 ($n=14$)	24.4 ∓ 0.4 ($n=9$)	9.8 ∓ 0.6 ($n=28$)	6.0 ∓ 0.3 ($n=15$)
Controls	10.0 ∓ 0.4 ($n=7$)	50.9 ∓ 4.0 ($n=6$)	9.1 ∓ 0.4 ($n=5$)	20.3 ∓ 0.5 ($n=17$)	3.7 ∓ 0.2 ($n=28$)	3.6 ∓ 0.3 ($n=7$)
Δ %	+44.0% $p<0.001$	+47.8% $p<0.01$	+118.2% $p<0.001$	+20.5% $p<0.001$	+164.0% $p<0.001$	+65.5% $p<0.05$

tion give relative values, because of the uncertainty of the estimation of L. Using the values from Table 1, one obtains the data given in Table 2.

Table 2 shows that the proximal tubular volume flow, under DNP, is the same as in control animals. The proximal tubular reabsorption, on the other hand, is depressed by 34%. GFR must, thus, have been depressed by the same fraction. In agreement with this conclusion we measured in 3 animals a 34% decrease of C_{In} (C-14-Inulin) under the influence of DNP. The decrease of GFR may in part be due to an increase of intratubular pressure. An increase of intratubular pressure was suggested by an increase of the proximal tubular diameter and directly demonstrated by measurement of intratubular pressure in 16 experiments under DNP as 20.1 ± 0.6 mm Hg (see also [7]).

Table 2

	Proximal tubular volume flow $10^{-5} \cdot L$ [mm³/sec]	Proximal tubular reabsorption $10^{-5} \cdot L$ [mm³/sec]
2,4 DNP 2×20 mg/kg per day i.p.	36.7 ± 2.4 ($n=8$)	25.7 ± 2.6 ($n=8$)
Controls	36.8 ± 2.5 ($n=17$)	41.4 ± 3.2 ($n=13$)
Δ %	-0.01 $p>0.1$	-37.8 $p<0.001$

The increase of the proximal intratubular pressure is caused by the inhibition of the proximal tubular reabsorption, presumably due to a metabolic failure of tubular cells under the influence of DNP, histologically seen as tubular distension and mainly proximal tubular cellular changes. The inhibition of the proximal tubular reabsorption leads to an increase of the volume flow in the collecting ducts without a corresponding decrease of the flow resistance there. So far, our results are in agreement with recently published observations of KOCH et al. [2], who showed a decrease of GFR by increased intratubular pressure under mannitol diuresis. The results are also in agreement with recently published investigations of CHERTOK et al. [1], who demonstrated an inhibition of proximal tubular fluid reabsorption under DNP in split drop experiments.

We thus conclude that 2,4-DNP, in sublethal doses, given subchronically, may induce a disturbance resembling the polyuric phase of acute renal failure.

The influence of the renin-angiotensin-system on the decrease of GFR under DNP needs further investigation.

Summary

The effect of intravenous and intraperitoneal administration of 20 mg/kg 2,4-DNP, given twice daily for several days, on renal histology and renal functions was investigated. Histologically the epitheloid cells of the vasa afferentia were degranulated. The proximal tubules were dilated. Proximal tubular cells were vacuolized and sometimes dehydrated or necrotic. The passage time of lissamine-green measured in incident light was prolonged by 44%, the "collapse time" after clamping the renal artery was prolonged by 118%, while urine flow was increased by 164%. These data indicate a depression of tubular reabsorption presumably due to metabolic failure caused by 2,4-dinitrophenol. A decrease of the GFR is due to an increase of intratubular pressure, caused by an inhibition of the proximal tubular reabsorption.

References

1. CHERTOK, R. J., W. H. HULET, and B. EPSTEIN: Effects of cyanide, amytal and DNP on renal sodium reabsorption. Amer. J. Physiol. **211**, 1379—1382 (1966).
2. KOCH, K. M., TH. DUME, H. H. KRAUSE u. B. OCHWADT: Intratubulärer Druck, glomerulärer Kapillardruck und Glomerulumfiltrat während Mannit-Diurese. Pflügers Arch. ges. Physiol. **295**, 72—79 (1967).
3. LEYSSAC, P. P.: Dependence of glomerular filtration rate on proximal tubular reabsorption of salt. Acta physiol. scand. **58**, 236—242 (1963).
4. LOOMIS, W. F., and F. LIPMAN: Reversible inhibition of the coupling between phosphorylation and oxydation. J. biol. Chem. **178**, 807—808 (1948).
5. STEINHAUSEN, M., u. J. IRAVANI: Das Tubuluslumen der Ratte in vivo bei verschiedenen Diuresezuständen und post mortem. Free Comm. Intern. Congr. Physiol. Sci. 275, Leiden 1962.
6. — Eine Methode zur Differenzierung proximaler und distaler Tubuli der Nierenrinde von Ratten in vivo und ihre Anwendung zur Bestimmung intratubulärer Strömungsgeschwindigkeiten. Pflügers Arch. ges. Physiol. **277**, 23—35 (1963).
7. — Messungen des tubulären Harnstromes und der tubulären Reabsorption unter erhöhtem Ureterdruck. Intravital-mikroskopische Untersuchungen an der Nierenrinde von Ratten. Pflügers Arch. ges. Physiol. **298**, 105—130 (1967).

3. Natriuretic and Antinatriuretic Agents

3.1. Action of Diuretics in the Proximal Convoluted Tubule of Rat Kidney

H. HOLZGREVE and K. LOESCHKE [1]

With 3 Figures

After administration of diuretics no change in the concentrations of sodium and potassium was found in the proximal convoluted tubule of rat and dog kidney. Our experiments confirmed these observations. In addition it seemed advisable to investigate the reabsorption of anions under the same conditions.

Method

We performed experiments with hydrochlorothiazide (5 mg/kg body weight as a priming dose and 5 mg/kg·h as a sustaining infusion), furosemide (35 mg/kg and 55—190 mg/kg·h respectively) and acetazolamide (40 mg/kg and 25—70 mg/kg·h respectively). The fluid loss was precisely replaced with Ringer solution containing 7 mEq/l potassium, using two calibrated infusion pumps (Unita I, Braun-Melsungen). Plasma concentrations of sodium, potassium and chloride were determined after every other micropuncture sample. Following the administration of diuretics the concentration of sodium did not change; the potassium concentration declined in spite of the fact that potassium was replaced continuously by the intravenous infusion of potassium-rich Ringer solution, while the chloride concentrations increased after acetazolamide only.

Two types of micropunctures were performed: 1. Free flow samples were collected out of the last loop of the proximal convoluted tubule accessible to puncture and identified with Lissamine green; 2. Steady state concentrations were measured using the stationary microperfusion technique [5, 7, 11]. In principle this method consists of the intratubular deposition of an isotonic test solution containing nonreabsorbable polyethylene-glycol (Carbowax 4000, Union Carbide Chemicals, New York) between a split oil droplet. The volume of this solution remains constant; it has no contact with tubular fluid. After a few seconds a constant concentration gradient across tubular epithelium is established and the electrolyte concentrations in samples of this test solution are then measured. Sodium and potassium concentrations were determined using an ultramicro-flame-photometer [6]. Chloride concentrations were measured according to the method described by RAMSAY et al. [9].

Results

During free flow along the proximal convoluted tubule, concentrations of chloride in tubular fluid increased up to mean values of 144 mEq/l with a cor-

[1] Medizinische Universitäts-Poliklinik and Medizinische Klinik Köln-Merheim and Physiologisches Institut der Freien Universität Berlin, Germany.

responding TF/P-ratio of 1.24 (Fig. 1). After acetazolamide, the TF/P-ratio for chloride at the end of the proximal convolution reached a value of 1.04 only as a result of decreased bicarbonate reabsorption [1]. This effect is to be expected since acetazolamide is a typical inhibitor of carbonic anhydrase. After administration of hydrochlorothiazide and furosemide, however, TF/P-ratios for chloride at the same puncture site decreased to values of 1.15 and 1.14, respectively. This again must be interpreted in terms of decreased reabsorption of bicarbonate.

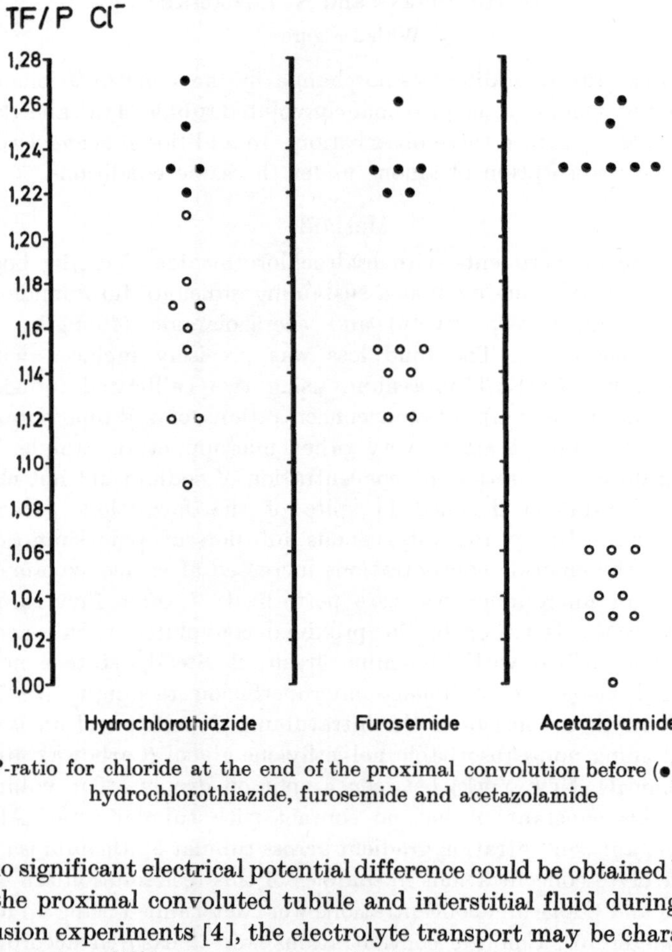

Fig. 1. TF/P-ratio for chloride at the end of the proximal convolution before (•) and after (○) hydrochlorothiazide, furosemide and acetazolamide

Since no significant electrical potential difference could be obtained between the lumen of the proximal convoluted tubule and interstitial fluid during stationary microperfusion experiments [4], the electrolyte transport may be characterized by the concentration difference between the peritubular compartment and the tubular lumen (concentration difference = concentration in plasma — concentration in tubular fluid). Therefore, the data presented in Figs. 2 and 3 are changes of this gradient after administration of diuretics as compared to control values. Each single point represents the results obtained in a single animal and is the mean of measurements in 3 to 4 micropuncture samples.

Fig. 2 shows the results for sodium, chloride and bicarbonate (calculated), Fig. 3 the results for potassium. After administration of hydrochlorothiazide there was a mean decrease of the sodium concentration difference of 2.5 mEq/l in four rats. The mean difference which was 38.5 mEq/l in the control experiments decreased by 6.5 mEq/l after furosemide and by 10.5 mEq/l after acetazolamide. The changes following the application of furosemide and acetazolamide were statistically significant ($P < 0{,}001$, calculated from all control and experimental values). The concentration difference for chloride showed a decrease of

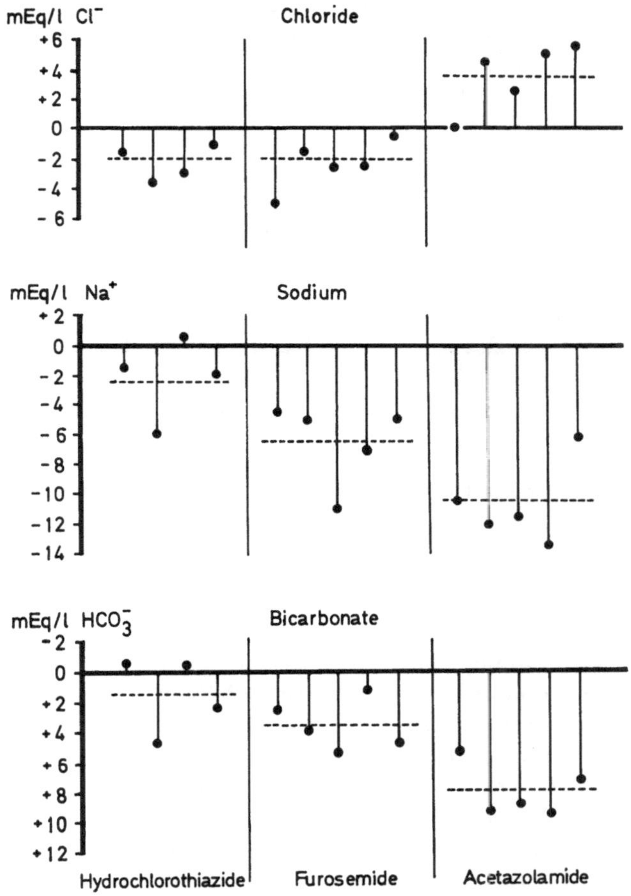

Fig. 2. Change of the Na^+- and Cl^--concentration difference (P-TF) and of the calculated HCO_3^--steady state concentration after hydrochlorothiazide, furosemide and acetazolamide. The concentration difference of the control period is taken as zero, a decrease of the difference is recorded downwards, an increase upwards. Mean values are represented by broken horizontal lines. P and TF = concentrations in plasma and tubular fluid respectively

2 mEq/l both after hydrochlorothiazide and furosemide but increased by 3.5 mEq/l after acetazolamide. The changes after furosemide and acetazolamide were statistically significant ($P < 0{,}02$ and $P < 0{,}001$ respectively). The concentration difference for potassium, on the other hand, did not change after hydrochlorothiazide and furosemide (Fig. 3), but showed a significant increase of 0.39 mEq/l following acetazolamide ($P < 0{,}01$).

The steady state concentration of bicarbonate was calculated according to the formula:

$$\mathrm{TF\,Na} + \mathrm{TF\,K} - (2 \cdot 2.66) - \mathrm{TF\,Cl}.$$

TF Na, TF K and TF Cl are the concentrations in tubular fluid of sodium, potassium and chloride respectively. The factor 2·2.66 takes into account the steady state concentration of calcium in the proximal tubule [3]. A possible change of the calcium concentration after diuretics was disregarded. Fig. 2 shows the values for bicarbonate calculated in this manner. Instead of the change of the concentration difference, this figure shows the change of the steady state

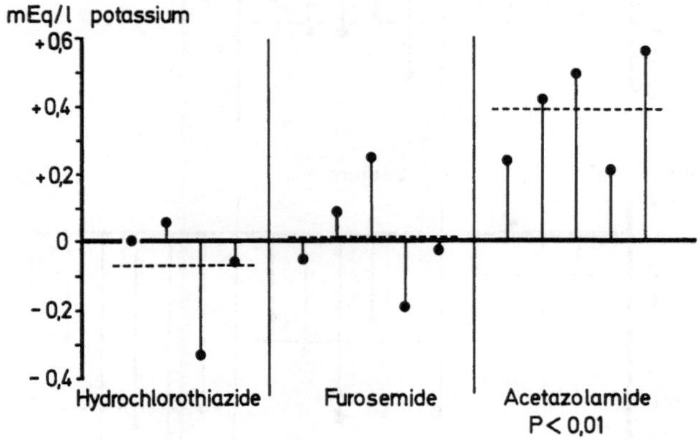

Fig. 3. Change of the K^+-concentration difference after hydrochlorothiazide, furosemide and acetazolamide. For explanation see Fig. 2

concentration after diuretics, since the bicarbonate concentration in plasma was not measured. Furthermore, since an increase of the steady state concentration corresponds to a decrease of the concentration difference in the presence of a constant plasma concentration, the scale of the ordinate is reversed. The mean bicarbonate steady state concentration increases in the following sequence: hydrochlorothiazide — furosemide — acetazolamide (1.5, 3.5 and 8 mEq/l respectively). These values correspond to the decrease of the bicarbonate concentration difference in the case of hydrochlorothiazide and furosemide since the plasma chloride concentrations did not change. Following acetazolamide the plasma chloride concentration increased and thus, a metabolic acidosis must be assumed and a decrease of bicarbonate concentration difference greater than 8 mEq/l must result.

Discussion

The decrease of the sodium and bicarbonate concentration differences are quantitatively correlated, the decrease being insignificant after hydrochlorothiazide, marked after furosemide and most pronounced after acetazolamide. On the other hand, the chloride concentration differences show no correlation to the sodium values. This is taken as evidence that the gradients resulting in the sodium and bicarbonate concentration differences are adjusted by the same active transport mechanism. In view of these results, the mechanism of sodium bicarbonate reabsorption via H^+-ion secretion under the influence of carbonic anhydrase first postulated by PITTS and ALEXANDER [8], appears to be the responsible transport system. This transport mechanism is inhibited to various extents by the diuretics studied. Generally it is assumed that the mode of action of the three diuretic agents differs. Our experiments, however, so far show no evidence that additional active electrolyte transport mechanisms other than the mechanism of sodium bicarbonate reabsorption are affected in the proximal convoluted tubules.

As found in earlier micropuncture studies, the potassium concentrations vary considerably [6, 7]. Following administration of hydrochlorothiazide and furosemide the potassium concentration difference does not change, while a significant increase was observed after acetazolamide. Thus, there is no parallelism between the changes of sodium and potassium concentration differences and it is suggested that sodium and potassium transport in the proximal convoluted tubule are different in respect to mode and/or number of mechanisms involved.

Summary

1. Hydrochlorothiazide, furosemide and acetazolamide inhibit the sodium bicarbonate reabsorption via H^+-ion secretion in the proximal convoluted tubule of the rat kidney as shown both in free flow and stationary microperfusion experiments.

2. In the proximal convoluted tubule the transport characteristics for sodium and potassium changed independently following the administration of the three diuretic agents.

References

1. CLAPP, J. R., J. F. WATSON, and R. W. BERLINER: Effect of carbonic anhydrase inhibition on proximal tubular bicarbonate reabsorption. Amer. J. Physiol. **205**, 693—696 (1963).
2. DIRKS, J. H., W. J. CIRKSENA, and R. W. BERLINER: Micropuncture study of the effect of various diuretics on sodium reabsorption by the proximal tubules of the dog. J. clin. Invest. **45**, 1875—1885 (1966).
3. FRICK, A., G. RUMRICH, K. J. ULLRICH, and W. E. LASSITER: Microperfusion study of calcium transport in the proximal tubule of the rat kidney. Pflügers Arch. ges. Physiol. **286**, 109—117 (1965).
4. FRÖMTER, E.: Personal communication.
5. HIERHOLZER, K., M. WIEDERHOLT, H. HOLZGREVE, G. GIEBISCH, R. M. KLOSE, and E. E. WINDHAGER: Micropuncture study of renal transtubular concentration gradients of sodium and potassium in adrenalectomized rats. Pflügers Arch. ges. Physiol. **285**, 193—210 (1965).
6. MALNIC, G., R. M. KLOSE, and G. GIEBISCH: Micropuncture study of renal potassium excretion in the rat. Amer. J. Physiol. **206**, 674—686 (1964).
7. MARSH, D. J., K. J. ULLRICH, and G. RUMRICH: Micropuncture analysis of the behavior of potassium ions in rat renal cortical tubules. Pflügers Arch. ges. Physiol. **277**, 107—119 (1963).
8. PITTS, R. F., and R. S. ALEXANDER: The nature of the renal tubular mechanism for acidifying the urine. Amer. J. Physiol. **144**, 239—254 (1945).
9. RAMSAY, J. A., R. H. J. BROWN, and P. C. CROGHAN: Electrometric titration of chloride in small volumes. J. exp. Biol. **32**, 822—829 (1955).

10. RECTOR, F. C., JR., F. P. BRUNNER, J. C. SELLMAN, and D. W. SELDIN: Pitfalls in the use of micropuncture for the localization of diuretic action. Ann. N. Y. Acad. Sci. **139**, 400—407 (1966).

11. SHIPP, J. C., I. B. HANENSON, E. E. WINDHAGER, H. J. SCHATZMANN, G. WHITTEMBURY, H. YOSHIMURA, and A. K. SOLOMON: Single proximal tubules of the Necturus kidney. Methods for micropuncture and microperfusion. Amer. J. Physiol. **195**, 563—569 (1958).

Discussion

FRICK:

You found different changes in the proximal tubular TF/P-ratios for chloride under the influence of the three diuretics in free flow-conditions. Since you used supramaximal doses of all three agents, the different values obtained appear to point to different mechanisms of action.

FÜLGRAFF:

Did you measure proximal tubular luminal diameters and did you find differences between furosemide and acetazolamide?

HOLZGREVE:

The changes in the TF/P-ratios for chloride concentration in the proximal tubule after diuretics, in free-flow and stationary microperfusion conditions, were secondary to changes in bicarbonate concentration. We, therefore, conclude that the three diuretics studied inhibit the reabsorption of bicarbonate in the proximal convoluted tubule. The different magnitude of the changes in chloride concentrations with the three diuretics is interpreted as a quantitative difference in the ability of each diuretic to inhibit the transport mechanism.

Further evidence for a common mode of action of these diuretics was provided by the experiments using the shrinking drop method of GERTZ. If furosemide and acetazolamide inhibit different transport mechanisms in the proximal convoluted tubule, an additive effect would be expected during the simultaneous administration of these drugs. However, when furosemide and acetazolamide were given together the inhibition of the intrinsic reabsorptive capacity was no greater than when acetazolamide was given alone.

In a series of experiments the mean proximal tubular luminal diameters in the control and experimental periods were as follows: Furosemide 19.8 and 25.8 μ; acetazolamide 19.4 and 22.2 μ respectively.

3.2. Diuretic Effect of Ethacrynic Acid in the Rat: a Micropuncture Study concerning the Relationship of Site and Mode of Diuretic Action

P. Deetjen, W. E. Büntig, Karin Hardt and R. Rohde [1]

With 2 Figures

Ethacrynic acid (EA) and furosemide, are the most effective known natriuretic and diuretic agents. In contrast to furosemide, however, there have been no direct studies at the nephron level on the site and mode of action of ethacrynic acid. The reason for this discrepancy is that the earliest publication on the action of this substance showed no diuretic effect in the rat [13], the experimental animal on which micropuncture studies are most easily performed. Similarly, in the guinea pig and cat, also suitable subjects for renal micropuncture, early reports showed no diuretic effect [10]. Only in the dog has a diuretic effect comparable to that observed in man been demonstrated [2, 13].

We have repeated an experimental study of the renal effect of EA in the cat and in the rat and observed a marked diuretic effect which is not basically different, in respect to volume and composition of the urine formed, from observations in the dog and in man. We find, in addition, no adverse effect of anesthesia, or the surgical manipulations preparatory to micropuncture. The opportunity is thus afforded to study the site of action of EA by analysis of tubular fluid collected from various sites along the nephron.

Methods

Experiments were performed on Wistar rats weighing 210—290 g, anesthetized with Inactin (80 mg/kg b.w.). The animals lay on a heated operating board by which the body temperature was held constant at 37—38° C. In the right jugular vein, a double-barrelled catheter permitted the infusion of an inulin solution for the determination of glomerular filtration rate (GFR) and of salt solution for replacement of body fluids, as well as the injection of EA. This catheter was also used for the injection of lissamine green for measuring tubular fluid passage times. Blood samples were taken from a femoral artery catheter, by which blood pressure was also recorded by a strain gauge. Urine was collected via a ureteral catheter.

We determined inulin in plasma and urine by the anthrone method [5], and in tubular fluid by a micromodification of this method [8].

Micropunctures of proximal and distal convolutions were carried out under stereomicroscopic observation using glass capillary pipettes ground to an outer tip diameter of 6—10 µm. Since compression of the tubule, injection of large oil droplets or withdrawal of more than about 10% of tubular fluid into the sampling

[1] Physiologisches Institut der Universität München, West Germany.

pipette may considerably alter intratubular flow, care was taken to avoid any of these conditions. By injection of lissamine-green the dye passage-time through the proximal convolution and through the loop of Henle was measured to control the constancy of intratubular urine flow rate during the experiment. After sampling, the nephron was filled with latex and the puncture site localized by microdissection.

Although cats were studied in the same manner the results did not differ from those in the rat. Only the latter are discussed here.

Results

1. Clearance Data

A typical experiment is shown in Fig. 1. GFR and urine flow are plotted against time. Blood pressure remained constant at about 110 mm Hg throughout the 8 hours of the experiment. The arrows indicate 3 single injections of EA

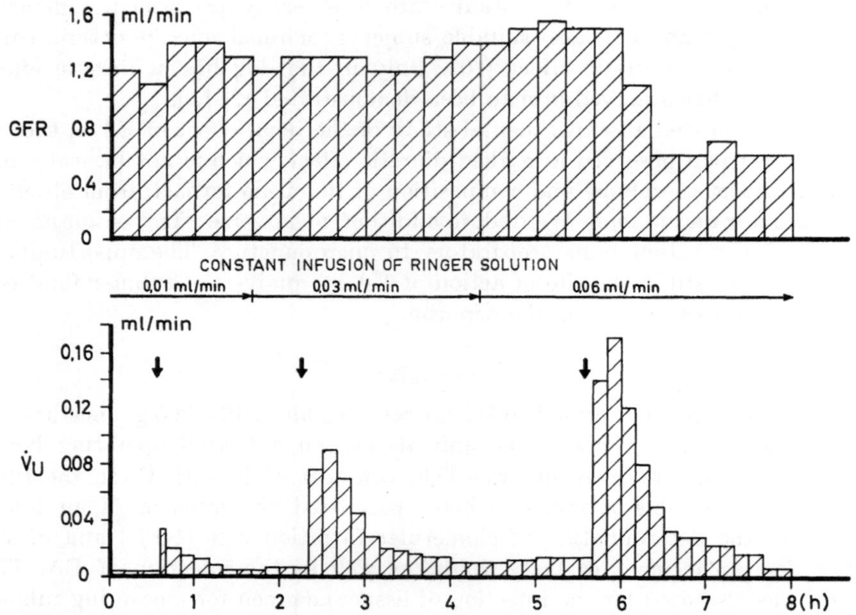

Fig. 1. Urine volume ($\dot{V}_u$) and glomerular filtration rate (*GFR*) in a 210 g rat. The weight of both kidneys was 1.65 gm. The constant infusion of Ringer solution was accelerated stepwise. At (↓) single doses of 60 μM/kg b.w. of ethacrynic acid were injected intravenously

(60 μM/kg b.w.). A diuretic effect followed each injection of the drug. The extent of this effect differed after the 3 injections and appeared to depend on the state of hydration of the animal. During the first control period, at the initial infusion rate of 0.01 ml/min the urine volume remained in the normal anti-diuretic range of 3 μl/min [11]. Following EA, urine-flow increased 10-fold for a short period of time; after 40 min normal flow rate was reestablished. The infusion rate was then increased to 0.03 ml/min with the effect of doubling the urine output. The same dose of EA now had a much more pronounced and

longer lasting diuretic effect. The infusion rate was again increased and at the new control level a still greater diuretic effect of EA was observed; 12% of the glomerular filtrate was excreted as final urine. If the infusion rate is kept constant, repeated injections of the same dose are followed by equal diuretic responses.

In other experiments the dose of EA was increased to 300 μM/kg, a level apparently well tolerated by the experimental animals as judged by constancy of GFR and arterial blood pressure. At this dose, up to 40% of the filtered volume is excreted in the final urine.

The GFR in the experiment depicted in Fig. 1 remained constant for more than 5 hrs. and fell only during the last two hours of the experimental period.

Each injection of EA was followed by an increase in sodium excretion during which sodium concentration of the urine rose to reach that of plasma.

The minimum effective dose of EA varied from one experimental animal to another. At times the first effect was noted after as little as 8 μM/kg. However in all experimental animals and at various states of hydration a dose of 60 μM/kg was invariably effective. This dose is clearly higher than that needed in man or dog; but it is known that with many diuretics a greater dose per body weight is required to produce an effect in the rat. With furosemide diuretic effects are occasionally observed with 6 μM/kg; while 30 μM/kg are effective in every case. In man a diuretic effect may follow a tenth of this dose.

2. *Micropuncture Data*

The relationship between the concentration of inulin in tubular fluid to that in plasma (TF/P_{In}) is a measure of the reabsorption of glomerular filtrate down to a given point in the tubule. In Fig. 2 TF/P_{In} ratios are plotted against the puncture sites. The shaded area comprises 90% of the control values in antidiuresis. Following EA the TF/P_{In} ratio along the proximal tubule is unquestionably below that of the controls. In these experiments an initial dose of 30 μ/kg b.w. EA was followed by the infusion of 0.5 μM/min·kg b.w. It should be pointed out that, in the course of the experiment, urinary losses of salt and water were replaced by infusion of Ringer's solution. The infusion rate was adjusted every 5 minutes to be slightly in excess of urine flow. In other studies in which no fluid replacement was given, end-proximal TF/P ratios up to 6.5 were found.

From the end of the proximal to the beginning of the distal convolution, i.e., during passage through Henle's loop, the increase in the inulin quotient is clearly less than in control animals. That a similar decrease in water reabsorption occurs in the collecting ducts is seen from the small difference in inulin ratios between the distal convolution and the pelvic urine.

In the micropuncture experiments in which EA was administered, the GFR ranged between 0.21 and 0.90 with a mean value of 0.60 ml/min·g kidney wt. During the control periods these measurements had a mean value of 0.71 ml/min·g.

The proximal tubular passage-time for lissamine-green during EA infusion had a mean and standard deviation of 13.0 ± 3.5 sec. Henle's loop passage time averaged 35.7 ± 13.3 sec. Comparable values under control conditions were 12.0 ± 2.4 sec for the proximal convolution and 38.9 ± 10.7 sec for Henle's loop.

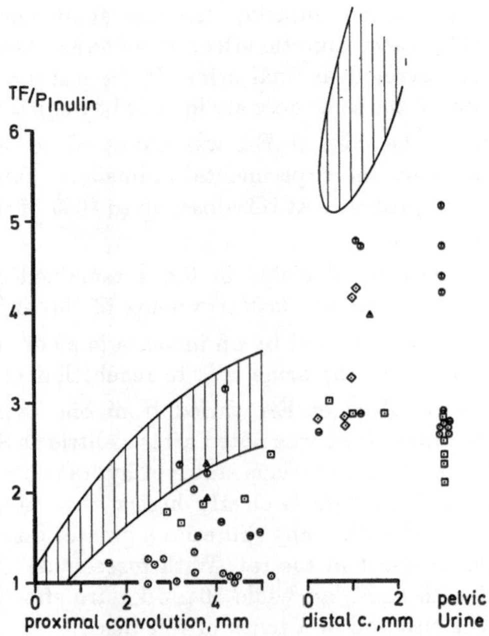

Fig. 2. TF/P_{In} quotients in proximal and distal convolutions of surface nephrons. Proximal puncture sites are given as distance from the glomerulum, distal puncture sites as distance from the end of Henle's loop. Different symbols refer to different animals undergoing ethacrynic acid diuresis. The shaded area includes 90% of control values in antidiuresis. The urine to plasma ratios of inulin concentration in the antidiuretic controls were higher than 190

Discussion

The marked natriuresis with excretion of urine at plasma sodium concentration leads to the conclusion that the diuretic effect of EA is mainly due to inhibition of active sodium reabsorption. Salt or water depletion maximally stimulates the mechanisms of sodium reabsorption which are then inhibited less aesily. The fact that in the first investigations no diuretic effect of EA was found in the rat [13], may have been due to a diminished sodium and water content of the animals at the time of study. In our experience no diuretic produces an appreciable effect in dehydrated or sodium-depleted animals. Furthermore, in studies on the conscious rat a diuretic period may be overlooked if, for technical reasons, long urine collection periods are selected. EA has its maximal effect 15 minutes after a single injection, an effect which rapidly diminishes with a half-time value of about 20 min. If no fluid replacement is given the diuresis is followed by an antidiuresis. Under these conditions protracted balance studies would not demonstrate the diuretic effect.

In micropuncture experiments the lesser increase in proximal TF/P_{In} than in controls is especially marked. This effect may be obscured by the opposite effects of dehydration in the rat as well as in dogs [1]. However, in well hydrated rats the reduced increase in TF/P ratios was significant and did not depend on GFR. This demonstrates an inhibition of proximal tubular reabsorption which distinguishes EA from all other diuretics. It is remarkable that in spite of this inhibition of proximal reabsorption not more than 40% of the GFR is excreted, either in our experiments or in the dog or in man [2].

In spite of different biochemical mechanisms the characteristic effects of diuretics are mainly determined by their site of action within the nephron. The case is best illustrated if we compare EA with other diuretics. Hydrochlorthiazide and furosemide will serve as examples, since sufficient information about their mode of action has been published.

The site of action of hydrochlorthiazide is almost exclusively in the distal convolution and collecting duct [9, 14]. It follows that not more than 25% of the GFR can be excreted during maximal hydrochlorthiazide activity, since no more than this fraction of GFR is delivered to the distal segment. An appreciable diuretic effect of such a diuretic can be observed, therefore, only if the reduction in GFR is not greater than 50%. With greater reductions of GFR the concentrating ability of the kidney is disturbed; a greater fraction of the volume reaching the distal segment must then be excreted (reduced U/P creatinine values). A diuretic which has its principle action on distal sites, thus, cannot be very effective.

With furosemide the situation is quite different. Here there is general agreement from both clinical and experimental studies that at normal or slightly reduced filtration rates up to 30% of the GFR may be excreted. On the other hand, with marked reduction in the filtered volume up to 80% of the filtrate may appear as final urine. This apparent paradox may be explained as follows: furosemide has, in addition to its inhibitory effect on distal reabsorption, including the loop of Henle, a demonstrable inhibitory effect on proximal reabsorption .The proximal effect, however, can be compensated for by another mechanism [3, 12]. During furosemide diuresis there is a marked increase in volume flow through the distal segment. This leads to an increase in intratubular pressure which is transmitted backward to the proximal segment and produces tubular dilatation. Because of the dependency of proximal reabsorptive capacity on the tubular geometry [6] this dilatation should produce an increase in the fractional reabsorption of NaCl and water. The later effect, however, is partially compensated for by the inhibitory action of furosemide. Therefore, the finding of TF/P_{In} ratios within the normal range during furosemide administration is not unexpected.

With reduction of GFR to less than half its normal value, the proximal effect of furosemide may be demonstrated by a reduction in the TF/P_{In} quotient. With a filtrate volume so greatly reduced, in spite of the continued action of the drug, distal flow is necessarily small and insufficient to produce proximal tubular dilatation. The less the intratubular flow rate, therefore, the more apparent will be the inhibitory effect of the diuretic.

In the case of EA, still other differences are apparent. Here we find TF/P_{In} ratios along the proximal convolution clearly smaller than those in controls, at all levels of filtration rate, provided that urinary losses of salt and water are carefully replaced. Since, at normal GFR, EA also induces widening of distal and proximal tubular lumina, the diminished TF/P_{In} quotients must, in the light of the above discussion, be interpreted as reflecting a still greater inhibition of proximal reabsorption.

From the end of the proximal to the beginning of the distal tubule (that is, over the course of Henle's loop) the increase in TF/P_{In} is smaller than seen in antidiuretic controls (Fig. 2). However, this reduced increase in TF/P_{In} does not mean that in this segment a smaller volume of filtrate has actually been reabsorbed.

The volume of filtrate delivered to Henle's loop may be shown to be greater than in controls. This is true even though GFR in the treated group is reduced by 12% in our experiments. In spite of this greater inflow to Henle's loop, the fraction appearing in the distal segment does not exceed 40%. It follows that in Henle's loop approximately the same volume of filtrate is reabsorbed in the diuretic and antidiuretic state.

The increase in the average tubular flow rate in the proximal convolutions and Henle's loops, in spite of the reduced filtration rate, explains why the dye passage time in these segments is not prolonged. The increased flow rate is compensated by an increase of the tubular diameter so that the linear velocity, in these segments, is unchanged.

The volume of fluid did not decrease in the distal convolution and collecting ducts of the animals treated with EA. The drug, thus appears to inhibit reabsorption at these sites. This finding, however, does not necessarily mean that an inhibiting effect on active transport exists in these distal segments. If the osmotic concentration in the medulla is reduced to isosmotic values, then the main operating force for the removal of water from collecting ducts no longer exists. This is to be expected following EA because of the increased volume flow through the medulla and has indeed been demonstrated [7]. By analogy, it has been shown that during "pressure diuresis" the same sort of increase in intratubular flow rate and comparably shortened contact time in the distal segment may lead to an excretion of the greater part of tubular fluid reaching this site, and, even in the presence of ADH, may result in an increased excretion of free water [15].

These findings and considerations agree well with published data on the effect of EA on osmolar clearance in man and dog [4, 14]: during maximal EA diuresis, osmotically free water may still be excreted. This is only possible if the function of the thick, ascending limb of Henle's loop is not substantially affected.

Summary

The effects of the diuretic ethacrynic acid (EA) were studied by clearance and micropuncture experiments in rats. The following conclusions were reached:

1. In contrast to the experience of others we have found that EA produces a definite diuretic effect in the rat. — 2. EA inhibits volume reabsorption in the proximal tubule. Sodium reabsorption in the thick ascending limb of Henle's loop is not comparably affected. — 3. In the distal convolutions and collecting ducts, volume reabsorption is markedly reduced by EA. It is possible that this latter effect is not due to a direct action of the drug on these segments but to

an increase in tubular flow rate. — 4. Differences in the type of diuretic action of EA, furosemide and hydrochlorthiazide may be explained by their different sites of action.

References

1. Berliner, R. W., J. H. Dirks, and W. J. Cirksena: Action of diuretics in dogs studied by micropuncture. In: The physiology of diuretic agents. Conference monograph, N.Y. Acad. Sci., 1966, p. 424—432.
2. Beyer, K. H., J. E. Baer, J. K. Michaelson, and H. F. Russo: Renotropic characteristics of ethacrynic acid: A phenoxyacetic saluretic-diuretic agent. J. Pharmacol. expl. Ther. **147**, 1—22 (1965).
3. Deetjen, P.: Micropuncture studies on site and mode of diuretic action of furosemide. In: The physiology of diuretic agents. Conference monograph, N.Y. Acad. Sci., 1966, p. 408—415.
4. Edel, H. H., J. Eigler u. E. Renner: Zum Wirkungsmechanismus der Ethacrynsäure. II. Der Einfluß der Ethacrynsäure auf das distale Nephron des Menschen. Klin. Wschr. **44**, 421—424 (1966).
5. Führ, J., J. Kaczmarczyk u. C. D. Krüttgen: Eine einfache kolorimetrische Methode zur Inulin-Bestimmung für Nieren-Clearance-Untersuchung bei Stoffwechselgesunden und Diabetikern. Klin. Wschr. **33**, 729—730 (1955).
6. Gertz, K. H., J. A. Mangos, G. Braun, and H. D. Pagel: On the glomerular tubular balance in the rat kidney. Pflügers Arch. ges. Physiol. **285**, 360—372 (1965).
7. Goldberg, M.: Ethacrynic acid: Site and mode of action. In: The physiology of diuretic agents. Conference monograph. N.Y. Acad. Sci., 1966, p. 443—452.
8. Hilger, H. H., J. D. Klümper u. K. J. Ullrich: Wasserrückresorption und Ionentransport durch die Sammelrohrzellen der Säugetierniere. Pflügers Arch. ges. Physiol. **267**, 218—237 (1958).
9. Meng, K.: Mikropunktionsuntersuchungen über die saluretische Wirkung von Hydrochlorothiazid, Acetazolamid und Furosemid. Naunyn-Schmiedebergs Arch. Pharmak. exp. Path. **257**, 355—371 (1967).
10. Merck, Sharp, and Dohme: Research Laboratories (Edit.) Synopsis of clinical experience with Edecrin (Ethacrynic acid). West Point, Pa.: Merck, Sharp and Dohme 1964.
11. Radford, E. P.: Factors modifying water metabolism in rats fed dry diets. Amer. J. Physiol. **196**, 1098—1108 (1959).
12. Rector, F. C., F. J. Brunner, and D. W. Seldin: Pitfalls in the use of micropuncture for the localization of diuretic action. In: The physiology of diuretic agents. Conference monograph, N.Y. Acad. Sci. 1966, p. 400—407.
13. Schultz, E. M., E. J. Cragoe, J. B. Bickins, W. A. Bohlhofer, and J. M. Sprague: d,β-unsaturated ketone derivatives of aryloxyacetic acids, a new class of diuretics. J. med. pharm. Chem. **5**, 660—662 (1962).
14. Seldin, D. W., G. Eknoyan, W. N. Suki, and F. C. Rector: Localization of diuretic action from the pattern of water and electrolyte excretion. In: The physiology of diuretic agents. Conference monograph, N.Y. Acad. Sci. 1966, p. 328—343.
15. Thurau, K., u. P. Deetjen: (mit einem theoretischen Beitrag von H. Günzler): Die Diurese bei arteriellen Drucksteigerungen. Pflügers Arch. ges. Physiol. **274**, 567—580 (1962).

3.3. The Efficacy of Ethacrynic Acid in the Treatment of Chronic Renal Failure

E. QUELLHORST, F. SCHELER and I. STEGEMANN[1]

With 5 Figures

Patients with chronic renal failure often retain much sodium and water though they only have a moderate depression of GFR. Particularly in cases complicated by hypertension and heart failure an augmentation of natriuresis appears desirable. Sometimes natriuretic treatment may temporarily obviate the need for treatment by dialysis in cases of severe renal failure. On the other hand, the loss of potassium during a forced diuresis may be dangerous in cases of heart failure caused by hypertension and chronic renal failure.

In this paper the efficacy of ethacrynic acid (E.A.), a strong diuretic and natriuretic agent [1, 4—12, 14, 15, 18, 21, 23] in the treatment of renal failure of different degrees will be demonstrated. Under these conditions the two anti-kaluretic drugs spironolactone and amiprazide (Amiloride) [22] proved useful. We attempted to ascertain the degree of renal failure compatible with a diuretic action of E.A. We furthermore studied the merits of amiprazide and of spironolactone in depressing the potassium-loss induced by E.A.

E.A. appears to possess properties which could be particularly useful in patients with renal failure:

1. After the administration of E.A. the excretion of H^+-ions is increased while bicarbonate is retained [3, 13, 17—20].

2. The carbohydrate-tolerance, which often is disturbed in renal failure [24], is not influenced by E.A. [18, 21].

Methods and results

19 patients with chronic renal failure, who were free of edema, were treated in the following manner:

1500 ml of a 5.25% fructose solution containing 100 mEq NaCl and 40 mEq potassium-lactate were infused within 6 hours on each of four days. On the second and fourth day of the study the patients received 10 mg of amiprazide 4 hours before the beginning of the infusion. On the third and fourth day 100 mg of E.A. were injected i.v. at the beginning of the infusion.

Fig. 1 shows the changes of urine volume, osmolar clearance and free water clearance induced by amiprazide, E.A. and E.A. combined with amiprazide. The groups consist of patients with similar degrees of renal failure. Whereas amiprazide did not cause a significant augmentation of urine flow, there was a considerable increase after E.A. This effect is known to occur in patients with

[1] Medizinische Universitätsklinik Göttingen, West Germany.

renal failure [13]. The additional administration of amiprazide does not further increase urine flow. The extent of the increase of osmolar clearance and the clearance of free water depends on the degree of renal failure.

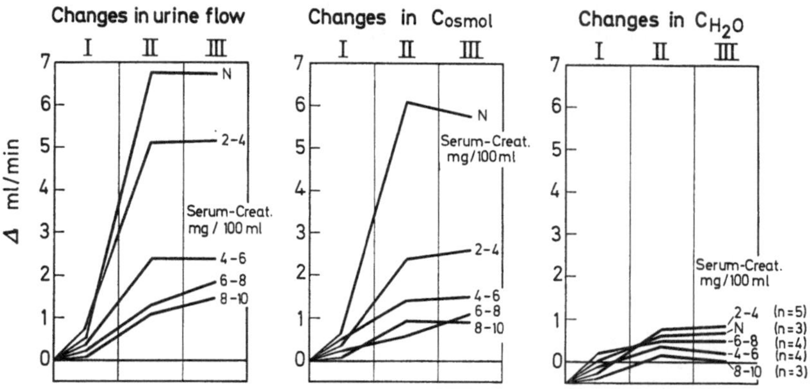

Fig. 1. Increase of urine flow, osmolar clearance and clearance of free water after administration of amiprazide, ethacrynic acid and ethacrynic acid in combination with amiprazide. *I* Amiprazide 10 mg orally; *II* Ethacrynic acid 100 mg i.v.; *III* Ethacrynic acid 100 mg i.v. + Amiprazide 10 mg orally

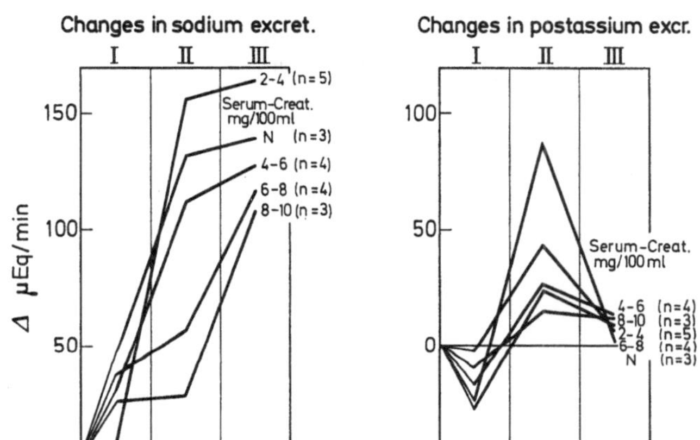

Fig. 2. Changes of sodium and potassium excretion after administration of amiprazide, ethacrynic acid and ethacrynic acid in combination with amiprazide. *I* Amiprazide 10 mg orally; *II* Ethacrynic acid 100 mg i.v.; *III* Ethacrynic acid 100 mg i.v. + Amiprazide 10 mg orally

Fig. 2 shows the changes of renal sodium and potassium excretion caused by amiprazide alone or in combination with E.A. Sodium excretion is considerably increased by E.A. with serum creatinine values lower than 6 mg-%. If renal function is markedly reduced the natriuretic effect of E.A. is improved by the additional administration of amiprazide. Patients with lower levels of serum creatinine show maximal natriuresis after injection of E.A. alone. Potassium excretion is reduced by amiprazide: the reduction is most pronounced at serum creatinine levels of 1 to 4 mg-%. As expected, E.A. alone induced an increase of potassium excretion. Additional amiprazide reduces potassium excretion to the control levels.

An increase of BUN after the administration of E.A., as reported by some authors [2, 14, 15, 20], was not observed in our patients. The excretion of urea and creatinine was not influenced by E.A. (Fig. 3).

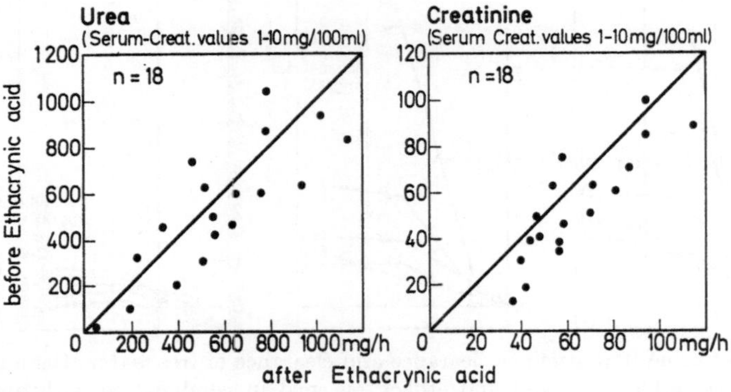

Fig. 3. Excretion of urea and creatinine before and after administration of 100 mg of ethacrynic acid

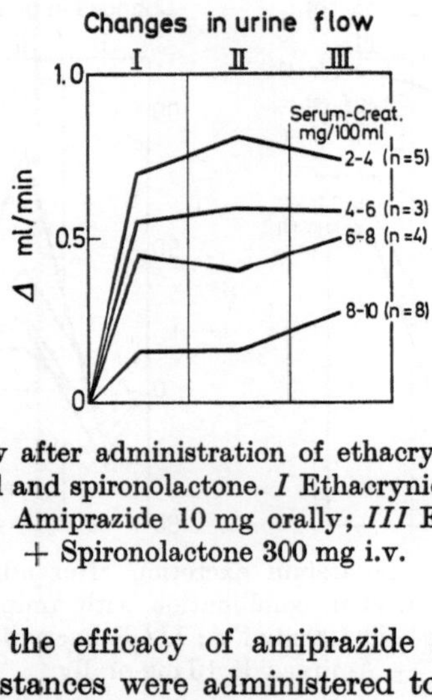

Fig. 4. Increase of urine flow after administration of ethacrynic acid, ethacrynic acid and amiprazide or ethacrynic acid and spironolactone. *I* Ethacrynic acid 100 mg orally; *II* Ethacrynic acid 100 mg orally + Amiprazide 10 mg orally; *III* Ethacrynic acid 100 mg orally + Spironolactone 300 mg i.v.

In order to compare the efficacy of amiprazide and spironolactone, when added to E.A., these substances were administered to 20 patients with chronic renal failure and edema on 6 consecutive days. After a control period of 3 to 4 days without diuretic treatment, 100 mg of E.A. were given orally on each of 6 consecutive days. On the third and fourth day of this treatment 10 mg of amiprazide, and on the fifth and sixth day 300 mg of spironolactone were given i.v. in addition to oral E.A. The diuretic effect of E.A. was not improved by either amiprazide or spironolactone (Fig. 4). On the other hand, sodium excretion was increased by the combined treatment (Fig. 5). Even if the renal functions were markedly reduced (serum creatinine levels from 6 to 10 mg-%) sodium excretion could be increased by combination of amiprazide and E.A. At serum creatinine levels between 2 to 6 mg-% a combination of spironolactone and E.A. was more effective. There was a marked retention of potassium at all degrees of renal failure when E.A. was combined with amiprazide. Hyperkalemia was observed in two cases.

Summarizing our results we may state that E.A. is an effective diuretic even with marked reduction of GFR. TRF values may be increased by 10 to 30%. The greatest increase is observed at the lowest values of GFR. A further augmentation of urine flow is not achieved by either amiprazide or spironolactone.

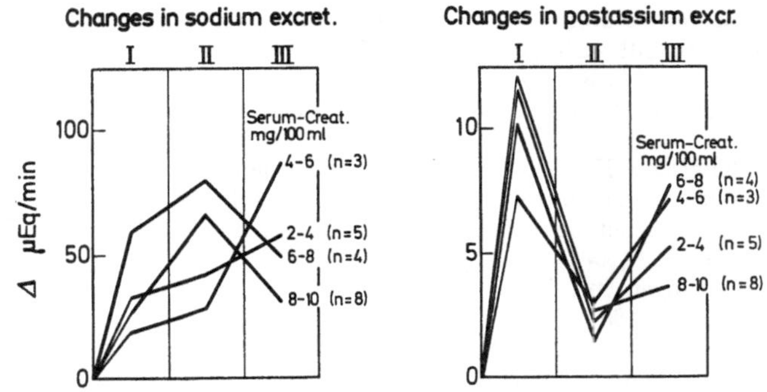

Fig. 5. Changes of sodium and potassium excretion after administration of ethacrynic acid, ethacrynic acid and amiprazide or ethacrynic acid and spironolactone. *I* Ethacrynic acid 100 mg orally; *II* Ethacrynic acid 100 mg orally + Amiprazide 10 mg orally; *III* Ethacrynic acid 100 mg orally + Spironolactone 300 mg i.v.

On the other hand, sodium excretion is increased, even, in severe renal failure by the administration of E.A. and amiprazide. Two types of side-effects may occur with the drugs used:

1. At reduced values of GFR, amiprazide may dangerously increase the plasma potassium concentration.

2. Accumulation of the diuretics and their metabolites could occur and produce toxic effects.

References

1. Bojs, G., and O. Lundvall: Effects of ethacrynic acid on renal function in man. Acta med. scand. **179**, 95—100 (1966).
2. Cannon, P. J., R. P. Ames, and J. H. Laragh: Methylenebutyryl phenoxyacetic acid. J. Amer. med. Ass. **185**, 854—863 (1963).
3. — H. O. Heinemann, M. S. Albert, J. H. Laragh, and R. W. Winters: "Contraction" alcalosis after diuresis of edematous patients with ethacrynic acid. Ann. intern. Med. **62**, 979—983 (1965).
4. — — W. B. Stason, and J. H. Laragh: Ethacrynic acid. Effectiveness and mode of diuretic action in man. Circulation **31**, 5—12 (1965).
5. Earley, L. E., and R. M. Friedler: Renal tubular effects of ethacrynic acid. J. clin. Invest. **43**, 1495—1506 (1964).
6. — J. A. Martino, and R. M. Friedler: Factors affecting sodium reabsorption by the proximal tubule as determined during blockade of distal sodium reabsorption. J. clin. Invest. **45**, 1668—1684 (1966).
7. — Diuretics. New Engl. J. Med. **276**, 966—968, 1023—1025 (1967).

8. Edel, H. H., J. Eigler u. E. Renner: Zum Wirkungsmechanismus der Ethacrynsäure. II. Der Einfluß der Ethacrynsäure auf das distale Nephron des Menschen. Klin. Wschr. **44**, 421—429 (1966).

9. Eigler, J., H. Carl u. H. H. Edel: Zum Wirkungsmechanismus der Ethacrynsäure. I. Der Einfluß von Ethacrynsäure und Furosemid auf Membranpotential und Kurzschlußstrom an der Krötenhaut. Klin. Wschr. **44**, 417—421 (1966).

10. Flanigan, W. J., and G. L. Ackerman: Site of action of ethacrynic acid. Arch. intern. Med. **118**, 117—122 (1966).

11. Foltz, E. L.: Preliminary clinical observations with an aryloxyacetic acid diuretic. Fed. Proc. **22**, 598 (1963).

12. Goldberg, M., D. K. McCurdy, E. L. Foltz, and L. W. Bluemle Jr.: Effects of ethacrynic acid (a new saluretic agent) on renal diluting and concentrating mechanisms. J. clin. Invest. **43**, 201—216 (1964).

13. Hagedorn, C. W., A. A. Kaplan, and W. H. Hulet: Prolonged administration of ethacrynic acid in patients with chronic renal disease. New Engl. J. Med. **272**, 1152—1155 (1965).

14. Kayser, D.: Klinische Erfahrungen mit einem neuen, oral wirksamen Diureticum (Aethacrynsäure). Arzneimittel-Forsch. (Drug Research) **14**, 949—953 (1964).

15. — Die Kurz- und Langzeitbehandlung kardialer Ödeme mit Ethacrynsäure. Dtsch. med. Wschr. **92**, 823—829 (1967).

16. Kopp, H.: Erfahrungen mit Ethacrynsäure, einem neuen Diureticum. Münch. med. Wschr. **108**, 2461—2465 (1966).

17. Krück, F.: Renale Acidose. Entstehungsmechanismen. In: Peritonealdialyse, S. 52—66. München-Berlin-Wien: Urban & Schwarzenberg 1967.

18. Ledigham, J. G. G., and R. I. S. Bayliss: Ethacrynic acid: Two year's experience with a new diuretic. Brit. med. J. **1965 II**, 732—735.

19. Maher, J. F., and G. E. Schreiner: Studies on ethacrynic acid in patients with refractory edema. Ann. intern. Med. **62**, 15—29 (1965).

20. Müller, P., u. F. Schaub: Experimentelle und klinische Untersuchungen mit Ethacrinsäure, einem chemisch neuartigen Diureticum. Klin. Wschr. **42**, 958—965 (1964).

21. Özen, M. A., Ö. Sandalci, and F. Berker: Ethacrynic acid and carbohydrate metabolism. Amer. J. med. Sci. **252**, 558—563 (1966).

22. Singh, B. N., D. E. Richmond, J. D. Wilson, H. A. Simmonds, and J. D. K. North: Evaluation of MK — 870: A new potassium sparing diuretic. Brit. med. J. **1967 I**, 143—146.

23. Stewart, J. H., and K. D. G. Edwards: Clinical comparison of frusemide with bendrofluazide, mersalyl and ethacrynic acid. Brit. med. J. **1965 II**, 1277—1281.

24. Willms, B., E. Quellhorst u. H.-V. Henning: Kohlenhydratstoffwechsel bei Niereninsuffizienz. In: Peritonealdialyse, S. 75—87. München-Berlin-Wien: Urban & Schwarzenberg 1967.

3.4. Biochemical Studies on Mechanisms of Action of Compounds Influencing Tubular Na^+ Transport: I. Aldosterone, Amiloride, Triamterene

W. LOSERT, R. SITT, G. SENFT †, K. v. BERGMANN and A. ZESCH [1]

With 5 Figures

It is generally accepted that aldosterone increases tubular sodium transport by inducing enzyme protein synthesis [6, 15]. With respect to the function of these enzymes two theories have been established. LEAF and his colleagues [16], on the basis of their experiments on the urinary bladder of the toad, have postulated that aldosterone increases the synthesis of an enzyme system which facilitates the diffusion of Na^+ into the epithelial cells across the mucosal surface leading to an increase in intracellular Na^+ concentration. Consequently more sodium ions are made available for active transport across the serosal cell membrane. This theory implies that the active transport system itself is not influenced by the action of the hormone.

There is no difficulty in applying this mechanism to tissues exhibiting unidirectional Na^+ transport, e.g. the urinary bladder of the toad or the mammalian kidney. However, aldosterone has been shown to exert extrarenal actions, as e.g. depressing intracellular Na^+ concentration, most evidently in the liver [5, 13]. It is difficult to conceive that this effect results from an increase in the permeability of the cellular membranes to Na^+. It has also been shown that the actions of aldosterone on renal tubules and liver cells show common features with respect to inhibition by actinomycin D, and the latent period which elapses between application of aldosterone and onset of its action [2, 17].

Provided that the mechanism of aldosterone action in the liver is identical with that in kidney a theory established by EDELMAN and his colleagues [7—9] seems more attractive, as it is applicable to both tissues. This theory is based on the findings that in substrate depleted toad bladders aldosterone does not augment Na^+ transport unless either oxaloacetate or pyruvate or β-hydroxybutyrate or their precursors have been added to the incubation medium. Succinate, α-ketoglutarate and propionate, a precursor of succinyl-CoA, have been found ineffective. Moreover, oxygen is required to obtain a response to aldosterone (Fig. 1). From these findings it has been concluded that aldosterone induces the synthesis of one or several enzymes in the pathway from oxaloacetate to α-ketoglutarate, thereby channeling metabolism to provide more energy for active Na^+ transport. To test this assumption the mitochondrial activities of citrate-synthetase, aconitase, isocitrate-dehydrogenase, glutamate-dehydrogenase, α-keto-

[1] Pharmakologisches Institut der Freien Universität Berlin, Germany.

Dr. W. LOSERT, Abteilungs für allgemeine Pharmakologie, Hauptlaboratorium, Schering AG, Berlin, Germany.

glutarate-dehydrogenase, succinate-dehydrogenase and $NADH_2$-cytochrome$_c$-reductase have been measured in the kidney of intact rats, adrenalectomized rats and adrenalectomized rats treated with aldosterone in doses comparable to the daily secretion rate of this hormone [3].

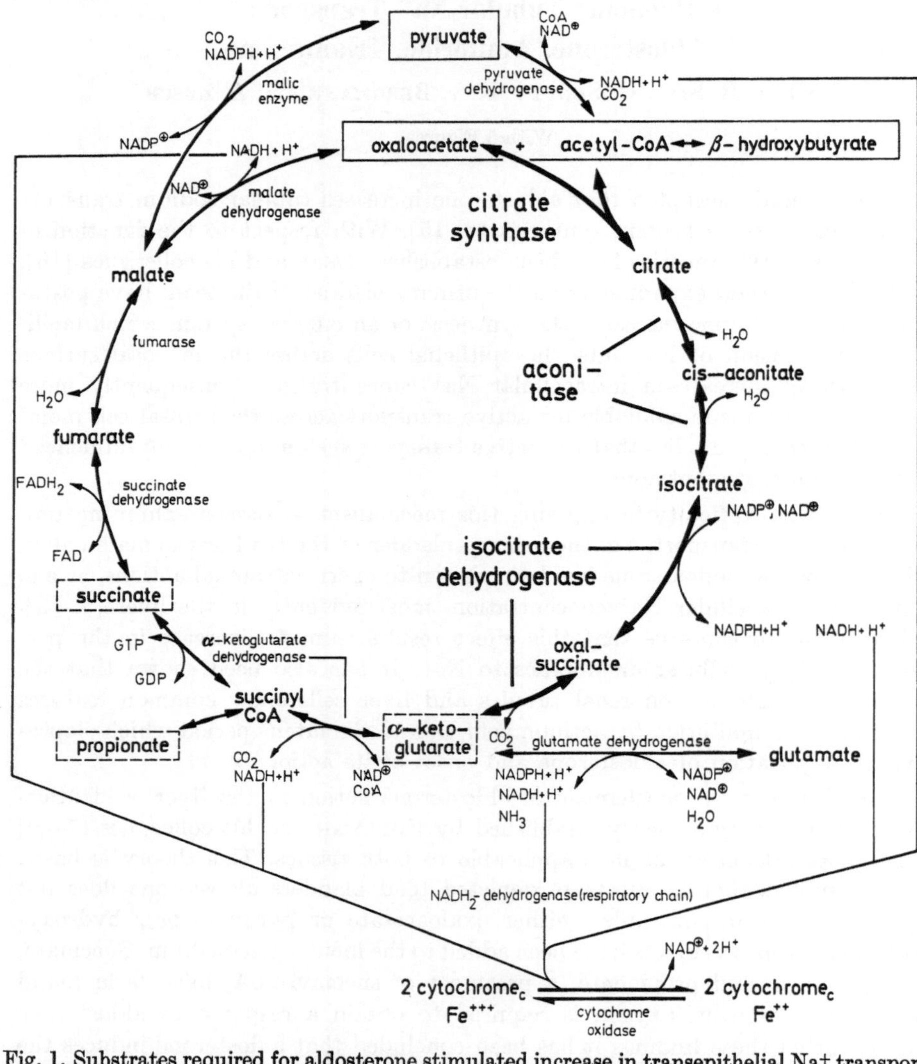

Fig. 1. Substrates required for aldosterone stimulated increase in transepithelial Na^+ transport in the urinary bladder of Bufo marinus. ▭ Substrates required for aldosterone stimulated Na^+ transport. ⬚ Substrates without influence on aldosterone stimulated Na^+ transport. (Data form Edelman [6, 7] and Fimognari, Porter, and Edelman [9])

Adrenalectomy resulted in a decreased activity of mitochondrial citrate-synthetase, NADP-isocitrate-dehydrogenase, succinate-dehydrogenase and $NADH_2$-cytochrome$_c$-reductase. Treating adrenalectomized animals with a single dose of D-aldosterone reversed within 90 minutes the decrease in NADP-isocitrate-dehydrogenase induced by adrenalectomy. The activity of the other enzymes reduced by adrenalectomy was not or only partially restored by a single injection of aldosterone; in the case of $NADH_2$-cytochrome$_c$-reductase and succinate-dehydrogenase chronic treatment prevented the decrease observed in adrenalectomized rats (Fig. 2). As a single injection of aldosterone suffices to accelerate Na^+ transport, the changes in the activity of these two enzymes are likely to be consequences rather than mechanisms of the hormone-stimulated electrolyte transport.

NADP-isocitrate-dehydrogenase catalyzes a reaction linked with the formation of $NADPH_2$ which may be used for reductive processes, e.g. the synthesis of fatty acids or amino-acids via the reductive amination of α-ketoglutarate [10, 11]. It is noteworthy that the aldosterone-dependent changes in the activity of this enzyme are restricted to the mitochondrial form only. Extramitochondrial NADP-isocitrate-dehydrogenase does not exhibit statistically significant changes. Glucose-6-phosphate dehydrogenase is another hyaloplasmic enzyme which catalyzes a reaction linked with the formation of $NADPH_2$. The activity of this enzyme has been found increased in adrenalectomized rats. Administration of aldosterone did not reduce enzymatic activity to control levels (Fig. 2). Similar results have been published by DIES and LOTSPEICH [4]. As the activity of this enzyme has also been found increased in salt-depleted animals the adrenals of which had not been removed [4], it seems justified to relate the adrenalectomy-induced change to the renal Na^+ loss known to occur in the absence of mineralocorticosteroids.

Although the enzymes shown to be influenced by aldosterone are located within the metabolic pathway, which is suggested to be linked with aldosterone-accelerated Na^+ transport by EDELMAN, our findings should not be interpreted to provide substantial support to this theory. This reservation is due to our ignorance of the significance of the altered enzymic activities, and to the finding that aldosterone influences the activity of at least one enzyme not located in the mitochondria.

Microsomal $NADPH_2$-cytochrome$_{(c)}$-reductase activity has been found decreased by 20% in adrenalectomized animals. Injection of aldosterone leads to an increase in enzymic activity which, however, does not attain the values measured in intact rats (Fig. 2). With respect to this result it should be mentioned that there is an increased incorporation of ^{14}C-orotate into microsomal RNA coincident with aldosterone-induced Na^+ retention as shown by CASTLES and WILLIAMSON [3a]. Moreover, DIES and LOTSPEICH [4] have speculated that reoxydation of $NADPH_2$ by $NADPH_2$-cytochrome$_{(c)}$-reductase could provide free hydrogen ions that would be available for tubular secretion and exchange for Na^+.

Triamterene and amiloride have been shown to exert tubular effects resembling those of adrenalectomy. It must be emphasized, however, that these compounds cannot be classified as specific aldosterone antagonists as their action can also be demonstrated in the absence of the hormone [1, 12, 14]. A tentative approach to elucidate the mode of action of these diuretics has been made by examining whether or not these drugs inhibit enzymes whose activities have been found to decrease owing to the lack of aldosterone in adrenalectomized rats. Such an inhibitory effect, if at all related to the tubular action of these compounds, ought to occur also in adrenalectomized rats.

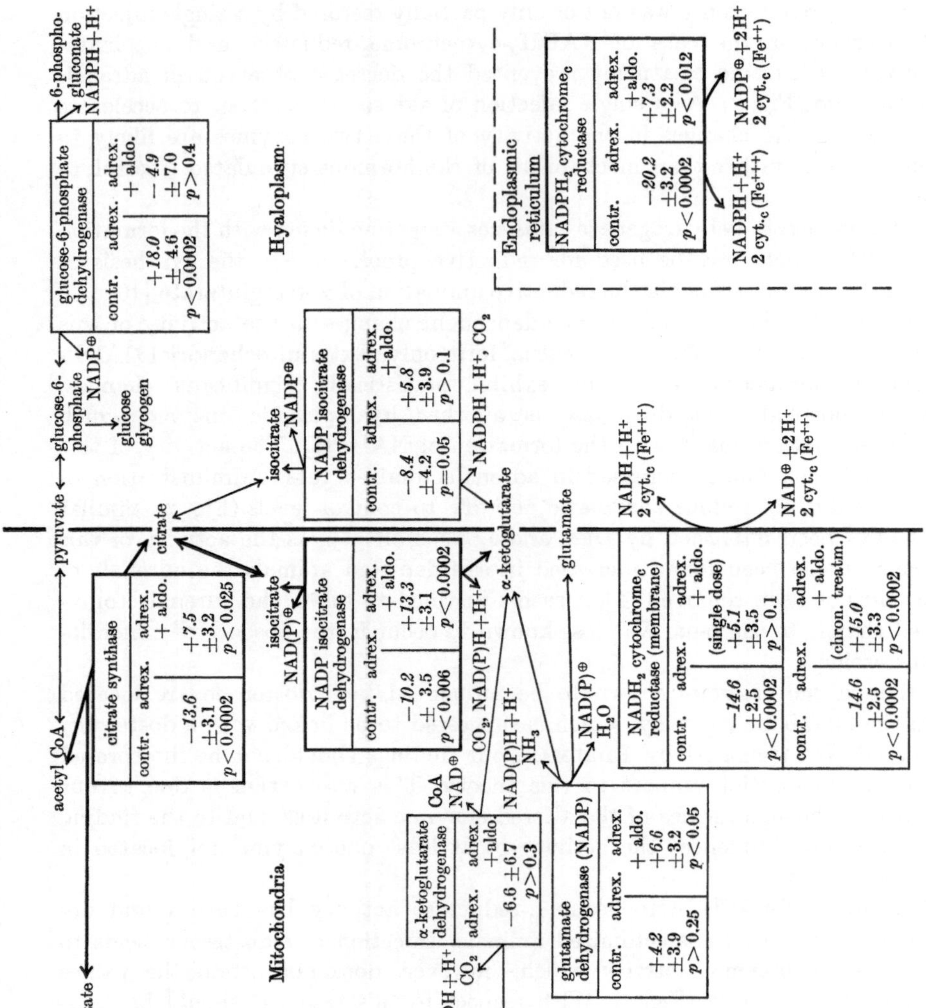

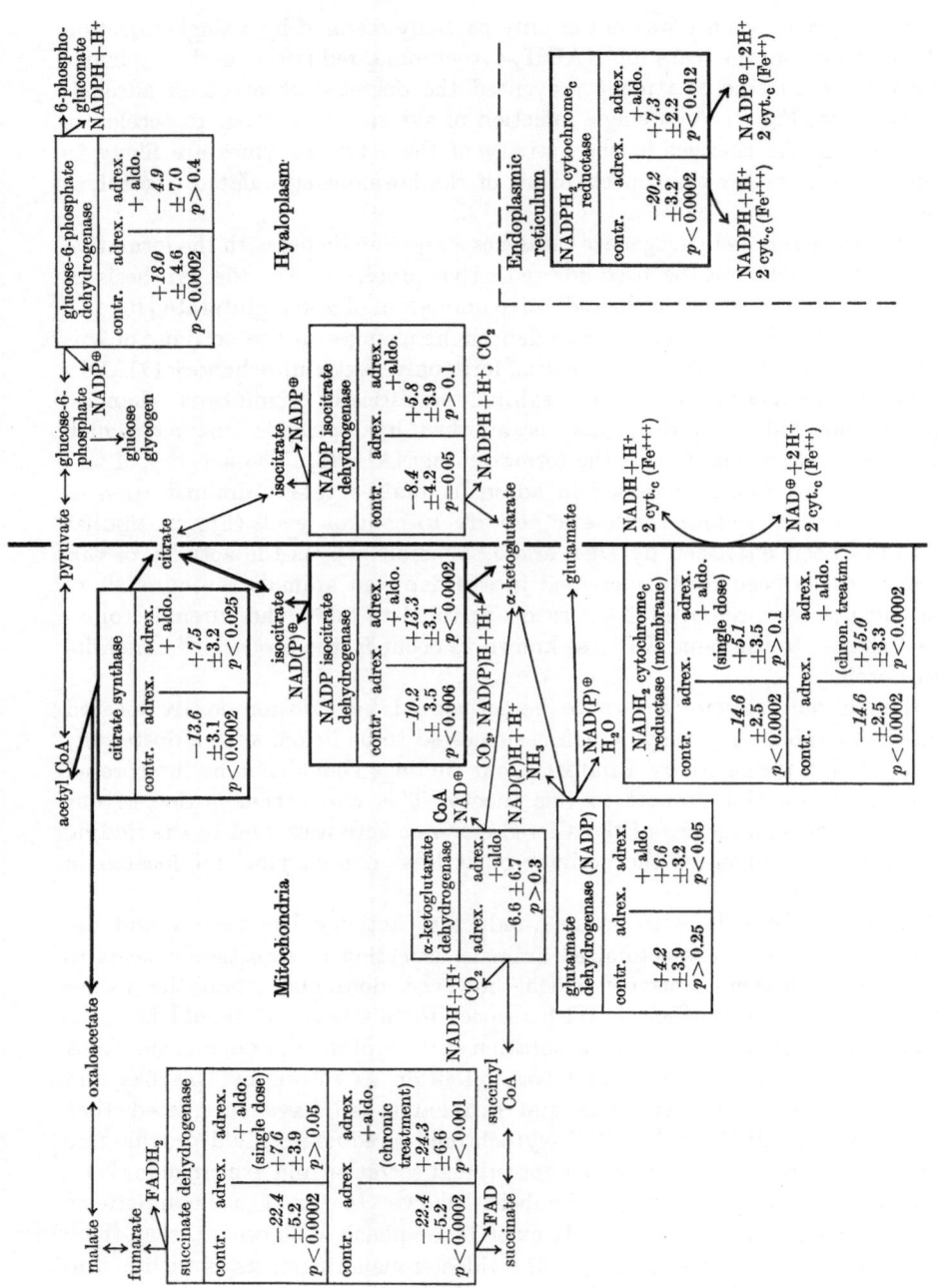

Fig. 2. Influence of aldosterone on the activity of enzymes in the rat kidney (values given as % decrease and % increase in enzymatic activity calculated on a protein basis). Contr.: intact controls, adrex.: adrenalectomized rats, adrex.+aldo: adrenalectomized rats given D-aldosterone (single dose: 15 μg/rat, 90 min; chronic treatment: 20 μg/rat und day)

As amiloride has been shown to induce a maximal increase in Na^+ excretion within the first hour after i.v. injection of the drug (Fig. 3), the enzymic activities have been measured in the kidney 60 minutes after application of the diuretics.

The activity of the two enzymes shown to be reduced in adrenalectomized animals and increased by aldosterone, namely mitochondrial NADP-isocitrate-dehydrogenase and microsomal $NADPH_2$-cytochrome$_{(c)}$-reductase, was found unchanged in rats treated with 10 mg triamterene/kg b.w. or 2 mg amiloride/kg b.w. Mitochondrial $NADH_2$-cytochrome$_c$-reductase and succinate dehydrogenase, whose activity has been shown to decrease in adrenalectomized rats but to attain normal values only in the case of chronic treatment with aldosterone, showed a decreased activity after both diuretics. As this effect did

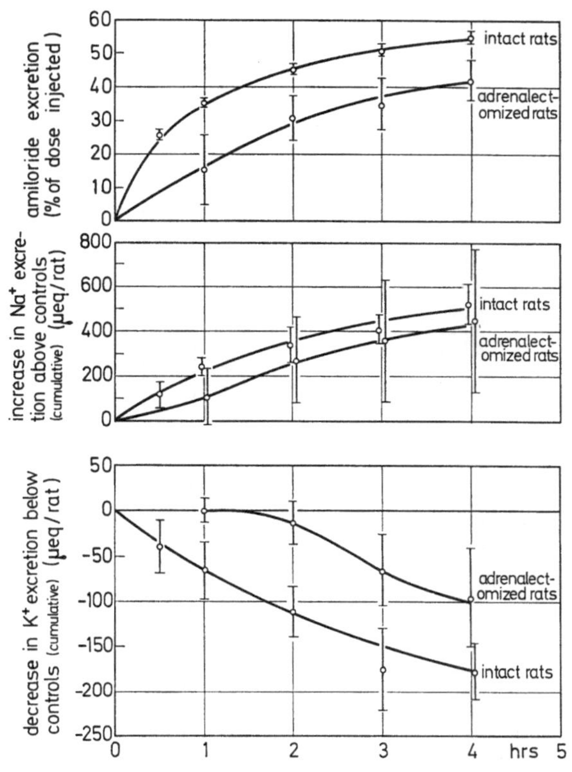

Fig. 3. Influence of amiloride (2 mg/kg i.v.) on renal Na^+ and K^+ excretion

not occur in adrenalectomized rats, it cannot be related to a direct interaction between the drugs and the enzymes. The activity of α-ketoglutarate-dehydrogenase, not influenced by aldosterone, was reduced by triamterene and amiloride both in intact and adrenalectomized animals. Simultaneously, there was an increase in instantaneous pyruvate concentration. Studies as to whether this increase is related to an inhibition of pyruvate-dehydrogenase, an enzyme system similar in function and components to α-ketoglutarate-dehydrogenase, are in progress (Fig. 4).

An inhibitory influence of amiloride on α-ketoglutarate-dehydrogenase prepared from mitochondria of rat kidney has been demonstrated in vitro. There is a non-competitive inhibition by amiloride with respect to α-ketoglu-

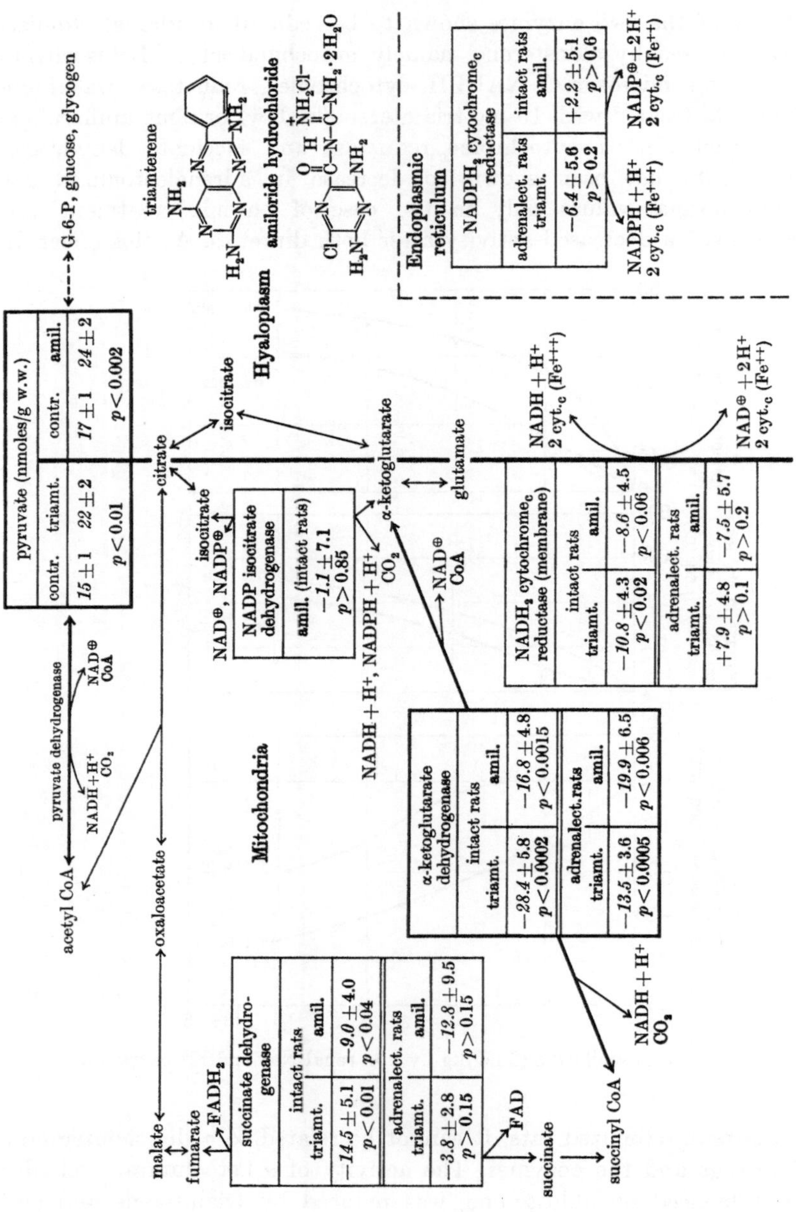

Fig. 4. Influence of triamterene and amiloride on the activity of enzymes in the rat kidney. (values given as % decrease or % increase of the enzymatic activity of untreated rats.). Triamt.: 10 mg triamterene/kg b.w., orally, 60 min. amil.: 2 mg amiloride/kg b.w., i.v., 60 min

tarate; 50% inhibition is achieved with approximately $9 \cdot 10^{-5}$ M (Fig. 5). This concentration is in the order of magnitude of that measured in the tissue water of rat kidneys one hour after i.v. injection of 2 mg amiloride/kg b.w. (Table). A non-competitive inhibition of α-ketoglutarate 1-dehydrogenase has also been found with respect to CoA and NAD ($K_I = 13.5 \cdot 10^{-5}$ M and $11 \cdot 10^{-5}$ M, respectively). We do not know the concentration of the drug in the tubular cells. As the concentration in the tissue water is much higher than in plasma and the distribution volume of amiloride larger than the total body water space, the intracellular concentration in some cells must be assumed to be higher than that measured in the tissue water. From this it can be concluded that the intracellular concentration necessary for inhibition of α-ketoglutarate 1-dehydrogenase may be attained in vivo.

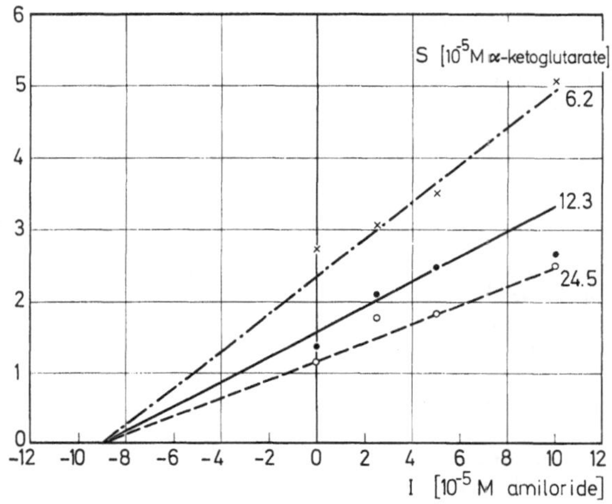

Fig. 5. Inhibition of α-ketoglutarate-dehydrogenase[2] by amiloride in vitro

Table. *Amiloride concentration in kidney and plasma of rats 1 hr after i.v. injection of 2 mg/kg*

		Intact rats $n = 5$	Adrenalectomized rats $n = 6$
Amiloride [10^{-5}M]	kidney (tissue H_2O)	*0.98* ± 0.17	*0.89* ± 0.17
	plasma	*0.056* ± 0.007	*0.062* ± 0.003
	kidney (tissue H_2O) / plasma	*18.5* ± 3.8	*14.1* ± 2.4
Amiloride distribution volume (% body weight)		*684* ± 91	*716* ± 31

References

1. Baer, J. E.: Pharmacology of diuretics. Renal and Diuretic Symposium, Rotterdam, Netherlands, October 15, 1966. Medicina scientia donat, **1** (2), 14—20 (1968).
2. Bartelheimer, H. K., W. Losert, G. Senft u. R. Sitt: Hemmung der extrarenalen Wirkung von d-Aldosteron durch Actinomycin D. Naunyn-Schmiedebergs Arch. Pharmak. exp. Path. **258**, 372—382 (1967).
3. Cade, R., and T. Perenich: Secretion of aldosterone by rats. Amer. J. Physiol. **208**, 1026—1030 (1965).
3a. Castles, T. R., and H. E. Williamson. Mediation of aldosterone induced anti-natriuresis via RNA-synthesis de novo. Proc. Soc. exp. Biol. (N.Y.) **124**, 717—719 (1967).
4. Dies, F., and W. D. Lotspeich: Hexose monophosphate shunt in the rat kidney during acid-base and electrolyte imbalance. Amer. J. Physiol. **212**, 61—71 (1967).

[2] Prepared from mitochondria of rat kidney.

5. DULCE, H.-J., and TH. GÜNTHER: Steuerung des cellulären Elektrolyt- und Wassergehaltes durch Hormone. Naunyn-Schmiedebergs Arch. exp. Path. Pharmak. **238**, 368—390 (1960).
6. EDELMAN, I. S.: Subcellular distribution and mode of action of aldosterone. In: Steroid dynamics, edit. by G. PINCUS, T. NAKAO, and J. F. TAIT, p. 551. New York and London: Academic Press 1966.
7. — Molecular process in steroid regulation of sodium transport. In: Second Internat. Congr. on Hormonal Steroids, Milan, Italy, May, 23—28, 1966, p. 43. Amsterdam-New York-Milan-Tokyo-Buenos Aires: Excerpta-Medica Foundation 1966.
8. — Action of aldosterone on sodium transport. Abstract, Internat. Congr. of Nephrology, Washington, D. C., September, 25—30, 1966, p. 67.
9. FIMOGNARI, G. M., G. A. PORTER, and I. S. EDELMAN: The role of the tricarboxylic acid cycle in the action of aldosterone on sodium transport. Biochim. biophys. Acta (Amst.) **135**, 89—99 (1967).
10. GOEBELL, H., u. D. PETTE: Die intracelluläre Verteilung von DPN- und TPN-spezifischer Isocitratdehydrogenase. Enzymol. biol. clin. **8**, 161—175 (1967).
11. KLINGENBERG, M., and D. PETTE: Proportions of mitochondrial enzymes and pyridine nucleotides. Biochem. biophys. Res. Commun. **7**, 430—438 (1962).
12. LIDDLE, G. W.: Specific and non-specific inhibition of mineralocorticoid activity. Metabolism **10**, 1021—1030 (1961).
13. LOSERT, W., C. SENFT, and G. SENFT: Extrarenale Wirkungen des Aldosterons und der Spirolactone. Naunyn-Schmiedebergs Arch. exp. Path. Pharmak. **248**, 450—463 (1964).
14. SENFT, G.: Über den Mechanismus und die Lokalisation der renalen Wirkung von 2-, 4-, 7-Triamino-6-phenylpteridin. Naunyn-Schmiedebergs Arch. exp. Path. Pharmak. **243**, 352 (1962).
15. SHARP, G. W. G., and A. LEAF: Mode of hormone action: Studies on the mode of action of aldosterone. In: Recent Progr. Hormone Res., vol. 22, p. 431, edit. by G. PINCUS. New York and London: Academic Press 1966.
16. — C. H. COGGINS, N. S. LICHTENSTEIN, and A. LEAF: Evidence for a mucosal effect of aldosterone on sodium transport in the toad bladder. J. clin. Invest. **45**, 1640—1647 (1966).
17. WIEDERHOLT, M.: Mikropunktionsuntersuchungen am proximalen und distalen Konvolut der Rattenniere über den Einfluß von Actinomycin D auf den mineralocorticoidabhängigen Na-Transport. Pflügers Arch. ges. Physiol. **292**, 334—342 (1966).

3.5. Biochemical Studies on Mechanisms of Action of Compounds Influencing Tubular Na^+ Transport: II. 6-Aminonicotinamide, Furosemide

A. ZESCH, G. SENFT† and W. LOSERT [1]

With 6 Figures

6-Aminonicotinamide (6-AN) produces a series of metabolic disturbances, among which a decrease in tubular Na^+ reabsorption has gained special interest [4, 7]. The site of the 6-AN induced impairment of tubular function has been localized by micropuncture studies in the distal convoluted tubules of the kidney [6].

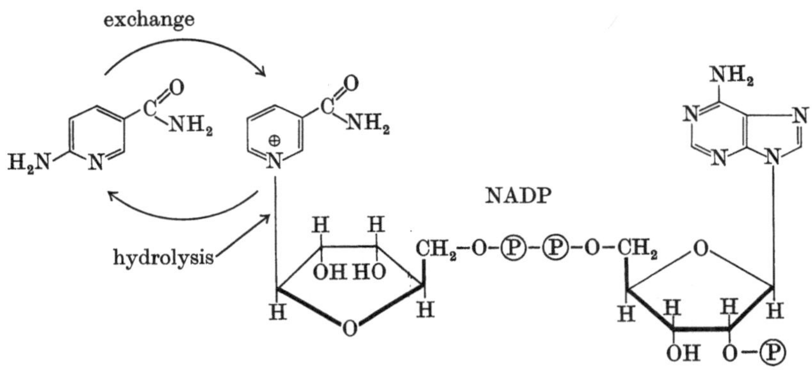

Fig. 1a. Formation of 6-aminonicotinamide-adenine-dinucleotide-phosphate (6-ANADP) by exchange of nicotinamide for 6-aminonicotinamide (6-AN). (DIETRICH, FRIEDLAND and KAPLAN, 1958)

6-AN is exchanged for nicotinamide by the action of NAD(P) glycohydrolase, thereby catalyzing the formation of 6-aminonicotinamide-adenine-dinucleotide (-phosphate) [6-ANAD(P)] [3] (Fig. 1a). The abnormally structured nucleotide does not function as hydrogen acceptor. Moreover, it acts as an inhibitor of hydrogen transfer in the presence of $NADPH_2$. This has been shown for the reduction of oxidized glutathione (GSSG) by the enzyme $NADPH_2$-glutathione-oxydoreductase (glutathione reductase). With a ratio $\frac{6\text{—ANADP}}{NADPH_2} = \frac{5}{1}$, 40% less reduced glutathione (GSH) is formed than in the absence of 6-ANADP [2] (Fig. 1b).

These in vitro studies prompted us to investigate if the application of 6-aminonicotinamide leads to a decrease in renal GSH concentration coincident with a decrease in tubular Na^+ transport.

[1] Pharmakologisches Institut der Freien Universität Berlin, Germany.

Dr. W. LOSERT, Abteilung für allgemeine Pharmakologie, Hauptlaboratorium, Schering AG, Berlin, Germany.

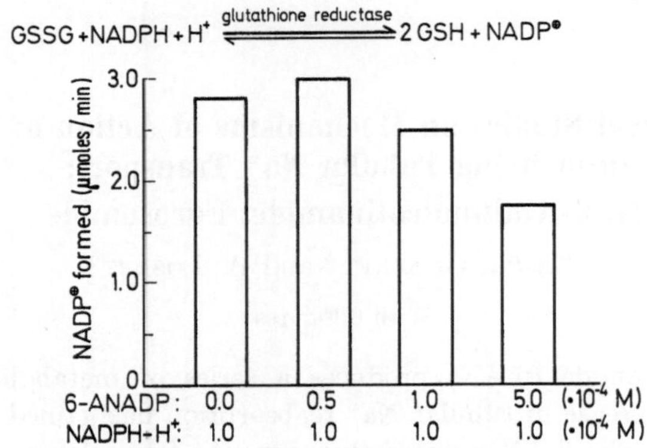

Fig. 1b. Inhibition of glutathione reductase by 6-ANADP in vitro (COPER and NEUBERT, 1964)

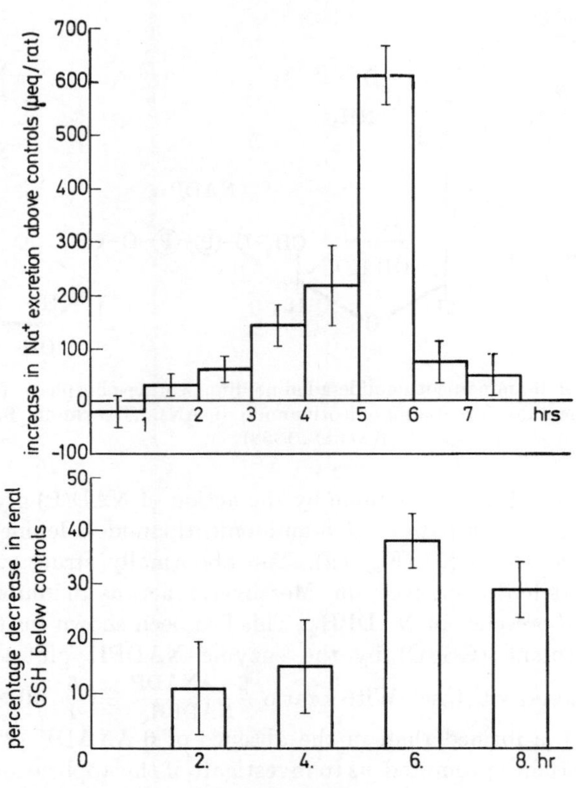

Fig. 2. Influence of 6-AN (50 mg/kg i.p.) on renal Na^+excretion and GSH concentration

As shown in Fig. 2, there is a decrease in renal GSH concentration following injection of 6-aminonicotinamide. The peak of the GSH-decrease is coincident with the peak of Na^+ excretion. When GSH concentration increases again, the diuretic effect of 6-AN decreases.

One is tempted to speculate that there might be a causal relationship between GSH concentration and Na^+ transport, especially, as this assumption has been supported by recent work of AVIRAM, SCHALITT, KASSEM and GROEN [1]. These authors showed that incubation of the isolated bovine lens in an N-ethylmaleimide containing medium results in a decrease in lens-GSH, accompanied by an increase in Na^+ concentration, e.g. in an inactivation of Na^+ transport.

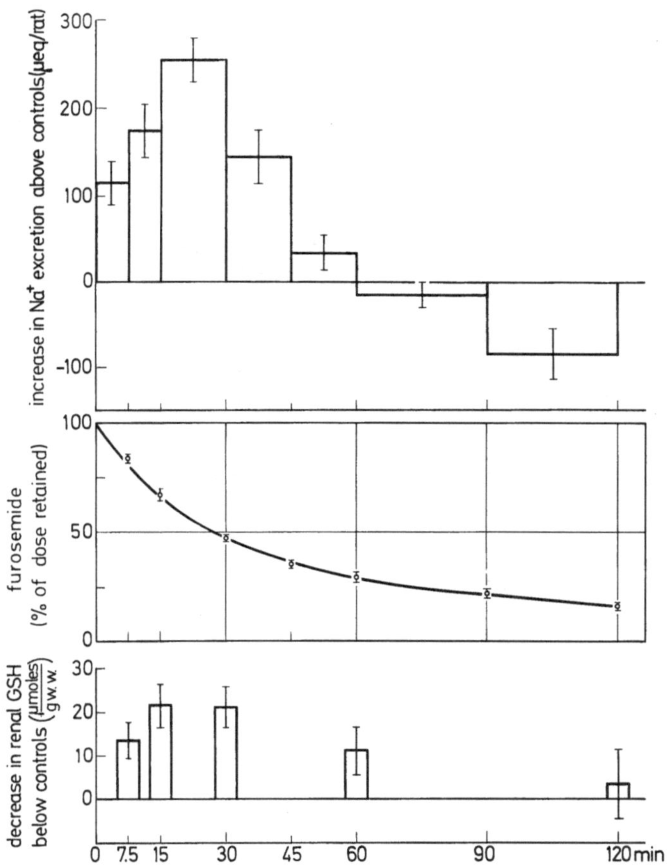

Fig. 3. Influence of furosemide (5 mg/kg i.v.) on renal Na^+ excretion and GSH concentration

Further support to this theory has been provided by the observation that furosemide leads to a decrease in renal GSH content. The peak of the GSH-decrease is coincident with the peak of Na^+ excretion. As the GSH concentration increases again simultaneously with the decline of the diuretic effect and with the decrease of the amount of furosemide present in the animal, it has been suggested that the reduction of renal GSH may be related to a direct action of the drug (Fig. 3).

This assumption is supported by the inhibition of glutathione reductase by furosemide. An analysis of enzyme kinetics was performed by plotting S/v on the ordinate against S on the abscissa [5]. With increasing concentrations of furose-

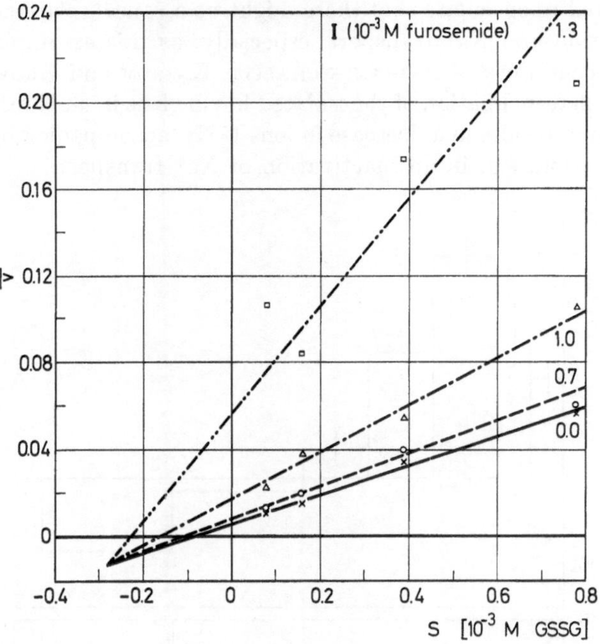

Fig. 4. Inhibition of glutathion reductase by furosemide in vitro

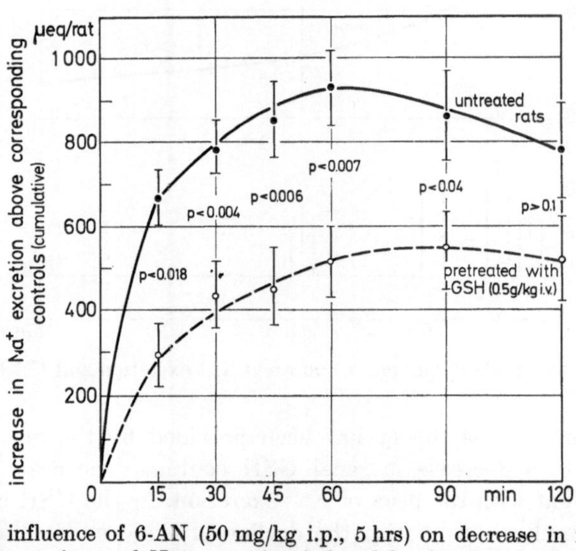

Fig. 5. Lack of influence of 6-AN (50 mg/kg i.p., 5 hrs) on decrease in renal GSH concentration and increase in renal Na^+ excretion induced by furosemide. * 5 mg furosemide/kg b.w., 15 min; ** 5 mg furosemide/kg b.w., 120 min

mide, the enzymic reduction of GSSG decreased. The diagram resulting from the plot S/v against S appears to represent a mixed (competitive/non competitive) type of inhibition (Fig. 4).

Further studies revealed a distinct difference between the action of furosemide and that of 6-AN on renal GSH content and tubular Na^+ transport. The latter compound lowers renal GSH by decreasing the availability of $NADPH_2$ for enzymic reduction of GSSG and by inhibiting the reaction between glutathione reductase and $NADPH_2$. Furosemide lowers renal GSH concentration apparently by inhibiting the reaction between glutathione reductase and GSSG. The action

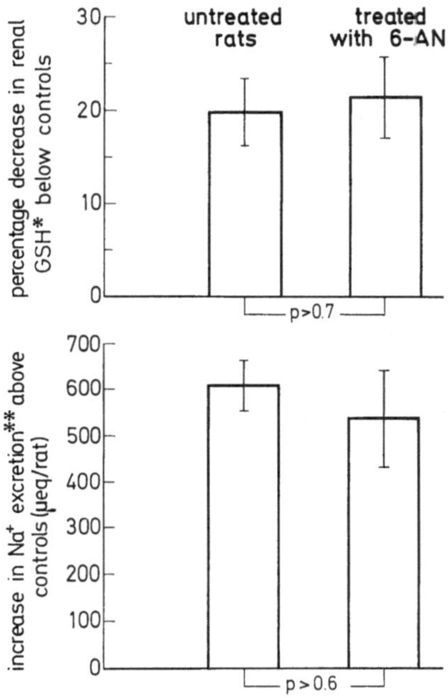

Fig. 6. Reduction of furosemide (5 mg/kg i.v.) induced natriuresis by pretreatment with GSH

of 6-AN was, therefore, expected to be additive to that of furosemide. As shown in Fig. 5 this has been found to be true with respect to the decrease in renal GSH as well as to the increase in urinary Na^+ excretion.

The assumption that the furosemide-induced decrease in renal GSH content is related to the natriuretic effect of the drug is in accordance with the finding that pretreatment with GSH leads to a reduction of the furosemide-induced increase in Na^+ excretion (Fig. 6).

References

1. Aviram, A., M. Schalitt, N. Kassem, and J. J. Groen: Glucose utilisation, glutathione, potassium and sodium content of the isolated bovine lens. Clin. chim. Acta **14**, 442—449 (1966).
2. Coper, H., u. D. Neubert: Einfluß von NADP-Analogen auf die Reaktionsgeschwindigkeit einiger NADP-bedürftiger Oxydoreduktasen. Biochim. biophys. Acta (Amst.) **89**, 23—32 (1964).
3. Dietrich, L. S., I. M. Friedland, and L. A. Kaplan: Pyridine nucleotide metabolism. Mechanism of action of the niacin antagonist 6-aminonicotinamide. J. biol. Chem. **233**, 964—968 (1958).

4. Herken, H., G. Senft u. B. Zemisch: Einschränkung des tubulären Natrium- und Kaliumtransports durch Biosynthese 6-Aminonicotinsäureamid enthaltender Nucleotide. Naunyn-Schmiedebergs Arch. exp. Path. Pharmak. **249**, 54—70 (1964).
5. Webb, J. L.: Enzyme and metabolic inhibitors, vol. I, General principles of inhibition. New York and London: Academic Press 1963.
6. Wiederholt, M., K. Hierholzer, G. Senft u. H. Herken: Lokalisation der natriuretischen Wirkung von 6-Aminonicotinamid in der Rattenniere. Naunyn-Schmiedebergs Arch. exp. Path. Pharmak. **261**, 143—151 (1968).
7. Zemisch, B.: Störungen des Elektrolyt- und Wasserhaushalts nach Bildung abnorm strukturierter NAD- bzw. NADP-Analoga. Inaug.-Diss. (Thesis), Medizinische Fakultät der Freien Universität Berlin, 1964.

3.6 Submicroscopic Alterations of Tubular Epithelia Induced by Furosemide

H.-J. MOHR [1]

With 6 Figures

Furosemide (Lasix) is a derivative of anthranilic acid and is used therapeutically as a diuretic agent. It has a rapid effect which lasts 3 to 4 hours allowing dimetic effects to be obtained at favorable times of the day and furthermore, it causes a high urinary Na/K excretion ratio. In addition furosemide is devoid

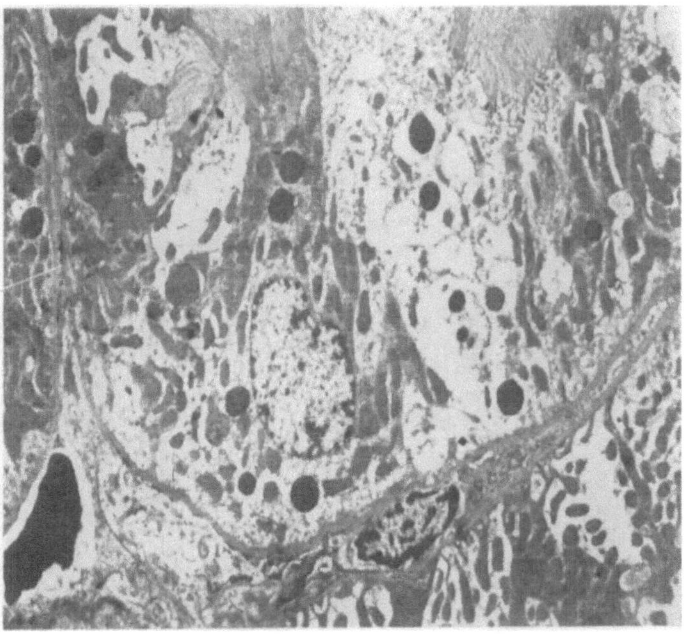

Fig. 1. Tubular epithelial cells one hour after furosemide with suppression of the basal labyrinths, rounding of mitochondria, displacement of mitochondria towards the middle of the cell and near to the brush border, increased transparency of the cytoplasm and partial disappearance of the brush border. Guines-pig (Ultrotom section contrasted by uranyl-lead-acetate). Zeiss EM 9, enlargement 10,800 times

of diabetogenic effects [2, 5, 7, 17, 33, 34, 36, 41]. The renal excretion of furosemide occurs by glomerular filtration as well as by tubular secretion. At therapeutic plasma levels, tubular secretion predominates. Its site is the proximal tubule. Clearance studies by GAYER [5] confirmed the assumption that furosemide is transported slowly through tubular cells and accumulates in the

[1] Pathologisches und Gewerbepathologisches Institut Gelsenkirchen, West Germany.

cells. Cellular accumulation may be assumed to be related to the rapidity of the inception of the diuretic effect. Since the morphological substrate of action of furosemide in the tubular cells does not appear to have been investigated, we studied the influence of the drug on the kidneys of mice, rats and guinea-pigs using light microscopic, histochemical and electronmicroscopic methods.

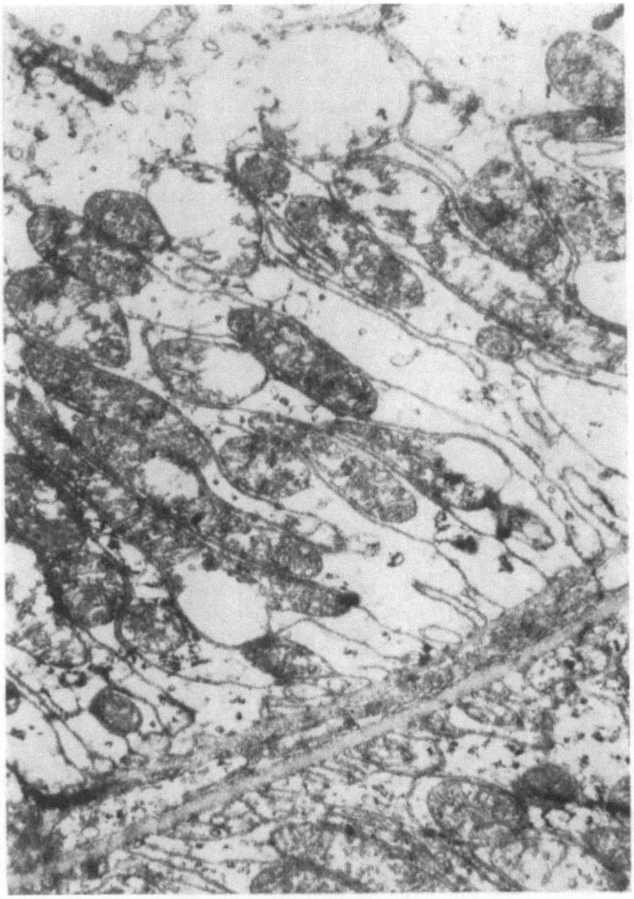

Fig. 2. Disappearance of the basal labyrinth, displacement of mitochondria, incipient vacuolization of mitochondria and pronounced increase of the translucency of the cytoplasm 2 hours after furosemide in Guinea-pig (Ultrotom section, uranyl-lead-acetate contrasting). Zeiss EM 9, enlargement 16,800 times

Material and Methods

Adult NMRI-mice, Wistar-rats and mongrel guinea-pigs of both sexes were injected s.c. with 6 mg/kg b.w. of furosemide and were killed 1, 2, 3, 4, 5, 6, or 24 hours later by a blow on the neck. Control animals were killed simultaneously in the same manner. The kidneys were removed immediately and were fixed in 4% neutral formalin for light microscopy, or in a 1% isotonic osmiuin tetroxide solution at pH 7,2 for electronmicroscopy, usually by perfusing the fixing agent through the renal vessels. Histochemical studies were done on cryostat sections. Material for light microscopy was embedded in paraffin for electron microscopy in methacrylate and epon. Histochemical investigations comprised staining for acid phosphatase, leucinaminopeptidase and succino-dehydrogenase, using the methods described by GOMORI and NACHLAS et al. and by MOHR [23, 24]. Succino-dehydro-

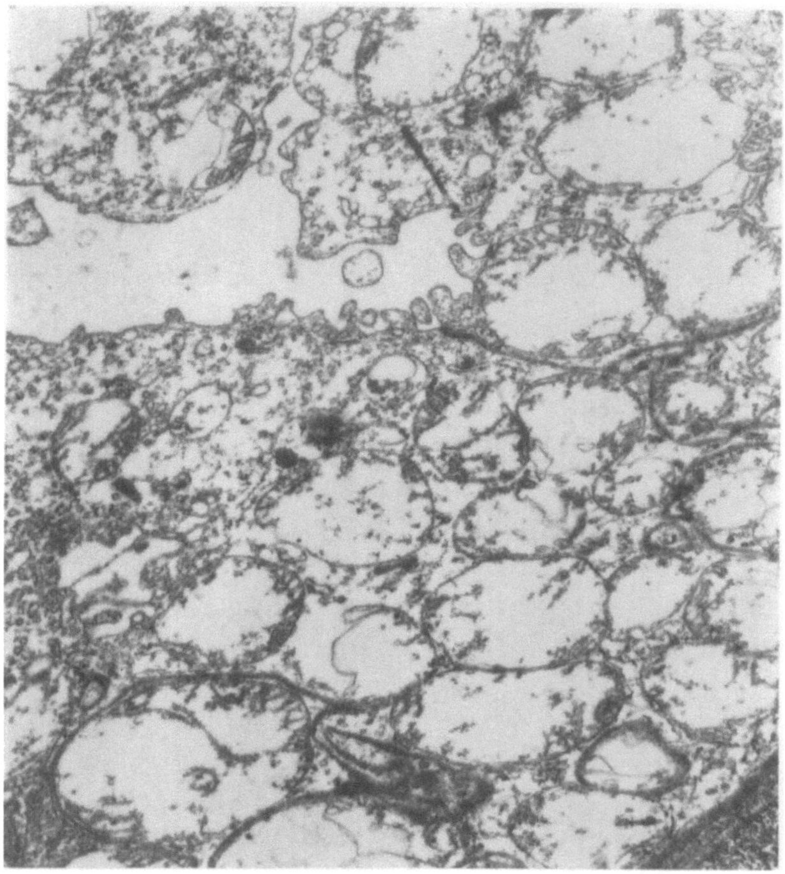

Fig. 3. Pronounced vacuolization of mitochondria by subtotal loss of cristae. The mitochondrial membranes are preserved and are connected with remnants of the cristae. Suppression of the basal labyrinth, increased translucency of the cytoplasm, rounding and strangulation of the brush border. 3 hours after furosemide in Guinea-pig (Ultrotom section, uranyl-lead-acetate contrasting). Zeiss EM 9, enlargement 20,000 times

genase activity was estimated in the conventional manner. Sections for electronmicroscopy were prepared with an Ultrotom 3, contrasted with lead acetate and uranyl acetate, and investigated and photographed with a Zeiss EM 9 electronmicroscope.

Discussion

According to clinical data and to our own experience, furosemide diuresis after a single dose reaches its maximum within 2—4 hours and ceases in 4—6 hours.

Diuresis in all 3 species investigated is accompanied by characteristic submicroscopic and histochemical changes in the cell organelles and in the cytoplasm. In the first hour the main changes were an increased translucency of the cytoplasm, a disappearance of the basal labyrinth and rounding and displacement of mitochondria from the base of the cell to its middle or its luminal surface

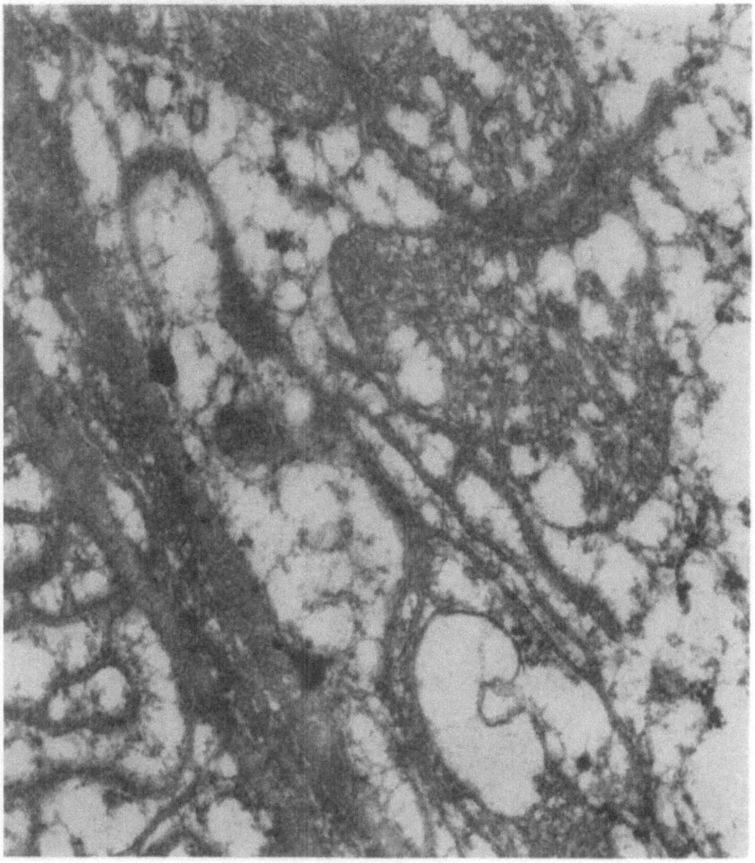

Fig. 4. Beginning regeneration of the basal labyrinths and of the michondrial cristae 4 hours after furosemide in Guinea-pig (Ultrotom section, contrasting by uranyl-lead-acetate). Zeiss EM 9, enlargement 56,000 times

(Fig. 1). With increasing diuresis there was, at first, a focal destruction of mitochondrial cristae and then a transformation of mitochondria to vacuoles containing a transparent mitochondrial matrix. The mitochondria were not actually destroyed (Fig. 2). The mitochondrial membranes were preserved and remained connected to remnants of the cristae which looked like strings on the membranes. These changes reached their maximal degree 3 hours after furosemide, i.e. at the time of maximal diuresis and progressively reverted to normal in the following hours (Fig. 3). The basal labyrinths and the mitochondrial cristae were partly regenerated 4 hours after injection (Fig. 4). 6 hours after injection, when the urine flow had fallen back to its initial value, the submicroscopic structures of the tubular epithelial cells and their organelles were completely normalized and did not differ any more from those observed in control animals (Fig. 5 and 6).

The electron microscopic pictures show that the mitochondria, particularly the mitochondrial cristae, may be considered as the site of action of furosemide within tubular epithelial cells. Furosemide induces at first a partial, and later

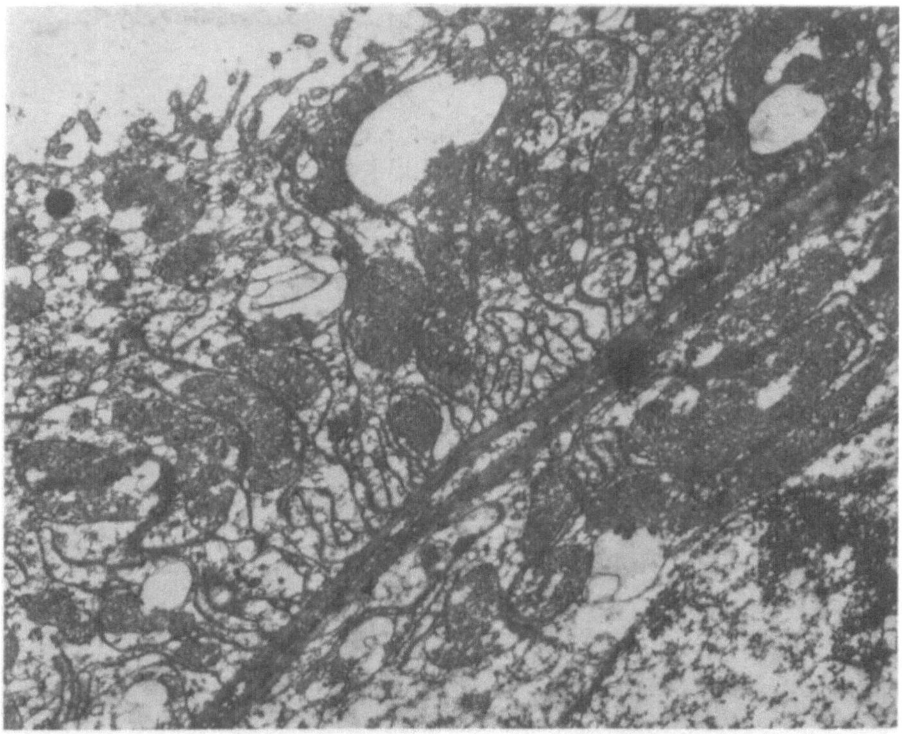

Fig. 5. A later stage of regeneration of the submicroscopic structures. Small defects in mitochondrial cristae and incomplete regeneration in the basal labyrinths 5 hours after furosemide in Guinea-pig (Ultrotom section contrasted by uranyl-lead-acetate). Zeiss EM 9, enlargement 16,000 times

a subtotal, disappearance of the cristae and transient transformation of mitochondria into vacuoles accompanied by a transient disappearance of the basal labyrinths within the first 3 hours after injecting the drug. The increased rate of urine flow may therefore be interpreted as the consequence of metabolic failure of tubular epithelial cells due to mitochondrial changes. Healing of the mitochondrial lesions between the 4th and 6th hours after a single dose is followed by re-establishment of normal fluid reabsorption. The regeneration of mitochondria and of basal labyrinths re-establishes normal metabolic functions and thereby a normal transport function of the tubular epithelial cells. Simultaneously with the occurrence of the submicroscopic mitochondrial changes, the acid phosphatase, succinodehydrogenase and leucinaminopeptidase activities of the tubular cells were depressed. All enzyme activities recovered simultaneously with the recovery of the normal aspect of the mitochondria.

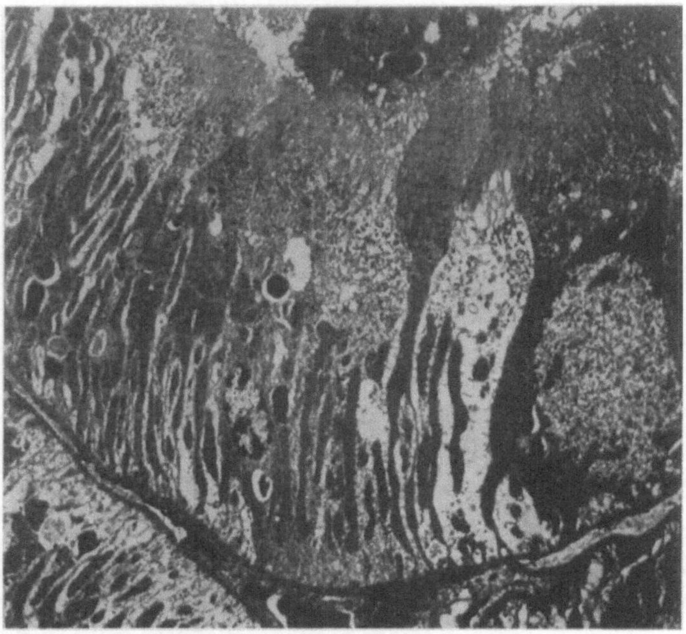

Fig. 6. Tubular epithelial cells with a regenerated subcellular structure. Picture seen 6 hours after furosemide aud similar to that found in normal control Guinea-pig (Ultratom section, contrasted by uranyl-lead-acetate). Zeiss EM 9, enlargement 10,800 times

Summary

Electron and light microscopic, as well as histochemical investigations on the kidney of mice, rats, and guinea-pigs showed that the intracellular site of action of furosemide is the tubular epithelial mitochondria. A single dose of furosemide causes a transient loss of mitochondrial cristae and a transformation of mitochondria into vacuoles accompanied by suppression of the basal labyrinths within the first 3 hours. These changes are correlated with the phase of increasing water excretion and/or the peak of diuresis. Simultaneously, there is a pronounced loss of acid phosphatase, succino-dehydrogenase and leucinaminopeptidase activities from tubular cells. When the diuretic effect ceases between the 4th and 6th hour after a single dose, the mitochondria are regenerated, the enzyme activities become normal again and the labyrinths reappear. The morphological aspect and the histochemical data are normal by the 6th hour after injection. The conclusion is reached that furosemide causes a mitochondrial blockade of 2—3 hours' duration responsible for metabolic failure of the cells. The metabolic failure, in turn, inhibits the reabsorption of sodium and of tubular fluid.

References

1. Ambrosoli, S., V. E. Andreucci, G. Baronio, G. C. Carrara, V. Ferioli, F. Pecchini, G. Prati e L. Scarpioni: Ricerche cliniche sull'attività diuretica del Furosemide. Minerva nefrol. **11**, 56—63 (1964).
2. Buchborn, E., u. S. Anastasakis: Angriffspunkt und Wirkungsmechanismus von Furosemid am distalen Nephron des Menschen. Klin. Wschr. **42**, 1127—1131 (1964).
3. Burgdorf, W.: Erfahrungen mit Furosemid. Med. Klin. **59**, 2027—2029 (1964).
4. Deetjen, P.: Mikropunktionsuntersuchungen zur Wirkung von Furosemid. Pflügers Arch. ges. Physiol. **284**, 184—190 (1965).
5. Gayer, J.: Die renale Exkretion des neuen Diuretikum Furosemid. Klin. Wschr. **43**, 898—902 (1965).
6. Gladtke, E.: Veränderungen des extrazellulären Flüssigkeitsraumes bei Kindern unter Furosemid. Z. Kinderheilk. **93**, 236—241 (1965).
7. Godwin, T. F., and R. W. Gunton: Clinical trial of a new diuretic, furosemide. Canad. med. Ass. J. **93**, 1296—1300 (1965).
8. Häussler, A.: Zur Pharmakodynamik von Furosemid. Podiumgespr. 25. 11. 1964, Dortmund.
9. Heidland, A., K. Klütsch u. F. Suzuki: Nierenhämodynamik, Wasser- und Elektrolytausscheidung nach 4-Chlor-N-(2-furylmethyl)-5-sulfamoyl-anthranilsäure. Arzneimittel-Forsch. **6**, 713—716 (1964).
10. Heller, J., V. Skrhová, and J. Vostal: The effect of various diuretic agents on renal electrolyte and urea concentration gradients in rats. Experientia (Basel) **21**, 454 (1965).
11. Hirsch, W., u. G. Woschee: Zur Diagnostik und Therapie des Symptoms: Lungenödem. Ther. d. Gegenw. **104**, 387—395 (1965).
12. Hoechst: Lasix, klinisch-experimentelle Ergebnisse. Internist. prax. **5**, 147—148 (1965).
13. Holzgreve, H., A. Frick, G. Rumrich, M. Wiederholt u. K. J. Ullrich: Wirkungsweise von Diuretika auf den transtubulären Transport von Natriumchlorid. 3. Symp. d. Ges. f. Nephrologie, Berlin 1964. In: Normale und pathologische Funktionen des Nierentubulus, hrsg. von K. J. Ullrich und K. Hierholzer, S. 147—154. Stuttgart: Huber 1965.
14. Hook, J. B., and H. E. Williamson: Lack of correlation between natriuretic activity and inhibition of renal Na-K-activated ATPase. Proc. Soc. exp. Biol. (N.Y.) **120**, 358—360 (1965).
15. Jänner, M.: Das Salidiuretikum Furosemid bei der Behandlung von Folgezuständen der venösen Insuffizienz. Münch. med. Wschr. **107**, 1420—1423 (1965).
16. Kiessling, J.: Praktische Erfahrungen mit Lasix, einem neuen Saluretikum. Münch. med. Wschr. **107**, 95—97 (1965).
17. Kleinfelder, H.: Experimentelle Untersuchungen und klinische Erfahrungen mit einem neuen Diuretikum. Dtsch. med. Wschr. **88**, 1695—1702 (1963).
18. Klütsch, K., A. Heidland e F. Suzuki: Cambiamenti comparativi nelle clearance dell'acqua libera dopo somministrazione di Idroclorotiazide, Politiazide e Fursemid. Atti Accad. med. lombarda **18**, 1255 (1963).
19. Königstein, R. P.: Die Anwendung von Furosemid (Lasix) in der Geriatrie. Wien. klin. Wschr. **77**, 93—97 (1965).
20. Kramer, G.: Zur medikamentösen Regulierung des Wasserhaushaltes beim Hirnödem. Med. Welt **42**, 2238—2244 (1964).
21. Larizza, P., P. Brunetti, G. Nenci u. L. Coli: Klinische Erfahrungen mit dem neuen Diuretikum Fursemid. Med. Klin. **59**, 1284—1287 (1964).
22. Lederbogen, Kl., u. M. Hüdepohl: Erfahrungen mit Fursemid (Lasix) bei Ödemen verschiedener Genese. Med. Welt **3**, 182—185 (1965).
23. Mohr, H.-J.: Histochemische Darstellung und feincytologische Lokalisation der L-Leucinaminopeptidase (LAP) im Nierengewebe. Beitr. path. Anat. B **134**, 52—64 (1966).
24. — Histochemie und submikroskopische Lokalisation der Aminopeptidase im Nierengewebe. Verh. dtsch. Ges. Path. **50**, 405—412 (1966).
25. Moll, H. Ch.: Kaliummangel. Münch. med. Wschr. **107**, 839—846 (1965).
26. Morrin, P. A. F.: The effect of furosemide, a new diuretic agent, on renal concentrating and diluting mechanism. Canad. J. Physiol. Pharmacol. **44**, 129—137 (1966).

27. Mühlbächer, W.: Zur Austreibung erkennbarer und verborgener Ödeme. Landarzt **40**, 1043—1044 (1964).
28. Muschaweck, R., u. P. Hajdu: Die salidiuretische Wirksamkeit der Chlor-N-(2-furyl-methyl)-5-sulfamyl-anthranilsäure. Arzneimittel-Forsch. **14**, 44—47 (1964).
29. Peltola, P.: Furosemide (Lasix) as a diuretic. Acta med. scand. **177**, 777—782 (1965).
30. Pupita, F., E. Bartoli, M. Molaschi, G. Bert, P. Dessy e B. Migheli: Ricerche sperimentali sul meccanismo d'azione e sugli effetti metabolici del furosemide. Clin. ter. **30**, 709 (1964).
31. Reimold, E.: Untersuchungen und klinische Erfahrungen mit Furosemid bei Säuglingen und Kindern. Arch. Kinderheilk. **172**, 6—18 (1965).
32. Robson, A. O., D. N. S. Kerr, R. Ashcroff, and G. Teasdale: The diuretic response to frusemide. Lancet **1964** I, No 7369, 1085—1087.
33. Rosenkranz, A.: Die renale Wasser- und Elektrolytausscheidung unter Fursemid beim Kind. Wien. med. Wschr. **114**, 236 (1964).
34. Schaefer, H.-F.: Moderne Diuretika und ihre Nebenwirkungen beim Diabetes mellitus. Med. Welt **16**, 922 (1964).
35. Schirmeister, J., u. H. Willmann: Über die Harnsäure- und andere Clearances nach intravenöser Gabe von Fursemid beim Menschen. Klin. Wschr. **42**, 623—628 (1964).
36. Schnack, H.: Therapeutische Erfahrungen mit einem neuen Saluretikum. Wien. klin. Wschr. **76**, 476 (1964).
37. Senft, G.: Tubuläre Wirkungen der Diuretika. Münch. med. Wschr. **108**, 2564—2571 (1966).
38. — Membrantransport und Pharmaka. In: Normale und pathologische Funktionen des Nierentubulus, hrsg. von K. J. Ullrich und K. Hierholzer, S. 63—81. Stuttgart: Huber 1965.
39. Small, A., and E. J. Cafruny: The renal sites of action of furosemide. Pharmakologist **7**, 165 (1965).
40. Thoms, R. K., F. R. Springman, and H. E. Wilson: A toxicological evaluation of furosemide: a new diuretic agent. Farmaco **19**, 544—549 (1964).
41. Timmerman, R. J., F. R. Springham u. R. K. Thoms: Beurteilung von Fursemid, einem neuen Diuretikum. Curr. ther. Res. **6** (1964).
42. Vorburger, C.: Fursemid, ein neuartiges Diuretikum. Rev. méd. Suisse rom. **4**, 1—12 (1964).
43. —, u. A. Huber: Fursemid, ein neues Diuretikum. Ther. Umsch. **21**, 486—491 (1964).

Discussion

Dubach:

Did the intranephronic sites of the lesions in your experiments coincide with the known sites of action of furosemide?

Heidland:

Do you think that the changes observed were due to a pharmacological effect of furosemide or were they the consequences of the hypovolemia induced by furosemide? Even after extremely high doses of furosemide (1,000 mg i.v.) in patients with terminal renal failure (GRF 3—4 ml/min) the drug, in our experience, did not interfere with proximal tubular excretion. In 4 such patients C_{PAH} increased from 5.6 ± 1.6 to 7.1 ± 2.6 ml/min within 45 minutes after furosemide.

Helmchen:

Single or repeated administration of high doses (50—100 mg/kg) of furosemide by the i.p. route induces extensive tubular cell necrosis mainly in the pars recta of the proximal tubules of the rat kidney. These lesions can be seen by light microscopy.

MOHR:

The intranephronic sites of the lesions were identical with the known sites of action of furosemide.

We think that the changes observed were, in fact, due to pharmacological effects of furosemide.

The lesions mentioned by HELMCHEN are similar is those observed in our experiments. Low doses of the drug caused minor changes in the mitochondria, high doses induced distinction of mitochondria and even necrosis, of tubular epithelial cells.

3.7. Studies on Oxygen Consumption and Changes of Tissue Cation Concentrations in K^+-Depleted Rabbit Kidney Slices, under the Influence of Diuretic Agents, p-Chloromercuribenzoate and N-Ethylmalemide*

W. Herms and F. Kersting [1]

With 3 Figures

One of the essential features of mammalian cells is their ability to maintain a high intracellular concentration of K^+ in the presence of a low extracellular K^+-concentration. The exact mechanism, by which the living cell is able to accumulate a high intracellular K^+-concentration, is unknown. Though the extent to which the K^+-transport is linked to other transport phenomena (notably an outward transport of Na^+) is equally unknown, there is considerable evidence, that both cation transport processes are performed at the expense of energy derived from cell metabolism. In the renal cortex, active cation transport is almost totally dependent on oxidative metabolism.

Apart from cell metabolism as the source of energy needed to establish and maintain the intracellular cation concentrations, the permeability characteristics of the cell membrane also determine the final Na^+ and K^+-concentration by influencing the passive movements down electro-chemical gradients which occur at the cell membrane both for K^+ and Na^+-ions.

Some years ago Mudge, in an extensive study on rabbit kidney cortex slices, described an *in vitro* technique which permits the simultaneous study of K^+-accumulation and the rate of metabolic activity [1, 2]. It was found, that rabbit kidney cortex slices readily lose K^+ when prepared and kept in K^+-free media, and that the reaccumulation of K^+ from a low external K^+ concentration in the bathing medium depends upon metabolic activity as measured by oxygen consumption. The K^+ uptake can be modified by such variables as oxygen tension, temperature and the addition of suitable substrates. Furthermore it could be demonstrated that K^+ accumulation is associated with a reciprocal change in Na^+ concentration. In a further study, Mudge examined the effect of certain metabolic inhibitors on this system. All compounds which decrease oxygen consumption (e.g. anoxia, cyanides) likewise prevented the uptake of K^+ [2].

We used the experimental procedure devised by Mudge in order to obtain information on the effect of diuretic agents, which might contribute to the understanding of their mechanism of action. Four diuretic agents were studied at different concentration ranges: mersalyl, hydrochlorothiazide, furosemide and ethacrynic acid. In addition p-mercuribenzoate (PMB) and N-ethylmalemide (NEM) were studied as nondiuretic compounds.

* Supported by Deutsche Forschungsgemeinschaft.

[1] I. Medizinische Klinik der Universität Düsseldorf, West Germany.

The initial tissue concentrations of K^+ and Na^+, expressed as mEq/kg dry weight, were approximately equal. The tissue slices were then leached for $2^1/_2$ hours at 15° C in a K^+-free 0.15 M NaCl solution, which was aerated and constantly stirred by a low speed mechanical stirrer. By this time, the K^+ concentrations had fallen from an initial value of about 450 mEq/kg dry weight to about 200 mEq/kg dry weight, and the Na^+ concentration had risen from 400 mEq/kg dry weight to about 710 mEq/kg dry weight. The slices were then immersed

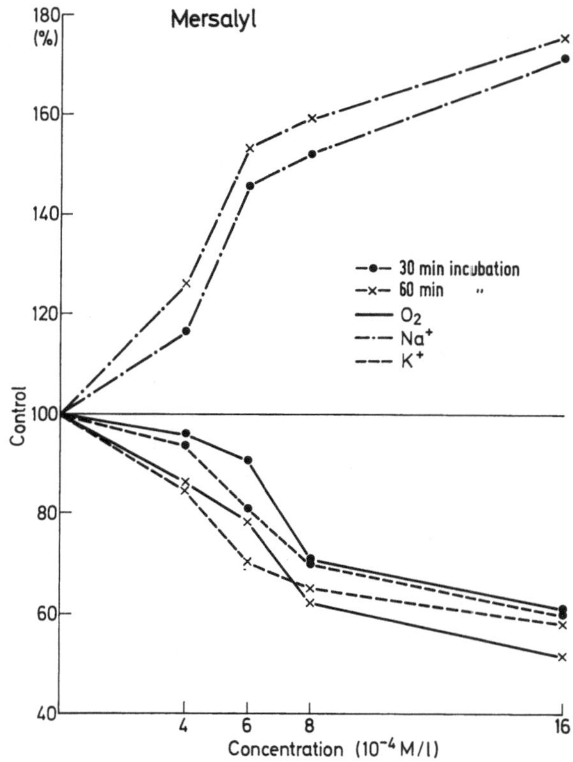

Fig. 1. Effect of mersalyl on changes of respiration; K^+ and Na^+ tissue concentrations in K^+ depleted kidney slices, as compared with control slices = 100%

in chilled saline and transferred to Warburg vessels. They were incubated in a Ringer solution with a K^+ concentration of 10.0 mEq/l and glucose (2 mg/ml). The osmolality was 310 mosm/l and the pH about 7.4. K^+ accumulation and O_2 consumption were measured under the influence of various diuretic agents which were added to the incubation medium at different concentrations. The oxygen consumption was measured at intervals of 15 minutes in 6 vessels containing the incubated slices plus the diuretic agent and in 6 control vessels. O_2 consumption was 8.0 ± 0.4 µl/mg dry weight per 60 min in the control vessels. After drying at 90° for 24 hrs. the slices were ashed with HNO_3. Tissue concentrations of Na^+ and K^+ were determined after 30 minutes and 60 minutes of Warburg incubation.

The observed effects on tissue concentration of Na^+ and K^+ and respiration of kidney slices incubated with mersalyl at different concentrations are given in Fig. 1, which shows the mean values of Na^+ and K^+-concentrations as well as an O_2 consumption, each obtained from at least 6 Warburg vessels, expressed as fractions of the control values = 100%. With increasing doses of the diuretic agent a decrease in O_2 consumption and tissue K^+-concentration and an increase in tissue Na^+-concentration was observed. Similar results were obtained with the other compounds studied.

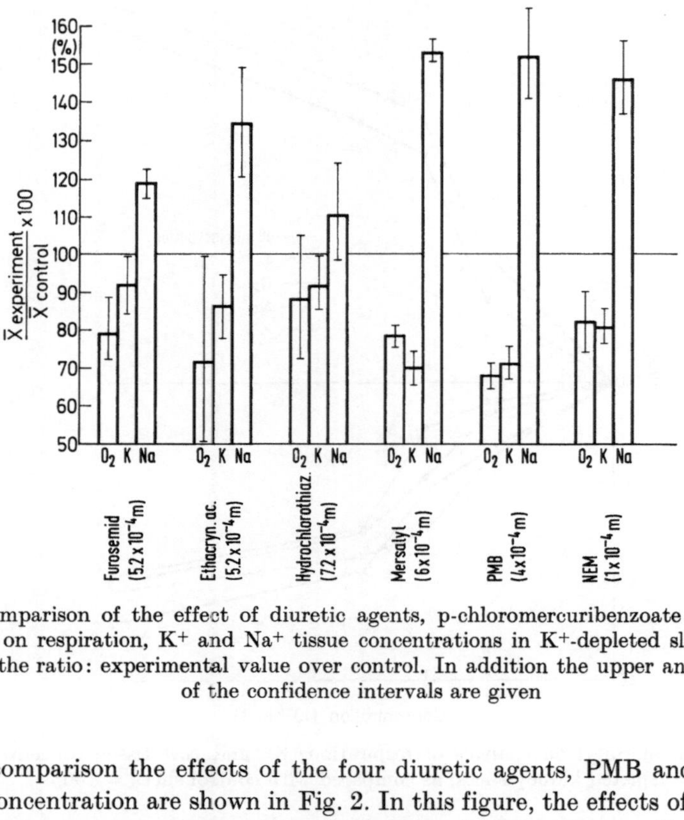

Fig. 2. Comparison of the effect of diuretic agents, p-chloromercuribenzoate and N-ethylmalemide on respiration, K^+ and Na^+ tissue concentrations in K^+-depleted slices. The bars represent the ratio: experimental value over control. In addition the upper and lower limits of the confidence intervals are given

For comparison the effects of the four diuretic agents, PMB and NEM at a similar concentration are shown in Fig. 2. In this figure, the effects of the various substances are expressed as ratios of slices incubated with the diuretic agents divided by the control values. If the upper limits of the confidence intervals for O_2 consumption- and K^+ tissue concentration ratios are below 100% and the lower limits for tissue Na^+ concentration ratios are above 100%, the observed effects are significant. There was no close relationship between the rate of depression of respiration and the decrease in K^+-uptake for the majority of the substances studied, with the exception of hydrochlorothiazide. With furosemide and ethacrynic acid, the decrease in O_2 consumption was larger than the decrease in tissue K^+ reaccumulation, whereas with mersalyl the inhibition of K^+-uptake was larger than the inhibition of respiration. Fig. 2 also demonstrates that the alterations in tissue Na^+ concentrations did not parallel the changes in K^+ concentrations. Nondiuretic substances like PMB and NEM had an analogous effect; when compared on a molar basis, these two agents were more potent than the diuretic agents.

In order to investigate whether blocking of SH-groups is responsible for the action of the 6 drugs, we studied the effect of adding cysteine chloride in twice the molar concentration to the inhibitory agents. The results of this series

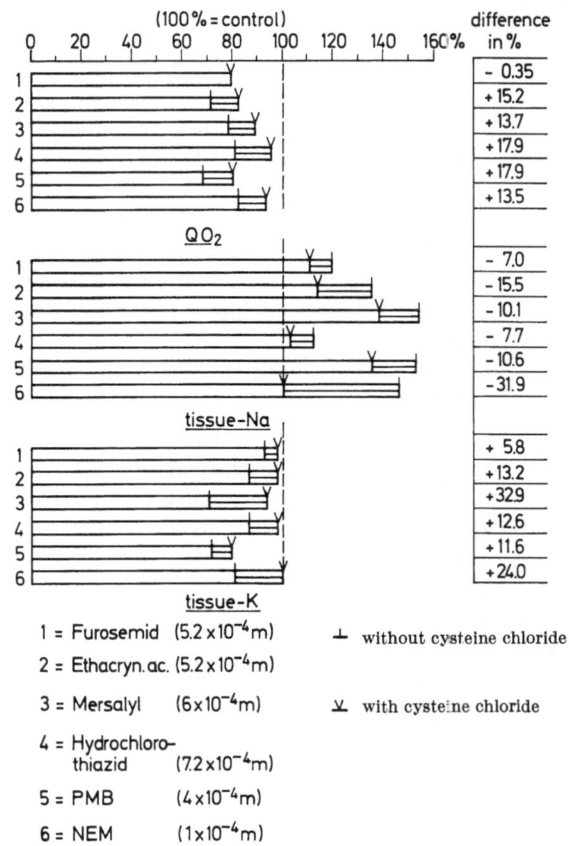

Fig. 3. Effect of cysteine on the observed effects of the inhibitory agents. 100% = control value without the inhibitory agent. The difference in percent given at the right hand side represents the alterations observed after adding cysteine to the diuretic agents, to PMB and to NEM

of experiments are listed in Fig. 3; the effect of NEM on tissue respiration and Na^+ and K^+ concentration could be reversed, whereas cysteine had only a small effect on depression by p-chloromercuribenzoate, hydrochlorothiazide and mersalyl and almost none on inhibition by furosemide.

Discussion

Mudge [2], observed an inhibition of K^+-uptake without any alteration in respiration when kidney slices were incubated with a mercurial compound. In contrast, we found that all diuretic agents influenced tissue respiration. The decrease in respiration was accompanied by a decrease in K^+-uptake of previously K^+-depleted kidney slices. The depression of K^+ reaccumulation is taken as an indication of inhibition of active K^+ transport. However, there was no close relationship between the depression of respiration and the inhibition of K^+-uptake. Therefore, it is suggested that active K^+-uptake is not closely linked to respiration. With all diuretics studied, an increase in tissue Na^+ concentration was observed. The change in tissue Na^+ did not closely parallel the change in tissue K^+ concentrations. Especially with ethacrynic acid, the relative increase in tissue Na^+ exceeded the decrease in tissue K^+, at a given value for tissue oxygen consumption. These agents, thus, might also exert some effect on membrane permeability of the cells.

The effect on oxygen consumption and tissue cation concentrations could be partially reversed by adding cysteine chloride. However the addition of SH-groups had the most pronounced protective effect in the experiments with non-diuretic agents like PMB and NEM. Inhibition of SH-groups, thus, is one, but not the main mechanism of diuretic action [3].

The different effects of the various diuretic compounds might partially be due to differences in lipid solubility [4]. Thus drugs with poor lipid solubility like furosemide may take a longer time before exerting an effect on cellular metabolism.

Changes in tissue cation concentrations may be considered as the net-result of changes in active transport and passive diffusion, and, furthermore, do not permit any differentiation between intra- or extracellular compartments. *In vivo* other factors, as e.g. changes in flow rates may be important. However, the present *in vitro* experiments demonstrate that the inhibitory effect on tissue respiration of various diuretic agents can only be observed by using comparatively high concentrations and that the depression in O_2 consumption does not parallel the alterations in tissue cation concentrations. Thus one might tentatively conclude, that apart from their inhibitory effect on tissue respiration, these agents also may act by altering some permeability characteristics of the cells.

References

1. MUDGE, G. H.: Studies on potassium accumulation by rabbit kidney slices: Effect of metabolic activity. Amer. J. Physiol. **165**, 113—127 (1951).
2. — Electrolyte and water metabolism of rabbit kidney slices: Effect of metabolic inhibitors. Amer. J. Physiol. **171**, 207—223 (1951).
3. —, and J. M. WEINER: The mechanism of action of mercurial and xanthine diuretics. Ann. N.Y. Acad. Sci. **71** (A), 344—354 (1958).
4. DE STEVENS, G.: Diuretics, chemistry and pharmacology. New York: Academic Press 1963.

Discussion

BURCK:

I doubt whether pre-incubation for $2^1/_2$ hours did not considerably damage your tissue slices. Together with F. PETRUCH, we investigated the influence of 1 µg or of 100 µg/ml of furosemide on the oxygen uptake of renal cortical slices from rabbits, incubated in a Krebs-III-solution. Furosemide did not cause any depression of the respiration of the cortical slices, even when the sodium concentration was increased to 350 mEq/l. With slices from the outer medullary zone, Q_{O_2} was depressed by the same doses of furosemide with 150 mEq Na^+/l or with 350 mEq Na^+/l of sodium in the incubation medium.

HERMS:

Preincubation of the slices might have depressed the metabolic activity. However we were interested in whether diuretics influence the capacity of K^+-depleted slices a) to reaccumulate K^+ and b) to consume oxygen. These values were compared to the controls without the diuretic agents added and the results in fact show significant differences. Our studies were done with cortical slices. I cannot comment on your remark concerning the influence of increasing NaCl in the incubation solution nor the difference in the effect of cortical and medullary slices.

3.8. The Effect of Amiprazide on Sodium and Water Flux Across Frog Skin

J. Eigler, J. Kelter and E. Renner [1]

With 1 Figure

In preliminary observations [3] amiprazide (MK 870, Amiloride HCl), a new diuretic agent [2], had been found to cause a profound but reversible decrease in short circuit current (SCC) and potential difference (PD) across the isolated frog skin. In view of newer concepts regarding the mucosal permeability barrier [6] it seemed of interest to evaluate the effect of this substance on sodium transport and water flux.

Our results indicate that: 1. the drop in short circuit current is accounted for by a diminished influx of sodium while the efflux of sodium remains unaltered. 2. The ADH mediated increase in water permeability is unaffected by the addition of amiprazide, while — at the same dose level — the influx of sodium is greatly decreased.

Methods

All experiments were carried out during the summer months of 1967. The isolated ventral skin of Rana temporaria was mounted between two halves of a Lucite chamber, each half containing 10 ml of frog Ringer's solution as bathing medium. The cross-sectional area of the skin exposed was 3,14 cm^2. SCC and PD were recorded according to conventional techniques as described by Ussing and Zerahn [7]. The frog Ringer's solution had the following composition: Na: 115 mEq/l; K: 2 mEq/l; Ca: 1 mEq/l; HCO_3: 2,5 mEq/l; pH after aeration: 7,8—8,1.

Sodium fluxes using Na^{22} [7] were measured during 3 consecutive 60 min periods. Samples were taken in duplicate and the radioactivity was measured in a well scintillation counter. The influx of water was measured using tritiated water during four consecutive periods with no osmotic gradient present. The radioactivity was determined in a Packard Tricarb liquid scintillation spectrometer.

According to Hays and Leaf the permeability coefficient for water

$$K_{\text{trans}} = \frac{Q_W}{(C_1 - C_2) \cdot A}$$

Q_W = Net increase of isotopic water per unit time on the unlabeled side.
C_1 = mean concentration of isotope on the labeled side during the 30 min periods of measurement.
C_2 = mean concentration of isotope on the unlabeled side during the 30 min periods of measurement.
A = Cross sectional area of the chamber (3.14 cm^2).

[1] Medizinische Universitäts-Poliklinik und Medizinische Klinik Köln-Merheim, West Germany.

was converted to a flux by multiplying K_{trans} by the molar concentration of water in the bathing medium (55,3 mM/ml of medium) times the partial molal volume of water (18 µl/mM), thus expressing the respective data as $\mu l \cdot cm^{-2} \cdot h^{-1}$ [4].

Amiprazid (N-amidino-3-amino-6-chloropyrazincarboxamide; Amiloride-HCl; molecular weight 268)[2] in this study was always used at a concentration of $4 \cdot 10^{-2}$ mM. The term ADH refers to commercial vasopressin (Pitressin or Tonephin)[3] and was always used in a concentration of 200 mU/ml in the inside bathing solution. Changes of bathing solutions were repeated twice in order to assure complete removal of the substance in question. The beginning of each experiment was preceeded by a period of equilibration lasting 1—2 hrs.

Results

As previously reported [3] amiprazid showed an effect on SCC and PD of the isolated frog skin only when added to the outside bathing solution. Over a wide range of concentrations it caused a dose related rapid drop of SCC and PD. At the high concentration used in our study the SCC dropped to low values (5—15 $\mu A/3.14\ cm^2$) within seconds. The fall was followed by a slight but insignificant rise during a 2 hour period of incubation (Fig. 1), while the PD, after its initial drop rose slowly up to about 50% of its value at zero time. After replacement of the bathing solution by normal frog Ringer's solution, SCC and PD rose rapidly again reaching values well above pretreatment level. The nature of this sort of rebound remains to be clarified. We have extended the period of observation after application of the agent up to three hours, and still obtained the same type of response, indicating that the viability of the skin apparently remained intact.

In view of the fact that such a marked drop of SCC and PD occurred after addition of amiprazide, it seemed advisable to determine whether the SCC recorded still represented the net sodium flux across the skin. The results of six experiments measuring Na influx and of three experiments measuring Na efflux are presented in Table 1. Within the limits of experimental error there was good agreement between SCC and sodium influx during the control period (since under normal conditions SCC equals Na influx minus Na efflux, the SCC usually is 5—10% lower than the Na influx). After application of amiprazide, both the Na influx and the SCC dropped to low values although the Na influx remained almost 50% higher than the SCC. If the measurements of the Na-efflux are taken into account, it becomes apparent that the SCC still represents the net flux of sodium after exposure of the skin to amiprazide, because the Na-efflux seems unaffected by the drug.

Following the addition of ADH the well known rise of the SCC by about 65% was observed (Fig. 1). This normal response to ADH was altered significantly when ADH and amiprazide were added at the same time (Fig. 1). Under these conditions there was a drop in SCC of the same order of magnitude as in experiments in which amiprazide alone was added. The initial decrease in SCC was

[2] Kindly furnished by Sharp u. Dohme GmbH, Munich.

[3] Pitressin was kindly supplied by Parke Davis u. Co., Munich. Tonephin was kindly supplied by Farbwerke Hoechst, Frankfurt.

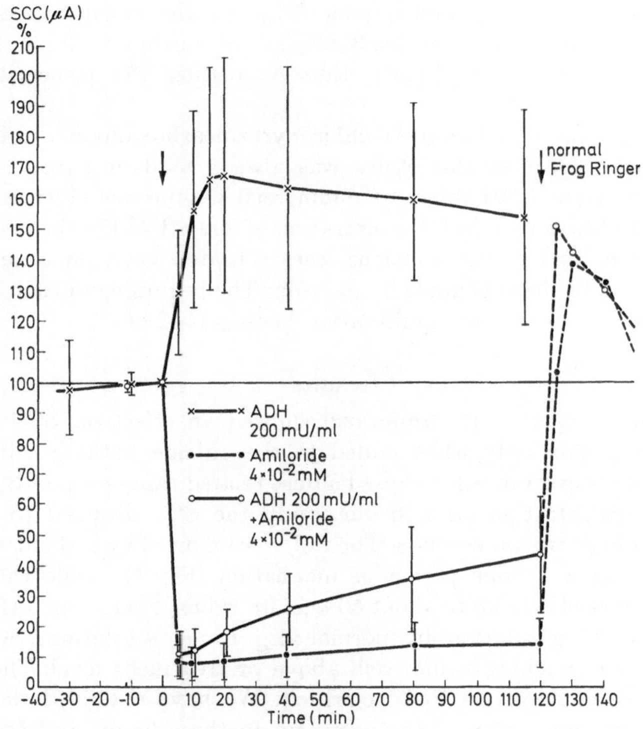

Fig. 1. The effect of vasopressin (ADH) and amiprazide on the short circuit current across frog skin. All values (mean ±1 SD) are given as percentage changes of the value at zero time. All drugs were added at zero time and replaced by normal frog Ringer's solution 2 hrs later. ×—×—× ADH ($n = 20$); ●—●—● Amiprazide ($n = 8$); ○—○—○ Amiprazide + ADH · ($n = 15$)

Table 1. *Comparison of mean short circuit current with Na influx (1—6) and Na efflux (7—9) across isolated frog skin during three consecutive 60 min periods before (1 hr) and after (2 hrs) addition of amiprazide. Values are given as* 10^{-11} *Eq/sec*

Before (1 hr)				After (1st hour)			After (2d hour)		
exper. No.	mean SCC	mean Na influx	mean Na efflux	mean SCC	mean Na influx	mean Na efflux	mean SCC	mean Na influx	mean Na efflux
1	122.4	120.0	—	12.3	13.6	—	12.3	12.3	—
2	138.8	131.6	—	13.4	27.4	—	18.5	18.0	—
3	117.3	131.6	—	13.4	25.7	—	16.4	36.0	—
4	145.0	130.4	—	11.3	25.4	—	11.3	7.8	—
5	98.7	111.7	—	3.1	13.0	—	4.1	7.2	—
6	145.0	129.0	—	18.5	26.1	—	19.5	33.4	—
7	132.7	—	7.2	8.2	—	8.2	9.2	—	9.7
8	131.6	—	11.2	15.4	—	7.2	19.5	—	11.7
9	108.0	—	18.7	7.2	—	20.5	9.2	—	14.5

then followed by a slow but steady rise of the SCC resulting in a different pattern of response and reaching, after two hours, a mean of 44% (±19% SD) of the value recorded at zero time. These findings indicate that the ADH-mediated characteristic increase in SCC (i.e. net sodium flux) is diminished when $4 \cdot 10^{-2}$ mM amiprazide are added to the outside bathing solution.

Our previously published observation (3) needs to be corrected in this respect: the pattern of response to ADH after exposure of the skin to amiprazide varies with the dose of the agent in relation to the natural electrical activity of the skin. Thus, skins of winter frogs (with frequently low PD and SCC), on which our earlier observations were made, received doses too large for inducing an ADH effect within a 30 min period.

Table 2. *Measurement of the influx of tritiated water across isolated frog skin during four consecutive 30 min periods before and after addition of ADH (1—4) and after ADH plus amiprazid (5—10), respectively. Exposed area: 3,14 cm², 10 ml frog* Ringer's *solution bathing each surface. No osmotic gradient was present. Values are given as* $\mu l \cdot cm^{-2} \cdot h^{-1}$

Exp. No.	Control	periods	After ADH		After ADH + amiprazid	
	a	b	c	d	c	d
1	293	298	315	290	—	—
2	336	317	352	281	—	—
3	254	314	376	372	—	—
4	269	316	308	382	—	—
5	313	384	—	—	331	396
6	297	352	—	—	358	330
7	341	343	—	—	408	629
8	328	198	—	—	359	330
9	223	308	—	—	300	338
10	306	336	—	—	378	400
Mean	296	316	337	331	355	403

The influx of water, on the other hand, did not change significantly after addition of both amiprazide and ADH as compared to the addition of ADH alone; in both instances the ADH-mediated increase of water diffusion was about 10% (Table 2). These figures agree well with those found by Koefoed-Johnsen and Ussing [5]. Since Na influx was greatly depressed in these experiments the results confirm the fact [4] that water permeability is independent of sodium transport.

Discussion

According to presently held concepts [3, 6] transepithelial transport across the toad bladder is influenced by a mucosal permeability barrier consisting of a dense and a porous diffusion barrier, in series. The dense diffusion barrier hinders the entrance of sodium and most small molecules, while the porous barrier represents the major obstacle to the diffusion of water. Antidiuretic hormone is thought to have a dual site of action: on the dense diffusion barrier with respect to sodium and small molecules like urea, and on the porous barrier with respect to water, facilitating the passive entry of the respective substances into the cell.

Although the anatomic structure of amphibian skin is much more complex in comparison to the toad bladder — in principle — a similar system of diffusion barriers at the mucosal or outward facing cell membrane may exist.

Amiloride HCl depresses greatly the transepithelial influx of sodium across the frog skin, but leaves the efflux of Na as well as the diffusion of water, unaltered. This effect could be brought about by a) blocking the passive entry of sodium at the dense diffusion barrier or b) interfering directly with active transport mechanisms at or near the serosal (or inward facing) cell membrane. We are inclined to favour the first possibility because at constant low SCC a slow increase in PD was observed and because, SCC and PD rose immediately after changing the bathing solution, even after 3 hours of incubation.

Assuming that the mode of action of amiprazide is to block the passive entry of sodium at the dense diffusion barrier the drug may prove a suitable tool for further studies on the concept of a dual permeability barrier and on the site of action of antidiuretic hormone.

Summary

1. Amiprazide caused a profound drop in SCC and PD across frog skin when added to the outside bathing solution.

2. At high doses the effect on SCC remained unchanged for periods up to three hours without apparent damage to the skin.

3. After replacing the bathing solution by normal frog Ringer's solution a rapid rise of both SCC and PD was observed.

4. The drop in SCC is quantitatively accounted for by a decrease in sodium influx, the SCC still being a measure of the net sodium transport under these conditions.

5. At high doses of amiprazide the normal response of the SCC to ADH was abolished while the ADH mediated increase in water permeability (influx) was not affected.

Acknowledgement

The skillful technical assistence of Miss A. THOMAS is gratefully acknowledged.

References

1. ANDERSEN, B., and H. H. USSING: Solvent drag on non-electrolytes during osmotic flow through isolated toads skin and its response to antidiuretic hormone. Acta physiol. scand. **39**, 228—239 (1957).

2. BAER, J. E., C. M. MUCHA, S. A. SPITZER, and H. W. YEE: A K^+-sparing natriuretic. Pyrazinamide derivative. Fed. Proc. **25**, 197 (1966).

3. EIGLER, J., J. KELTER u. E. RENNER: Wirkungscharakteristika eines neuen Acylguanidins — Amiloride HCl (MK 870) — an der isolierten Haut von Amphibien. Klin. Wschr. **45**, 737—738 (1967).

4. HAYS, R. M., and A. LEAF: Studies on the movement of water through the isolated toad bladder and its modification by vasopressin. J. gen. Physiol. **45**, 905—919 (1962).

5. KOEFOED-JOHNSEN, V., and H. H. USSING: The contributions of diffusion and flow to the passage of D_2O through living membranes. Effect of neurohypophyseal hormone on isolated anuran skin. Acta physiol. scand. **28**, 60—76 (1953).

6. LICHTENSTEIN, N., and A. LEAF: The effect of Amphotericin B on the permeability of the toad bladder. J. clin. Invest. **44**, 1328—1342 (1965).
7. USSING, H. H., and K. ZERAHN: Active transport of sodium as the source of electric current in the short-circuited isolated frog skin. Acta physiol. scand. **23**, 110—121 (1951).

Discussion

KRUECK:

A dissociation of short circuit current and potential difference, as observed in the second half of your experiments in the presence of amiprazide, suggests a change in membrane resistance as the basic phenomenon of the second phase, which could follow, or be additive to, an inhibition of active sodium transport during the first phase.

EIGLER:

A change in resistance may play a role, but the dissociation between potential difference and short circuit current is rather small so that the basic phenomenon still would be a marked inhibition of sodium transport.

4. Renin, Angiotensin, Aldosterone

4.1. A Light and Electron Microscopic Investigation of the Juxtaglomerular Apparatus of the Kidneys of Patients with Conn's Syndrome*

A. Bohle, A. Helber, D. Meyer, J. Schürholz and H. P. Wolff [1]

With 6 Figures

We studied the morphology of the juxtaglomerular apparatus on wedge excisions of the kidney, obtained in the course of operations, on 3 patients with primary hyperaldosteronism, using light as well as electron microscopy.

The case histories may be summarized as follows:

1. 38 year old man with hypertension for 2 years (BP 220/110 and 170/100 mm Hg). Serum potassium 2.6—3.6 mEq/l. Serum sodium 141—150 mEq/l. Total exchangeable potassium decreased to 126 g (normal 140 g). Aldosterone secretion increased to 69.7 μg/24 hrs. Plasma renin concentration between 12.5 and 30.3 U/l. At operation an adrenal adenoma weighing 12.5 g was removed.

2. 38 year old woman with hypertension for 7 years (BP between 220/160 and 140/110 mm Hg). Serum potassium: 8 mEq/l, serum sodium 153 mEq/l, total exchangeable potassium 67.3 ± 5 g (normal 84 g). Aldosterone secretion 50.6 to 76.6 μg/24 hrs. Renin activity in plasma: 3.6 to 11.1 U/l. At operation, a left-sided cortical adrenal adenoma was found.

3. 42 year old man hypertensive for 15 years (BP between 240/120 and 210/130 mm Hg). Serum potassium: 3.4 mEq/l, serum sodium: 142 mEq/l, total exchangeable potassium: 125 to 135 g (normal value: 135 to 140 g). Aldosterone secretion rate: 426 μg/24 hrs, plasma renin activity: 3.1 to 27.5 U/l. Operation revealed a diffuse hyperplasia of the adrenal cortex on both sides and a hemorrhage into the adrenal medulla on one side.

Results

At light microscopy, typical changes were observed in the cortex and sometimes also in the outer strip of the outer medulla which had been excised by chance, in all 3 patients. The glomeruli and tubules appeared quite normal. In the renal arterioles the intima and the media showed pronounced focal sclerosis. Counts of the cells of the juxtaglomerular apparatus, done for each patient on 300 randomly sectioned glomeruli, without distinguishing smooth muscle cells, epitheloid cells and Goormaghtigh's cells, showed values within or at the lower limit of the normal range (case 1: 883 cells; case 2: 1,252 cells; case 3: 1,436 cells; normal controls: 891 to 1,772 cells).

Since many investigators assume an intimate relationship between the juxtaglomerular apparatus and the macula densa (MD) [9, 10, 13, 14, 18], we also investigated the early distal tubules attached to 300 glomeruli. In the kidneys

* Supported by Deutsche Forschungsgemeinschaft.

[1] Pathologisches Institut der Universität Tübingen and II. Medizinische Universitätsklinik und Poliklinik Homburg/Saar, West Germany.

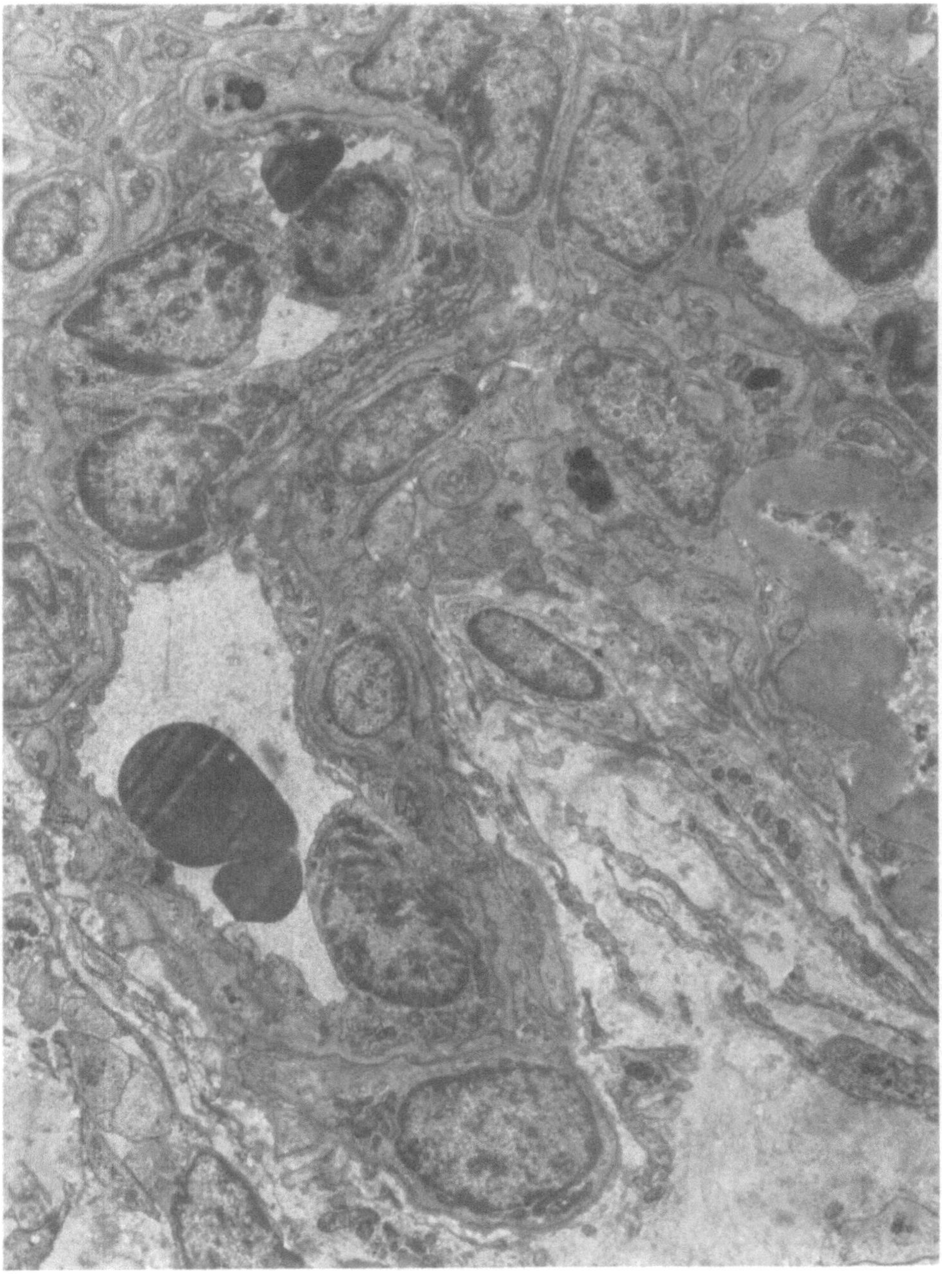

Fig. 1. (Case No 1, male, 38 years.) Partially tangential section through a vas afferens with smooth muscle cells in the media embedded in basal membrane-like structures. The cytoplasm of the smooth muscle cells contains lipofuscin-like granules. Enlargement at electron microscopy: 1,600 times. Final enlargement: 4,000 times

of the patients with Conn's syndrome, 8 to 8.6% of these sections showed the typical MD structure, while a similar count in normal subjects showed typical MD structures in 10 to 18%. The electron microscopic study of at least 4 vascular poles of glomeruli per kidney showed that the media cells of the vasa afferentia,

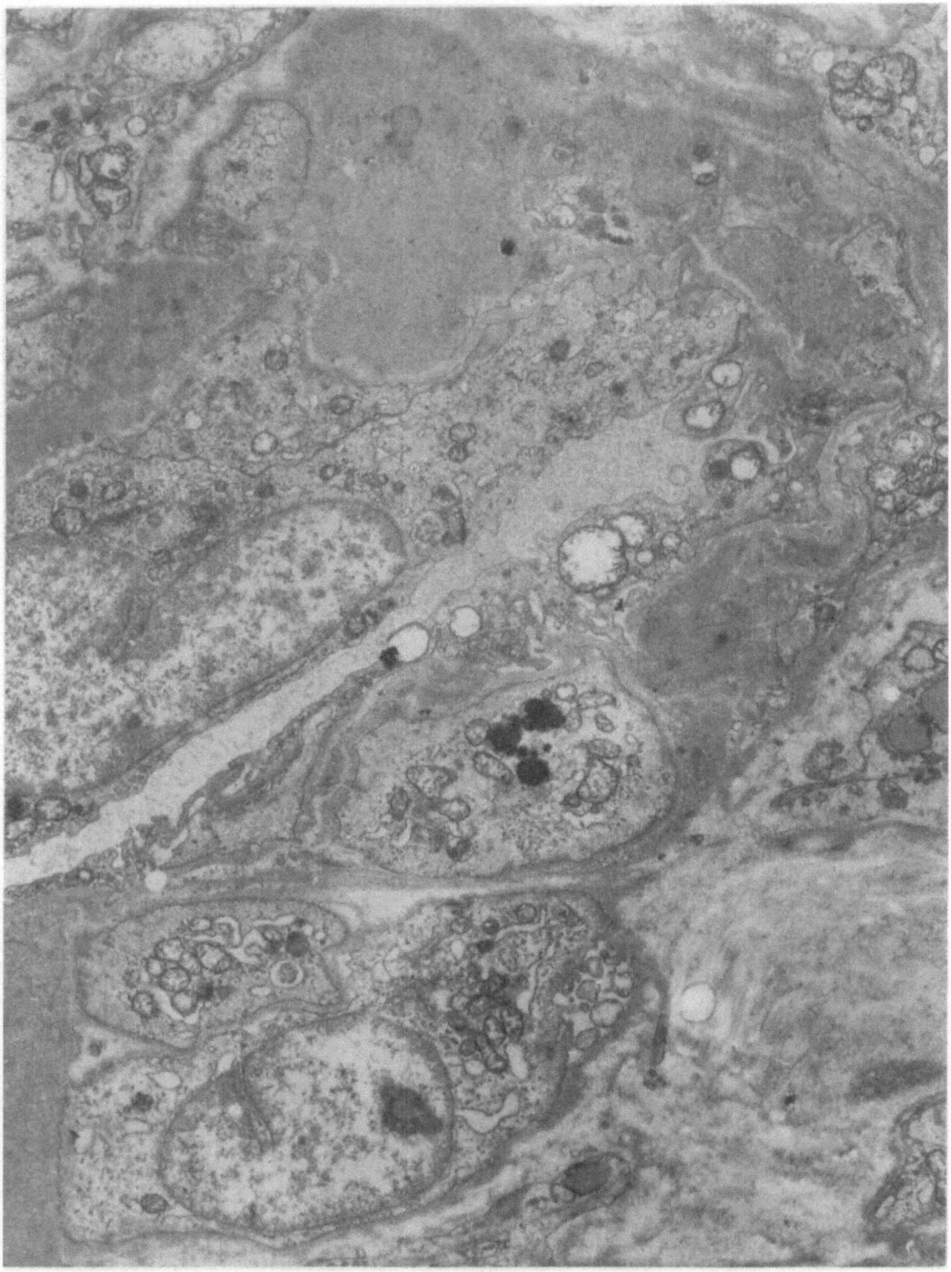

Fig. 2. (Case No 3, male, 42 years.) In the middle of the picture a vas afferens containing a smooth muscle cell and a transitional cell between smooth muscle and epitheloid cell, containing a well-developed endoplasmatic reticulum and Golgi apparatus and a decreased number of smooth muscle fiber filaments. The cytoplasm of this cell contains a few small pale granules (presumably true secretory granules), which differ clearly from the lipofuscin-like granules in the cytoplasm of the smooth muscle cell in the middle of the picture. The media of the arteriole contains fine granular material due to focal arteriosclerosis. Enlargement at electron microscopy: 3,200 times. Final enlargement: 8,000 times

even when cut quite close to the vascular poles, were typical smooth muscle cells (Fig. 1), with muscle fiber filaments, a sparse endoplasmatic reticulum, few mitochondria and plasma vacuoles of varying sizes. These smooth muscle cells were embedded in structures resembling basal membranes and were separated from the endothelial cells by such structures. The cytoplasm of the media cells contained granular fragmented or droplike inclusions which looked like lipofuscin [2, 3, 5].

Only very rarely media cells of afferent arterioles showed the structural characteristics of either epitheloid cells or of stages of transition between smooth muscle and epitheloid cells (Fig. 2). In the latter, the endoplasmic reticulum was more developed, the number of muscle fiber filaments was reduced and there was an accumulation of ribosomes. Even in such cells, so-called secretory granules were extremely rare.

Between MD structures and the juxtaglomerular apparatus the tubular basal membranes looked like a seam of fiber filaments spread between the distal tubules and the juxtaglomerular apparatus (Fig. 3). Similar findings have been reported by other authors [1, 7]. More frequently, we found that the tubular basal membrane between distal tubule and juxtaglomerular apparatus was split into fibers on both sides of the membrane and extended continuously into the thick mesh of basal membrane-like fibers around Goormaghtigh's cells (Fig. 4). Like Thoenes [21] we did not see any capillaries at the point of closest contact between MD and juxtaglomerular apparatus. There were, however, some capillaries quite near to that point (Fig. 3). In the kidneys from patients with Conn's syndrome, as in normal kidneys, the epithelial cells of the MD differed from those of the remaining early distal tubule by their height [6, 21], and by their sparse and low basal membrane folds. Mitochondria were found in the apical part of the cell and at the side and base of the nucleus (Fig. 4). We did not yet quantitate the mitochondria. Like other observers [6, 20] we found that the Golgi apparatus was usually situated either at the same height as the nucleus or nearer to the base of the cell. Goormaghtigh's cells (Fig. 4) were surrounded by basal membrane-like structures [5, 6, 17]. Their nuclei were of variable shape, usually within small rims of cytoplasm containing mitochondria and a Golgi apparatus. The endoplasmatic reticulum of the Goormaghtigh's cells was slightly more developed in the 3rd patient, than in the two others. The cytoplasm of Goormaghtigh's cells contained inclusions which looked like lipofuscin (Figs. 4 and 5). In the Goormaghtighs cells from the 3rd case, there were a few true secretory granules (Fig. 5). The cytoplasm of some Goormaghtigh cells contained isolated small muscle fibre filaments. As described previously [5], in four epitheloid cells we also found synapses of non-myelinated nerves located between some Goormaghtigh's cells (Fig. 6).

Summarizing the results, we may state that there were very few signs of secretory activity in the cells of the juxtaglomerular apparatus of 3 patients with Conn's syndrome: the few secretory signs were seen in only one of the patients (case No 3). If the juxtaglomerular apparatus is considered as the source of renin, these findings are in agreement with the clinical observation of low plasma renin activities. The morphological findings are quite similar to those of Fisher et al. [11] and Biava and West [4] in patients with essential hypertension.

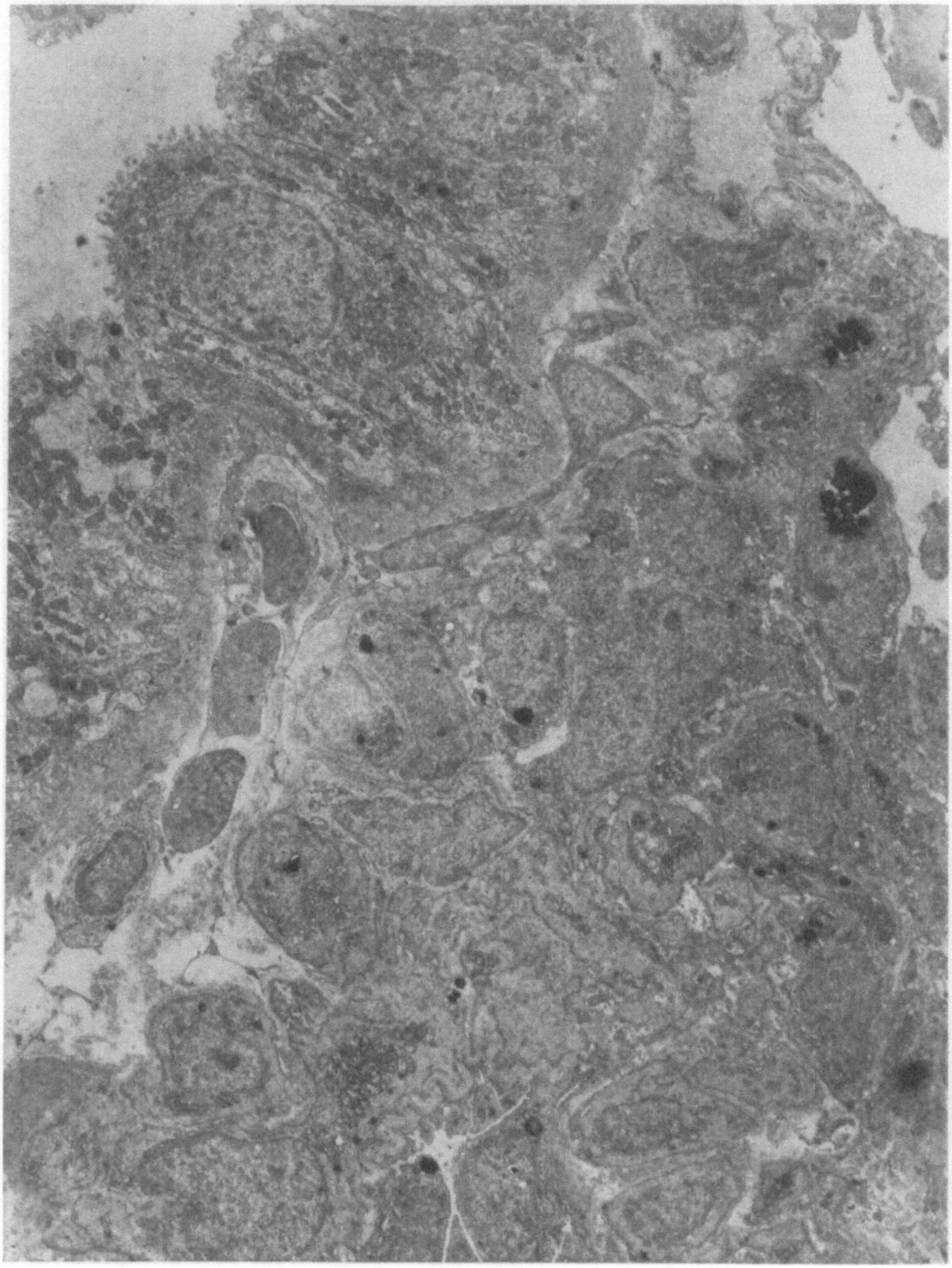

Fig. 3. (Case No 3, male, 42 years.) Juxtaglomerular apparatus and macula densa. The lower margin of the picture shows an open vas afferens with smooth muscle cells in the medial layer. In the middle of the picture Goormaghtigh's cells, some of which contain lipofuscin granules. Continuous tubular basal membrane between macula densa and Goormaghtigh's cells. Capillary vessels on both sides of the touching point of MD and juxtaglomerular apparatus. Enlargement at electron microscopy: 1,200 times. Final enlargement: 3,000 times

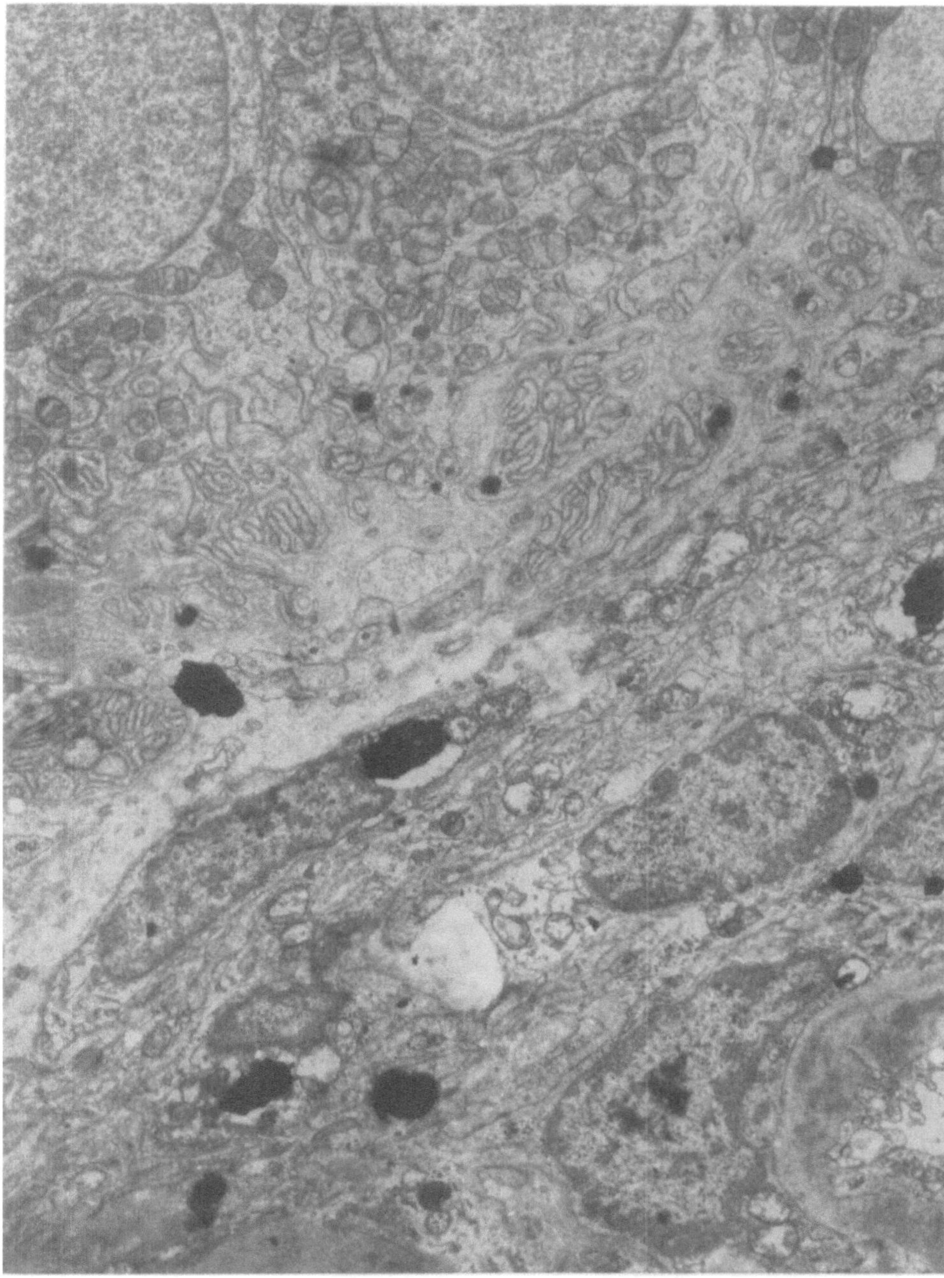

Fig. 4. (Case No 1, male, 38 years old.) Contact zone between macula densa (upper half) and Goormaghtigh's cells, with a clearly split tubular basal membrane extending into the mesh around the Goormaghtigh's cells. Lipofuscin granules in the cytoplasm of Goormaghtigh's cells. In the lower third of the picture one Goormaghtigh cell between the parietal leaves of Bowman's capsule as they reach the glomerular capillaries. The Goormaghtigh cell contains smooth muscle fibers. In the upper third of the picture a macula densa cell with a Golgi-apparatus at the right side of the nucleus. Enlargement at electron miscroscopy: 2,900 times. Final enlargement: 9,860 times

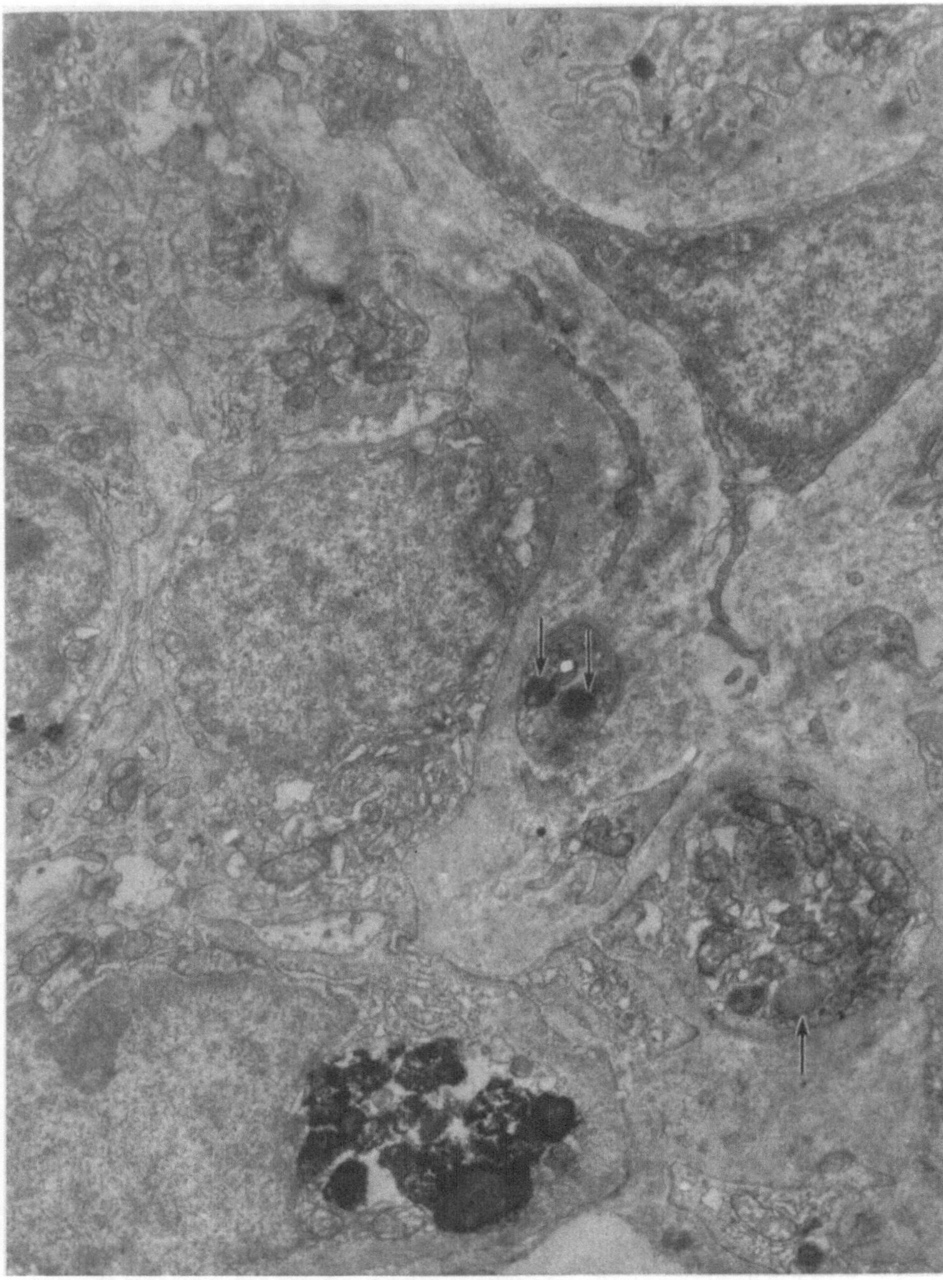

Fig. 5. (Case No 3, male, 42 years.) Goormaghtigh's cells with highly developed endoplasmatic reticulum, Golgi-apparatus and lipofuscin granules (lower margin of the picture) and cytoplasmatic inclusions looking like true secretory granules (arrows). At the upper margin of the picture, the macula densa with its subepithelial basal membrane. Enlargement at electron microscopy: 5,500 times. Final enlargement: 13,750 times

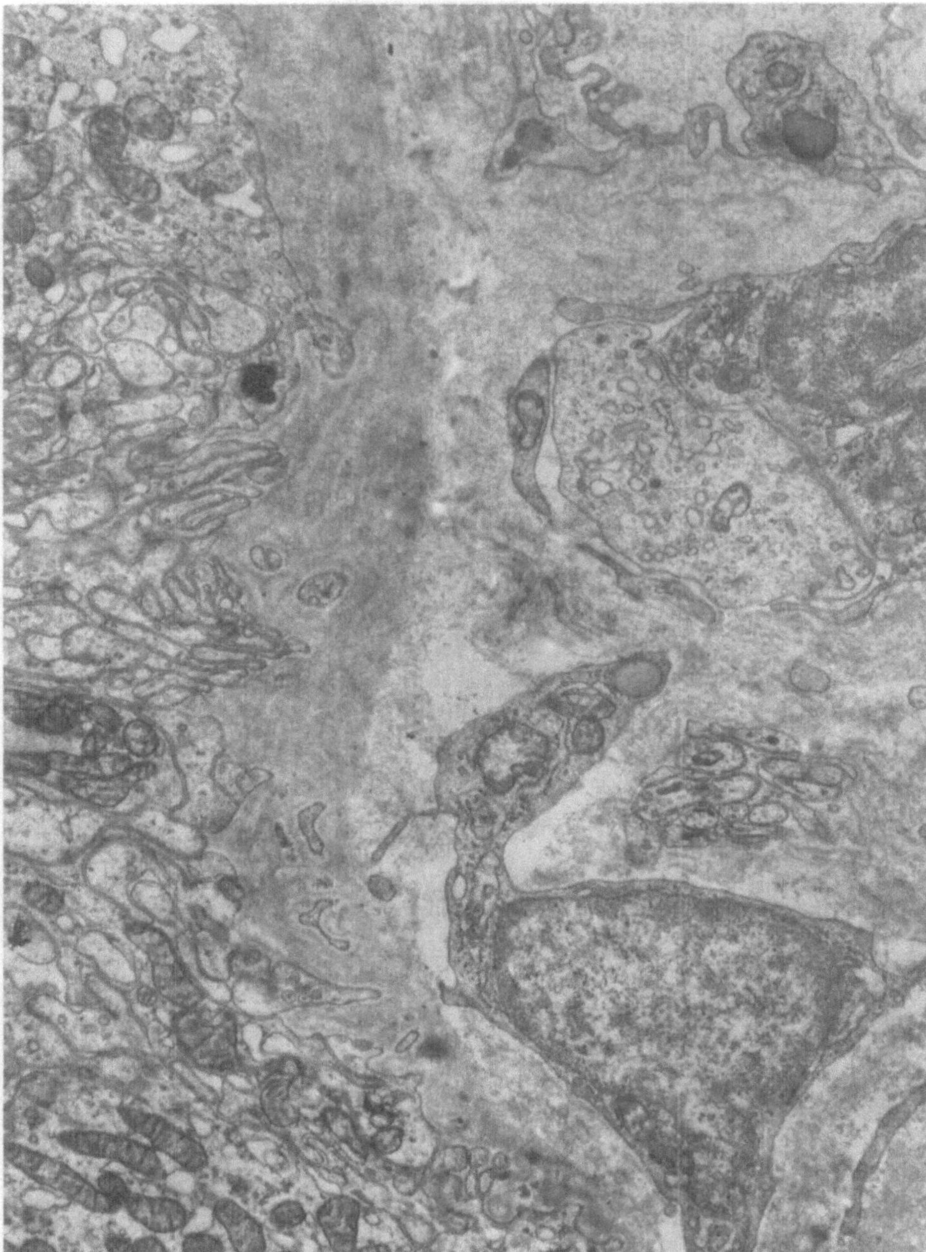

Fig. 6. (Case No 3, male, 42 years.) Basal parts: of macula densa cells with their tubular basal membrane and Goormaghtigh's cells. Between 2 Goormaghthigh's cells a synapsis of a nonmyelinated nerve. Enlargement at electron microscopy: 6,000 times. Final enlargement: 15,000 times

The apparent atrophy of the juxtaglomerular apparatus in the light microscopic picture is explained by the absence of typical epitheloid cells as revealed by electron microscopy. In contrast to a case described by Cohen et al. [8], but supported by inadequate illustrations, the number of juxtaglomerular cells did not appear to be markedly diminished in our cases. The atrophy of the juxtaglomerular apparatus may be the expression of an atrophy by inactivity as a consequence of the increase in blood pressure, since the juxtaglomerular apparatus may contain baroreceptor cells.

It is not clear, in 2 of our cases, how far the increase in the serum sodium concentration or the increased level of circulating aldosterone [12] may have influenced the functional state of the juxtaglomerular apparatus. It is furthermore not clear, why MD structures were seen more rarely in our patients with Conn's syndrome than in normal subjects, though this finding was expected after the reports of other investigators [1, 9, 10, 13, 14, 18].

Summary

Light and electron microscopic investigations of the juxtaglomerular apparatus and the macula densa in biopsy material from 3 patients with Conn's syndrome demonstrate an atrophy of the juxtaglomerular apparatus possibly due to "inactivity". Furthermore, typical macula densa structures were observed more rarely in distal tubules of these patients than in those of normal subjects.

References

1. BARAJAS, L., and H. LATTA: The juxtaglomerular apparatus in adrenalectomized rats. Light and electron-microscopic observations. Lab. Invest. **12**, 1046—1059 (1963).
2. BIAVA, C., and M. WEST: Lipofuscin-like granules in vascular smooth muscle and juxtaglomerular cells of human kidneys. Amer. J. Path. **47**, 287—313 (1965).
3. — — Fine structure of normal human juxtaglomerular cells. II. Specific and nonspecific cytoplasmic granules. Amer. J. Path. **49**, 955—979 (1966a).
4. — — Fine morphology of human juxtaglomerular cells in patients with benign essential hypertension. Lab. Invest. **15**, 1902—1920 (1966b).
5. BOHLE, A., H. SITTE u. S. HELBER: Der juxtaglomeruläre Apparat der Niere. In: Aktuelle Probleme der Nephrologie. IV. Symposion der Ges. f. Nephrologie, S. 3—17 u. 765—775. Berlin-Heidelberg-New York: Springer 1966.
6. BUCHER, O., u. B. RIEDEL: Der juxtaglomeruläre Apparat der Niere. Hippokrates (Stuttg.) **36**, 857 (1965).
7. —, et E. ZIMMERMANN: A propos de la macula densa du rein. Acta anat. (Basel) **42**, 352—371 (1960).
8. COHEN, R. J., R. C. SEVERANCE, E. G. WHITING, and G. D. LUNDBERG: A study of the juxtaglomerular body in primary aldosteronism. Ann. intern. Med. **62**, 569—575 (1965).
9. FISHER, E. R.: Correlation of juxtaglomerular granulation, pressor activity, and enzymes of macula densa in experimental hypertension. Lab. Invest. **10**, 707—718 (1961).
10. —, and H. Z. KLEIN: Effect of sodium on reactivity of renal juxtaglomerular cells and adrenal zona glomerulosa. Proc. Soc. exp. Biol. (N.Y.) **121**, 142—146 (1966).
11. — E. PEREZ-STALDE, and V. PARDO: Ultrastructural studies in hypertension. I. Comparison of renal vascular and juxtaglomerular cell alterations in essential and renal hypertension in man. Lab. Invest. **15**, 1409—1433 (1966).
12. —, and M. TAMURA: Effect of aldosterone on juxtaglomerular index and zona glomerulosa of normotensive and hypertensive rats. Proc. Soc. exp. Biol. (N.Y.) **118**, 402—405 (1965).
13. HESS, R., and F. GROSS: Glucose-6-phosphate dehydrogenase and renin in kidneys of hypertensive or adrenalectomized rats. Amer. J. Physiol. **197**, 869—872 (1959).
14. —, and A. G. E. PEARSE: Mitochondrial alpha-glycerophosphate dehydrogenase activity of juxtaglomerular cells in experimental hypertension and adrenal insufficiency. Proc. Soc. exp. Biol. (N.Y.) **106**, 872—895 (1961).

15. MEYER, D., and P. J. MITTMEYER: Relationship between serum-sodium concentration, hematocrit and juxtaglomerular granulation index of the mouse kidney. In: Progress of nephrology, p. 322—326, Berlin-Heidelberg-New York: Springer 1969.
16. OTTO, H., u. M. GEMÄHLICH: Studien über die Macula densa. Frankfurt. Z. Path. **67**, 232—246 (1956).
17. OBERLING, C., et P. Y. HATT: Étude de l'appareil juxtaglomérulaire du rat au microscope électronique. Ann. Anat. path. **5**, 441—474 (1960).
18. REEVES, G., L. M. LOWENSTEIN, and SH. C. SOMMERS: The macula densa and juxtaglomerular body in cirrhosis. Arch. intern. Med. **112**, 708—715 (1963).
19. —, and SH. C. SOMMERS: Sensitivity of the renal macula densa to urinary sodium. Proc. Soc. exp. Biol. (N.Y.) **120**, 324—326 (1965).
20. RIEDEL, B., u. O. BUCHER: Die Ultrastruktur des juxtaglomerulären Apparates des Meerschweinchens. Z. Zellforsch. **79**, 244—258 (1967).
21. THOENES, W.: Zur Feinstruktur der Macula densa im Nephron der Maus. Z. Zellforsch. **55**, 486—499 (1961).

4.2. Light and Electron Microscopic Investigations of the Juxtaglomerular Apparatus in a Patient with a "Pseudo-Bartter"-Syndrome*

J. SCHÜRHOLZ, H. J. SCHMID, D. MEYER and A. BOHLE [1]

With 5 Figures

A few years ago, BARTTER and his collaborators [4, 7] observed 3 patients with a disease entity apparently due to secondary hyperaldosteronism as a consequence of increased plasma renin activity. The typical signs of the disease were normal or lowered blood pressure, hypokalemic alkalosis and partial vascular refractoriness against angiotensin II. Renal tissue obtained by percutaneous biopsy or by operative excisions showed hyperplasia of the juxtaglomerular apparatus, and sometimes also hyperplasia of the macula densa.

In the German literature, several reports of a similar disease entity have been published [1, 9, 11]. While HÄNZE et al. demonstrated hyperplasia of the juxtaglomerular apparatus in 4 glomerular vascular poles [9], no hyperplasia of the juxtaglomerular apparatus was found by ALEXANDER and PRAETORIUS [1]. We could not demonstrate any juxtaglomerular hyperplasia in biopsy material from a patient of A. F. MULLER in Geneva, who had kaliopenic nephropathy, and several other features of the Bartter-syndrome [11].

We now investigated renal tissue of a 34 year old female patient who had been observed at the Kantonsspital of Lucerne, Switzerland, and had been considered as a case of the Bartter-syndrome.

The patient was well until the age of 23 years, when she first complained of attacks of tiredness and general weakness accompanied by headache as well as by polyuria and polydipsia (1956).

One year later she had paresthesia in both hands, tetanic contractions and transient hirsutism. In 1959, she was found to have hypernatremia, hypochloremia and hypokalemia with an increased potassium excretion in the urine. She, furthermore, had renal glycosuria. Renal concentrating ability was normal, the clearance of PAH (325 ml/min) slightly decreased and the plasma creatinine concentration in the normal range. In 1965 the sodium excretion in urine also increased above normal while the serum sodium values were normal or low. The urinary excretion of aldosterone was increased to 75 μg/day, while the urinary excretion of 17-hydroxyketosteroids was normal. The vascular response to angiotensin was depressed, huge doses of Hypertensin (1,000 ng/kg/min) were needed to elevate the blood pressure. In 1966, MULLER and VEYRAT found the plasma renin activity and the secretion of aldosterone increased at a normal salt intake.

* Supported by Deutsche Forschungsgemeinschaft.

[1] Pathologisches Institut der Universität, Tübingen, West Germany, and Medizinische Klinik des Kantonsspitals, Lucerne, Switzerland.

In the following 2 years, the patient suffered continuously from tetany. It became increasingly difficult to maintain normal plasma potassium concentrations. She was, therefore, submitted to subtotal adrenalectomy on February 2, 1967. At this occasion, wedge excisions were done on both kidneys.

Light microscopic investigation of the renal tissue showed pronounced interstitial fibrosis, mainly in the capsular and middle cortical zone without inflammatory changes, but accompanied by partial atrophy of the tubules. The glomeruli appeared normal with a slight homogenous enlargement of the mesangium. The renal vessels appeared normal. The juxtaglomerular apparatus was very well developed. Counts of all cells in the juxtaglomerular apparatus in 300 randomly sectioned glomeruli yielded a number of 2,072 cells. In normal renal tissue, analogous counts yielded figures from 891 to 1,772 cells. In about 21% of these glomeruli a typical MD structure was found (in normal cases: in 10 to 18%. mean: 14%).

At electron microscopy the media cells of the vasa afferentia in the vicinity of the glomeruli differed markedly from each other (Fig. 1). A number of these cells could not be distinguished from smooth muscle cells, while in others the endoplasmic reticulum was more developed than in smooth muscle cells and the number of myofibrils was diminished. The cytoplasm of the cells contained varying amounts of lipofuscin granules [5]. Other media cells contained so-called true secretory granules [3] within the cisternae of a highly developed endoplasmic reticulum. At some vascular poles, all afferent media cells belonged to the second cell type (Fig. 2) and contained varying amounts of "true secretory" and lipofuscin granules. Finally, some epitheloid cells contained rhomboid, cristalloid, granules, as first described and called protogranules by Barajas and Latta [3].

The morphologic relation between the juxtaglomerular apparatus and the macula densa, in this case of Bartter's syndrome, was the same as in normal kidneys. In the contact zone, the tubular basal membrane could clearly be recognized and was split at its outer border into a mesh of basal membrane-like strings which enveloped the Goormaghtigh cells (Fig. 3). The Goormaghtigh cells showed a very well developed rough endoplasmic reticulum when compared to similar cells as seen in cases of Conn's syndrome [6]. The cytoplasm of these cells also contained lipofuscin granules as well as granular inclusions corresponding to "true secretory granules" or, at least, resembling them. The cytoplasm of the epithelial cells of the macula densa near the vascular poles showed a dense cytoplasm with a Golgi-apparatus situated at the side of the nucleus or between the base of the cell and the nucleus, and a well developed endoplasmic reticulum. Their cytoplasm sometimes contained round to oval homogenous inclusions. At the basal side of the cells the invaginations of the cytoplasm were as sparse as in normal kidneys.

Discussion

Most of the cases of Bartter's syndrome reported until now were observed in children who were dwarfs and had chronic hypokalemia with metabolic alkalosis, normal blood pressure, an increased plasma renin and aldosterone concentration as well as decreased vascular response to angiotensin [4, 7, 8, 18, 19].

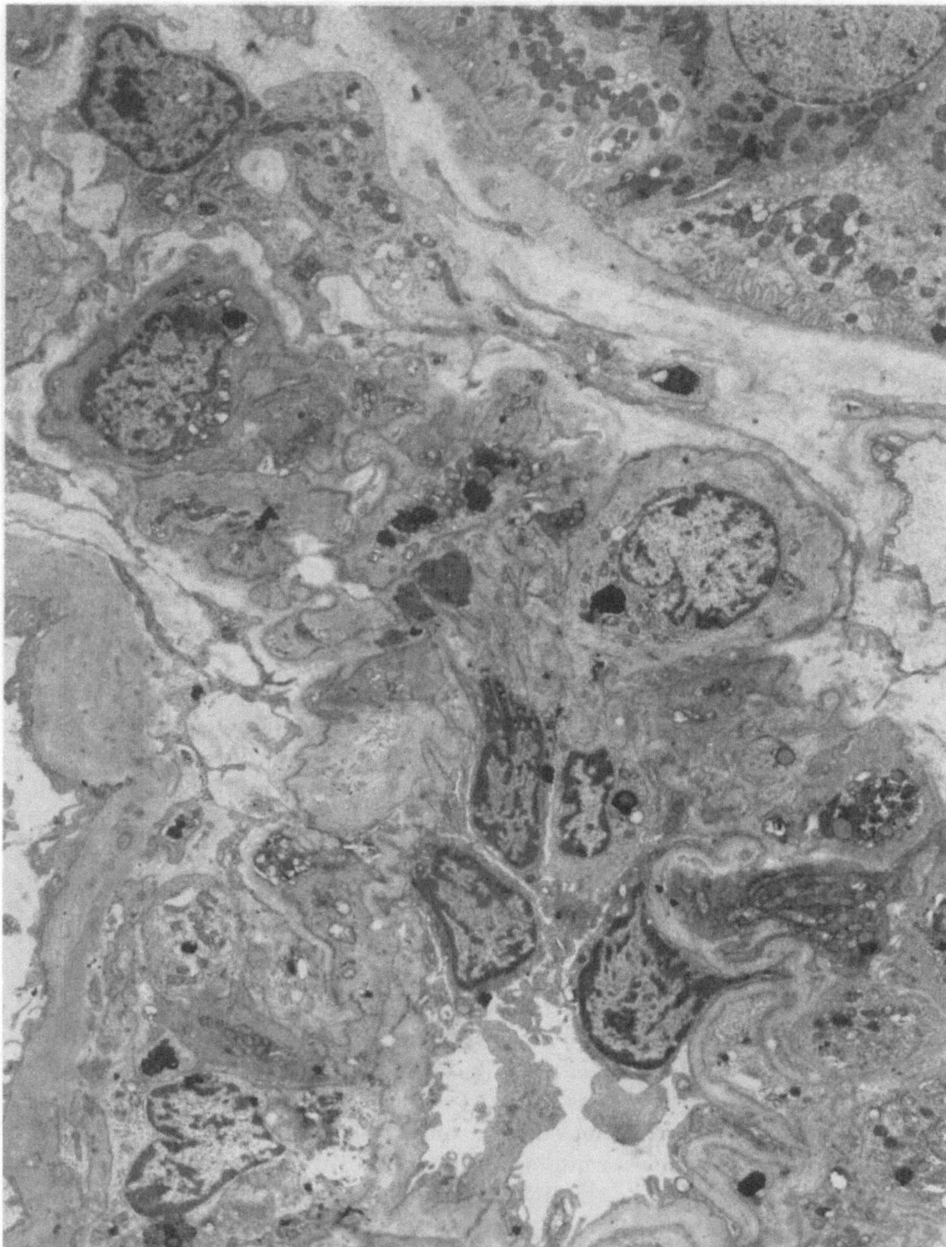

Fig. 1. Section through a vas afferens in a case of "Pseudo-Bartter" syndrome with smooth muscle cells, some of which contain lipofuscin granules. At the right lower border, an epitheloid cell with a well developed endoplasmic reticulum and so-called true secretory granules. Enlargement at electron microscopy: 1,800 times, final enlargement 4,00 times

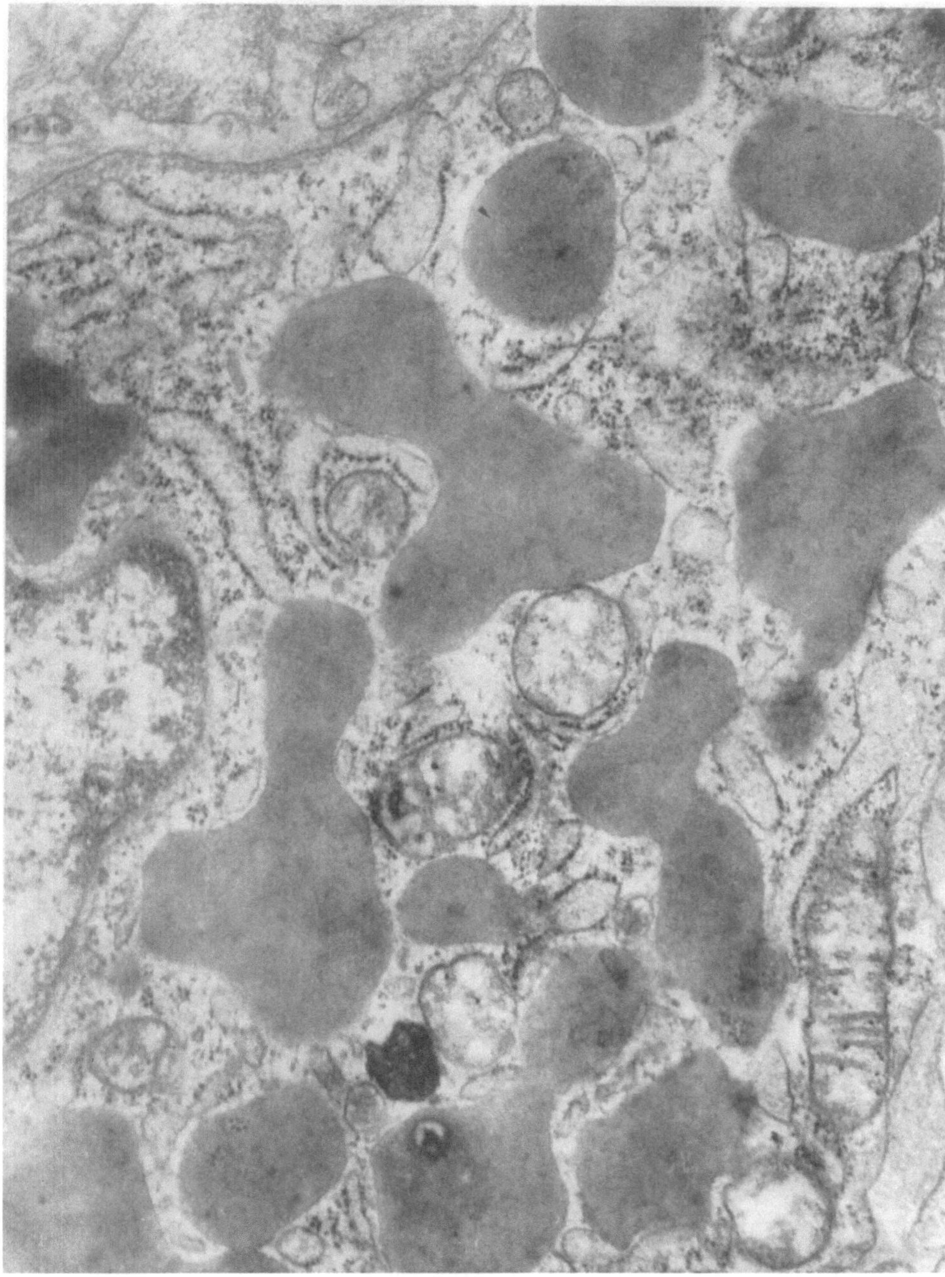

Fig. 2. Section through an epitheloid cell of the vas afferens in a case of "Pseudo-Bartter" syndrome. Highly developed rough endoplasmic reticulum with numerous round or oval polyedric so-called secretory granules in the cytoplasm. Enlargement electron microscopy: 1,500 times. Final enlargement: 37,500 times

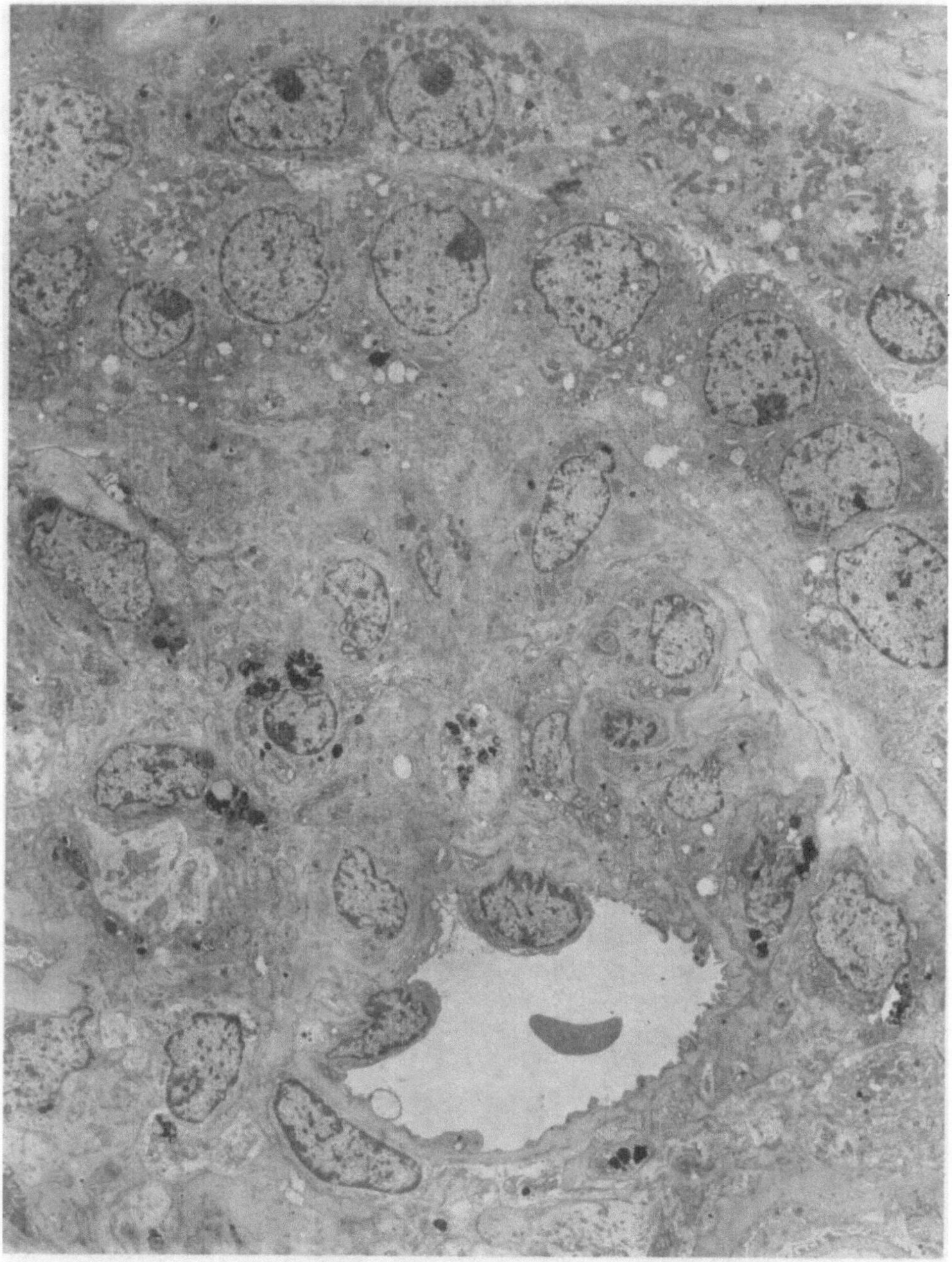

Fig. 3. Juxtaglomerular apparatus with a macula densa in the kidney of a patient with a "Pseudo-Bartter" syndrome. The tubular basal membrane between the macula densa and the Goormaghtigh cells is partially well separated, partially difficult to delimit, because of splitting at the external border and participation in the mesh surrounding Goormaghtigh cells. In the Goormaghtigh cells and in some afferent medial cells there are lipofuscin granules. At the right lower border an epitheloid cell contains so-called secretory granules in its cytoplasm. Enlargement at electron microscopy: 1,000 times. Final enlargement: 2,500 times

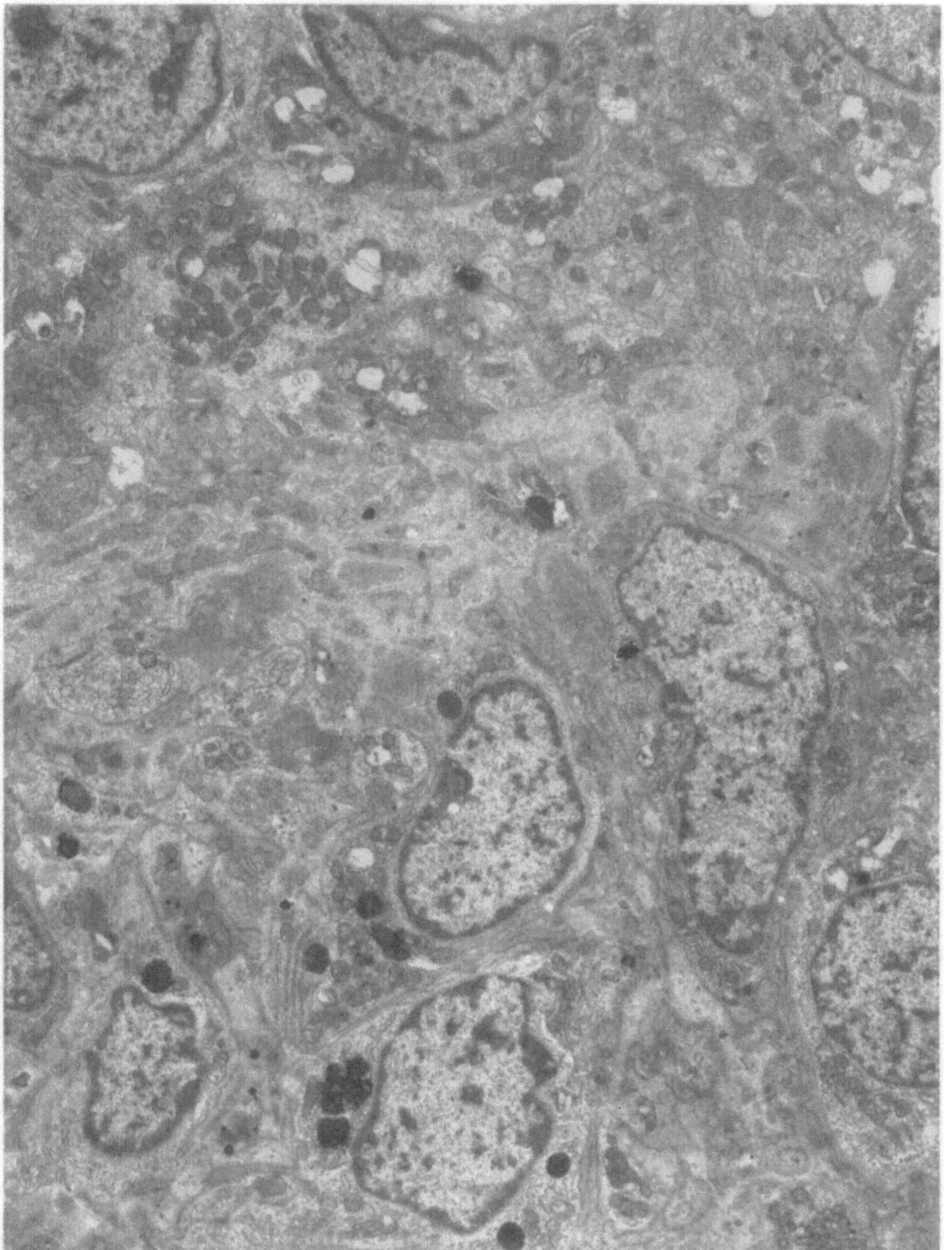

Fig. 4. Zone of contact between the macula densa and Goormaghtigh's cells in a case of "Pseudo-Bartter" syndrome with evident splitting of the tubular membrane. Well-developed rough endoplasmic reticulum in Goormaghtigh's cells which contain lipofuscin granules and some so-called secretory granules. Enlargement at electron microscopy: 2,800 times. Final enlargement: 7,000 times

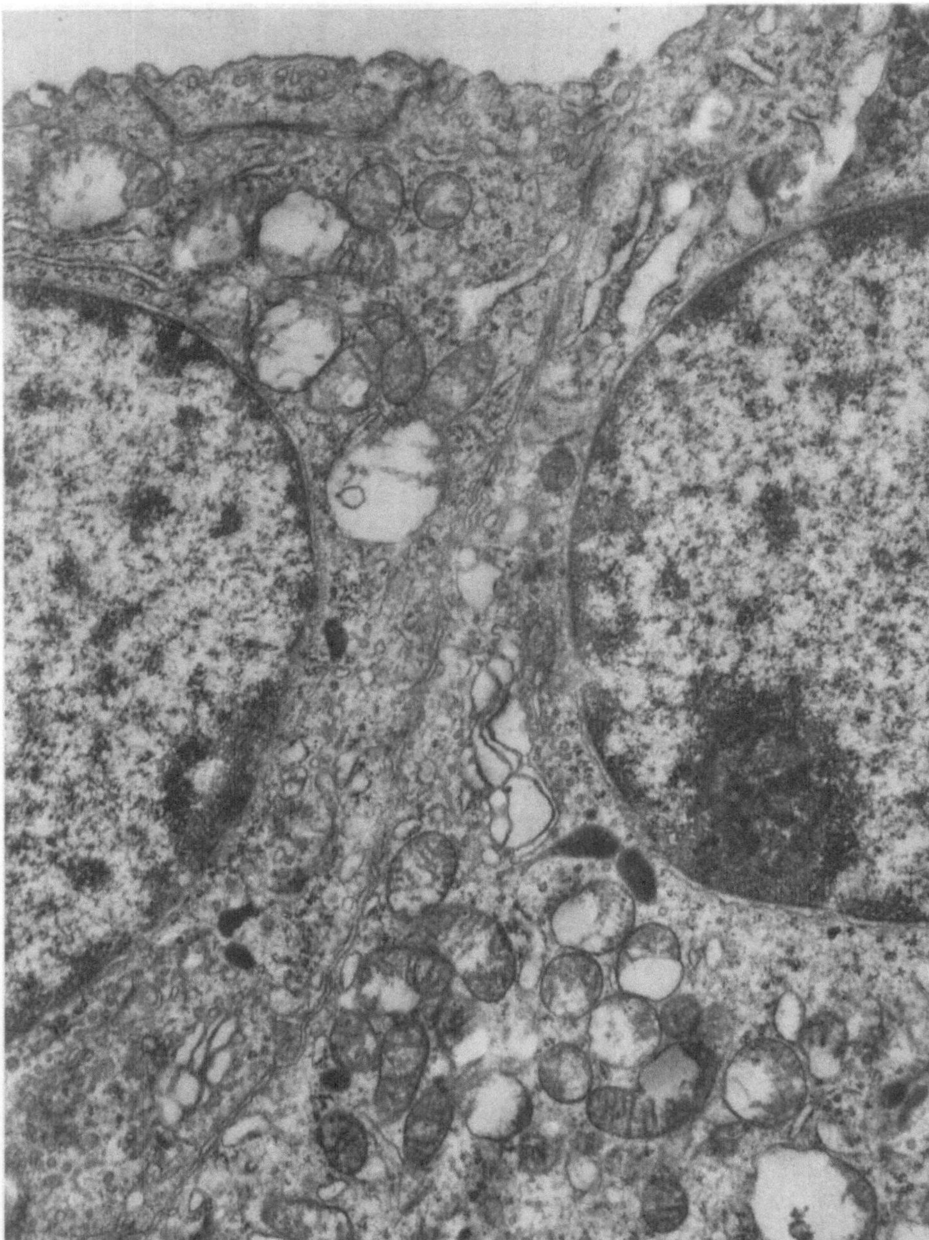

Fig. 5. Section from the macula densa with parts of 2 epithelial cells. At the side of the nucleus or near to the base of the nucleus a Golgi apparatus. The cytoplasm of the epithelial cells contains some dense inclusions, numerous small vacuoles and a well developed rough endoplasmic reticulum. Enlargement at electron microscopy: 8,000 times. Final enlargement: 20,000 times

The cases reported in the German literature refer to quite a different group of patients. The patients observed by MULLER et al. [11] as well as by ALEXANDER and PRAETORIUS [1] occurred in adult nurses. The case described by HÄNZE et al. [9] concerned a 41 year old woman. In all these cases there were clinical signs of hypokalemia, hypokalemic alkalosis, secondary hyperaldosteronism with increased plasma renin activity at normal or low blood pressure and a partial vascular resistance against the blood pressure increasing effect of angiotensin II.

While BARTTER et al. [4] considered the vascular resistance against the constrictor effect of angiotensin as an important and characteristic feature of the syndrome, HÄNZE et al. [9] as well as VISSER et al. [19] point out that a similar decrease in vascular response of arteries and arterioles to angiotensin is also found in liver failure due to cirrhosis of the liver with ascites, or in patients with Addison's disease. Investigations by LARAGH et al. [10] and by AMES et al. [2] showed that a decrease of the serum-sodium concentration is generally associated with a depressed vascular response to angiotensin. This particular sign may, therefore, be secondary in cases of Bartter's syndrome.

It has been suggested by others [19] that the syndrome could be due to a hereditary deficiency of the proximal nephron which would interfere with the conservation of sodium and would, thus, depress the vascular response to angiotensin. The consequent fall in blood pressure, according to this idea, would induce a compensatory hyperplasia of the juxtaglomerular apparatus, which, in turn, would produce increased amounts of renin and of angiotension and a secondary stimulation of the secretion of aldosterone. Secondary hyperaldosteronism would entail accelerated sodium-potassium exchanges in the distal tubules and, thereby, cause potassium losses which finally result in potassium depletion and hypokalemic alkalosis.

A careful distinction should be made between this group of patients in whom a Bartter's syndrome occurs independently of known causal factors, and another group of patients with the so-called "Pseudo-Bartter" syndrome. The latter was first described by WOLFF in 1967 [20] as "psychogenic potassium and sodium losses with secondary hypovolemia and secondary hyperaldosteronism". The disease entity observed by WOLFF occurs exclusively in women, and is characterized by potassium depletion with constipation and weakness, sometimes accompanied by kaliopenic edema, metabolic alkalosis, diminished circulating blood volume, increased plasma renin concentration, increased secretion of aldosterone and depressed responsiveness of the vascular system to angiotensin. According to WOLFF, the causes of the primary potassium losses vary from one subject to the next and may be the following: anorexia, psychogenic vomiting or chronic abuse of laxatives or natriuretic agents. According to WOLFF, the renin-angiotensin-aldosterone system is activated in these patients by primary hypovolemia.

When the present investigations were completed, we were surprised to learn that our patient, who had always denied any use of laxatives during her various stays in hospitals, in fact possessed a great number of packages of laxatives found after her death. It, therefore, appears probable that she abused laxatives for a number of years.

The case described should, therefore, probably be considered as an example of the Pseudo-Bartter's syndrome as described by WOLFF. The same conclusion probably applies to the other cases published in the German literature. For the present case, this diagnosis is based on the late manifestation of the clinical symptoms between the 20th and 30th year of life, and the probable abuse of laxatives. The morphological findings, in our case, agree well with the clinically demonstrated increased secretion of renin.

Summary

In a case of "Pseudo-Bartter" syndrome with renal glucosuria, light and electron microscopic investigations showed hyperplasia of the juxtaglomerular apparatus with signs of an increased metabolic activity of epitheloid cells and Goormaghtigh cells, which agreed with the clinical finding of an increased secretion of renin. The differences between such cases and cases of the "true" Bartter's syndrome are discussed.

References

1. ALEXANDER, M., u. F. PRAETORIUS: Zur Abgrenzung des „Bartter-Syndroms". Dtsch. med. Wschr. **92**, 1022 (1967).
2. AMES, R. P., A. J. BORKOWSKI, A. M. SICINSKI, and J. H. LARAGH: J. clin. Invest. **44**, 1171 (1965). Zit. nach VISSER u. Mitarb.
3. BARAJAS, L., and H. LATTA: Structure of the juxtaglomerular apparatus. Circulat. Res. **21**, Suppl. II, 15 (1967).
4. BARTTER, F. C., P. PRONOVE, J. R. GILL, and R. C. MACCARDLE: Hyperplasia of the juxtaglomerular complex with hyperaldosteronism and hypokalemic alkalosis. Amer. J. Med. **33**, 811 (1962).
5. BIAVA, C. G.: Ultrastructural observations on the morphogenesis of nonspecific granules in human juxtaglomerular and renal vascular cells. Circulat. Res. **21**, Suppl. II, 47 (1967).
6. BOHLE, A., A. HELBER, D. MEYER, J. SCHÜRHOLZ u. H. P. WOLFF: (In press, 1968.)
7. BRYAN, G. T., R. C. MACCARDLE, and F. C. BARTTER: Hyperaldosteronism, hyperplasia of the juxtaglomerular complex, normal blood pressure, and dwarfism. Pediatrics **37**, 43 (1966).
8. CAMPBELL, R. A., H. R. BLAIR, H. D. KLEVIT, and S. H. GOODNIGHT: Abstracts Soc. Ped. Res., 35th Ann. Meeting (1965) 111. Zit. nach VISSER u. Mitarb.
9. HÄNZE, S., C. A. PIERACH u. G. STARK: Das Bartter-Syndrom. Dtsch. med. Wschr. **90**, 2041 (1965).
10. — Die endokrin bedingten hypokaliämischen Alkalosen. Dtsch. med. Wschr. **90**, 1033 (1965).
11. LARAGH, J. H., P. J. CANNON, and R. P. AMES: Canad. med. Ass. J. **90**, 248 (1964). Zit. nach VISSER u. Mitarb.
12. MULLER, A. F., E. L. MANNING u. J. HODLER: Hypokaliämie, Aldosteronausscheidung und primärer Hyperaldosteronismus. Schweiz. med. Wschr. **63**, 1265 (1963).
13. REUBI, F., A. CERUTTI, A. BOHLE u. R. VEYRAT: Kaliumverlierende Tubulopathie oder Bartter-Syndrom? Aktuelle Probleme der Nephrologie. IV. Symposium der Ges. f. Nephrologie 1965. Berlin-Heidelberg-New York: Springer 1966.
14. SKINNER, S. L., J. W. MCCUBBIN, and I. H. PAGE: Control of renin secretion. Circulat. Res. **40**, 64 (1964).
15. THURAU, K., J. SCHNERMANN, W. NAGEL, M. HORSTER, and M. WAHL: Composition of tubular fluid in the macula densa segment as a factor regulation the function of the juxtaglomerular apparatus. Circulat. Res. **21**, Suppl. II, 79 (1967).

16. VANDER, A. J., and J. R. LUCIANO: Effects of mercurial diuresis and acute sodium depletion on renin release in dog. Amer. J. Physiol. **212**, 651 (1967a).
17. — — Neutral and humoral control of renin release in salt depletion. Circulat. Res. **21**, Suppl. II, 69 (1967b).
18. VAN OLPHEN, A. H. F., P. J. J. VAN MUNSTER, and J. P. SLOOF: In: Water and electrolyte metabolism II. Proc. 2nd Symp., eds. F. DE GRAEFF and B. LEYNSE, p. 134. Amsterdam: Elsevier Publ. 1963. Zit. nach VISSER u. Mitarb.
19. VISSER, H. K. A., H. J. DEGENHART, E. DESMIT, and W. S. COST: Mineralocorticoid excess in two brothers with dwarfism, hypokalaemic alkalosis and normal blood pressure. Acta endocr. (Kbh.) **55**, 661 (1967).
20. WOLFF, H. P.: Intern. Klausurgespräch am 21./22. 4. 1967 in Titisee/Schwarzw. über „Probleme der renovaskulären Hypertonie“. In: KAUFMANN, KLAUS, NIETH, SCHUBERT u. THIEL, Renovaskuläre Hypertonie. Arzneimittel-Forschg. **17**, 1065 (1967).

4.3. Relationship between Serum-Sodium Concentration, Hematocrit and Juxtaglomerular Granulation Index of the Mouse Kidney*

D. MEYER and P. J. MITTMEYER[1]

With 1 Figure

The question whether the functions of the juxtaglomerular apparatus of the kidney depend on the presence of a baroreceptor, a volume receptor or a chemoreceptor has not been satisfactorily answered by the many investigations published in the course of the last few years [11].

The present experiments were done in order to investigate possible correlations between serum-sodium concentration, plasma volume and the activity of epitheloid cells (E.C.) of the juxtaglomerular apparatus (JGA).

We determined the juxtaglomerular granulation index (JGI) in 61 female albino mice in their normal state, in conditions of abnormal sodium exchanges, or after lowering or increasing the hematocrit value by dietary measures with or without additional intraperitoneal injections of furosemide (Lasix) or cortexone (Percorten).

JGI values were estimated according to HARTROFT and HARTROFT [9] on 5 μ thick paraffin-embedded sections fixed in Schaffer's solution and stained with PAS-Alcian blue [8]. The hematocrit was measured in venous blood, taken simultaneously with the removal of the kidneys. The serum of the same blood sample was used for the flame photometric measurement of the sodium concentration.

Results (Table):

1. The JGI in 11 animals of normal standardized diet and given tap water was 38.76 ± 2.79 (mean $\pm$ SE).

In mice given a 2% NaCl-solution as drinking fluid for 20 days, together with the normal standard diet ($n = 15$), JGI fell to 23.50 ± 5.22.

After 20 days on a sodium poor diet (Altromin) with distilled water as drinking fluid the JGI increased to 53.30 ± 5.35 in 6 animals. The highest JGI of 93.10 ± 11.04 was found in mice given a sodium poor diet and treated during the last 5 days of the diet by daily interperitoneal injections of 1 mg furosemide.

Daily injections of 1 mg cortexone during the last 5 days, either in 6 animals given the sodium poor diet, or in 14 animals given a sodium poor diet and treated with furosemide, resulted in significant depressions of JGI to 48.18 ± 6.50 (sodium poor diet + cortexone), and 64.83 ± 4.73 (sodium poor diet + furosemide + cortexone).

---

* Supported by Deutsche Forschungsgemeinschaft.

[1] Pathologisches Institut der Universität Tübingen, West Germany.

2. In spite of considerable variations of the JGI, there was no statistically significant difference in the serum-sodium concentrations between the different groups of treated and untreated animals. The serum-sodium concentration in the untreated animals was 144.6 ± 0.9 mEq/l.

3. There were, however, considerable differences between the hematocrit values in the different groups of experimental animals. In the normal animals the hematocrit was 41.2 ± 0.7 vol.-%. In the animals overloaded with sodium, the hematocrit was significantly depressed to 39.1 ± 0.7 vol.-%. After 20 days of dietary sodium deprivation it increased significantly to 43.3 ± 1.1 vol.-%. The highest hematocrit values of 47.4 ± 0.7 vol.-% were observed in the sodium depleted, furosemide treated animals. Cortexone tended to depress the hematocrit values towards normal in the sodium depleted and in the sodium depleted furosemide treated animals.

Table. *Juxtaglomerular granulation index, hematocrit and serum-sodium concentration in different groups of mice*

Group	*n*	Juxtaglomerular granulation index (JGI)		Hematocrit (Vol-%)		Na-concentration in serum (mEq/l)	
		$\bar{x}$	*n*	$\bar{x}$	*n*	$\bar{x}$	*n*
I	11	38.76 ± 2.79	11	41.18 ± 0.66	11	144.63 ± 0.85	11
II	6	53.30 ± 5.35	6	43.33 ± 1.07	6	144.83 ± 1.37 [a]	6
III	6	48.18 ± 6.50	6	42.08 ± 0.84 [a]	6	145.66 ± 1.07 [a]	6
IV	9	93.10 ± 11.04	9	47.43 ± 0.67	8	143.37 ± 1.41 [a]	8
V	14	64.83 ± 4.73	14	44.70 ± 1.29	12	144.91 ± 2.45 [a]	12
VI	15	23.50 ± 5.22	15	39.14 ± 0.71	14	146.42 ± 3.80 [a]	14

I: Normal animals (normal standard food pellets and tap water). II: animals given a sodium poor diet (sodium poor diet Altromin), and distilled water as drinking fluid for 20 days. III: Dietary sodium depletion as in II + 1 mg cortexone per day i. p., during the last 5 days. IV: Dietary sodium depletion as in II + 1 mg furosemide (Lasix) per day during the last 5 days. V: Dietary sodium depletion as in II + 1 mg furosemide per day + 1 mg cortexone per day i. p. during the last 5 days. VI: Sodium loading (normal standard food pellets + 2% NaCl solution as drinking fluid), n = Number of animals per group. $\bar{x} = \pm$ SE.

[a] Not significantly different from mean value of normal animals ($p > 0{,}05$).

Our results, therefore, demonstrate a direct relationship between changes associated with the hematocrit value and JGI, but no relationship between serum-sodium concentration and JGI (Fig. 1).

In interpreting these findings, it should be remembered that a decreased ingestion of sodium induces a decrease in the total volume of extracellular fluid without necessarily influencing the serum-sodium concentration. Hypovolemia and a possible decrease in blood pressure may activate the JGA of the kidneys by depressing the tension of the walls of the afferent arterioles [19, 20]. The activation may induce an increase of JGI. An increase of JGI presumably occurs simultaneously with an increased secretion of renin [3, 6, 13] and an increased formation of angiotensin [2, 15]. Angiotensin, in turn, may depress glomerular filtration by a local vascular effect [22, 23] which may diminish renal fluid losses.

Furthermore, increased renin secretion stimulates aldosterone secretion from the adrenal cortex [1, 12] and may, thus, increase the tubular reabsorption of filtered sodium, and contribute to the constancy of the serum-sodium concentration.

The strong natriuretic effect of furosemide in sodium deprived animals, secreting increased amounts of renin, did not depress the serum-sodium concentration, while hematocrit and JGI increased to maximal values. Furosemide which causes an enhanced loss of sodium and water thus causes a still more pronounced hypovolemia, and therefore, presumably also a more pronounced

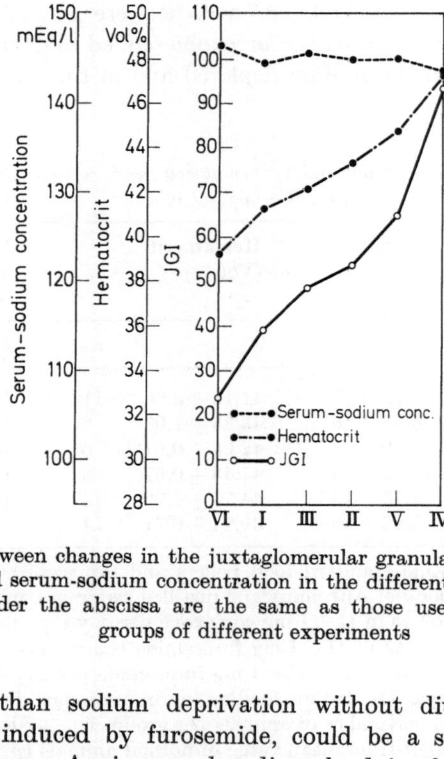

Fig. 1. Correlation between changes in the juxtaglomerular granulation index and hematocrit value with unchanged serum-sodium concentration in the different groups of animals shown on Table. Figures under the abscissa are the same as those used on Table indicating the groups of different experiments

counterregulation than sodium deprivation without diuretic treatment. The counterregulation, induced by furosemide, could be a still larger secretion of renin and aldosterone. An increased sodium load in the early distal tubules, as postulated by the Thurau hypothesis of a feedback role of the macula densa [16—18], may contribute to the more efficient counterregulation. The mineralocorticosteroid cortexone, which shares the effects of endogenous aldosterone, lowers the hematocrit value in sodium depleted and furosemide treated animals as a consequence of a repletion of the extracellular volume. At an unchanged serum-sodium concentration this results in a decrease of the JGI and presumably in a decrease in the secretion of renin. A similar correlation between degranulation and lowering of the hematocrit values was found in animals given 2% NaCl solution as drinking fluid with a normal diet.

If our interpretation is correct, the JGA contains a sensor element responding to volume or pressure changes [7, 14] rather than to changes in the serum sodium concentration [5, 9]. The function of this sensor system does not appear to need a stimulation of the macula densa by increasing sodium concentrations in tubular fluid, as seen from the observations on animals given a sodium poor diet, but not treated with diuretics. A similar conclusion was reached by TRIBE and HEPTINSTALL [21] who obtained changes in the JGA as a consequence of changes in blood pressure in rats in whom Henle's loops had been cut.

This conclusion does not mean that the JGA could not also be stimulated by increases of the early distal sodium concentration to values comparable to those found in plasma, as demonstrated by THURAU and SCHNERMANN [17]. This mechanism could contribute to the changes which we observe in the sodium depleted, furosemide treated animals, if furosemide is assumed to increase the early distal sodium concentration to values capable of influencing the JGA. If the renal arteriolar walls are considered as pressure or volume receptors, which trigger an increased secretion of renin as a response to diminished tension of the wall, as suggested by a series of clinical and experimental observations [4, 7, 14, 20, 22, 23], a stimulation of the JGA via the macula densa is not needed in order to explain our findings.

Summary

JGI, hematocrit and serum-sodium concentrations were investigated in normal mice as well as in animals given a sodium rich drinking fluid, and in animals given a sodium poor diet. Additional groups were given a sodium poor diet and furosemide, or a sodium poor diet and cortexone, or a sodium poor diet plus furosemide plus cortexone. The following results were obtained:

1. Sodium depletion causes a significant increase in JGI and hematocrit values. Additional i.p. treatment with furosemide causes a maximal increase of both parameters. Cortexone tends to depress JGI and hematocrit.

2. Additional sodium, given as 2% NaCl solution as drinking fluid, causes a decrease of JGI and the hematocrit values.

3. The variations in sodium intake and treatment with sodium retaining or natriuretic drugs did not cause any changes of the serum-sodium concentration.

The relationships between the functions of the JGA and the renin-angiotensin-aldosterone system are discussed.

References

1. BIRON, P., E. KOIW, W. NOWACZYNSKI, J. BROUILLET, and J. GENEST: The effects of intravenous infusion of valin-5-angiotensin II and other pressor agents on urinary electrolytes and corticosteroids including aldosterone. J. clin. Invest. **40**, 338 (1961).
2. BRAUN-MENENDEZ, E., J. C. FASCIOLO, L. F. LELOIR, and J. M. MUNOZ: Substances causing renal hypertension. J. Physiol. (Lond.) **98**, 283 (1940).
3. CHANDRA, S., J. CASTLEMAN HUBBARD, F. R. SKELTON, L. L. BERNARDIS, and S. KAMURA: Genesis of juxtaglomerular cell granules. A physiologic, light and electron microscopic study concerning experimental hypertension. Lab. Invest. **14**, 1834—1847 (1965).
4. COHEN, R. J., R. C. SEVERANCE, E. G. WHITING, and G. D. LUNDBERG: A study of the juxtaglomerular body in primary aldosteronism. Amer. J. Med. **62**, 569—575 (1965).
5. FISHER, E. R., and H. Z. KLEIN: Effect of sodium state on reactivity of renal juxtaglomerular cells and adrenal zona glomerulosa. Proc. Soc. exp. Biol. (N.Y.) **121**, 142—146 (1966).
6. — M. TAMURA, and G. M. C. MASSON: Renal renin in unilaterally nephrectomized hypertensive rats. Proc. Soc. exp. Biol. (N.Y.) **118**, 1191—1193 (1965).
7. GROSS, F., H. BRUNNER, and M. ZIEGLER: Renin-angiotensin system, aldosterone and sodium balance. Recent Progr. Hormone Res. **21**, 119—177 (1965).

8. HARADA, K.: Fixative-stain sequences for selective demonstration of juxtaglomerular cells. Stain Technol. **41**, 83—89 (1966).

9. HARTROFT, P. M., and W. S. HARTROFT: Studies on juxtaglomerular cells. I. Variations produced by sodium chloride and desoxy-corticosterone-acetate. J. exp. Med. **97**, 415—417 (1953).

10. — — Studies on renal juxtaglomerular cells. II. Correlation of degree of granulation of juxtaglomerular cells with the width of the zona glomerulosa of the adrenal cortex. J. exp. Med. **102**, 205—212 (1955).

11. HATT, P. Y.: L'appareil juxtaglomérulaire. Presse méd. **74**, 2269—2271 (1966).

12. LARAGH, J. H., M. ANGERS, W. G. KELLY, and S. LIEBERMAN: Hypotensive agents and pressor substances. The effect of epinephrine, nor-epinephrine, angiotensin II, and others on the secretory rate of aldosterone in man. J. Amer. med. Ass. **174**, 234—240 (1960).

13. MASSON, G. M. C., S. YAGI, CH. KASHII, and E. R. FISHER: Further observations on juxtaglomerular cells and renal pressor activity in experimental hypertension. Lab. Invest. **13**, 321—330 (1964).

14. MEYER, P., J. MENARD, J. M. ALEXANDRE, and B. WEIL: Correlation between plasma renin, hematocrit and natriuresis. Rev. canad. Biol. **25**, 111—114 (1966).

15. PAGE, I. H., and O. M. HELMER: Crystalline pressor substance (angiotensin) resulting from reaction between renin and renin activator. J. exp. Med. **71**, 29 (1940).

16. SCHNERMANN, J., W. NAGEL u. K. THURAU: Die frühdistale Natriumkonzentration in Rattennieren nach renaler Ischämie und hämorrhagischer Hypotension. Pflügers Arch. ges. Physiol. **287**, 296—310 (1966).

17. THURAU, K., u. J. SCHNERMANN: Die Natriumkonzentration an den Macula densa-Zellen als regulierender Faktor für das Glomerulumfiltrat. Klin. Wschr. **43**, 410—413 (1965).

18. — — W. NAGEL, M. HORSTER, and M. WAHL: Composition of tubular fluid in the macula densa segment as a factor regulating the function of the juxtaglomerular apparatus. Circulat. Res. **21**, Suppl. II, 79—90 (1967).

19. TOBIAN, L.: Interelationship of electrolytes, juxtaglomerular cells and hypertension. Physiol. Rev. **40**, 280—312 (1960).

20. — Renin release and its role in renal function and the control of salt balance and arterial pressure. Fed. Proc. **26**, 48—54 (1967).

21. TRIBE, C. R., and R. H. HEPTINSTALL: The juxtaglomerular apparatus in scarred kidneys. An experimental study into the nature of the stimulus causing hyperplasia of the juxtaglomerular apparatus in rats. Brit. J. exp. Path. **46**, 339—347 (1965).

22. VANDER, A. J., and J. R. LUCIANO: Effects of mercurial diuresis and acute sodium depletion on renin release in dog. Amer. J. Physiol. **212**, 651—656 (1967).

23. — — Neural and humoral control of renin release in salt depletion. Circulat. Res. **21**, Suppl. II, 69—75 (1967).

4.4. Normokalemic Primary Aldosteronism

H. P. Wolff, Ch. Barth, S. Roscher and P. Vecsei [1]
and J. B. Brown, G. Düsterdieck, A. F. Lever and J. I. S. Robertson [2]

With 2 Figures

In primary aldosteronism hypertension may exist many years before hypokalemia develops. In this normokalemic stage, primary aldosteronism is clinically indistinguishable from essential hypertension. Conn [1] has claimed that about 20% of all patients with the clinical diagnosis of "essential hypertension" harbor an aldosterone secreting tumor as its curable cause. To collect information on the relative frequency of normokalemic primary aldosteronism 75 normokalemic patients with arterial hypertension, in which primary renal or renovascular disease, pheochromocytoma, coarction of the aorta and Cushing syndrome had been excluded, were screened by the following procedures:

In a first period total body potassium, using endogenous K^{40}, urinary and erythrocyte Na/K ratio, plasma renin concentration in the recumbent state and the response of plasma renin to upright posture and/or i.v. injection of 20 mg furosemide were measured during intake of the standard diet containing 110 mEq Na and 68 mEq K per day. An i.v. glucose tolerance test and renal biopsy were performed. Thereafter treatment with a natriuretic agent was started and plasma potassium measured at regular intervals. Where suppression of plasma renin and/or latent potassium depletion or hypoplasia and hypogranularity of the juxtaglomerular cells were detected, secretion rates of aldosterone, corticosterone, cortexone and cortisol were measured in a second period. In 5 out of 75 patients normokalemic aldosteronism was discovered by the triad: suppres-

Table. *Laboratory findings in 5 patients with the clinical diagnosis "normokalemic primary aldosteronism" (1—5) and two suspects (6 and 7)*

Patient	Plasma-renin	SR Aldo	SR B	SR DOC	SR F
1. G. E., ♀, 51	n—↓	4—5 +	2 +	2 +	n
2. K. W., ♂, 43	n—↓	5 +	n	n	n
3. A. O., ♂, 46	n—↓	2—3 +	n	n	n
4. E. L., ♂, 49	↓↓	3 +	2 +	n	n
5. K. D., ♂, 46	↓	n—3 +	n	∅	2 +
6. M. Sch., ♀, 56	↓	—	—	—	—
7. R. P., ♀, 43	↓↓	—	—	—	—

[1] 2nd Medical Department of the University of the Saarland, Homburg-Saar, West Germany.

[2] Medical Research Council, Blood Pressure Research Unit, Western Infirmary, Glasgow, Scottland.

sed plasma renin, increased aldosterone secretion and early appearance of hypokalemia during diuretic therapy (Table 1). In 1 out of this 5, the secretion rates of aldosterone, corticosterone and desoxycorticosterone were elevated, suggesting the diagnosis of a mixed mineralocorticoid syndrome rather than that of primary aldosteronism. In two other patients suppressed plasma renin aroused suspicion of normokalemic aldosteronism; the secretion rates have still to be measured. In some patients hypoplasia and hypogranularity of the juxtaglomerular cells

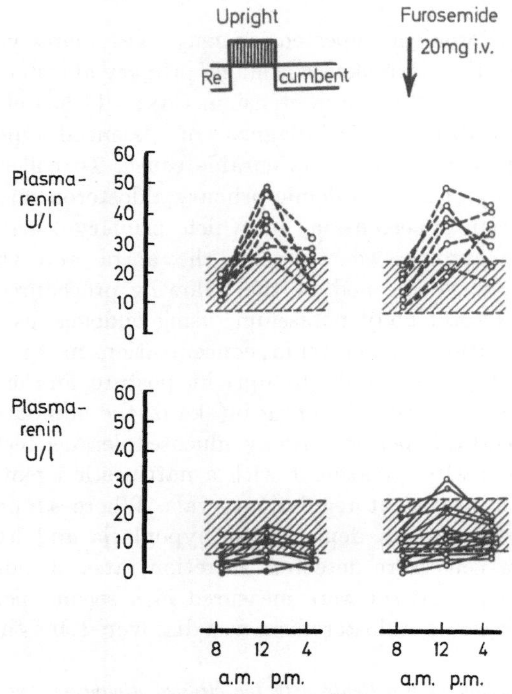

Fig. 1. Plasma renin concentration before and after stimulation by orthostasis or i.v. injection of furosemide. o- - - -o Normal individuals; •——• hypokalemic primary aldosteronism; o——o normokalemic primary aldosteronism in bilateral hyperplasia

could be detected. Occasionally the plasma renin concentration in the recumbent state was within the normal range, but the response to stimulation was almost always suppressed and did not differ significantly from that of 8 patients with hypokalemic primary aldosteronism studied at the same time. In the normokalemic group, serum sodium, chloride, bicarbonate and pH as well as total body potassium and erythrocyte and urinary Na/K ratios were within the normal range; only exchangeable sodium and blood volume were increased in 2 out of the 5.

In the patient with the mixed mineralocorticoid syndrome a small suprarenal tumor was demonstrated on the left side by selective arteriography. Surgical exploration revealed 1 large and 2 small adenomas together with nodular hyperplasia of the remaining cortex. Histologically, the adenomas showed the characteristic nests and columns of lipid-rich clear cells and scattered compact cells with granular cytoplasm; the surrounding tissue exhibited macro- and micronodules of similar structure. Incubation of the adenomatous and of the normal tissue with 4-C^{14}-progesterone revealed a significantly greater production of cortisol, cortison, 6-OH-corticosterone, desoxycorticosterone and aldosterone and a somewhat lower output of corticosterone by the tumor tissue. No detectable amounts of 18-OH-corticosterone and 18-OH-desoxycorticosterone were present.

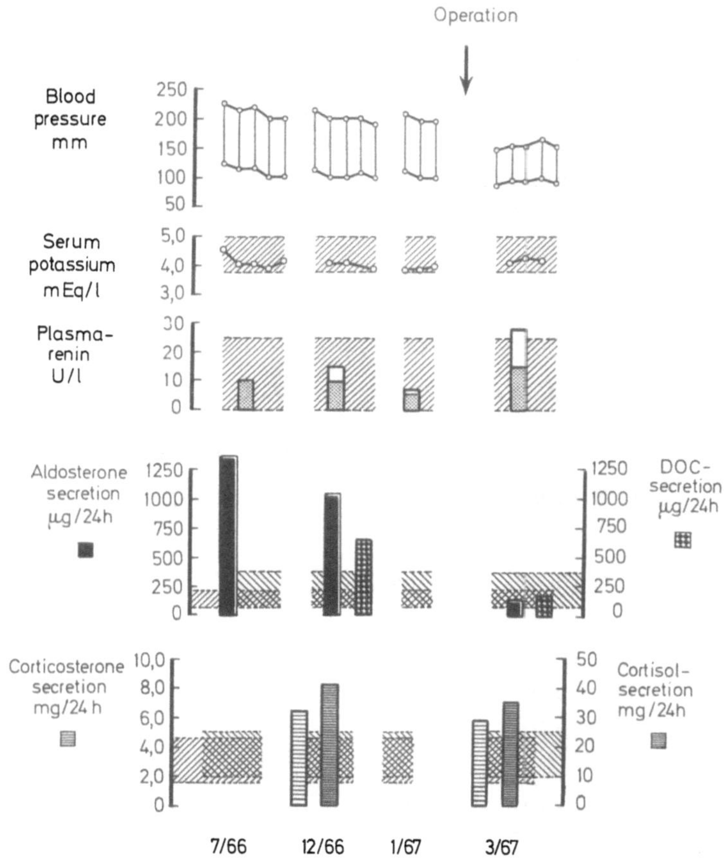

Fig. 2. Bilateral adrenal nodular hyperplasia with normokalemic aldosteronism, suppressed plasma renin and increased secretion of desoxycorticosterone and corticosterone before and after surgery

The strikingly low production of 18-hydroxylated compounds, aldosterone and desoxycorticosterone in vitro stood out in contrast to the marked hypersecretion of the latter two in vivo. After surgery, blood pressure, renin response and steroid secretion, with the exception of cortisol and corticosterone returned to normal. In patient 2 and 3 no radiologic diagnosis of a tumor could be made. Surgical exploration revealed micronodular hyperplasia in patient 2 and 3. After unilateral (case 2) and bilateral subtotal (case 3) adrenalectomy, respectively, blood pressure and aldosterone secretion returned to normal in both patients but later started to rise again. The remaining 4 cases await surgical exploration.

Hypertension with bilateral adenomatosis hyperplasia of the adrenal cortex can imitate the clinical features of classical primary aldosteronism due to a solitary adenoma. The combination of high aldosterone secretion with low plasma renin has been reported in several cases with bilateral adrenal hyperplasia (SUTHERLAND et al. [2], LEDINGHAM et al. [3], NEW and PETERSON [4]). In our own experience the incidence of nodular hyperplasia was surprisingly high. It was found in 5 out of 75 patients with the clinical diagnosis of essential hypertension, whereas no normokalaemic case of the classic Conn-Syndrome due to a solitary adenoma was detected. Clinical, biochemical and morphological differences, which will be discussed elsewhere, indicate that classic primary aldosteronism with solitary adrenal cortical adenoma(ta) and hypertensive disease with adrenal nodular hyperplasia represent syndromes with different etiology and a different meaning of mineralocorticoid excess in the pathogenesis of hypertension.

References

1. CONN, J. W., E. L. COHEN, D. R. ROVNER, and R. M. WESBIT: J. Amer. med. Ass. **193**, 200 (1965).
2. SUTHERLAND, D. J. A., J. L. ROSE, and J. C. LAIDLAW: Canad. med. Ass. J. **95**, 1109 (1966).
3. LEDINGHAM, J. G. G., M. C. BULL, and J. H. LARAGH: Circulat. Res., Suppl. II to Vol. XX and XXI, 177 (1967).
4. NEW, M. I., and R. E. PETERSON: J. clin. Endocr. **27**, 300 (1967).

Discussion

NIETH:

What do you think of Brown's "poor man's" test, i.e. sodium loading with 200 to 300 mEq per day for a few days? Does this test prove useful in clinical work?

RENSCHLER:

Do you have any experience about the significance of red blood cell Na^+/K^+ ratios in other diagnostic problems?

WOLFF:

The "poor men's test" was devised by F. C. BARTTER as a screening procedure for primary aldosteronism in hypokalemic hypertensives at a time when estimations of aldosterone were done by a few groups only and the assessment of plasma renin activity was impossible for technical reasons. It might be useful in the screening of patients with "essential hypertension" for normokalemic primary or acquired (bilateral nodular adrenal cortical hyperplasia with suppressed plasma renin and hypertension) aldosteronism, but, unfortunately, we have no experience in this field.

We could not detect any significant reproducible changes in erythrocyte Na^+/K^+ ratios in hypokalemic primary aldosteronism nor in hypertensives with increased aldosterone activity due to renal artery stenosis or bilateral nodular hyperplasia of the adrenal cortex.

4.5. Evaluation of Renal Hypertension with Special Reference to the Morphology of the Juxtaglomerular Apparatus*

P. Faarup[1], O. Munck[2], J. Ladefoged[2], F. R. Mathiesen[3], F. Pedersen[2] and P. A. Gammelgård[3]

With 4 Figures

Demonstration of an abnormally high production of renin or other pressor substances would a priori seem to be the best basis for describing a kidney as "probably responsible for hypertension." This approach has not been practicable for us until now, and we have, therefore, made a statistical analysis of the predictive value of a number of indirect diagnostic tests in 23 operated cases with hypertension and renovascular disease. The major part of the clinical investigations have recently been published in detail [3].

One of the most significant findings was that the juxtaglomerular apparatus was affected in a characteristic manner in most of those patients who became normotensive or improved after operation. Besides the morphology of the juxtaglomerular apparatus the tests found to be correlated with the operative result were: intravenous pyelography, renography, kidney size and heart size.

The purpose of the present paper is to show the results concerning the morphology of the juxtaglomerular apparatus (JGA), as they suggest that the function of the juxtaglomerular cells play an important part in sustained renovascular hypertension in man.

In 19 of the 23 patients the tissue from the operated kidney was histologically examined. The biopsies were fixed in Helly's fluid for 24—48 hours and tissue sections of a thickness of 4 microns were Bowie-stained.

In the JGA of the nephrons the content of juxtaglomerular granules was estimated using the juxtaglomerular index [5]. Besides, the number of epithelioid cells found in the JGA were counted, since it has previously been claimed — i.e. in this society [2] — that hyperplasia of this type of cell quite often could be found in the stenosed kidney from patients with renovascular hypertension. Fig. 1 shows a JGA containing several epithelioid cells in the afferent arteriole and in the place of the cell group of Goormaghtigh. Fig. 2 shows a JGA without epithelioid cells.

The juxtaglomerular index was correlated to the effect of the operative treatment (Fig. 3). In the majority of the cases the index values obtained were so small in the unchanged group as well as in the improved or normotensive group, that the use of the index as a diagnostic tool seems questionable.

* This work was supported by grants from "King Christian X's Foundation", "P. A. Brandts Legat", and from "Foreningen til Hjertesygdommenes Bekæmpelse".

[1] Institute for Experimental Medicine, University of Copenhagen.

[2] Dept. Clinical Physiology, Glostrup Hospital, Copenhagen.

[3] Dept. Surgery H, Gentofte Hospital, Copenhagen.

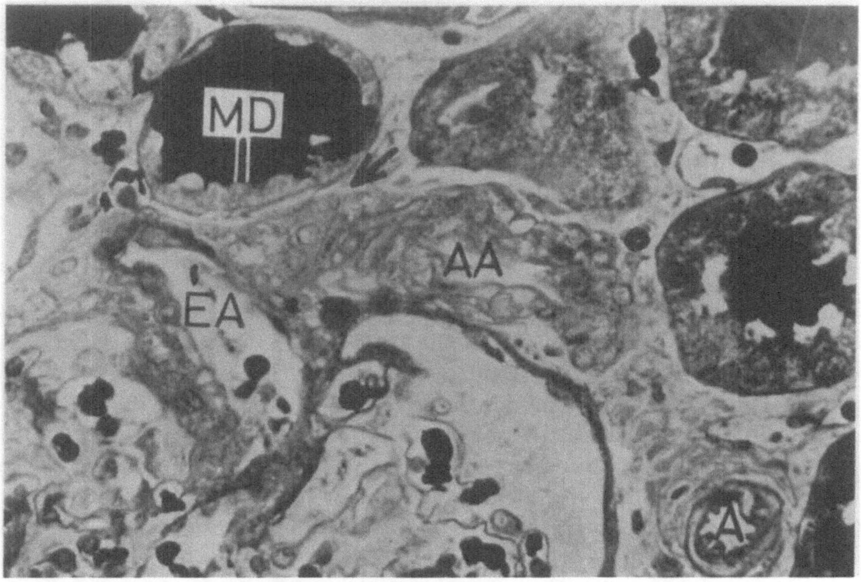

Fig. 1. In the juxtaglomerular apparatus several epithelioid cells can be seen in the wall of the afferent arteriole (*AA*) as well as in the place of the cell group of Goormaghtigh (arrow), beneath the macula densa (*MD*). *EA* Efferent arteriole. No juxtaglomerular granules are present. Smooth muscle cells are found in the wall of a small arteriole (*A*) outside the juxtaglomerular apparatus (Bowie stain, ×640)

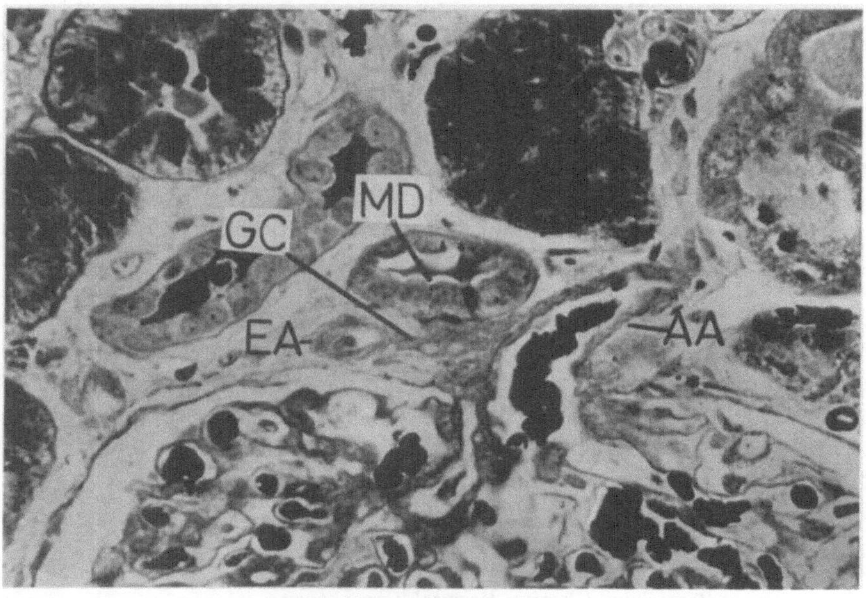

Fig. 2. In this juxtaglomerular apparatus no epithelioid cells or juxtaglomerular granules can be seen. Cells typical for the cell group of Goormaghtigh (*GC*) are present. *AA* Afferent arteriole; *EA* efferent arteriole; *MD* macula densa (Bowie stain, ×640)

The occurrence of epithelioid cells in the JGA was examined in 25 JGA in the total cortical area in each biopsy by counting the number of epithelioid cells with or without juxtaglomerular granules in nephrons in which at least one cross section of the afferent arteriole was seen. As previously stated [3] an epithelioid cell was defined as a cell larger than a smooth muscle cell, having a lighter cytoplasm and containing an enlarged, light nucleus, placed in the arteriolar media

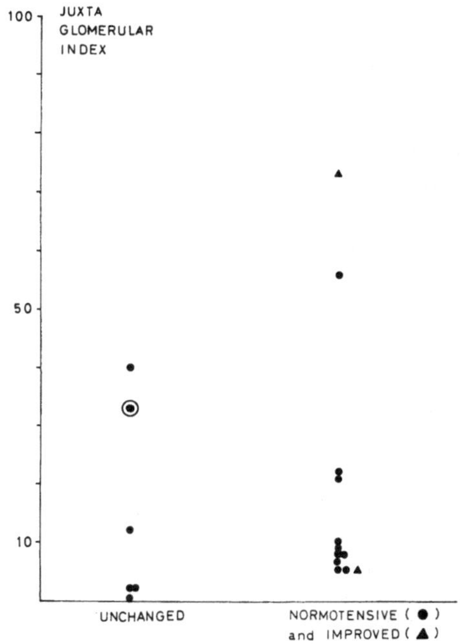

Fig. 3

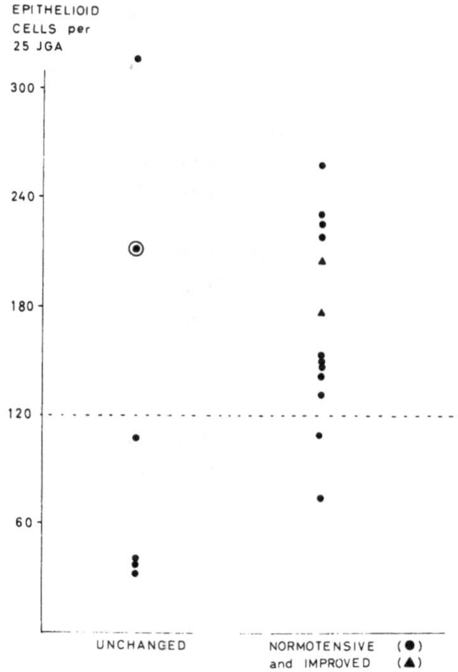

Fig. 4

Fig. 3. The juxtaglomerular index (ordinate) from the stenosed kidney of patients who were unchanged after the operation and who were normotensive or improved after the operation. As can be seen the index was of little help in assessing the outcome of surgery

Fig. 4. The number of epithelioid cells per 25 juxtaglomerular apparatus (ordinate) from the stenosed kidney of patients who were unchanged after the operation and who were normotensive or improved after the operation. This number correlated quite well to the outcome of surgery

or at the site of the cell group of Goormaghtigh. In Fig. 4 the quantitative expression of the hyperplasia thus obtained is given.

In the improved or normotensive group 11 of the 13 results exceeded 120 epithelioid cells per 25 JGA. Of the two cases with less than 120 cells per 25 JGA the one having the highest number would nevertheless have been selected for surgery according to our present approach, whereas the other would not have been operated to-day.

In the unchanged group 4 of the 6 results showed less than 120 epithelioid cell per 25 JGA. One of the 2 remaining cases, where the number of cells exceeded 120 per 25 JGA (encircled point in Figs. 3 and 4), had an infarction in the upper pole of the kidney where the biopsy was taken. In spite of the nephrectomy performed, the blood pressure remained unchanged postoperatively. This may indicate the existence of a non-renal hypertension in this case. In the last case, which had the greatest number of epithelioid cells found in this investigation, a heminephrectomy was made because of stenosis of a main branch of the renal artery. Further investigation or postoperative treatment were not wanted by the patient, and no information concerning the postoperative conditions is available.

It can, therefore, be summarized that in the present study the juxtaglomerular index was found of no value for the assessment of the outcome of the operation. On the other hand, it was found that the hyperplasia of the epithelioid cells in the juxtaglomerular apparatus was fairly well in accordance with the result of the operative treatment. In connection with the other tests, which we have found to be of predictive value, the degree of hyperplasia of the epithelioid cells thus seems to be applicable for deciding whether the renovascular hypertension in question is curable. In needle biopsies the examination of sections from different levels in the tissue block usually permits a quantitative estimation of the epithelioid cells found in the JGA. As indicated by Genest et al. [4] and by Barajas et al. [1] the degree of nephrosclerosis and of tubular atrophy in the stenosed kidney should also be taken into account. The close correlation between the result of the operative treatment and the number of epithelioid cells in the JGA suggests that the function of the JGA plays an important role in renovascular hypertension.

References

1. Barajas, L., A. N. Lupu, J. Kaufman, H. Latta, and M. H. Maxwell: The value of the renal biopsy in unilateral renovascular hypertension. Nephron **4**, 231—247 (1967).
2. Bohle, A., u. H. Sitte: Der juxtaglomeruläre Apparat der Niere. Aktuelle Probleme der Nephrologie, S. 3—17. New York 1966.
3. Gammelgaard, A., J. Ladefoged, P. Faarup, F. R. Mathiesen, F. Pedersen, and O. Munck: Selection of hypertensive patients with renovascular disease for surgical treatment. Proc. 14. Internat. Congr. Urol. München 1967, p. 339—353.
4. Genest, J., G. Y. Tremblay, R. Boucher, J. de Champlain, J. M. Rojo Ortega, R. Lefebvre, P. Roy, and P. Cartier: Diagnostic significance of humoral factors in renovascular hypertension. Antihypertensive Therapy, p. 518—540. 1966.
5. Hartroft, P. M., and W. S. Hartroft: Studies on renal juxtaglomerular cells. II. Correlation of the degree of granulation of juxtaglomerular cells with width of the zona glomerulosa of the adrenal cortex. J. exp. Med. **102**, 205—212 (1955).

Discussion

Tcherdakoff:

We are currently studying the morphology of both kidneys on biopsy specimens obtained by surgery in cases of renovascular hypertension; it is yet too early to state any results.

4.6. The Renin Activity of Rat Plasma* **

D. Regoli, G. Schaechtelin and G. Peters [1]

A method has been developed for measuring renin activity in small volumes of rat plasma:

Heparinized blood, drawn through polyethylene catheters from a carotid or a femoral artery or from the veins on the back of the paw, is collected in polyethylene tubes kept in ice. The blood is heparinized either by injecting 5 mg/kg of heparin i.v., or by using heparinized tubes for collection. The refrigerated tubes are centrifuged at 800 g for 20 min at a temperature of 2° C. They are then again refrigerated to 0° C, and the pH is lowered to 3.5 by adding 1.2 N HCl; the volume needed is usually 0.05 ml per ml of plasma. After thirty minutes the pH is again increased to 5.2 by adding 1.2 N NaOH (0,025 ml/ml of plasma).

The temporary acidification to pH 3.5 partially destroys the angiotensin-degrading peptidases ("angiotensinases") contained in blood, and irreversibly destroys a renin inactivating system contained in normal rat plasma [1].

0.2 or 0.1 ml of plasma at pH 5.2 are then mixed with 0.8 ml (0.4 ml) of a partially purified angiotensinase-free angiotensinogen preparation obtained from rat plasma [2]. The substrate and the plasma are incubated for two, or for four hours at 40° C at pH 5.2 after adding 20 mMol/l of Na_2-EDTA. The EDTA suppresses all residual "angiotensinase" activity which could still be present in plasma. The renin-angiotensinogen-reaction is then stopped by boiling for five minutes. In order to stabilize the angiotensin formed in the course of the reaction, the pH is then increased to 10.0 by adding 0.2 N NaOH (0.09 ml/ml of incubation mixture). The mixture is centrifuged at 2,000 g for twenty minutes at 20° C. The angiotensin contained in the supernatant is assayed on the blood pressure of the urethane-anaesthetized nephrectomized rat [2].

When a commercial standardized renin preparation (Renin N.B.C.) was incubated for 2 to 4 hours under the same conditions with the same amount of substrate, the formation of angiotensin occurred as a zero order reaction. For measuring plasma renin activities, the plasma sample-angiotensinogen mixture was always incubated simultaneously with mixtures of known amounts of standardized hog renin and angiotensinogen; the plasma renin activities could thus be expressed in Goldblatt units/ml of plasma, since the standard preparation was labelled in Goldblatt units.

---

* Supported by Fonds National Suisse de la Recherche Scientifique (Grant no 4190).

** Full report in preparation.

[1] Institut de Pharmacologie de l'Université de Lausanne, Switzerland.

The following table shows the influence of two types of anaesthesia on the renin activity of normal rat plasma:

Table

	n	Goldblatt units/L
Unanesthetized	16	7.4 ± 1.0
Pentobarbital 30 mg/kg i.p.	6	8.4 ± 1.2
Urethane 1.4 g/kg i.p.	10	11.5 ± 0.9

Unanesthetized vs. Pentobarbital: N.S.
Unanesthetized vs. Urethane: $p < 0.01$

References

1. Schaechtelin, G., et D. Regoli: Inactivation de la rénine par le plasma de rat. J. Physiol. (Paris) **59**, 500 (1967).
2. —, Françoise Chométy, D. Regoli et G. Peters: Dosage de l'activité réninique d'extraits tissulaires par incubation avec un substrat naturel purifié. Helv. physiol. pharmacol. Acta **24**, 89—105 (1966).

Discussion

Renner:

Was there any angiotensinase activity present in your final incubation mixture?

Schaechtelin:

No measurable destruction of synthetic angiotensin-II-amide occurred, when the final incubation mixture was incubated with the peptide for four hours.

4.7. Preparative Methods to Purify Renin Substrate*

H. DAHLHEIM, P. WEBER, I. HEROLD, K. PETSCHAUER and K. THURAU[1]

With 4 Figures

The present studies were carried out to identify the naturally occurring renin substrate and to recover sufficient amounts of the pure substrate for investigative work. Such a pure and concentrated substrate is essential not only for the characterization of individual steps in the formation of angiotensin but also for the accurate assay of renin content of a single juxtaglomerular apparatus (JGA). Hog serum was first fractionated by a salting-out technique and subsequent centrifugation, following a modified method of LEVER et al. [1]. Fig. 1a shows the serum fractions so obtained. Corresponding to the increasing amounts of NaCl added to the serum, as shown on the abscissa, the bars represent the percentage of precipitated protein and the curve represents the substrate content per mg protein (specific substrate activity) at each NaCl increment. The specific substrate activity was determined from the velocity of angiotensin formation after incubation with a known amount of renin (0.01 Goldblatt units/ml at low substrate concentrations). The quantity of angiotensin formed was determined by the rat assay method.

The highest specific substrate activity, 30-times that of the natural serum, was found in the salt fraction of 180—200 g NaCl, and only this fraction was employed in the following purification steps using Sephadex-gels. The highest substrate concentration, which was 30 times greater than that of the above-described salt separated fraction, was obtained with Sephadex gel G-75, as shown in Fig. 1b.

Thus, the use of both the salt precipitation method and Sephadex Gel filtration technique (G 75) results in a substrate concentration approximately 1,000 times greater than that found in the original material. The renin substrate thus obtained is free of renin and angiotensinase. This follows from two observations. First, after 48 hours of incubation at 37° C, the substrate did not produce any angiotensin activity and second, after incubation of substrate with renin, angiotensin remained stable for at least five days.

Fig. 1b also demonstrates the results where Gel-25 and Gel-50 are employed. The maxima of substrate activity are found in the fractions indicated by the arrows. Since protein concentrations in these fractions are higher than at Gel 75, the resulting substrate activity is less.

Following the use of salt fractionation and gel filtration, further attempts at substrate concentration were carried out by the use of preparative free curtain electrophoresis. This resulted in a further separation of the remaining non-renin-substrate proteins. Preliminary observations indicate the ensuing increase of

* Supported by the Deutsche Forschungsgemeinschaft.

[1] Physiologisches Institut der Universität München, West Germany.

specific activity to be about double. Although the use of sucrose density gradient ultracentrifugation after salting out, resulted in less specific activity than that obtained with gel filtration, it did reveal the distribution of the specific substrate activity into several maxima. Similarly, corresponding maxima were obtained when the total substrate activity was considered.

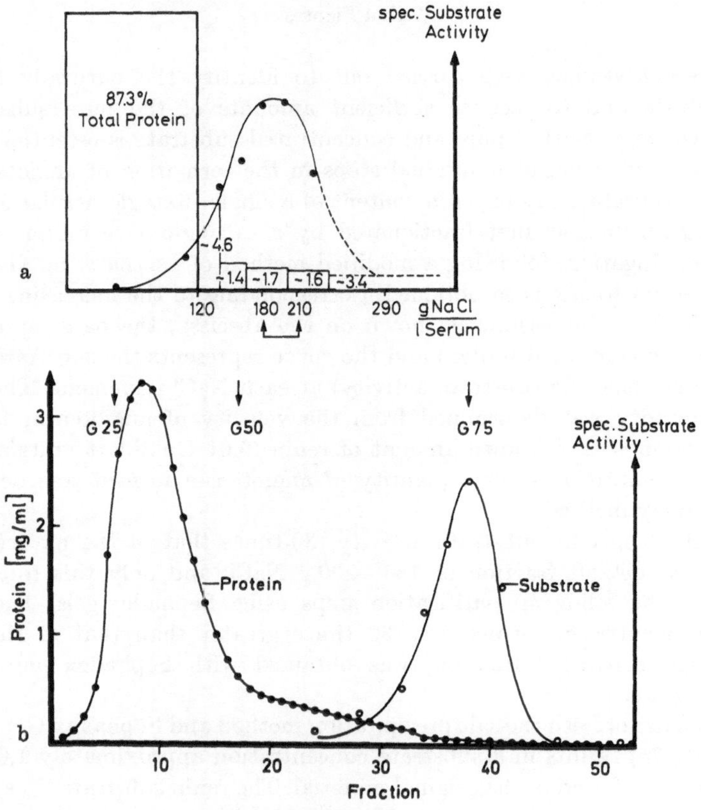

Fig. 1a and b. Purification of renin substrate. a) Upper panel: by NaCl precipitation. b) Lower panel: by gel filtration following NaCl precipitation. The salt fraction (180—200 g NaCl/l serum) which had the highest substrate concentration, was used as starting material. (See text for details)

As shown in Fig. 2, the maxima of specific substrate activity are at 3, 9 and 13% sucrose concentrations. This demonstration of several substrates of different density may be consistent with the results of SKEGGS et al. [2], implying a heterogenous renin substrate with respect to density. As shown in the lower part of Fig. 2 this heterogeneity is not caused by prior salt fractionation at pH 3.1. In the experiments represented here, salt precipitation is replaced by gel filtration without acidification and the sucrose density ultracentrifugation results in similar maxima, consistent with the above noted heterogeneity.

The concentrated substrate so obtained was used in the determination of renin content of single juxtaglomerular apparatus (Fig. 3). Single rat glomeruli

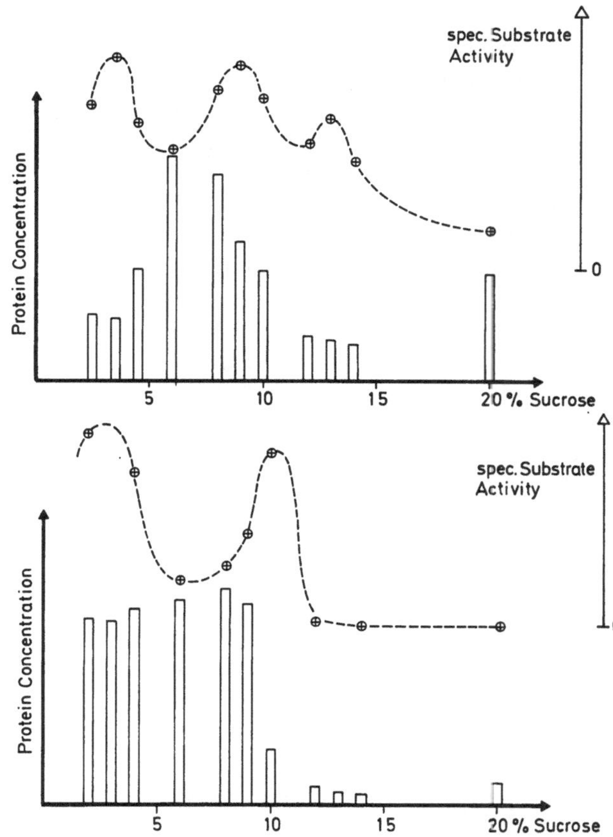

Fig. 2. Distribution pattern of renin substrate following sucrose density ultracentrifugation. Upper panel: after salt precipitation at pH 3.15. Lower panel: without prior salt precipitation at pH 7

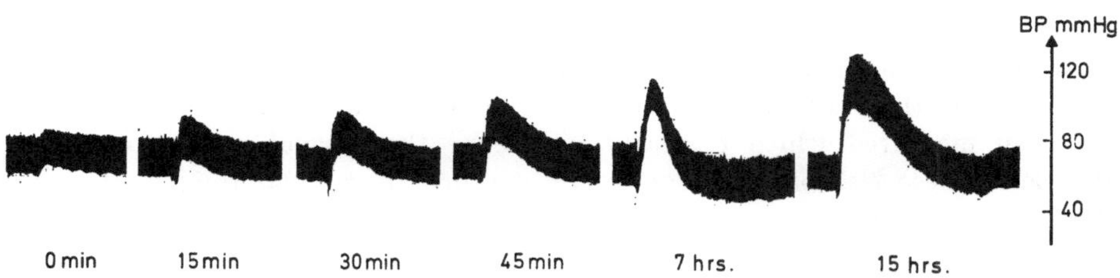

Fig. 3. Renin assay of single JGA's. BP of the assay rat following injection of glomerular homogenate-substrate mixture at different times of incubation

with the attached JGA were dissected[2] and homogenized. The homogenate was incubated with the substrate at 37° C, and the time course of angiotensin formation was determined. Fig. 3 shows the original B.P. response to the i.v. injection of 0.05 ml incubate at different incubation times. Because of the high concentration of the substrate the reaction velocity can be measured in 6 hours.

[2] We are indebted to Mr. M. WAHL who did the dissections.

In the course of these investigations an interesting observation was made of possible relevance to the understanding of the regulation of angiotensin formation in vivo. The rate of angiotensin formation by the substrate-renin mixture was found to depend critically upon the sodium concentration of the medium, as demonstrated in Fig. 4. On the ordinate is plotted the reaction velocity and the abscissa shows the sodium concentrations of the medium, using chloride or bromide as the anion at each level. Angiotensin formation was decreased at increasing sodium concentrations, irrespective of the anion. Of interest is the fact that the steepest part of the slope, and therefore the most pronounced

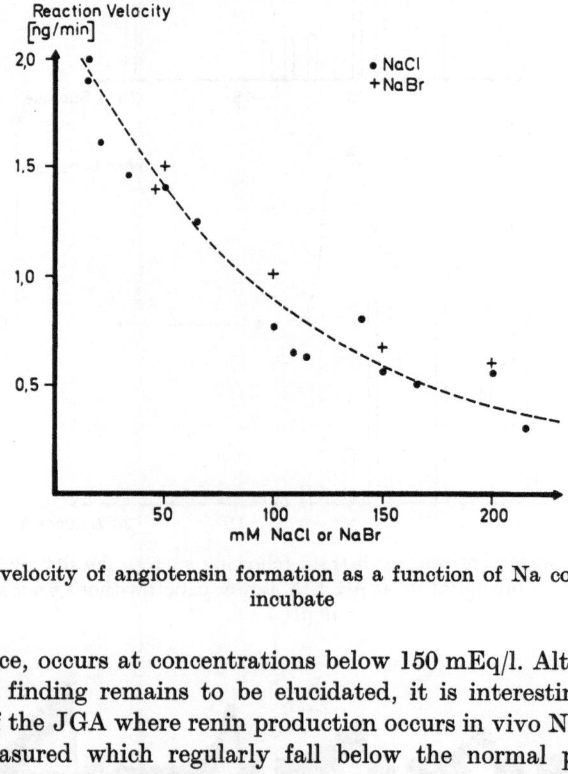

Fig. 4. Reaction velocity of angiotensin formation as a function of Na concentration in the incubate

sodium influence, occurs at concentrations below 150 mEq/l. Although the significance of this finding remains to be elucidated, it is interesting to note, that in the region of the JGA where renin production occurs in vivo Na concentrations have been measured which regularly fall below the normal plasma value of 150 mEq/l. These Na concentrations were measured in tubular fluid at the site of the macula densa by micropuncture techniques.

Of course, the relevance of these sodium influences demonstrated in vitro to the in vivo situation is tentative. However, one may speculate that the well-known relationship between sodium and the release of angiotensin may be determined by the local [Na] concentration in the fluid space where the enzyme reaction occurs.

References

1. Lever, A. F., J. I. S. Robertson, and M. Tree: The estimation of renin in plasma by an enzyme kinetic technique. Biochim. J. **91**, 346 (1964).
2. Skeggs, L. T., K. E. Lentz, H. Hochstrasser, and J. R. Kahn: The chemistry of renin substrate. Canad. med. Ass. J. **90**, 185 (1964).

4.8. Enzyme Activity in Isolated Glomeruli of Rats with Renal Hypertension

M. NAGANO[1]

With 1 Figure

In previous studies on Masugi's nephritis a correlation was found between enzyme activity in the isolated glomerulus and the development of immunological reactions [6, 11]. Because of a close relationship between glomerular damage and changes in carbohydrate metabolism it was of interest to study the activity of enzymes in the isolated glomerulus of rats with experimental renal hypertension.

Renal hypertension was induced in rats by constricting the left renal artery with a silver clip, either without (Group A) or with simultaneous contralateral nephrectomy (Group B). The blood pressure was measured in each rat under light ether anesthesia using the tail plethysmographic method [3]. After direct blood pressure measurement in the abdominal aorta with a mercury manometer the kidney was perfused with a 0.4 m sucrose solution until it appeared blood-free. Glomeruli were isolated by a modification of our previous method [7].

By this technique, the renal cortex was immersed in a 0.4 m sucrose solution and crushed by hand in a Potter-homogenizer. The cortex suspension was filtered with a fine mesh nylon stocking net. Relatively larger particles of the cortex which remained on the net were again ground by the same technique and were re-filtered.

This suspension was layered on a sucrose density-gradient (spec. gravity: 1.137, 1.146, 1.156, 1.187, 1.197) in a 100 ml cylinder glass which was kept in a refrigerator for 2—3 hours.

The particles in the suspension sank down to each layer according to their proper specific gravities. Upper layer: fine homogenized material; 2nd layer: cellular components; 3rd layer: destroyed tubules; 4th layer: glomeruli. The 4th layer and the layer between the 3rd and 4th were again filtered with a double-folded nylon net, and then centrifuged at 1,200—1,500 rpm for 5 minutes. The collected sediment was dispersed with 44% sucrose solution (spec. gravity 1.197) before it was layered over 46% sucrose solution in a centrifuge glass tube. This was centrifuged at 600—800 rpm for 5 minutes, so that the glomeruli were on the wall of the centrifuge glass and in the sediment (Fig. 1).

The activities of 6 enzymes in the isolated glomeruli were determined. The results are summarized in the Table. The enzyme activities in the glomeruli of group A show distinct changes as compared with normal findings; hexokinase

[1] Medizinische Universitätsklinik Würzburg, West Germany.

(HK), fructose-1,6-diphosphate aldolase (ALD) and lactate dehydrogenase (LDH) exhibit a lower activity in group A than those in the controls, whereas they have a higher value in rats with Masugi's nephritis.

The activities of malate dehydrogenase (MDH) and isocitrate dehydrogenase (ICDH) were lower than those in the controls, and this tendency was identical to that observed in Masugi's nephritis.

The previous study on Masugi's nephritis showed that anaerobic glycolysis was accelerated in the glomeruli and the enzyme activities related to the citric acid cycle were lower. These data seem to confirm a speculation that cellular

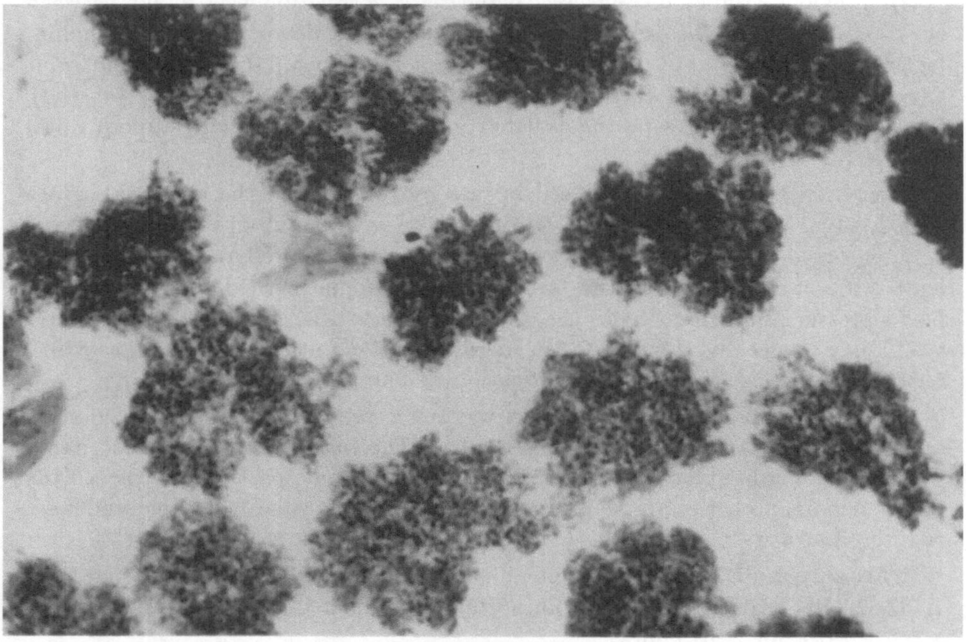

Fig. 1

damage in the glomerular basement membrane is caused by hypoxia during the immunological process of Masugi's nephritis. There was no statistically significant difference in enzyme activities between the clamped side and the non-clamped side of the kidney in this particular group.

BOGATZKI [1] reported that simple compensatory renal hypertrophy was observed in unilaterally nephrectomised rat, in which an increase in urinary excretion of enzymes was noted simultaneously with increased proteinuria. She also indicated that this was much more apparent when the blood flow of the remaining kidney was diminished.

Decreased enzyme activities in glomeruli in group A as observed in this study may have occurred as a result of circulatory change in the kidney leading to increased glomerular filtration of enzymes. If one assumes that enzymes are excreted in parallel with protein, an increase in enzyme excretion can be expected in Masugi's nephritis in which massive proteinuria is noted.

Table. *Enzyme activity in isolated glomerulus of rat with renal hypertension*

	Control $n = 5$	Group A		Group B $n = 5$
		clamped side (left kidney) $n = 10$	non-clamped side (right kidney) $n = 8$	
Blood pressure (mm Hg)	83 ± 11	154 ± 20	156 ± 19	169 ± 36
HK	7.94 ± 0.95	5.40 ± 2.47	5.01 ± 2.25	8.06 ± 1.88
	└ $0.02 > p > 0.01$ ┘ (Control–clamped)	└ n.s. ┘ (clamped–non-clamped)		
	└ $0.02 > p > 0.01$ ┘ (Control–non-clamped)			
	└ n.s. ┘ (Control–Group B)			
FDP-ALD	62.8 ± 4.7	45.2 ± 13.1	45.7 ± 8.8	63.8 ± 19.3
	└ $0.01 > p > 0.001$ ┘ (Control–clamped)	└ n.s. ┘ (clamped–non-clamped)		
	└ $0.001 > p$ ┘ (Control–non-clamped)			
	└ n.s. ┘ (Control–Group B)			
LDH	403 ± 45	248 ± 67	190 ± 81	247 ± 67
	└ $0.001 > p$ ┘ (Control–clamped)	└ n.s. ┘ (clamped–non-clamped)		
	└ $0.001 > p$ ┘ (Control–non-clamped)			
	└ $0.01 > p > 0.001$ ┘ (Control–Group B)			
MDH	1,125 ± 204	742 ± 219	615 ± 240	734 ± 217
	└ $0.01 > p > 0.001$ ┘ (Control–clamped)	└ n.s. ┘ (clamped–non-clamped)		
	└ $0.01 > p > 0.001$ ┘ (Control–non-clamped)			
	└ $0.02 > p > 0.01$ ┘ (Control–Group B)			
ICDH	20.4 ± 1.9	7.3 ± 4.2	7.8 ± 4.1	
	└ $0.001 > p$ ┘ (Control–clamped)	└ n.s. ┘ (clamped–non-clamped)		
		$0.01 > p > 0.001$		
GOT	363 ± 99	213 ± 70	209 ± 39	254 ± 73
	└ $0.02 > p > 0.01$ ┘ (Control–clamped)	└ n.s. ┘ (clamped–non-clamped)		
	└ $0.01 > p > 0.001$ ┘ (Control–non-clamped)			
	└ n.s. ┘ (Control–Group B)			

Actually, however, there was no evidence of a parallel relationship between enzyme and protein excretion [5, 6, 11]. Rats in group B showed no statistically significant difference in activities of such enzymes as HK, ALD and GOT, and therefore, the decreased enzyme activity observed can hardly be explained by the above speculation of increased enzyme excretion into the urine.

As previously reported [2, 9, 10, 12, 13], the renin content in the kidney and the concentration of renin-like-substance in blood of animals with hypertension showed no correlation with each other. Artificial renal arterial stenosis with contralateral nephrectomy, as made in group B, did not lead to an increase in pressor substance in blood, while an increase of this substance was detected in group A. Because of this, it is suspected that the metabolic change in group A occurred in relation with the renin-angiotensin-system, whereas other factors contributed to that in group B.

References

1. BOGATZKI, M.: Fortschr. Med. **83**, 859—862 (1965).
2. BROWN, J. J., G. CHAPUIS, and J. J. S. ROBERTSON: Lancet **1963 I**, 1356—1357.
3. BYROM, B., and C. WILSON: J. Physiol. (Lond.) **93**, 301—304 (1938).
4. DUBACH, U. C., u. L. RECANT: Klin. Wschr. **40**, 333—337 (1962).
5. FRANZ, H. E., M. FRANZ u. R. KLUTHE: Klin. Wschr. **40**, 646—648 (1962).
6. NAGANO, M., u. H. E. SCHÄFER: In: Das Nephrotische Syndrom, hrsg. von F. REUBI u. H. G. PAULI, S. 185. Stuttgart: Georg Thieme 1963.
7. — — Klin. Wschr. **41**, 1203—1207 (1963).
8. — M. KAWAMURA, T. KOGURE, and H. E. SCHÄFER: Jap. J. Nephrol. **8**, 94—95 (1966).
9. REGOLI, D., R. HESS, H. BRUNNER, G. PETERS, and F. GROSS: Arch. int. Pharmacodyn. **140**, 416—426 (1962).
10. SCHAECHTELIN, G., D. REGOLI, and F. GROSS: Amer. J. Physiol. **205**, 303—306 (1963).
11. SCHÄFER, H. E.: Z. klin. Med. **158**, 221—298 (1964).
12. WOLLHEIM, E.: Die essentielle Hypertonie und andere Hochdruckformen, Klinik, Differentialdiagnose und Pathogenese. Invited Lecture bei japan. Med. Kongr. in Nagoya/Japan 1967.
13. ZIEGLER, M., u. G. SCHAECHTELIN: Verh. d. Dtsch. Ges. f. Urol. 21. Tagg 1965, S. 225. Berlin-Heidelberg-New York: Springer 1966.

4.9. Renal Effects of Angiotensin and of Postpituitary Peptides*

G. Peters, J. Ph. Bonjour and D. Regoli[1]

The type and the intensity of the renal responses evoked by angiotensin or postpituitary peptides in rats, depend to a large extent on the experimental conditions [1, 2]. Thus, angiotensin enhances sodium and water excretion in unanesthetized rats loaded with hypotonic or isotonic saline solutions, while a marked antidiuretic effect is observed when the peptide is infused into rats anesthetized with ethanol and in water diuresis [1, 2]. Moreover the antidiuretic effect of vasopressin is about 10 times stronger in rats anesthetized with ethanol than in the unanesthetized animals [2]. Little is known about the effects of oxytocin in these different experimental conditions.

The present communication deals with the renal effects of angiotensin and oxytocin in hydrated rats, anesthetized with ethanol (Table 1), or unanesthetized (Table 2). The methods used have been fully described elsewhere [2].

In hydrated rats anesthetized with ethanol val_5 angiotensin II amide (Hypertensin Ciba), infused at a constant rate of 1.25 μg/kg·min, for 45 minutes, enhanced sodium excretion (UV_{Na^+}) and reduced free water clearance (C_{H_2O}). During

Table 1. *Renal effects of angiotensin and oxytocin in rats anesthetized with ethanol*

	Control period (30 min)	Angiotensin II-amide 1.25 μg/kg·min (15 min)	Angiotensin II-amide 1.25 μg/kg·min (30 min)	Control period (30 min)	Oxytocin 250 mU/kg → 50 mU/kg·min (30 min)
V (ml/kg·min)	0.71 ± 0.04	0.28^c ± 0.08	0.79 ± 0.07	0.70 ± 0.06	0.41^c ± 0.05
C_{H_2O} (ml/kg·min)	0.56 ± 0.04	0.07^c ± 0.03	0.24^c ± 0.05	0.49 ± 0.02	-0.02^c ± 0.02
C_{IN} (ml/kg·min)	8.1 ± 0.3	4.1^c ± 0.6	8.4 ± 0.8	7.34 ± 0.5	8.9^c ± 0.7
TRF_{Na^+} (%)	0.52 ± 0.15	3.17^a ± 0.91	5.60^c ± 0.98	0.75 ± 0.16	5.84^c ± 0.70

Groups of 10 to 15 rats. Experiments in ethanol anesthesia and water diuresis: two doses of 3% b. w. of 12% ethanol in water p. o., at a 30 min interval, followed by i. v. infusion of 0.08 M glucose + 0.03 M NaCl + 1 vol.-% ethanol at 0.15/ml/rat·min. — Data are means ± S.E. Superscripts indicate significance of differences between the treatment periods and the control period preceding the infusion of the drugs:

[a] $p < 0.05$.
[b] $p < 0.01$.
[c] $p < 0.001$.

* Supported by Fonds National Suisse de la Recherche Scientifique (Grant no 4190).

[1] Institut de Pharmacologie de l'Université de Lausanne.

the first 15 minutes of the infusion of angiotensin, glomerular filtration rate (GFR) and urine flow (V) fell significantly. Both GFR and V rose subsequently in spite of the continued infusion of angiotensin, while C_{H_2O} remained low.

Similar effects on C_{H_2O} and UV_{Na^+} were observed, when oxytocin (Syntocinon Sandoz) was given as a priming intravenous injection of 250 mU/kg followed by a constant infusion of 50 mU/kg·min. In contrast to angiotensin, oxytocin depressed V during the whole period of infusion and significantly increased GFR.

The most important difference in the action of the two peptides in the water loaded rat anesthetized with ethanol is the "vascular" antidiuretic effect of angiotensin. Oxytocin, to the contrary, increases GFR. Under the same experimental conditions much smaller doses of vasopressin reduce V and C_{H_2O} without modifying GFR or UV_{Na^+} [2].

Table 2. *Renal effects of angiotensin and oxytocin in unanesthetized rats*

	Control period (30 min)	Angiotensin II-amide 1.25 μg/kg·min (15 min)	Control period (30 min)	Oxytocin 250 mU/kg → 50 mU/kg·min (15 min)
V (ml/kg·min)	0.62 ± 0.06	1.26[b] ± 0.18	0.74 ± 0.05	0.67 ± 0.07
H_2O (ml/kg·min)	0.51 ± 0.06	0.54 ± 0.08	0.43 ± 0.03	−0.02[c] ± 0.05
C_{IN} (ml/kg·min)	7.2 ± 0.3	9.6[b] ± 0.5	7.1 ± 0.5	8.2[a] ± 0.5
TRF_{Na+} (%)	2.5 ± 0.33	19.4[c] ± 1.37	3.2 ± 0.40	7.9[c] ± 0.80

Groups of 10 to 15 rats in water diuresis: 50 ml/kg of water per stomach tube followed by infusion of 0.17 M glucose + 0.008 M NaCl at a rate of 0.2 ml/rat·min. — Data are means ± S.E. Superscripts indicate significance of differences between the treatment period and the control period preceding the infusion of the drug:
[a] $p < 0.05$.
[b] $p < 0.01$.
[c] $p < 0.001$.

In unanesthetized rats (Table 2) both angiotensin and oxytocin enhanced sodium excretion and caused an increase of GFR. However the natriuresis elicited by angiotensin was not associated with any change of C_{H_2O}, while oxytocin had, in the unanesthetized animal, the same antidiuretic effect (reduction of C_{H_2O}) as under ethanol anaesthesia.

An inhibition of sodium reabsorption in the proximal tubule does not influence or even enhances the formation of free water in the diluting segment of the nephron. On the contrary inhibition of sodium reabsorption in the diluting segment depresses free water formation.

Our results suggest that angiotensin may have its site of action above the diluting segment; the natriuretic effect is accompanied by a slight increase of C_{H_2O}. The effects of oxytocin could be referred to a block of the sodium reabsorption in the diluting segment, because the natriuresis is associated with a fall of C_{H_2O}.

Alternatively, and more probably, the effects of oxytocin are explained by assuming two different sites of action of the drug in the nephron: 1. a block of the reabsorption of sodium above or in the diluting segment and 2. a vasopressin-like effect on the collecting ducts.

References

1. Bonjour, J. Ph., D. Regoli, F. Roch-Ramel, and G. Peters: Prerequisites for the natriuretic effect of Val[5] angiotensin II amide in the rat. Amer. J. Physiol. **215**, 1133—1138 (1968).

2. — G. Peters, F. Chomety, and D. Regoli: Renal effects of Val_5 angiotensin II amide, vasopressin and diuretics in the rat, as influenced by water diuresis and by ethanol anesthesia. Europ. J. Pharmacol. **2**, 88—105 (1967).

3. Eknoyon, E., W. N. Suki, F. C. Rector, and D. W. Seldin: Functional characteristics of the diluting segment of the dog nephron and the effect of extracellular volume expansion on its reabsorptive capacity. J. clin. Invest. **46**, 1178—1188 (1967).

5. Urinary Concentration and Dilution

5.1. Micropuncture Study of Tubular Sodium and Water Reabsorption in Rats with Hereditary Hypothalamic Diabetes insipidus

J. Schnermann, H. Valtin, H. Fischbach, W. Nagel, M. Horster, G. Liebau, M. Tabor, A. Geltinger, and K. Thurau[1]

With 5 Figures

Micropuncture experiments [9] and studies on isolated renal tubules [5] have demonstrated that ADH influences final urine concentration by increasing the water permeability of the epithelium of the distal convolution and collecting duct. However, it is unclear whether a possible ADH-mediated enhancement of sodium reabsorption in the loop of Henle also participates in the concentrating mechanism [4, 8]. This is worthy of serious consideration in view of the demonstration of the stimulation of sodium transport of toad bladder epithelium by ADH [6, 7].

To clarify this question we carried out micropuncture experiments on rats with hereditary hypothalamic diabetes insipidus [11]. Previous experimental preparations of diabetes insipidus in the rat were made possible by creating hypothalamic lesions [1]. However, this led to diabetes insipidus of variable severity and resulted in an average GFR of about 50% of normal under micropuncture conditions [3]. Both of these limitations were avoided by the use of rats, first introduced by Valtin et al. [11], which have a hereditary defect in ADH synthesis.

8 male rats of 250—330 g were used. The rats were pretreated with 2×3 mg cortisone i.m. and 3×10 ml water p.o. at intervals of 60 min and 30 min respectively, before being anaesthetized with 120 mg/kg Inactin. Water lost during the experiment was replaced by infusing 2% glucose at a rate of 0.2 ml/min. During ADH administration this infusion rate was reduced to correspond to the decreased urine flow. In view of the minimal measured urinary loss of Na during the experiment (about 0.24 μEq/min) no replacement was undertaken other than the saline (0.02 ml/min) used for the inulin infusion. Micropuncture experiments were carried out in each experiment during the water diuresis normally found in these rats and, subsequently, during ADH induced antidiuresis. In some studies, when the ADH protocol was completed, more tubular samples were collected after the water diuresis had spontaneously resumed. Recollections of early distal segments — identified by i.v. injections of lissamine-green — were performed during the different experimental periods. The fractional net sodium and water reabsorption of a single loop of Henle was calculated by subtracting the fraction of sodium and water present at early distal tubular puncture sites

[1] Physiologisches Institut der Universität München.

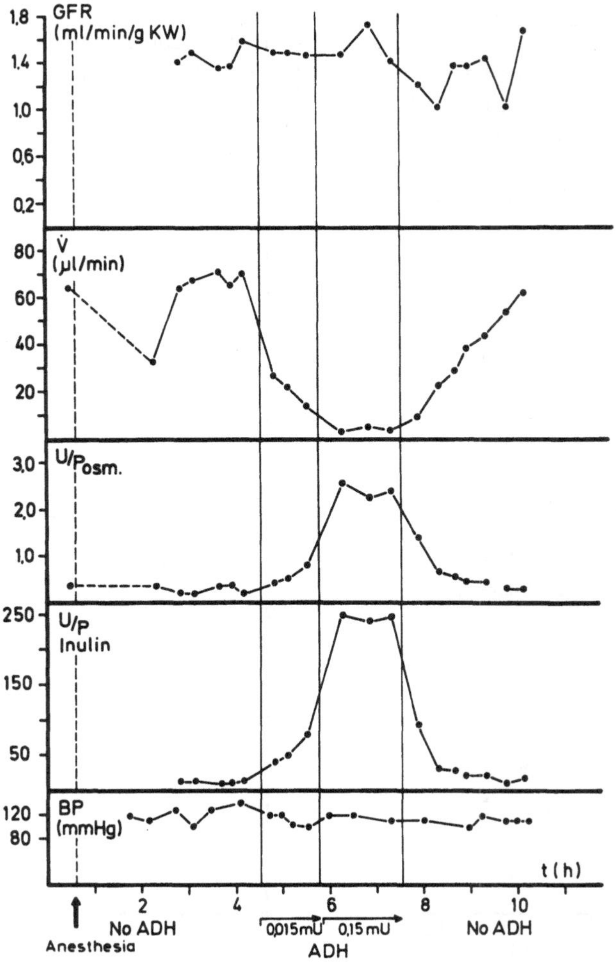

Fig. 1. Glomerular filtration rate, excretory functions, and blood pressure in diabetes insipidus rats before, during, and after ADH-infusion in a single experiment. The dose of ADH is given in mUnits/min (Pitressin, Parke-Davis)

from the corresponding values obtained from puncturing late proximal convolutions, according to

$$\% \; H_2O_{\text{reabs. (loop)}} = \left(\frac{1}{\text{TF/P In. prox.}} - \frac{1}{\text{TF/P In. dist.}}\right) \times 100$$

$$\% \; Na_{\text{reabs. (loop)}} = \left(\frac{1}{\text{TF/P In. prox.}} - \frac{\text{TF/P Na dist.}}{\text{TF/P In. dist.}}\right) \times 100$$

Data from one of these experiments are presented in Fig. 1, which shows approximately the same GFR during the periods of ADH infusion, at doses of 0.015 mU/min and 0.15 mU/min, and in water diuresis. Experiments in which GFR was variable were discarded. The urine volume of about 60 μl/min and the osmolarity of about 100 mosm/l were essentially the same as in the unanesthetized animal and correspond to data of VALTIN [10]. The dose of ADH required to produce a maximal urine concentration of up to 1250 mosm/l, without simultaneous elevation of blood pressure, was 0.15 mU Pitressin/min.

The average late proximal tubular TF/P Inulin ratios, as well as the proximal passage times (Table) during the different procedures, show no significant dif-

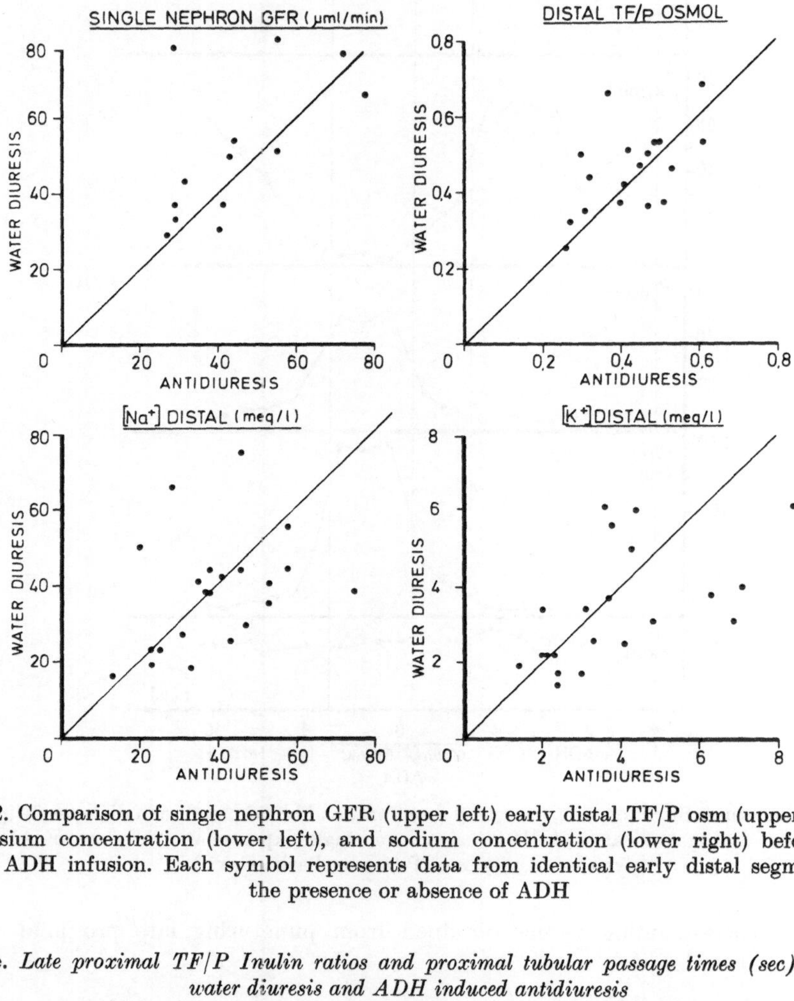

Fig. 2. Comparison of single nephron GFR (upper left) early distal TF/P osm (upper right), potassium concentration (lower left), and sodium concentration (lower right) before and after ADH infusion. Each symbol represents data from identical early distal segments in the presence or absence of ADH

Table. *Late proximal TF/P Inulin ratios and proximal tubular passage times (sec) during water diuresis and ADH induced antidiuresis*

	Initial H_2O diuresis	ADH 0.015 mU/min	0.15 mU/min	Return to H_2O diuresis
Late proximal TF/P Inulin	2.53 $\pm$ 0.58 ($n = 20$)	2.26 $\pm$ 0.17 ($n = 8$)	2.27 $\pm$ 0.46 ($n = 11$)	2.32 $\pm$ 0.42 ($n = 4$)
	$p < 0.2$			
Proximal passage time	11.3 $\pm$ 2.1	10.1 $\pm$ 2.0	10.6 $\pm$ 1.6	12.6 $\pm$ 3.0

ferences. This indicates that ADH administration does not influence proximal tubular reabsorptive capacity $\left(\frac{C}{\pi r^2}\right)$ for sodium as already suggested by GERTZ et al. in rat studies [3] and by DAVIS et al. in dog experiments [2].

The results from re-puncturing the same distal tubule during water diuresis and antidiuresis are presented in Fig. 2. The GFR of single punctured nephrons

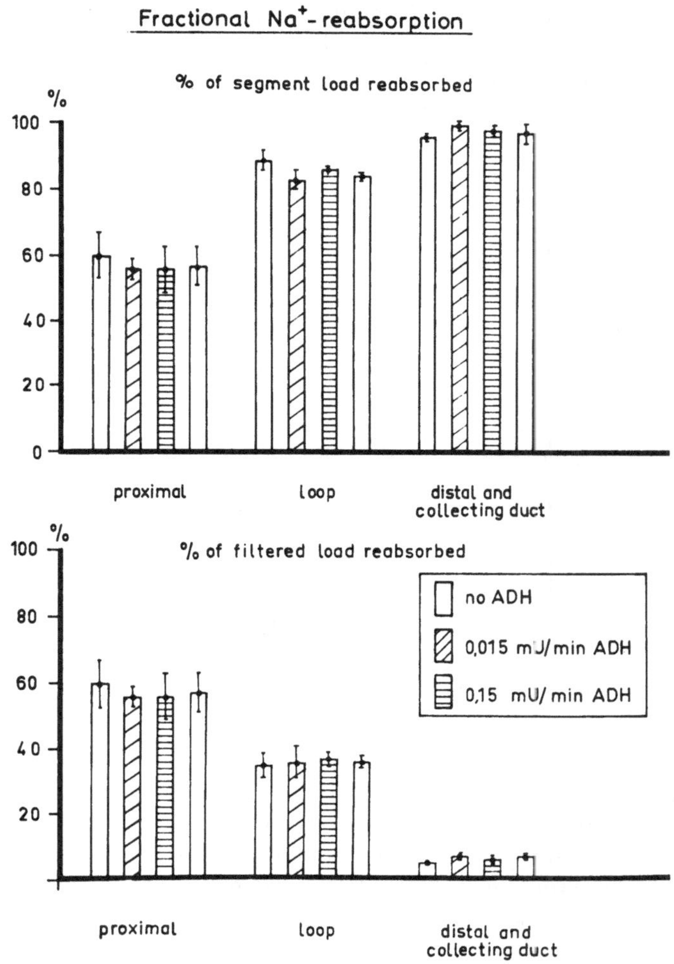

Fig. 3. Tubular reabsorption of sodium as fraction of segmental (upper part) or filtered load (lower part) for different nephron segments in the presence or absence of ADH

was calculated from the early distal TF/P Inulin and the timed tubular volume collection. Single nephron GFR showed no dependency on the diuretic state, which is consistent with the demonstrated constancy of the whole kidney GFR. Similarly, the concentrations of Na^+, K^+, and the osmolarity in the early distal tubular fluid were not significantly influenced by ADH.

The present data bear critically on the question as to whether ADH has an effect on the sodium transport in the short loops of Henle. Since the constancy of GFR and of late proximal TF/P Inulin implies an unchanged sodium and water inflow into the loop, the calculation of fractional sodium reabsorption within the loop is alone sufficient to reveal such an influence of ADH. Indeed, these calculations show that sodium transport in the short loops of Henle is not altered by ADH (Fig. 3). Thus, it appears unlikely that the increase in tissue osmolality observed in antidiuresis is the result of an increase of sodium reabsorption in the loops of Henle. Also shown in Fig. 3, is the constancy of fractional sodium reabsorption along the distal convolution and the collecting ducts with and without ADH administration.

Fig. 4 shows that the early distal tubular TF/P inulin ratios from repunctured nephrons, generally fell above the line of identity, i.e. the fractional water reabsorption along the short loops of Henle during water diuresis is higher than

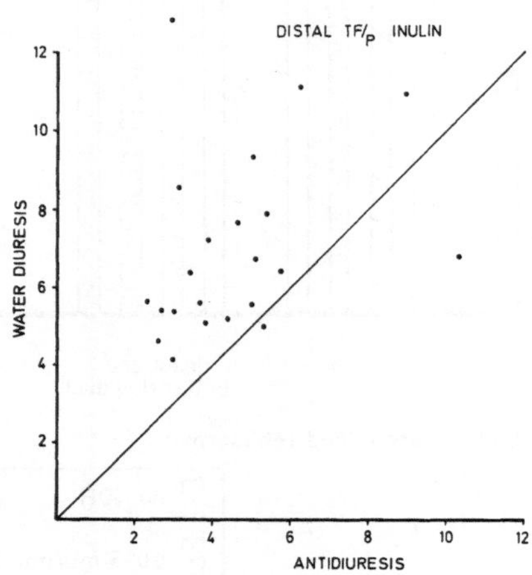

Fig. 4. Comparison of early distal TF/P Inulin ratios in water diuresis and ADH induced antidiuresis

in antidiuresis. During water diuresis an average TF/P inulin of 6.46 ± 2.1 was obtained in contrast to 4.56 ± 1.8 during ADH infusion. This difference is significant ($p < 0.01$). As expected, fractional water reabsorption along the distal convolution and collecting duct was greatly decreased during water diuresis (Fig. 5). This surprising finding of a lower rate of water reabsorption in the short loops of Henle during antidiuresis cannot be attributed to a direct effect of ADH on the water permeability of the loop epithelium. This would necessitate the implausible assumption that ADH administration simultaneously decreases the permeability of the loop of Henle while increasing the permeability to water of the distal tubular epithelium. A more attractive hypothesis is that the determination of the fractional water reabsorption across the short loops of Henle is dictated by the degree of permeability of the collecting duct epithelium with reference to that of the loop. Under the influence of a fixed outer medullary osmotic driving force [10], loop and collecting duct epithelium will compete for available water to satisfy this stimulus to water movement. Thus, in antidiuresis more water will be reabsorbed across the loops than occurs in water diuresis because the more permeable collecting duct epithelium permits greater delivery of water to the medulla. And, conversely, in water diuresis more water will be reabsorbed from the loop because of the relative impermeability of the collecting duct epithelium.

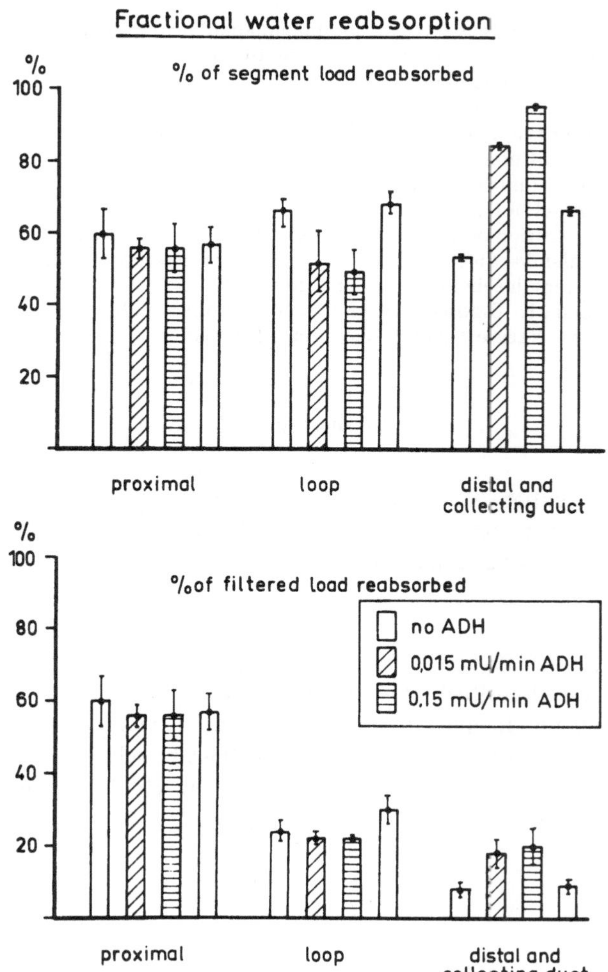

Fig. 5. Tubular reabsorption of water as fraction of segmental (upper part) of filtered load (lower part) for different nephron segments in the presence or absence of ADH

References

1. Bruce, H. M., and G. C. Kennedy: The central nervous control of food and water intake. Proc. roy. Soc. B **138**, 528—532 (1951).
2. Davis, B. B., F. G. Knox, and R. W. Berliner: The effect of vasopressin on proximal tubule sodium reabsorption in the dog. Amer. J. Physiol. **212**, 1361—1364 (1967).
3. Gertz, K. H., G. C. Kennedy u. K. J. Ullrich: Mikropunktionsuntersuchungen über die Flüssigkeitsrückresorption aus einzelnen Tubulusabschnitten bei Wasserdiurese (Diabetes insipidus). Pflügers Arch. ges. Physiol. **278**, 513—519 (1964).

4. GOTTSCHALK, C. W.: Osmotic concentration and dilution of the urine. Amer. J. Med. **36**, 670—685 (1964).
5. GRANTHAM, J. J., and M. B. BURG: Effect of vasopressin and cyclic AMP on permeability of isolated collecting tubules. Amer. J. Physiol. **211**, 255—259 (1966).
6. LEAF, A., J. ANDERSON, and L. B. PAGE: Active sodium transport by the isolated toad bladder. J. gen. Physiol. **41**, 657—668 (1958).
7. —, and E. F. DEMPSEY: Some effects of mammalian neurohypophyseal hormones on metabolism and active transport of sodium by the isolated toad bladder. J. biol. Chem. **235**, 2160—2169 (1960).
8. ULLRICH, K. J., K. KRAMER, and J. W. BOYLAN: Present knowledge of the counter-current system in the mammalian kidney. Progr. cardiovasc. Dis. **3**, 395—431 (1961).
9. — G. RUMRICH u. G. FUCHS: Wasserpermeabilität und transtubulärer Wasserfluß corticaler Nephronabschnitte bei verschiedenen Diuresezuständen. Pflügers Arch. ges. Physiol. **280**, 99—119 (1964).
10. VALTIN, H.: Sequestration of urea and nonurea solutes in renal tissues of rats with hereditary hypothalamic diabetes insipidus: effect of vasopressin and dehydration on the counter-current mechanism. J. clin. Invest. **45**, 337—345 (1966).
11. — H. A. SCHROEDER, K. BENIRSCHKE, and H. W. SOKOL: Familial hypothalamic diabetes insipidus in rats. Nature (Lond.) **196**, 1109—1110 (1962).

Discussion

WIEDERHOLT:

Unanesthetized diabetes insipidus-rats are usually dehydrated. In your experiments, the animals were copiously hydrated. Did you also succeed in inducing water diuresis in anesthetized dehydrated rats ?

BRODEHL:

Three years ago [J. BRODEHL, K. GELLISSEN and W. HAGGE: Klin. Wschr. **43**, 72 (1964)], we described the effects of vasopression in children with nephrogenous diabetes insipidus. In these children vasopressin considerably increased the clearance of free water. Could this effect be related to the depression of water reabsorption from the ascending limbs of Henle's loops which you described ?

5.2. The Effect of Elevated Plasma Calcium Concentrations on Renal Concentrating and Diluting Mechanisms

G. Fülgraff, G. Heinz, A. Herzfeld and O. Heidenreich[1]

Calcium ions have a diuretic action in dogs and rats. Elevated Ca concentration in plasma or tubular fluid diminishes the intrinsic reabsorptive capacity of the proximal tubular wall. However, fractional proximal reabsorption of Na and fluid remains constant, since the tubules dilate, and the contact time of tubular fluid with epithelium increases. The diuresis after infusion of Ca ions observed by us and by others must be due to an action on a more distal part of the nephron [1].

We investigated the effect of calcium on renal diluting and concentrating mechanisms in dogs. In water diuresis (7 experiments), an infusion of $CaCl_2$ depressed C_{H_2O} significantly, while C_{osm} and the excretion of Na, K, Ca and chloride were enhanced. In hydropenic dogs an elevated plasma calcium concentration resulted in a significant fall of urine osmolarity and Tc_{H_2O}.

We further investigated the tissue concentrations of solutes, Na, K and water of the renal cortex, medulla and papilla following acute and chronic hypercalcemia in hydropenic dogs. Both, acute (infusion of $CaCl_2$ in one renal artery for 20 min) and chronic (elevation of P_{Ca} for at least one week) hypercalcemia lowered tissue osmolality and sodium concentration in medulla and papilla. Papillary osmolality decreased to about 730 mosm/kg, as compared to 1,200 mosm/kg in controls. Potassium and water contents were unchanged.

These results give some evidence, that sodium reabsorption in the loop of Henle may be impaired by elevated Ca concentrations.

Reference

Fülgraff, G., u. O. Heidenreich: Naunyn-Schmiedebergs Arch. Pharmak. exp. Path. **258**, 440—451 (1967).

Discussion

Heidland:

We found that the response of GFR to experimental hypercalcemia depends on the plasma calcium concentration. GFR usually decreases at plasma concentrations above 16 mg-%.

How do you explain the decrease of urinary pH after the administration of calcium?

[1] Abteilung für Pharmakologie der Technischen Hochschule Aachen, West Germany.

Fülgraff:

As we have stressed in a previous paper GFR does not change significantly, when plasma calcium is elevated into the range of 7—10 mEq/l. Higher plasma calcium concentrations depress GFR [Fülgraff, Heidenreich, and Laaff: Naunyn-Schmiedebergs Arch. Pharmak. exp. Path. 257, 372—390 (1967)].

We also found a small and inconstant decrease of pH during the diuresis in hypercalcemia. Bicarbonate reabsorption is increased and urinary chloride concentration is equal or greater than the sum of Na and K. However we have no idea about the mechanism. Possibly H^+-excretion is enhanced as a consequence of increased distal Na-load in the same manner as in K-excretion.

5.3. The Localization of Chloride Ions in the Proximal Tubule, Studied by a Micropuncture Method*

W. Thoenes and K. H. Langer[1]

With 4 Figures

Using a cytochemical method based on the precipitation of chloride as silver chloride [2] Komnick and Komnick [3] found that the silver chloride precipitates in the salt gland of the sea gull are found almost exclusively between the cells, but never within the cells. Similar observations were made by Nolte [6] in the rat kidney. These investigators concluded that chloride ions pass through the epithelial layer by the intercellular clefts, in contrast to sodium ions which pass through the cells. Both investigations [3, 6] used excised pieces of tissue. In order to eliminate the possibility of supravital changes, we repeated similar experiments on proximal tubules of the rat kidney, introducing the histochemical reagent into the living kidney by micropuncture.

Methods

Three male Sprague-Dawley rats were anesthetized with Inactin (80 mg/kg b.w.). The left kidney was prepared for micropuncture, immobilized in a plexiglass cup, and superfused with prewarmed mineral oil. The surface of the kidney was observed by a stereoscopic microscope (Leitz). Microphotographs were taken with a Leica camera through this microscope. Leitz micromanipulators and sharpened glass capillaries made of pyrex glass with a tip diameter of 10—12 μm were used for micropuncture.

9 proximal tubules were perfused with a solution containing 1% osmium tetroxide + 0.25% silver lactate, neutralized to pH 6.8 by adding a 0.01 M borax solution [2]. The perfusion was continued for no more than 1 to 2 min; after this time, the lumen of the glass capillary in the tubule was usually blocked by salt precipitates (a). In 4 other proximal tubules, the same solution was injected between 2 columns of oil, as in the split drop method [1] (b).

With both methods of preparation, the pieces of tissue containing the intravitally perfused tubules were removed from the kidney and were again fixed in 1% osmium tetroxide at pH 6.8.

Pieces of control tissue of similar size (1 mm^3) were excised from the control i.e. not perfused kidney, and were immediately fixed for 1—2 hours at 4° C in the silver lactate solution used for microperfusion (c). The tissues were handled in red light in order to avoid photochemical reactions. At the 50% ethanol stage of dehydration, the pieces of tissue were bathed in nitric acid (0.1 N). They were finally embedded in Epon. 1—2 μm slices were stained in concentrated

* Supported by Deutsche Forschungsgemeinschaft.

[1] Pathologisches Institut der Universität Würzburg, West Germany.

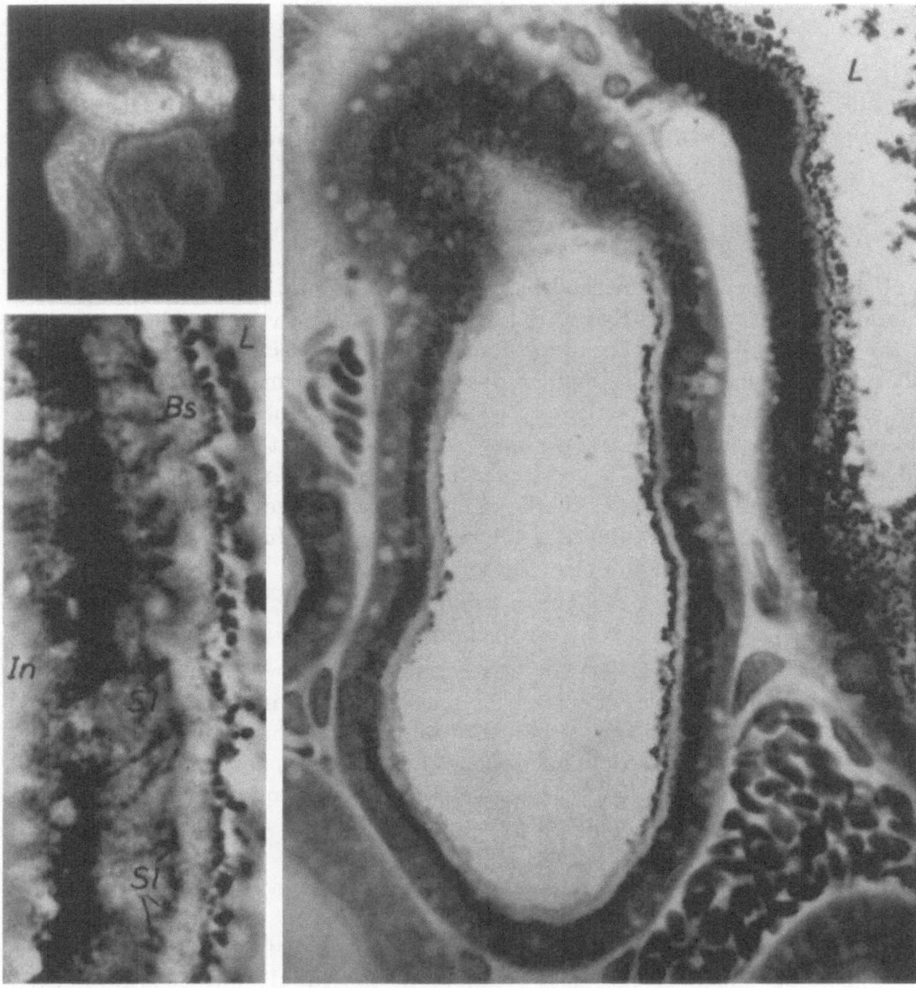

a c b

Fig. 1a—c. Proximal tubules of the rat kidney perfused in vivo under free-flow conditions with a silver lactate-osmium tetroxide solution. a) Proximal convolutions marked by white silver chloride precipitates, as seen within an Epon block. b) Light microscopy: precipitates in the tubular lumen (right upper corner), on the brush border and within the epithelial wall. Terminal bars are clearly visible in the flat part of the section (upper part of left tubule). Giemsa. Enlargement: 735 times. c) Greater magnification demonstrates the precipitates in the terminal bars and stripes in the basal part of the cell. Giemsa. Magnification 2,700 times. *L* tubular lumen; *BS* brush border; *Sl* terminal bars; *In* interstitium

Giemsa solution for light microscopy [8]. Thin slices for electron microscopy were cut with a Porter-Blum microtome. The electron microscope used was an Elmiskop I (Siemens).

Results

At incident light microscopy of the living kidney, the infusion of a silver lactate solution into open (a) or oil blocked (b) tubules rapidly caused the appearance of thick white precipitates in the tubular lumen and within the epithelial cells. The simultaneous fixation of the tissue by osmium tetroxide entailed a brown to black coloration of the surrounding cells. As another consequence of fixation, the tubular lumens remained open, i.e. did not collapse.

At light microscopy of the embedded tissue, the perfused tubules were immediately recognized by their whiteness in contrast to the surrounding tissue blackened by osmium tetroxide (Fig. 1a). In stained sections precipitates were

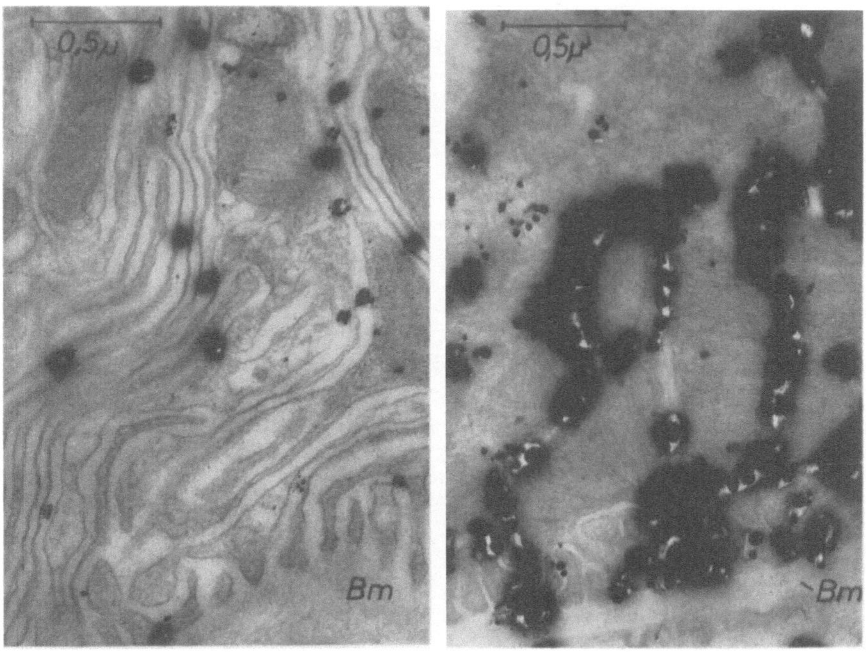

Fig. 2a and b. Electron microscopic picture of the base of the tubular epithelial cell layer. Histochemical chloride reactions: a) on an excised portion of tissue, showing silver chloride precipitates only in the intercellular spaces; b) on a living tubular epithelium after microperfusion of silver lactate and osmium tetroxide, showing dense intercellular and sparse intracytoplasmatic precipitates. *Bm* peritubular basal membrane. Enlargement: 34,000 times

seen in the lumens, at the brush borders and within the epithelial wall (Fig. 1b). Particularly striking features were stripes near to the base of the cell (Fig. 1c) and intensely accumulated precipitates at the terminal bars which in flat cuts appear like ornamental meanders (Fig. 1b). Their shape did not differ from the classical pictures obtained by the Swiss anatomist ZIMMERMANN [11] by iron-hematoxylin staining.

The electron microscopic pictures fully confirmed the occurrence of precipitates in the intercellular clefts (Fig. 2b) as described by other investigators [3, 6] in the salt gland of the silver gull and in the rat kidney. The stripes in the light-microscopic pictures represent such intercellular clefts which extend into the cytoplasm near to the basal labyrinth [7, 9]. Furthermore, there always were thick silver precipitates near to the terminal bars. Inasfar as such a conclusion

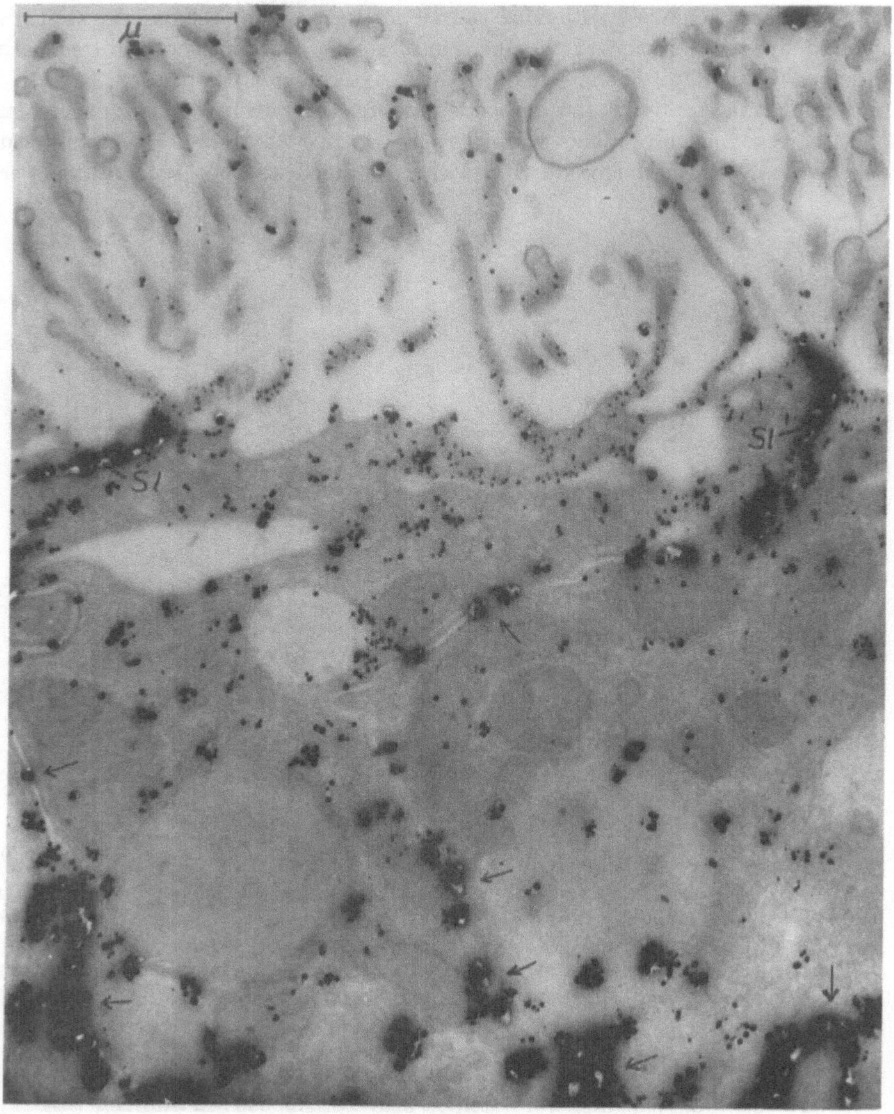

Fig. 3. Proximal tubule after vital perfusion with silver lactate-osmium tetroxide. Dense precipitates at the terminal ridges (*Sl*) and along the intercellular clefts (→). Sparse precipitates in and along the microvilli of the brush-border, as well as in the cytoplasm. Magnification: 28,000 times

is not excluded by the site of the precipitates, they appear to be related predominantly to the cement substance of the intercellular clefts. Komnick observed similar precipitates in the salt gland of the silver gull and considered their localization as a consequence of the removal of silver precipitates by filtration of the fluid streaming through the intercellular clefts through the cement substance.

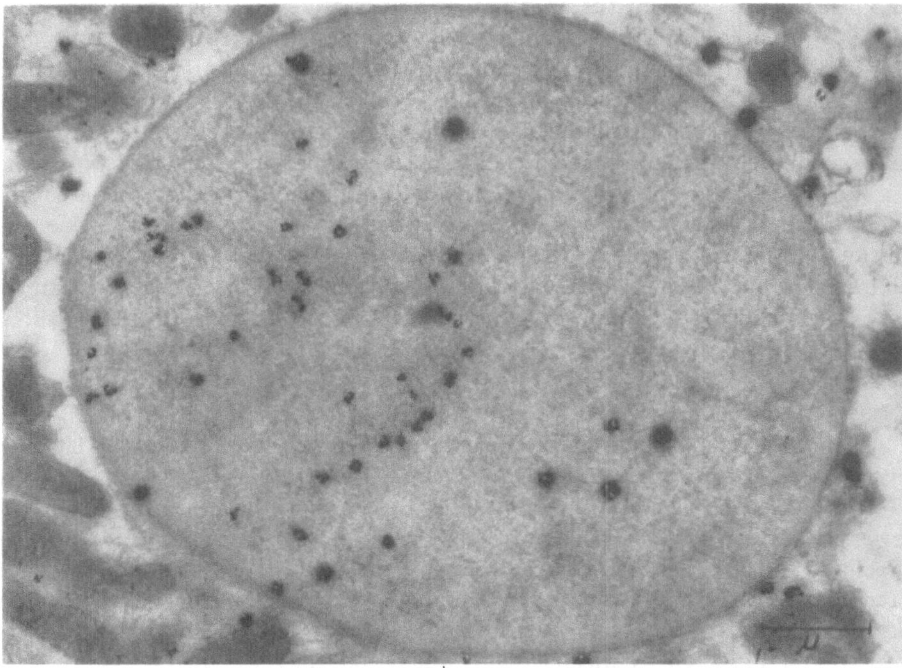

a

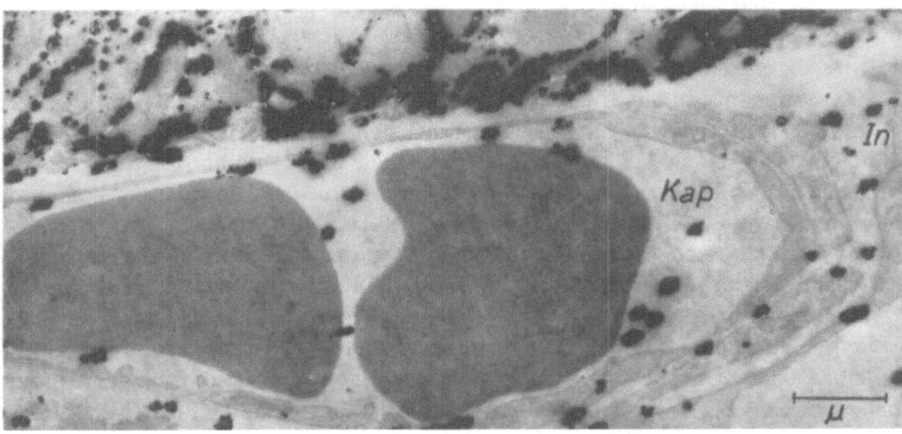

b

Fig. 4a and b. Proximal tubule after microperfusion with chloride reagent: a) Nucleus of a tubular cell with silver precipitates in the caryoplasma. Magnification: 14,000 times. b) Base of a tubular epithelium cell with dense intercellular and sparse intracellular silver precipitates, as well as medium density precipitations in the interstitial space (*In*) and within the blood capillaries (*Kap*). Enlargement: 12,000 times

When using the in vitro incubation procedure in silver lactate solution, like previous investigators [3, 6], we found silver chloride precipitates only outside the cells. In contrast, in tubules perfused by the micropuncture technique, we also succeeded regularly in demonstrating the presence of finely dispersed silver chloride precipitates within the tubular cells, particularly in the microvilli of the brush border and in the subapical region of the cell. Somewhat larger precipitates occurred in the remainder of the tubular cells. The precipitates thus were distributed throughout the whole cytoplasm without a preferential localization. They occurred in the cytoplasma as well as in mitochondria, in absorption vacuoles as well as in the nucleus (Fig. 4a). The occasional occurrence of large amounts of precipitates within the nucleus appeared interesting when compared to biochemical observations of Langendorf et al. [5]. While these authors found that the nuclei of liver cells contained up to 10 times more chloride than the cytoplasm, we could not regularly demonstrate a greater density of precipitates in nuclei. The silver chloride precipitates were also seen in the interstitia and in blood capillaries where the reagents diffused across the epithelial wall (Fig. 4b).

Discussion

The problem of the specificity of the histochemical chloride reaction has been discussed by Komnick [2, 3]; with the technical precautions taken, the formation of precipitates is probably highly specific for chlorides, when a nitric acid bath is used as described [4]. The most important initial reaction is probably the precipitation of silver chloride, as seen by the immediate formation of white precipitates in the microperfusion experiments. In drops of liquid in the tubular lumen (Gertz' "split drop" procedure) the formation of silver chloride precipitates, as observed by incident light microscopy in the living animal, is comparable to that seen in the electron microscopic preparations. We, therefore, think, like previous investigators, that the precipitates seen with our technique indicate the presence of chloride ions.

The occurrence of silver chloride precipitates within the cytoplasm of tubular cells demonstrated with a microperfusion method, and their absence after incubation of excised tissue in silver lactate solution, could be due to a postmortem extrusion of chloride from cells. Another explanation, however, seems more convincing: when comparing pictures obtained with Komnick's original method [3] on excised tissue with those obtained by microperfusion of tubules with a silver lactate solution (Fig. 2a and b), one is struck by the much greater density of precipitates in the whole picture and particularly in the intercellular space in the perfusion experiments, though the perfusions were done for only 1—2 min, while the excised tissues were bathed in the silver lactate solution for 2 hours. Our pictures, obtained with in vitro incubation in silver lactate (Fig. 2a), are strictly comparable to those published by Komnick and Komnick [3] as well as by Nolte [6]. We, therefore, think that the diffusion of the silver lactate reagent occurs much more slowly in the excised tissue. The small amounts of silver ions reaching the tissue can, thus, only demonstrate the presence of large concentrations of chloride while small amounts escape detection.

The demonstration of intracellular chloride ions in tubular cells, as opposed to the older findings, may be consistent with the assumption of a transcellular transport of chloride.

The high concentration of chloride responsible for the density of silver chloride precipitates in the intercellular clefts, in the intercellular labyrinth and in the terminal ridges appears as striking in our experiments as in those of earlier investigators. The density of precipitates at these sites is much higher than in the interstitial space known to be rich in chlorides (Fig. 4b). These findings raise the question whether certain, presumably organic substances in the intercellular spaces [10] contribute to the preferential deposition of silver chloride. We assume that the very marked precipitation at the terminal bars is due to the diffusion of chloride ions within the intercellular space towards the tubular lumen in the beginning of the tubular microperfusion with silver lactate. Here, at the terminal bars, the chloride ions are accumulated and lead to the heavy precipitate observed.

Summary

A method of cytochemical localization of chloride described by KOMNICK [2] was applied to proximal tubules of rat kidneys in vivo. After micropuncture, a solution of silver lactate (0.25% +1% OsO_4) was injected into proximal tubules both in free-flow conditions and by the "split oil drop method". With both methods white precipitates immediately occur within the lumen, as well as in the tubular epithelial wall. Precipitates can be demonstrated, by light microscopy, in the lumen, adjacent to the brush border, and within the epithelial wall. Electron microscopy confirms dense precipitations within the intercellular spaces (including the basal labyrinth) and at the terminal bars. In contrast to previous results, precipitates were also found within the cells (cytoplasma, mitochondria, absorption vacuoles and nuclei). — Considering the specificity of the reaction for chloride, our results suggest that chlorides occur not only in the intercellular spaces but also (in lower concentrations) within the cells of the tubular epithelium. An unknown intercellular organic substance might be the cause for the dense precipitation within the intercellular spaces and specially at the terminal bars.

References

1. GERTZ, H.: Transtubuläre Natriumchloridflüsse und Permeabilität für Nichtelektrolyte im proximalen und distalen Konvolut der Rattenniere. Pflügers Arch. ges. Physiol. **276**, 336—356 (1963).
2. KOMNICK, H.: Elektronenmikroskopische Lokalisation von Na^+ und Cl^- in Zellen und Geweben. Protoplasma **55**, 414—418 (1962).
3. —, u. U. KOMNICK: Elektronenmikroskopische Untersuchungen zur funktionellen Morphologie des Ionentransportes in der Salzdrüse von Larus Argentatus. Z. Zellforsch. **60**, 163—203 (1963).
4. — Zur funktionellen Morphologie der Salzsäureproduktion in der Magenschleimhaut. Histochemischer Chloridnachweis mit Hilfe der Elektronenmikroskopie. Histochemie **3**, 354—378 (1963).
5. LANGENDORF, H., G. SIEBERT, K. KESSELRING, and R. HANNOVER: High nucleo-cytoplasmic concentration gradient of chloride in rat liver. Nature (Lond.) **209**, 1130—1131 (1966).
6. NOLTE, A.: Elektronenmikroskopischer Nachweis und die Lokalisation von Natrium- und Chlorionen im proximalen Tubulusepithel der Rattenniere. In: Normale und pathologische Funktionen des Nierentubulus. III. Symp. Ges. Nephrologie, S. 299. Bern: Huber 1965.
7. RHODIN, H.: Anatomy of kidney tubules. Int. Rev. Cytol. **7**, 485—534 (1958).
8. THOENES, W.: Giemsafärbung an Geweben nach Einbettung in Poyester („Vestopal") und Methacrylat. Z. wiss. Mikr. **64**, 406—413 (1960).

9. THOENES, W.: Transportwege in den Harnkanälchen der Säugerniere. In: Funktionelle und morphologische Organisation der Zelle. Sekretion und Exkretion. 2. Wiss. Konf. Ges. Dtsch. Naturforscher und Ärzte, S. 315—341. Berlin-Heidelberg-New York: Springer 1965.

10. — Neue Befunde zur Beschaffenheit des basalen Labyrinthes im Nierentubulus. Z. Zellforsch. **86**, 351—363 (1968).

11. ZIMMERMANN, K. W.: Zur Morphologie der Epithelzellen der Säugetierniere. Arch. mikr. Anat. **78**, 199—231 (1911).

Discussion

HEIDENREICH:

I doubt, whether you may actually discuss "chloride ions" when interpreting your findings. Single ions or molecules cannot be visualized at electron microscopy. I, therefore, wonder, what threshold concentration of chloride is needed for producing the precipitates seen in your preparations? Could your precipitates be chloride-containing vacuoles or similar structures?

NOLTE:

If you had attempted a simultaneous histochemical demonstration of sodium ions, you would have found a much greater intracellular concentration of sodium as compared to chloride.

I readily admit that my observations suggest intercellular passage of chloride ions, but do not prove it. Neither do your observations prove, that this intercellular passage of chloride ions doesn't exist.

THOENES:

Our histochemical reaction is based on the precipitation of AgCl: the silver ion of this compound strongly deflects electrons. Of course, precipitates must contain much more than one molecule of AgCl to become visible at electron microscopy. The threshold sensitivity of the in vitro precipitation of Cl^- by Ag^+ has been studied to be approximately 1.0 μg Cl^-/100 ml. Our electron-microscopic finding exclude the occurrence of precipitates within vacuoles.

Miss NOLTE's objection emphasizes the difficulty of reaching conclusions on transport processes from electron-microscopic pictures. Her own conclusion as to an exclusively intercellular passage of chlorid ions was based on the absence of precipitates within the cells. In our own pictures such precipitates were found within cells, though at a much lower density and frequency than outside the cells. This leads to the conclusion that chloride ions may pass the tubular walls across the cells, but does not prove the occurrence of a transcellular passage. Our findings, thus, are compatible with the assumption of coupling of chloride fluxes to active sodium transport.

5.4. Human Renal Oxygen Comsumption and its Determinants in Intact and Impaired Function*

P. SCHOLLMEYER and H. NIETH[1]

With 3 Figures

The oxygen consumption may be considered as a measure of the energy requirement of an organ. It is exceptionally high for the kidney.

The original investigations of renal oxygen consumption in man were performed by WARREN, BRANNON and MERRILL [16], BRADLEY and HALPERIN [2] and CARGILL and HICKAM [4]. Comparing measurements of the oxygen content in renal venous blood with that in arterial blood showed a difference of 1.42—2.3 vol.-%. In spite of this small extraction, the calculated oxygen consumption is 12—20 ml/min or 4.1—6.2 ml $(100\,g\cdot min)^{-1}$ [5, 6], since there is a large renal blood flow.

In confirmation of animal experiments, results from the human kidney also show that under most conditions the arteriovenous oxygen difference remains constant. If the renal oxygen extraction varies very little, this implies that, in the human kidney also, the oxygen uptake is determined by the blood flow [2—4].

ZEHRAN's investigations [18] on frog shed light on the problem of which partial function of the tubule cells determines renal oxygen consumption. He found a stoichiometric relationship between transmembrane sodium transport and oxygen consumption. Using dog kidney DEETJEN and KRAMER [7], LASSEN, MUNCK and THAYSEN [10], KIILL et al. [9] and THURAU [15], at the same time and independently of each other, demonstrated a relation between sodium reabsorption and oxygen consumption.

A similar relationship between sodium reabsorption and oxygen consumption was sought in the present experiments in the human kidney with intact and with impaired function.

Method and Patients

The following test subjects were examined under conditions of basal metabolism: 46 healthy male volunteers between 21 and 25 years old with intact renal functions, and 74 patients with various types of impairment of renal function due to glomerulonephritis with vascular and nephrotic courses, pyelonephritis, malignant hypertension and heart failure.

Following catheterization of the renal vein, in the middle period of a standard clearance of 3×15 minutes, blood samples were taken simultaneously from the brachial artery and the right renal vein for oxygen determination. Oxygen analyses were carried out according to VAN SLYKE [14a]. Plasma and urinary sodium was determined for the corresponding period. The indications of WOLF [17] were taken into account in the calculation of renal blood flow.

* Supported by Deutsche Forschungsgemeinschaft.

[1] Medizinische Universitätsklinik Tübingen, West Germany.

Results and Discussion

The mean arteriovenous oxygen difference (AVD-O_2) for subjects with healthy kidneys was 1.57 vol.-%, corresponding to 0.699 ± 0.170 mmol/l. This gives an oxygen consumption of 0.82 ± 0.28 mmol/min. Assuming a total weight of 300 g for both kidneys, one obtains an oxygen consumption of 0.274 mmol $\cdot$ (100 g $\cdot$ min)$^{-1}$ for the healthy human kidney. This value correlates well with data given in the literature: 0.181 to 0.310 mmol $\cdot$ (100 g $\cdot$ min)$^{-1}$ [2, 4—6a].

In the group with impaired renal function, the mean AVD-O_2 was found to be 1.71 vol.-% (0.91—3.66 vol.-%), corresponding to 0.60 mmol/min. In this group, the mean kidney weight is certainly lower, but cannot be estimated.

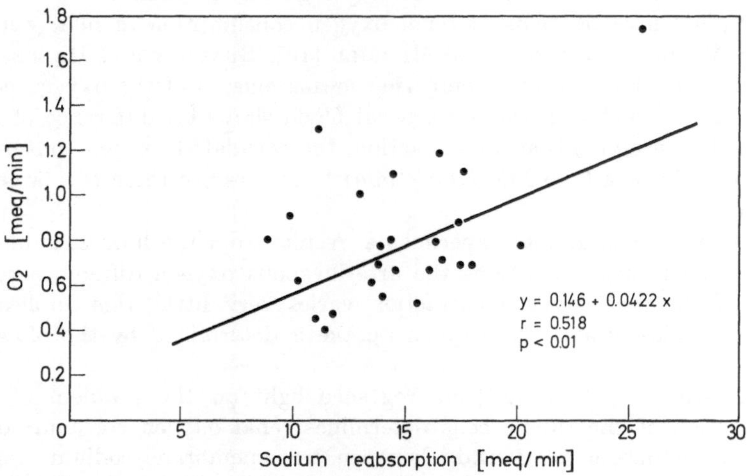

Fig. 1. Relation between sodium reabsorption and oxygen consumption in subjects with healthy kidneys. There is statistically significant difference between *r* and zero

The highest values for renal AVD-O_2 were found in patients with only one kidney, in the early recovery phase following acute renal failure, and in heart failure.

Both in the group with intact renal function and in the group with impaired renal function, there is a linear, statistically significant correlation between the renal blood flow and the oxygen uptake per minute. This result confirms those obtained in the human kidney by CARGILL and HICKAM [3] and refutes those of CROSLEY et al. [6a].

The relation between sodium reabsorption and oxygen consumption, which so far has only been demonstrated in animal experiments, is also valid for the human kidney. Fig. 1 shows this correlation for the group with healthy kidneys. One value was obtained from each experiment. We obtained reliable data from 26 experiments. Although for both sodium reabsorption and for oxygen consumption the points are grouped around a mean value, there is a statistically significant difference between the slope of the regression line and zero. The same relation is more apparent in the group of patients with impaired renal function (Fig. 2). In this group too, the correlation between sodium reabsorption and oxygen consumption is statistically significant, but the individual results show a much wider scattering comparable to that observed in animal experiments. This is due to the different experimental conditions. It is easier to keep initial and experimental conditions constant in anaesthetised animals than in test subjects who are awake. The data do not differ in distribution, even though there are different types of disorders of renal function in individual disease-group.

Assuming that the regression line is linear even for very small sodium values, its point of intersection with the ordinate gives the basal renal oxygen consumption, i.e. the oxygen used by the kidneys when no glomerular filtrate is formed and there is no absorptive activity. In the group with healthy kidneys, the basal oxygen consumption is 0.15 mmol/min, while for the group with impaired renal function it is 0.25 mmol/min. It is certainly possible that there is a higher oxygen consumption in the "diseased" kidney as a result of inflammatory

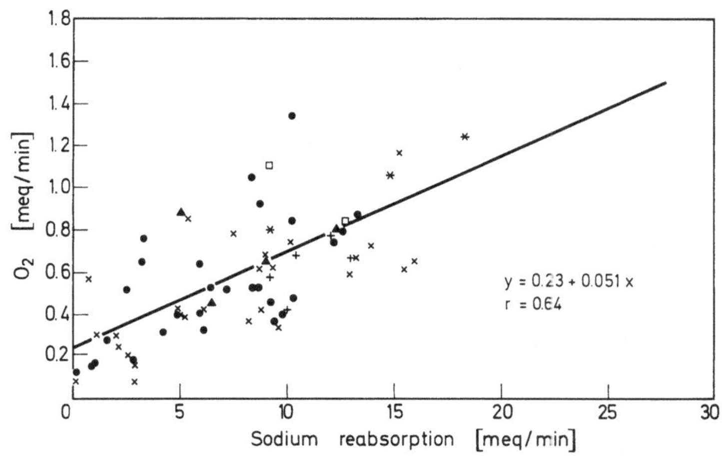

Fig. 2. Relation between sodium reabsorption and oxygen consumption in patients with diseased kidneys. There is statistically significant difference between r and zero

and reparative processes. In spite of this, this latter value seemed more reliable, because of the larger number of individual values and their distribution. This basal oxygen consumption corresponds approximately to the value of 100—110 μmol (100 g·min)$^{-1}$ obtained by LASSEN et al. [10] and DEETJEN and KRAMER [7] for the dog's kidney.

Fig. 2 also gives the quotient sodium reabsorption/oxygen consumption. In the dog's kidney this figure was found to be 6.0—8.0 [1, 7, 9, 10, 15]. From our data, after subtracting the basal oxygen consumption, Q is 5.4 for the group with impaired renal function; the quotient is 7 for the group with healthy kidneys. 1 mEq O_2 is necessary for the reabsorption of 5.4 mEq Na or 7 mEq Na. Thus, this value also corresponds approximately to the results obtained in animal experiments. It is only in the human kidney with impaired function that sodium reabsorption seems to go hand in hand with a higher oxygen consumption. This could be due to anatomical changes of the "diseased" kidney.

However, the relation between sodium reabsorption and oxygen consumption in the kidney is only indirect, since the renal oxygen uptake is governed by the substrate oxidation by which the chemical energy (probably in the form of energy-rich phosphate bonds) necessary for sodium reabsorption is made available.

As substrates the human kidney assimilates free fatty acids, lactate, pyruvate and citrate, and the oxidation of these substances supplies the energy for the transport process [11—14].

In Fig. 3 we have attempted to demonstrate that to a large extent the oxygen assimilated by the kidney is used for the oxidation of free fatty acids, lactate and pyruvate. For this purpose, in each case the oxygen required for complete oxidation of the named substrates was calculated from the amounts of substrate assimilated per unit time, and this was compared with the measured oxygen consumption. This shows there is a significant relationship between the oxygen value calculated for the substrate oxidation and the measured oxygen uptake. However, it is not known which energy-rich phosphate bond is produced by substrate oxidation in the kidney, and in what form it is involved in the process of sodium reabsorption.

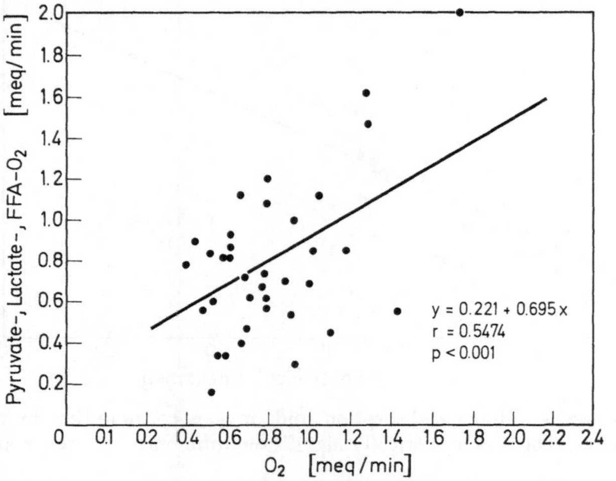

Fig. 3. Relation between oxygen consumption and substrate oxidation. Abscissa: measured oxygen consumption of kidney. Ordinate: calculated oxygen consumption necessary for complete oxidation of the assimilated free fatty acids, lactate and pyruvate. The relation is statistically significant. r differs significantly from zero

Summary

1. In 46 healthy test subjects, the renal oxygen uptake was 0.82 mmol/min. In a second group of 74 patients with impaired renal function, an oxygen consumption of 0.60 mmol/min was determined.

2. There is a linear and statistically significant relation between oxygen consumption and renal blood flow for both groups investigated.

3. That sodium reabsorption determines oxygen consumption is also valid for the human kidney. The quotient sodium reabsorption/oxygen consumption (in mEq) was 7 for subjects with healthy kidneys, and 5.4 for the group with impaired renal function.

4. In intact renal function, the basal renal oxygen consumption was determined as 0.15 mmol/min, in the group with impaired renal function it was 0.25 mmol/min.

We thank Mrs. B. HOPPE-SEYLER, Miss S. HEYL and Miss H. KUPPLER for their technical assistance.

References

1. Bálint, P., u. J. Forgacs: Natriumabsorption und Sauerstoffverbrauch der Niere bei osmotischer Belastung. Pflügers Arch. ges. Physiol. **288**, 332—341 (1966).
2. Bradley, S. E., and M. H. Halperin: Renal oxygen consumption in man during abdominal compression. J. clin. Invest. **27**, 635—638 (1948).
3. Bucht, H. L., L. Werkö, and B. Josephson: The oxygen consumption of the human kidney doing heavy tubular excretory work. Scand. J. clin. Lab. Invest. **1**, 277—280 (1949).
4. Cargill, W. H., and J. B. Hickam: The oxygen consumption of the normal and diseased human kidney. J. clin. Invest. **28**, 526—532 (1949).
5. Clark, J. K., and H. G. Barker: Studies of renal oxygen consumption in man. J. clin. Invest. **30**, 745—750 (1951).
6. Crosley, A. P., J. F. Brown, J. H. Huston, and D. A. Emanuel: The adaptation of the nitrous oxide method to the determination of renal blood flow and in vivo renal weight in man. J. clin. Invest. **35**, 1340—1344 (1956).
6a. — C. Castillo, and G. G. Rowe: The relationship of renal oxygen consumption to renal function and weight in individuals with normal and diseased kidneys. J. clin. Invest. **40**, 836—841 (1961).
7. Deetjen, P., u. K. Kramer: Die Abhängigkeit des O_2-Verbrauchs der Niere von der Na-Rückresorption. Pflügers Arch. ges. Physiol. **273**, 636—650 (1961).
8. Hess-Thaysen, J., N. A. Lassen, and O. Munck: Sodium transport and oxygen consumption in the mammalian kidney. Nature (Lond.) **190**, 919—921 (1961).
9. Kiil, F., K. Aukland, and H. E. Refsum: Renal sodium transport and oxygen consumption. Amer. J. Physiol. **201**, 511—516 (1961).
10. Lassen, N. A., O. Munck, and J. K. Thaysen: Oxygen consumption and sodium reabsorption in the kidney. Acta physiol. Scand. **51**, 371—384 (1961).
11. Nieth, H., and P. Schollmeyer: Substrate-utilization of the human kidney. Nature (Lond.) **209**, 1244—1245 (1966).
12. — — Citratstoffwechsel der menschlichen Niere. Verh. dtsch. Ges. inn. Med. **71**, 693—696 (1965).
13. Schollmeyer, P.: Untersuchungen über den Sauerstoffverbrauch und die Substratversorgung der gesunden und kranken Niere des Menschen. Habil.-Schr. Tübingen 1966.
14. —, u. H. Nieth: Untersuchungen über den Stoffwechsel der gesunden menschlichen Niere. In: Aktuelle Probleme der Nephrologie, S. 455. Berlin-Heidelberg-New York: Springer 1966.
14a. Slyke, D. D. van, and J. M. Neill: The determination of gases in blood and other solutions by vacuum extraction and manometric measurements. J. biol. Chem. **61**, 523—573 (1927).
15. Thurau, K.: Renal Na-reabsorption and O_2-uptake in dogs during hypoxia and hydrochlorothiazide infusion. Proc. Soc. exp. Biol. (N.Y.) **106**, 714—717 (1961).
16. Warren, J. V., E. S. Brannon, and A. J. Merrill: A method of obtaining renal venous blood in unanesthetized persons with observations on the extractions of oxygen and PAH. Science **100**, 108—110 (1944).
17. Wolf, A. V.: Total renal blood flow at any urine flow or extraction fraction. Amer. J. Physiol. **133**, 496—497 (1941).
18. Zehran, K.: Oxygen consumption and active sodium transport in the isolated and short-circuited frog skin. Acta physiol. scand. **36**, 300—318 (1956).

5.5. Incident-Light Microscopy of the Renal Surface During Stimulation of Sympathetic Renal Nerves*

M. Steinhausen, H. Weidinger, H. J. Ross and G. M. Eisenbach[1]

With 4 Figures

Renal nerves were first stimulated in the second half of the 19th century. This was done to clarify the role of the renal nerves in renal functions and in patho-physiological mechanisms [1, 4]. Continuing our incident-light microscopic measurements of the tubular volume flow [6, 7] we investigated the changes on the renal surface during stimulation of the renal nerves.

For this purpose the kidneys of rats or cats, anaesthetized with Inactin or pentobarbital, were fixed in a kidney container as used in micropuncture techniques. Using a stereo-microscope, a renal nerve was prepared and laid on stainless steel electrodes and was stimulated by rectangular impulses of different frequencies and voltages. An additional pair of recording electrodes was placed on the cat's renal nerves 2—5 mm distal to the stimulating electrodes. The recorder showed the spontaneous activity of the renal nerves [8] as well as the action potentials produced by electrical stimulation. Then, the renal surface was observed with a stereo-microscope (Zeiss) or with Ultropak objectives (Leitz) and microphotographed or microcinematographed. In addition, the color changes of the renal surface were recorded continuously by a microscopic photometer. For measuring the passage time of lissamine-green [5] the direct observation and the microphotometric technique were combined. The following results of our measurements on rats and cats were in close agreement with those of Block et al. [2]. The changes occurring on the renal surface after stimulation were biphasic. Initially, a pronounced vasoconstriction induced a blanching of the renal surface. The blanching was either complete or focal, depending on the distribution of the stimulated nerves and partly on the intensity of stimulation. The frequency of the stimulation determined the onset of the vasoconstriction which occured 1—2 sec after the onset of the stimulation. At increasing frequencies the onset of vasoconstriction occurred earlier and the brightness of reflected light increased, and in addition, the re-establishment of superficial blood flow was delayed (see Fig. 1). When lissamine-green was injected intra-arterially or intravenously during the blanching phase the dye reached neither the lumens of the blood vessels nor the renal tubules, as shown by cinematographic records.

The phase of blanching of the renal surface is only of short duration [2]. After 1—2 min the renal surface changed its color in spite of continuous stimulation. A similar change of color of the renal surface occurred, when the renal artery was clamped (see Fig. 2). It could be due to metabolic vasodilatation

* Supported by Deutsche Forschungsgemeinschaft.

[1] Physiologisches Institut der Universität Heidelberg, West Germany.

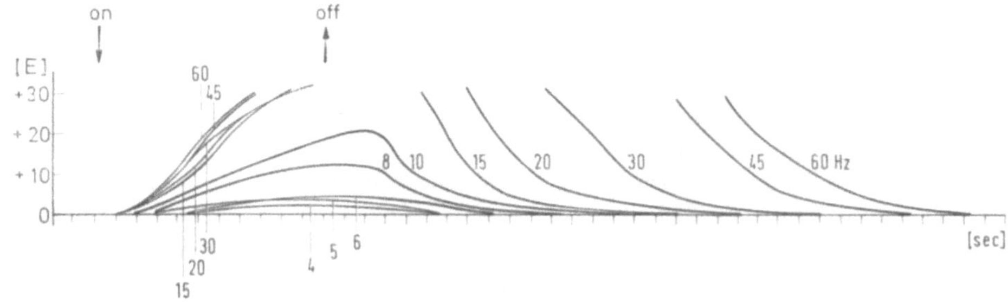

Fig. 1. Blanching of the kidney surface in relation to stimulation of kidney nerves at different frequences. Ordinate: blanching in photometer units (E); abscissa: time of blanching. The square wave pulse stimulation (1.2 V, 2 msec duration) was given between the arrows

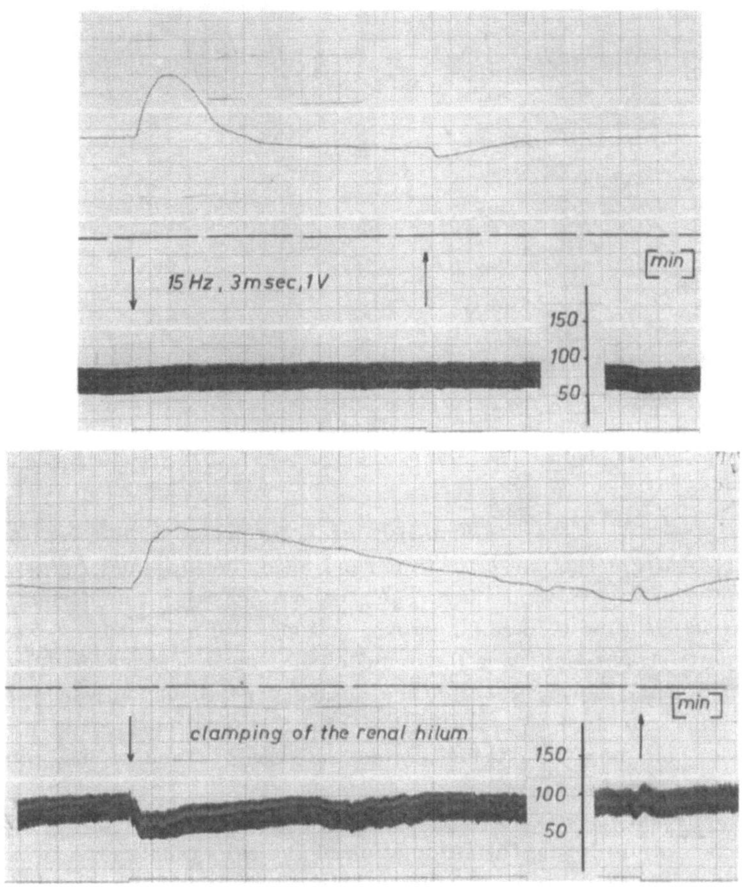

Fig. 2. Above: Reflected light recorded by microphotometry. Renal nerve stimulation between the arrows. Below: Same recording. Between the arrows clamping of the renal hilum. The beginning of the curves represents the brightness of reflected light of a normal kidney surface. Thick line: arterial blood pressure measured in carotid artery

with a consequent inflow of red blood cells containing reduced hemoglobin. In contrast to the effect of clamping of the renal artery, a true re-establishment of blood flow could be observed during the second phase of the stimulation of the renal nerves. At the beginning of this second phase (Fig. 2) red patches alternate on the renal surface with white patches, so that the total amount of light reflected from the renal surface appears normal.

If stimulation of the nerves is interrupted after 3 min, a normal circulation is rapidly re-established. However, the curve of Fig. 2 shows, that immediately after the end of the stimulus there is a transient decrease of intensity of reflected

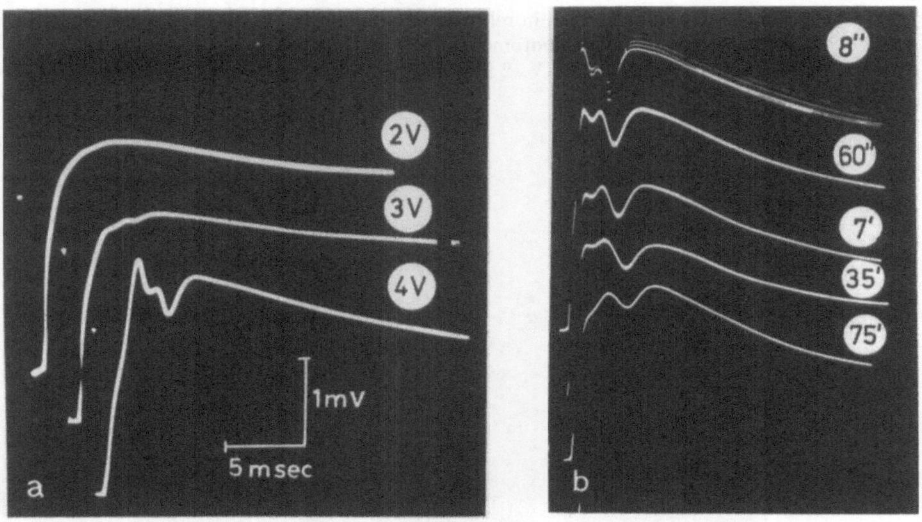

Fig. 3. Action potentials from the renal nerve after stimulation with square wave impulses (see text). Left side: Subthreshold and suprathreshold stimulation with 2, 3 and 4 V. Right side: Action potentials photographed during different times after beginning of stimulation

light. This means, that the less blanched areas are perfused with venous blood. During the return of the curve to its normal level the proximal tubules, which were collapsed in large areas, reopen. The renal surface attains its normal appearance; the passage time of lissamine-green becomes normal again.

Continuous stimulation caused an incomplete vasoconstriction during 1 to a maximum of 2 hrs. During this time the vasoconstriction response decreased continuously; the extent of the spotted areas on the renal surface, in which the tubules were collapsed, diminished, while the passage time of lissamine-green was gradually normalized.

An explanation of the shortness of the two phases was sought by recording the action potentials during the stimulation of the cat's renal nerve by a second pair of electrodes. The results are shown in Figs. 3a and b. Fig. 3a depicts the measurement of threshold intensity of stimulation (upper lines: subthreshold stimulation; middle: threshold stimulation; lower lines: suprathreshold stimulation; all stimulations at 15 Hz, 1 msec). An action potential occurred simultaneously with the beginning of the first phase of complete vasoconstriction. This phase, therefore, may be a consequence of the stimulation of the renal nerve. In Fig. 3b evoked action potentials are shown at different times after the beginning of the stimulation (to a max. of 75 min). During the first phase and during the beginning of the second phase of vascular response, the action potential showed no changes, consequently, the spontaneous activity of the renal sympathetic nerves was unchanged. The decreased vasoconstriction during this time therefore is not caused by local changes in the area of the stimulating electrodes. A change in the action potential (sometimes a complete loss in action potential) was observed near the end of the second phase of the microscopically visible vasoconstriction. One drop of a 0.5% solution of procaine blocked the action potential.

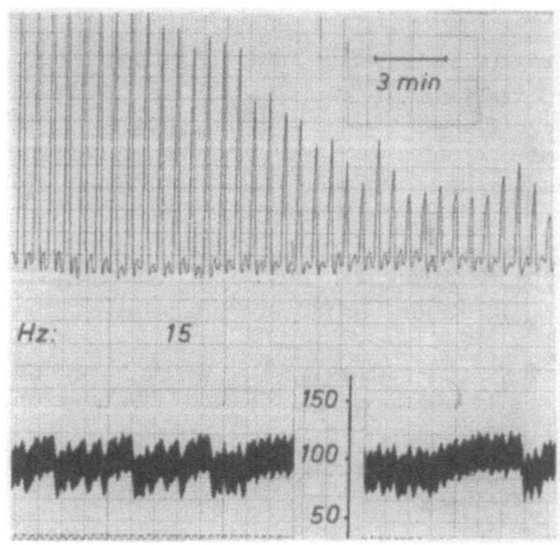

Fig. 4. Original recording of decrease of renal blanching (see Fig. 2) during repeated kidney nerve stimulation. Stimulation with alternating polarization and a duration of 10 seconds each, with a following pause of 10 seconds. Only when the cathode was proximal to the kidney, was the stimulation successful

In animals, reserpinized or applied with dibenzyline nerve stimulation did not induce vasoconstriction.

The first phase could not continously be repeated (Fig. 4). This depends on a deficiency of the transmitter substance but not on a failure of the receptors, because the application of noradrenaline before and after stimulation has the same blanching effect.

Summary

During renal nerve stimulation changes of tubular flow (passage time of lissamine-green) and renal blood flow on the renal surface of cats and rats were measured using incident-light microscopic and microphotometric techniques. 1—2 sec after the onset of the stimulation a complete vasoconstriction occurred, which induced a tubular collapse (first phase). In spite of continuous stimulation the amount of the vasoconstriction response decreased after approximately 1 min, but was still visible on the renal surface as spotted areas of collapsed tubules during 1 to a maximum of 2 hrs. In the first min of stimulation no changes in action potential were seen, but after this time, while passage times of lissamine-green were normalized, changes in action potential occurred. In animals reserpinized or treated with dibenzyline, nerve stimulation did not induce vasoconstriction. The first phase could not often be repeated. This depends on a deficiency of the transmitter substance but not on a failure of the receptors.

References

1. BALINT, P.: Aktuelle Probleme der Nierenphysiologie. Berlin: VEB Verlag Volk und Gesundheit 1961.
2. BLOCK, M. A., K. G. WAKIM, and F. C. MANN: Circulation through kidney during stimulation of the renal nerves. Amer. J. Physiol. **169**, 659—669 (1952).
3. — — — Renal function during stimulation of renal nerves. Amer. J. Physiol. **169**, 670—677 (1952).
4. SARRE, H., u. A. MOENCH: Funktionelle und morphologische Veränderungen der Niere durch chronischen Nervenreiz. Z. ges. exp. Med. **117**, 49—95 (1951).
5. STEINHAUSEN, M.: Eine Methode zur Differenzierung proximaler und distaler Tubuli der Nierenrinde von Ratten in vivo und ihre Anwendung zur Bestimmung tubulärer Strömungsgeschwindigkeiten. Pflügers Arch. ges. Physiol. **277**, 23—35 (1963).
6. — Messungen des tubulären Harnstromes und der tubulären Reabsorption unter erhöhtem Ureterdruck. Pflügers Arch. ges. Physiol. **298**, 105—130 (1967).
7. — A. LORETH u. S. OLSON: Messungen des tubulären Harnstromes, seine Beziehungen zum Blutdruck und zur Inulin-Clearance. Pflügers Arch. ges. Physiol. **286**, 118—141 (1965).
8. WEIDINGER, H., L. FEDINA u. H. KEHREL: Der Einfluß von Adrenalin auf die Tätigkeit des „Sympathicus". Pflügers Arch. ges. Physiol. **278**, 229—240 (1963).

6. Miscellaneous

6.1. Balance of Electrolytes and Sodium Rejection after Sodium Depletion by Means of Peritoneal Dialysis or of Repeated Mannitol Infusions

D. W. BEHRENBECK, A. DÖRGE and H. W. REINHARDT[1]

With 3 Figures

The mode of sodium excretion responsible for the maintenance of sodium balance is still unknown. Changes in glomerular filtration, mineralocorticoid-activity or in plasma sodium concentration do not explain adequately the mechanism controlling balanced salt- and water-metabolism. LADD (1949), DE WARDENER (1961) and LEVINSKY (1963) suggest that an increase in the volume of ECF releases a natriuretic factor, and that sodium excretion is regulated by volume changes of ECF and not by the sodium-ion. In contrast to these results it was found that in dogs kept on low sodium diet the volume expansion of ECF which always follows ingestion of food does not induce an increase of sodium excretion (BEHRENBECK and REINHARDT, 1967). It was observed also that an increase of intracellular sodium concentration and of sodium rejection occurred after feeding of high sodium amounts (BEHRENBECK, LENGAS and KRAMER, 1966). The following experiments were done in order to investigate whether a depletion of intracellular sodium concentration causes a simultaneous decrease of renal sodium rejection.

Methods

As in previous experiments unanaesthetized female mongrel dogs received a standardized low sodium diet with 0.5 to 0.8 mEq sodium per kg body weight and per day (REINHARDT and BEHRENBECK, 1967). The sodium and potassium balances were controlled daily. 6 g-% mannitol were given to each dog intravenously (5 ml/min) for 3 hours on six consecutive days starting in the morning after feeding. During the time of infusion the urine volume, the GFR (by means of inulin clearance), the sodium concentration of plasma and the tubular sodium rejection were examined. In another experiment peritoneal dialysis with isotonic glucose-potassium solution was performed to produce a sodium depletion. This was followed by subsequent observation of the daily sodium and potassium balance. In some of these experiments the inulin space as an indicator of the physiological active volume of extracellular fluid, the GFR and the tubular sodium rejection were checked preprandially several days before and after dialysis.

Results

In three animals on a low sodium diet who received mannitol infusion on six days, a definite increase in urinary output up to 5.0 ml/min resulted as com-

[1] Physiologisches Institut der Universität München, West Germany.

pared to 1.68 ml/min in the previous control period without mannitol infusion (Fig. 1). There was an extracellular volume expansion and the fluid was hypotonic in respect to sodium. This was caused by the postprandial expansion as well as by osmosis. On the first day a remarkable increase in sodium excretion was noticed mainly during the mannitol infusion resulting in a negative sodium balance.

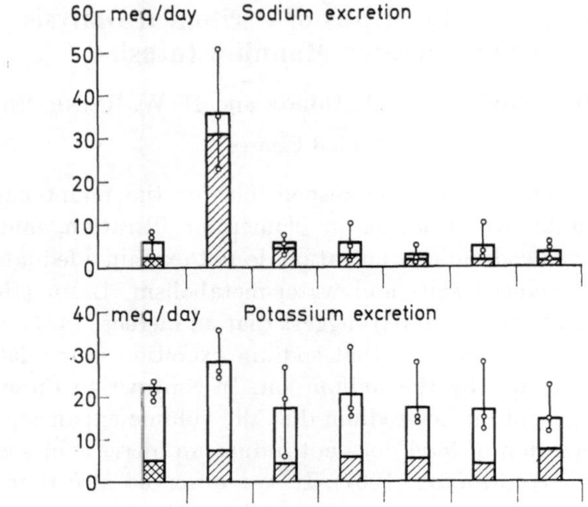

	Contr.	1st	2nd	3rd	4th	5th	6th
Urine volume ml/min	1.68	5.53	4.70	5.00	5.40	5.40	5.33
GFR ml/min	71.6	58.7	57.3	56.9	55.7	59.4	59.4
Plasma-Na meq/l	135.7	130.1	128.3	130.4	130.5	131.6	130.2
Na-rejection % of load	0.23	2.67	0.20	0.27	0.11	0.11	0.14

Day with mannitol infusion

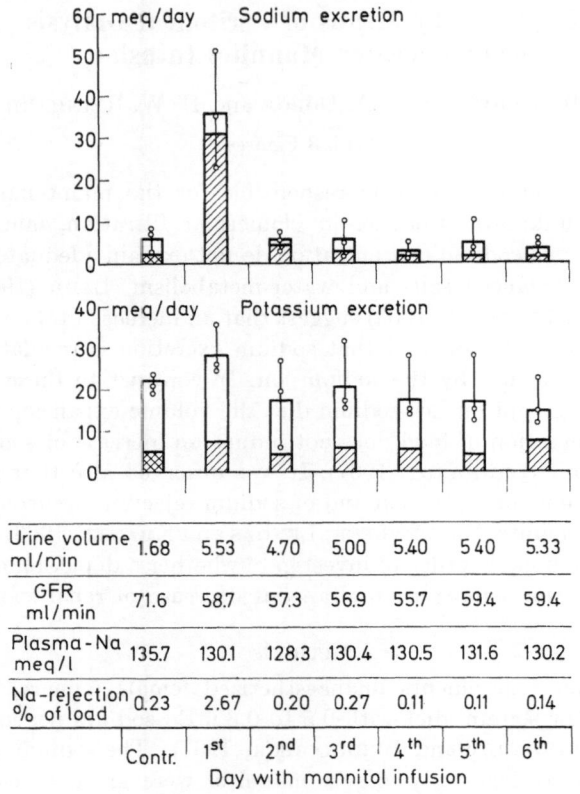

Fig. 1. Sodium and potassium excretion (mEq/day) during low sodium diet and daily postprandial administration of mannitol infusion (6 g-%; 5 ml/min; 3 hours). ▩ Sodium excretion during the control period. ▨ Sodium excretion during mannitol infusion. Urine volume, GFR, plasma sodium concentration and sodium rejection are measured during mannitol infusion or control period. (3 experiments)

In the subsequent days, the sodium balance as well as the sodium excretion during the osmotic diuresis was within the range of the control values. The potassium balance did not exhibit any changes except for a slightly increased excretion on the first day. During each period of infusion the GFR decreased (by about 20%) as well as the sodium load. The latter was caused by a slight decrease in the plasma sodium concentration. On the first day the rejection of sodium equaled the degree of its excretion. Subsequently the sodium rejection decreased, while the sodium excretion remained within the range of premannitol infusion values. In other words, no correlation could be established between the GFR and the sodium excretion on the basis of these results.

On the second day, and thereafter, the sodium excretion did not increase in spite of the osmotic diuresis. This might be caused by:

1. a decrease in total amount of body sodium resulting from the sodium loss on the first day due to osmotic diuresis. If this assumption is correct, it should be expected that the first mannitol diuresis performed after sodium depletion by peritoneal dialysis would not cause any further increase in sodium excretion.

2. An increased response to mineralocorticoids. This should be inhibited by spirolactone.

In order to investigate these possibilities two experiments were performed with unanaesthetized dogs (Fig. 2). 6.1 mEq sodium per kg body weight was with-

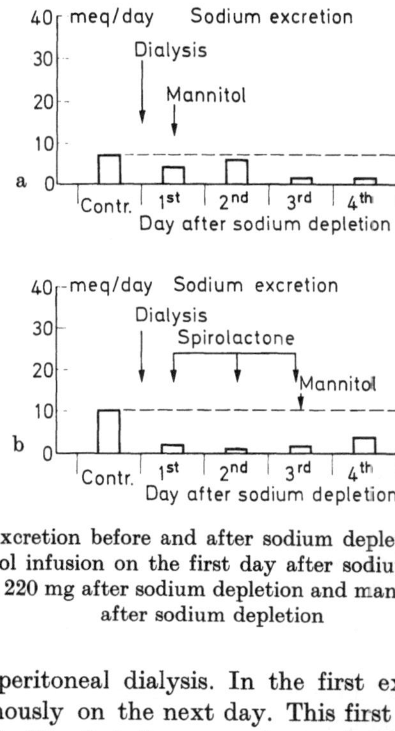

Fig. 2a and b. Sodium excretion before and after sodium depletion by means of peritoneal dialysis. a) With mannitol infusion on the first day after sodium depletion. b) With spirolactone at a daily dose of 220 mg after sodium depletion and mannitol infusion on the 4th day after sodium depletion

drawn by means of peritoneal dialysis. In the first experiment mannitol was administered intravenously on the next day. This first osmotic diuresis did not enhance the natriuresis (Fig. 2a). In a second experiment spirolactone was given at a daily dose of 220 mg after sodium depletion by peritoneal dialysis. However, it was not possible to shift the sodium excretion from the low rate to a high rate of excretion by spirolactone, although it is generally understood that spirolactone inhibits the tubular response to mineralocorticoids.

In another series of ten experiments the animals were kept on a low sodium diet and were depleted of sodium by dialysis. They lost $^1/_5$ of their total body sodium. After sodium depletion the renal sodium excretion decreased markedly from 8 mEq/day to 2 mEq/day. That means that there was a positive balance by a minimal sodium intake of 8 mEq/day. A loss of potassium did not occur. However, the potassium balance was sometimes positive (Fig. 3).

In three of the experiments just described GFR, volume of ECF, sodium load and tubular sodium rejection were determined (Table 1). The GFR increased while a distinct decrease in sodium excretion took place simultaneously. Here again no correlation can be seen between GFR and sodium excretion. Compared with the control period the sodium load remained constant after a slight increase on the first day. Because of that the decrease in excretion can be attributed only to the increase in tubular sodium reabsorption.

A quantitative estimation of the extracellular sodium before and after sodium depletion can be obtained by calculating the sodium balance and determining

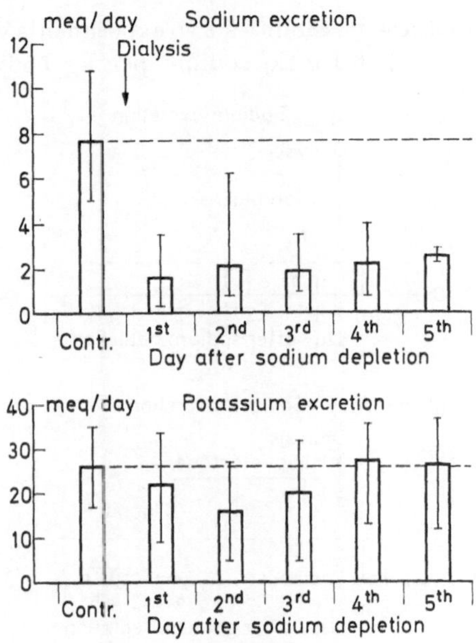

Fig. 3. Sodium and potassium excretion before and after sodium depletion (6.1 mEq/kg body weight) by means of peritoneal dialysis in 10 experiments

the volume of ECF and the plasma sodium concentration. 36 hours after sodium depletion an increase of extracellular sodium may be observed although there is no sodium intake at all (Table 2). This is probably due to a simultaneous decrease in intracellular sodium.

The sodium rejection after sodium loading increases to 1.5% and even 3.9% as compared to 0.1% of sodium load during low sodium diet. There is a simultaneous increase in intracellular sodium of 22 mEq max. 144 mEq (Table 3). On the

Table 1. *Sodium rejection values before and after sodium depletion by peritoneal dialysis in 3 experiments*

	Control	Days after sodium depletion			
Na-excretion (μEq/min)	9.8	3.0	4.3	3.6	4.2
GFR (ml/min)	66.0	76.3	71.1	67.8	61.8
Plasma-Na (mEq/l)	146.0	143.8	140.6	136.8	142.4
Na-load (mEq/min)	9.6	12.2	10.0	9.3	8.8
Na-rejection (% of load)	0.137	0.025	0.045	0.041	0.046

Table 2. *Sodium balance and changes of intracellular and extracellular sodium after sodium depletion by peritoneal dialysis in 3 experiments*

	Δ ECF-Na (mEq)	Na-balance (mEq)	Δ ICF-Na (mEq)
2 hours after sodium depletion	−105.3	−112.9	−7.9
36 hours after sodium depletion	+52.8	−3.5	−56.3

Table 3. *Changes in intracellular sodium and the rate of tubular sodium rejection during low sodium diet, after sodium loading and after sodium depletion*

	ICF-Na (mEq)	Na-rejection (% of load)
After Na-loading	+22 to +144	1.54 to 3.94
During low Na-diet	±0	0.071 to 0.231
After Na-depletion	−36.8 to −94.7	0.015 to 0.079

other hand, the sodium rejection is decreased after sodium depletion. In this event values of 0.015 to 0.079% of sodium load were found. At the same time a decrease in intracellular sodium amounting to between −36.8 and −94.7 mEq was observed in these experiments (Table 3).

In summary no significant correlation between GFR, mineralocorticoid-activity and extracellular volume on the one hand, and sodium excretion on the other hand, could be established after sodium depletion. There is some evidence, that a correlation between the intracellular sodium concentration and sodium rejection exists under the experimental conditions described. These experiments, however, do not explain which mechanism directly or indirectly controls the regulation of sodium excretion mediated by intracellular sodium concentration of the tubular cell.

References

1. Behrenbeck, D. W., u. H. W. Reinhardt: Untersuchungen an wachen Hunden über die Einstellung der Natriumbilanz. II. Mitt. Postprandiale Elektrolyt- und Wasserbilanzen bei unterschiedlicher Kochsalzzufuhr. Pflügers Arch. ges. Physiol. **295**, 280—292 (1967).
2. — A. Lengas u. K. Kramer: Die Einstellung einer ausgeglichenen Natriumbilanz bei wachen Hunden in Abhängigkeit von der Größe des Extrazellulärraumes und der extraintrazellulären Elektrolytverteilung. Pflügers Arch. ges. Physiol. **289**, 80 (1966).
3. Ladd, M.: Renal excretion of sodium and water in man as affected by prehydration saline infusion, pitressin and thiomerin. J. appl. Physiol. **4**, 602—619 (1952).
4. —, and L. G. Raisz: Response of the normal dog to dietary sodium chloride. Amer. J. Physiol. **159**, 149—152 (1949).
5. Levinsky, N., and R. C. Lalone: The mechanism of sodium diuresis after saline loading: evidence for a factor other than increased filtered sodium and decreased aldosteron. J. clin. Invest. **42**, 951 (1963).
6. Reinhardt, H. W., u. D. W. Behrenbeck: Untersuchungen an wachen Hunden über die Einstellung der Natriumbilanz. I. Mitt. Die Bedeutung des Extrazellulärraumes für die Einstellung der Natriumtagesbilanz. Pflügers Arch. ges. Physiol. **295**, 266—279 (1967).
7. Wardener, H. E. de, J. H. Mills, W. F. Clapham, and C. J. Hayter: Studies on the efferent mechanism of the sodium diuresis which follows the administration of intravenous saline in the dog. Clin. Sci. **21**, 249—258 (1961).

6.2. A Micropuncture Investigation of the Effect of Parathormone on Proximal Tubular Fluid Reabsorption in the Rat Kidney*

D. Gekle, D. Rostock and G. Kurth[1]

With 3 Figures

In spite of a great number of investigations on the mechanism of action of parathormone (PTH), its biochemical action and its site of impact within the cell are not yet fully understood.

Particularly, the renal actions of the hormone appear confusing. Its phosphaturic effect has been known for a long time [1, 12, 17]. Micropuncture investigations [3, 6] have shown that its mechanism is an inhibition of proximal tubular phosphate reabsorption. Contradictory conclusions were reached by different investigators [4, 9, 15, 18, 20] who tried to elucidate whether a secretory transport of phosphate occurs in mammals. Such a transport is known to occur in some species of fishes [19], reptiles [11] and birds [16]. There are, furthermore, reports [2, 5, 10] on an enhanced urinary excretion of sodium, potassium, citrate, chloride, bicarbonate, sulfate and water under the influence of PTH which is also said to enhance the urinary excretion of amino-acids [14] and of magnesium [8], to increase the urinary pH and to depress the renal excretion of calcium.

Since a possible influence of parathormone on the renal transport of sodium and of water would be important, this phenomenon was investigated in the present experiments, using micropuncture methods and studying fluid reabsorption from the proximal tubule of the rat.

Under conventional free flow micropuncture conditions, inulin-TF/P values were measured before and again 100—150 min after injecting 20 USP-U of parathormone (Para-Thor-Mone, E. Lilly) by the i.m. route. Inulin-I^{131} (Farbwerke Hoechst, A.G., Frankfurt, West Germany) was used. The animals were given an i.v. priming dose of 150 μC, followed by the infusion of 150 μC dissolved in 1,5 ml 0,9% NaCl per hour. Puncture sites were localized at the end of experiments by injection of latex and by measuring the length of the tubules from the glomeruli to the puncture sites.

Results are shown in Fig. 1. The ordinate gives the inulin TF/P ratios, while the abscissa shows the percent length of proximal tubules. Full dots represent specimens obtained before injecting parathormone, open circles specimens obtained under parathormone. The total ranges of variation are shown by the hand-drawn lines. It appears clearly that parathormone significantly depresses the figures around 1.5. The hormone thus appears to inhibit transtubular fluid reabsorption. Glomerular filtration rate did not change in the course of any

* Supported by the Deutsche Forschungsgemeinschaft.

[1] Universitäts-Kinderklinik Würzburg, West Germany.

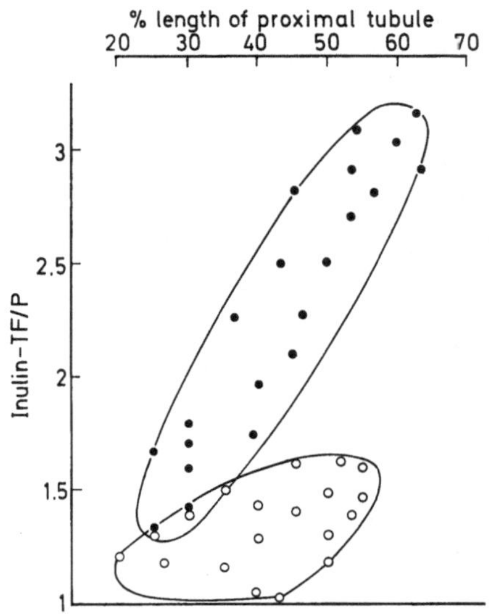

Fig. 1. Inulin TF/P ratios as a function of proximal tubular length. Full dots: values before parathormone, open circles: after injection of 20 USP units of parathormone

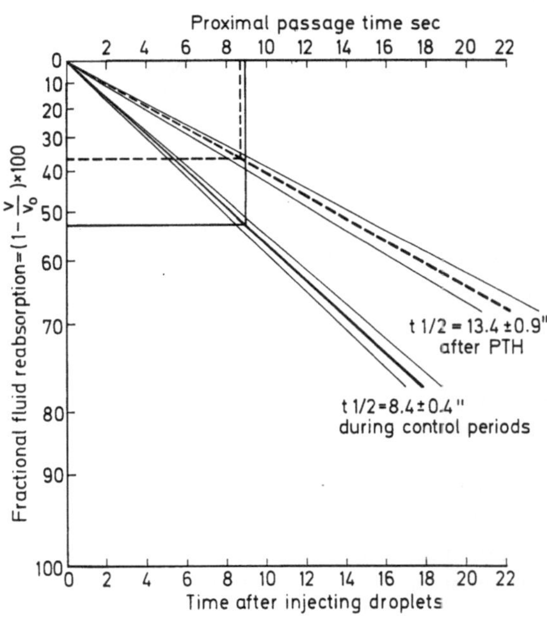

Fig. 2. Graphic measurement of proximal fractional fluid reabsorption. The lines shown are the absorption lines before and after injecting 20 USP units of PTH. If a vertical line is drawn from the passage time to the absorption line, the corresponding ordinate value shows the fractional reabsorption of fluid and sodium at the end of the proximal convolution

single experiment; its mean value was 6.6 ml/kg/min at the beginning of the experiments and 7.0 ml/kg/min under the influence of parathormone.

In another series of investigations, we studied the influence of parathormone on fluid reabsorption by the split oil droplet method of GERTZ. A droplet of isotonic NaCl solution was injected between two columns of oil and its rate of disappearance was measured. The half-time of disappearance [$(t/2)$ according to GERTZ [7] and HIERHOLZER et al. [13]] varies between 8 and 9 sec. In our

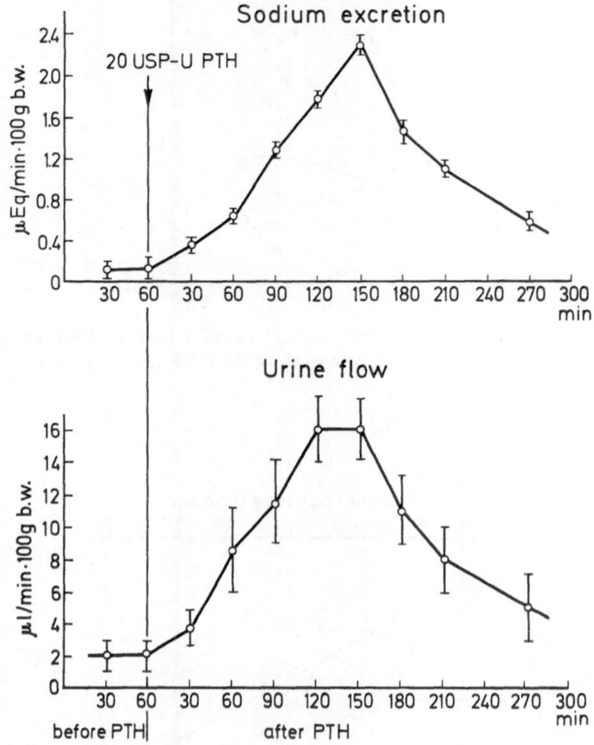

Fig. 3. The influence of parathormone (20 USP units) on urine flow and sodium excretion in normal rats

experiments, it was 8.4 ± 0.4 sec during the control periods and increased to $13.4 \pm 0{,}9$ sec under the influence of parathormone. The fluid reabsorption was thus clearly inhibited. As shown by GERTZ, the fractional reabsorption can be calculated from the half time of isotonic fluid in the split column-method and from the proximal tubular passage time as measured with lissamine-green. We used the graphic method proposed by HIERHOLZER et al .[13]. The results of such experiments are given in Fig. 2. The figure shows the reabsorption lines before and after the injection of 20 USP-units of parathormone. The ordinate shows the fractional reabsorption. During the control period the proximal passage time was 9.0 ± 0.8 sec and the proximal fractional reabsorption 52%. The passage time after parathormone did not change significantly (8.8 ± 0.9 sec) while the fractional reabsorption fell to 36%. These data confirm a depression of the reabsorptive capacity of the proximal tubules under the influence of parathormone. A fractional reabsorption of 36% at the end of the proximal convolutions corresponds roughly to an inulin-TF/P value of 1.5 which we measured independently. (An inulin TF/P value of 3.0 corresponds to the fractional reabsorption of 66% of GFR.)

Fig. 3 shows the influence of PTH on urine flow and on sodium excretion. The ordinate shows the urine flow in µl/min/100 g b.w. or the sodium excretion in µEq/min/100 g b.w., the abscissa the time in minutes. The urine flow before parathormone was 2.0 µl/min, sodium excretion 0.12 µEq/min. After 30 min, there was a significant increase in urine flow and sodium excretion; both reached their maximal value after 100—150 min and subsequently fell continuously. A slight effect persisted 5 hours after injection. The serum sodium concentration did not change in the course of these experiments.

These observations show that parathormone inhibits proximal tubular sodium and fluid reabsorption. In spite of the pronounced inhibition, only a relatively small function (2.2%) of filtered sodium is excreted at the peak of the diuretic response. The inhibition of proximal reabsorption must, therefore, be partially compensated distally. The data do not show whether the inhibition of reabsorption is due to a primary depression of the transport capacity for sodium ions or to a primary effect on membrane permeability. Investigations on renal mitochondria showed that parathormone alters the permeability of the inner mitochondrial membrane [2, 5]. It would, therefore, be conceivable that the hormone exerts an analogous effect on cell membranes.

Summary

Micropuncture investigations demonstrated an inhibitory effect of parathormone on proximal tubular sodium and fluid reabsorption. This effect results in an increase in urine flow and enhanced excretion of sodium. GFR is not influenced by parathormone.

References

1. Albright, F.: The parathyroids-physiology and therapeutics. J. Amer. med. Ass. **117**, 527—530 (1941).
2. Arnaud, C. D., A. M. Tenenhouse, and H. Rasmussen: Parathyroid hormone. Ann. Rev. Physiol. **29**, 349—372 (1967).
3. Carone, F. A.: Micropuncture study of renal phosphate excretion and action of parathyroid hormone. Clin. Res. **12**, 249 (1964).
4. Carrasquer, G., and W. A. Brodsky: Elimination of transient secretion of phosphate by alkalinization of plasma in dogs. Amer. J. Physiol. **201**, 499—504 (1961).
5. Fischer, J. A.: Die Wirkungsweise des Parathormons. Schweiz. med.Wschr. **96**, 273—278, 321—327 (1966).
6. Gekle, D., u. K. Kossmann: Der Einfluß von Thyreocalcitonin auf die Phosphatreabsorption der Niere (Mikropunktionsuntersuchungen). Mschr. Kinderheilk. **116**, 308—310 (1968).
7. Gertz, K. H., J. A. Mangos, G. Braun, and H. D. Pagel: On the glomerular tubular balance in the rat kidney. Pflügers Arch. ges. Physiol. **285**, 360—372 (1965).
8. Gill, J. R., N. H. Bell, and F. C. Bartter: Effect of parathyroid extract on magnesium excretion in man. J. appl. Physiol. **22**, 136—138 (1967).
9. Handler, J. S.: A study of renal phosphate excretion in the dog. Amer. J. Physiol. **202**, 787—794 (1962).

10. Hellman, D. E., W. Y. W. Au, and F. C. Bartter: Evidence for a direct effect of parathyroid hormone on urinary acidification. Amer. J. Physiol. **209**, 643—650 (1965).
11. Hernandez, T., and R. A. Coulson: Renal clearance in the alligator. Fed. Proc. **15**, 91—94 (1956).
12. Hiatt, H. H., and D. D. Thompson: The effects of parathyroid extract on renal function in man. J. clin. Invest. **36**, 557—572 (1957).
13. Hierholzer, K., M. Wiederholt u. H. Stolte: Hemmung der Natriumresorption im proximalen und distalen Konvolut adrenalektomierter Ratten. Pflügers Arch. ges. Physiol. **291**, 43—62 (1966).
14. Hillman, D. A., C. R. Scriver, S. Redvis, and J. Shragovitch: Neonatal familial primary hyperparathyroidism. New Engl. J. Med. **270**, 483—487 (1964).
15. Kleeman, C. R., and R. E. Cooke: The acute effects of parathyroid hormone on the metabolism of endogenous phosphate. J. Lab. clin. Med. **38**, 112—127 (1951).
16. Levinsky, N. G., and D. G. Davidson: Renal action of parathyroid extract in the chicken. Amer. J. Physiol. **191**, 530—536 (1957).
17. Pullman, T. N., A. R. Lavender, J. Aho, and H. Rasmussen: Direct renal action of a purified parathyroid extract. Endocrinology **67**, 570—582 (1960).
18. Samiy, A. H., P. F. Hirsch, and A. G. Ramsay: Localization of phosphaturic effect of parathyroid hormone in nephron of the dog. Amer. J. Physiol. **208**, 73—77 (1965).
19. Smith, W. W.: The excretion of phosphate in the dog fish, Squalus acanthias. J. cell. comp. Physiol. **14**, 95—98 (1939).
20. Strickler, J. C., D. D. Thompson, R. M. Klose, and G. Giebisch: Micropuncture study of inorganic phosphate excretion in the rat. J. clin. Invest. **43**, 1596—1607 (1964).

6.3. The Influence of an Intravenous Glucose Load on Renal Sodium Excretion*

H. E. Renschler, D. Jaenkner, E. Kammerer and R. Thoma[1]

With 2 Figures

Interrelationships between glucose and sodium transport have been demonstrated in many biological membranes. It was the purpose of the present experiments to investigate the influence of an increased glucose load on the urinary excretion of sodium and potassium. The experiments were done in the course of studies on the renal glucose threshold.

Methods

The experimental subjects were 21 healthy male volunteers, engaged in sport activities, and aged from 19 to 28 years. On the 3 days preceding the experiments, the subjects were given 250 g per day of glucose in addition to their normal diet. The experiments were done in the morning on an empty stomach. A rapid rate of urine flow was induced by giving tea at the rate of 12.5 ml per min, at equally spaced intervals. The rate of urine flow was always maintained above 10 ml/min. The subjects then received an intravenous injection of 0.5 g/kg of glucose given within 3—5 min. Urine was collected through an indwelling catheter, at 10 min intervals during the 1st hour, and at 15 min intervals during the 2nd hour after injecting glucose. Simultaneously, the plasma glucose concentration was measured in capillary blood plasma. Venous blood was obtained at 40 min intervals.

Glucose was assayed enzymatically by the hexokinase-glucose-6-phosphate-dehydrogenase method, creatinine by a modification of Løken's method [4, 5], sodium and potassium by flame photometry. Statistical computations were done on an IBM 360 computer belonging to the Recheninstitut der Universität Köln. One of the experiments had to be interrupted for technical reasons, so that the total number of subjects investigated was reduced to 20. In a control experiment, seven of the subjects were submitted to a similar procedure in which the glucose solution was replaced by a 20% mannitol solution.

Results

The mean rates of urine flow and urinary excretion of glucose, sodium and potassium are shown in Fig. 1. The timing of the glucose injection, after the beginning of an experiment, varied from one subject to the next; for this reason, all timings were related to the time of the glucose injection. Whenever urine

* Supported by Deutsche Forschungsgemeinschaft and grants-in-aid of C. F. Boehringer Söhne, Mannheim, and Deutsche Maizena Werke GmbH, Hamburg.

1 Medizinische Universitätsklinik Köln, West Germany.

collection periods before the injection of glucose differed from 15 min, they were transformed, by interpolation, into 15 min periods.

As shown in Fig. 1, urine flow rose progressively in the pre-injection periods and reached, at the time of injection, a mean value of 14.6 ml/min, with an SD of 4.0 ml/min. 20 min after the injection of glucose the urine flow decreased

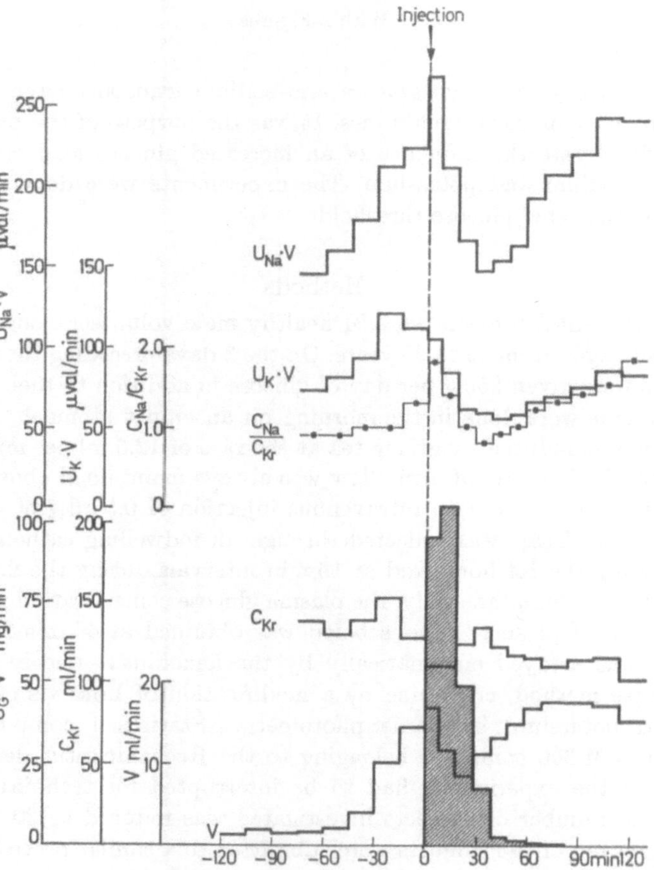

Fig. 1. Urinary excretion of sodium and potassium, fractional excretion of sodium, urinary clearance of creatinine, and urine flow before and after the i.v. injection of glucose in 20 healthy subjects. The figure shows mean values at times calculated backward and forward from the time of injection

transiently, presumably as a consequence of the secretion of vasopressin induced by the hyperosmolar glucose solution. Glucose excretion, as shown by the gray surface, began immediately after the injection and was terminated 60 min later. The clearance of creatinine rose for a very short time, presumably by a washout-effect, and remained stable thereafter. The most surprising finding was, however, the change in urinary excretion of sodium shown in the uppermost tracing of Fig. 1. With a progressively increasing rate of urine flow, in the pre-injection period, the excretion of sodium increased. The injection of glucose was followed by a pronounced fall of the sodium excretion rate which lasted longer than the transient antidiuresis.

When sodium excretion was expressed as a fraction of the filtered sodium load (computed by assuming that the clearance of creatinine was identical with the GFR), it became clear that the progressive decrease in sodium reabsorption under continuous hydration, was interrupted and reversed after an i.v. injection of glucose.

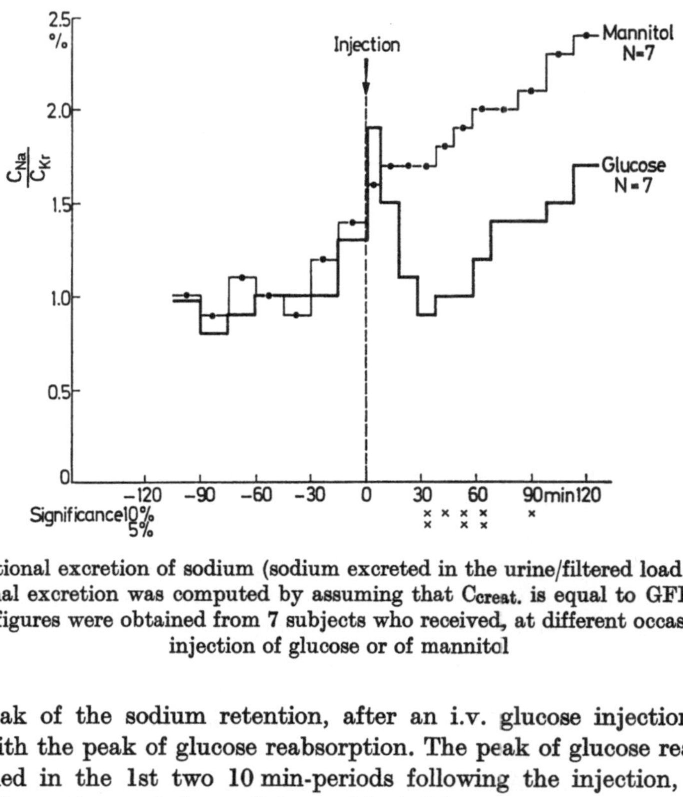

Fig. 2. Fractional excretion of sodium (sodium excreted in the urine/filtered load of sodium). The fractional excretion was computed by assuming that $C_{creat.}$ is equal to GFR. The data used in the figures were obtained from 7 subjects who received, at different occasions, an i.v. injection of glucose or of mannitol

The peak of the sodium retention, after an i.v. glucose injection, did not coincide with the peak of glucose reabsorption. The peak of glucose reabsorption was attained in the 1st two 10 min-periods following the injection, while the sodium reabsorption peak began later and lasted longer.

In 7 control experiments, 0.67 ml/kg b.w. of a 20% mannitol solution were injected instead of the glucose solution. The depression of urine flow was the same as that observed after a glucose injection. The response of the sodium excretion, however, differed totally. Fig. 1 shows the mean values of the sodium excretion (μEq/min) in seven experimental subjects who received an injection of glucose, and, at another occasion, an injection of mannitol. The fall in the sodium excretion rate observed after glucose did not occur after mannitol. The renal excretion of sodium continued to rise progressively throughout the pre- and post-injection time, and did not appear to be influenced by the injection of mannitol in spite of a transient fall in urine flow. The difference between the 2 groups of experiments was significant at the 0.05 level during 3 collection periods following the glucose injection. These results became still clearer when the sodium excretion was shown as a fraction of the filtered sodium load ($C_{Na^+}/C_{creat.}$). As shown in Fig. 2, there was a progressive decrease of sodium reabsorption which was not interrupted by an i.v. injection of mannitol, but interrupted and reversed by an i.v. injection of glucose. The figure also shows clearly that the antinatriuretic action of glucose outlasts the glucosuria.

In addition we investigated the response of the renal excretion of potassium. Comparing the glucose, and the mannitol series, a highly significant decrease in the renal excretion of potassium could be demonstrated after a glucose load but not after a mannitol load.

It thus appears that an i.v. injection of glucose causes a pronounced transient enhancement of tubular sodium reabsorption and either an enhancement of potassium reabsorption or a decrease of potassium secretion.

Mean values were compared by judging linear contrasts according to SCHEFFE [7]. The small number of seven samples is responsible for the fact that differences significant at $p<0.05$ can only be recognized with differences between true sample means larger than 1.4 times the SD.

The antinatriuretic effect of glucose observed in the present experiments contrasts with the natriuretic effect in the course of osmotic diuresis induced by a large dose of glucose observed by SELDIN and TARAIL [6] and by WRIGHT et al. [8]. A sodium retaining effect of glucose, on the other hand, had been previously observed by BLOOM [1], who recorded sodium excretion in 24 hour periods and found that 150 g of glucose in previously fasting subjects caused a decrease in sodium excretion, while other nutritive materials with the same caloric value had no influence.

Different mechanisms could be responsible for the depression of sodium excretion after an i.v. glucose injection observed in the present experiments: 1. The enhanced tubular reabsorption of glucose could entail an enhanced reabsorption of sodium. After glucose, the sodium excretion was depressed, on the average, by 140 μEq/min. The glucose reabsorption after the i.v. injection of glucose increased by a maximum of 1 mMol/min, i.e. by an amount sufficiently large to explain an enhancement of sodium reabsorption. An argument against this explanation is that the peaks of the glucose and the sodium reabsorptions do not occur simultaneously. 2. I.v. injections of glucose could stimulate the secretion of aldosterone. Against this interpretation is the immediate occurrence of sodium retention without a latent period, as well as the simultaneous retention of potassium. — 3. Since the i.v. injection of glucose was followed for the first 10—20 min by a brief manifestation of osmotic diuresis and a slight loss of sodium, the ensuing antinatriuretic phase could be explained as a phase of compensatory retention. This explanation appears improbable in view of the large amount of sodium retained, in comparison with the small amount excreted during the osmotic diuresis. — 4. Since the antinatriuretic effect of the i.v. injection of glucose was observed under the artificial conditions of imposed water diuresis and, furthermore, in the course of a diurnal rise of sodium excretion in the morning hours [2], the whole phenomenon could be considered as an artefact. We found, however, in 4 unpublished experiments, that glucose injections caused a decrease in the nonreabsorbed fraction of sodium in normal subjects who were not in water diuresis. On the other hand, the mechanisms of the rise in sodium excretions with water diuresis or of the diurnal rise in sodium excretion during the morning hours are unknown [2, 3]. — 5. The simultaneous decrease in sodium and in potassium excretion may point to a biochemical effect of the intravenously injected glucose on the tubular epithelial cells. The nature of this effect remains unexplained.

Summary

20 healthy students received an i.v. injection of 0.5 g/kg of glucose, in the course of water diuresis in experiments originally designed to measure glucose excretion thresholds. The clearances of creatinine, sodium potassium and glucose were measured. In some of the subjects, control experiments were done with a rapid i.v. injection of 0.13 g/kg of mannitol. Intravenous injection of mannitol was followed by an increase of the absolute and the fractional sodium excretion. After i.v. injection of glucose there was a significant decrease in the absolute and in the fractional excretion of sodium as well as of potassium which may be due to a metabolic effect of glucose.

References

1. Bloom, W. L.: Inhibition of salt excretion by carbohydrate. Arch. intern. Med. **109**, 80—86 (1962).
2. De Vries, L. A., S. P. Ten Holt, J. J. van Daatselaar, A. Mulder, and J. G. G. Borst: Characteristic renal excretion patterns in response to physiological, pathological and pharmacological stimuli. Clin. chim. Acta **5**, 915—937 (1960).
3. Krück, F., and H. J. Krecke: The renal sodium excretion during oral hydration in man. Nephron **2**, 321—333 (1965).
4. Løken, F.: On the determination of creatinine in plasma by the Jaffe reaction after absorption to Lloyd's reagent. Scand. J. clin. Lab. Invest. **6**, 325—334 (1954).
5. Renschler, H. E.: Der Einfluß der Nierenfunktion auf die Glukoseausscheidung Gesunder. Habil.-Schr. Heidelberg 1964.
6. Seldin, D. W., and R. Tarail: Effect of hypertonic solutions on metabolism and excretion of electrolytes. Amer. J. Physiol. **159**, 160—173 (1949).
7. Scheffe, H.: The analysis of variance, 3. edit., p. 66. New York: John Wiley & Sons Inc. 1963.
8. Wright, H. K., D. S. Gann, and K. Albertsen: Effect of glucose on sodium excretion and renal concentration ability after starvation in man. Metabolism **12**, 804—811 (1963).

Discussion

Ludwig:

In split renal function studies on patients with pyelonephritis of different severity on both sides, infused with glucose intravenously, we did not observe any sodium retention at plasma glucose concentrations of 100 or 500 mg-%, in a steady state. The infusion of glucose, in both kidneys of these patients, caused a clear-cut osmotic diuresis with an increased sodium excretion. The fractional sodium excretion ($U/P_{Na}/U/P_{In}$) was always higher in the kidney with the lower value of GFR. These data show that the sodium retention observed by you after single intravenous injections does not occur with continuous intravenous infusion of glucose.

6.4. Influence of Acute Metabolic Changes in Acid-Base-Balance on the Renal Sodium Excretion in Man*

D. P. Mertz and F. Schindera[1]

The effects of metabolic acidosis or alkalosis on renal sodium excretion were examined in comparative studies in hydropenic hypertensive subjects. The subjects first received an intravenous infusion of 5 per cent sodium chloride and later of 5 per cent sodium lactate solutions at rates between 2 and 10 ml/min. At comparable rates of osmolar clearance (to 20 ml/min and more), glomerular filtered sodium load (to 32 mEq/min) and excreted sodium load (to 2.5 mEq/min or 9.5 per cent of the filtered load) there is no indication for a different fate of sodium in different segments of the nephron under the two conditions. Potassium excretion was also similar under both conditions. The results are discussed in regard to the high sodium permeability of proximal tubular walls.

---

* Abstract. The full paper will appear in Klinische Wochenschrift.

[1] Medizinische Poliklinik der Universität Freiburg i. Br., West Germany.

6.5. The Renal Clearance of Lissamine Green in the Rat

D. F. GROSSMANN and J. FREY[1]

With 3 Figures

Lissamine green[2] is currently used in nephrology for the measurement of the velocity of flow of tubular fluid since its introduction by STEINHAUSEN [1]. Lissamine green is usually assumed to reach tubular fluid exclusively by glomerular ultrafiltration. The present experiments were done in order to confirm or to disprove this assumption by measuring the renal clearance of the dye.

Methods

Lissamine green SF (obtained from Chroma-Gesellschaft, Stuttgart-Untertürkheim, West Germany) as a 7% solution in either unbuffered Ringer's solution, or after neutralization with NaOH to pH 7.4, was given in single intravenous injections of 0.1 to 0.2 ml, or continuously by an infusion pump through a tail vein, to female Wistar rats weighing 180—200 g. Mannitol (10%) or urea (1—2 M) were added to the injected or the infused solution in order to obtain adequate rates of urine flow.

The concentration of lissamine green in urine was estimated, after dilution with a 0.2 M acetate buffer of pH 4.5—5.0 and centrifugation, by photometry of the supernatant at 578 nm at a temperature of 21—24° C.

The concentration of lissamine green in serum was assayed after dilution of the serum with a mixture of 0.2 M acetate + 0.2 M trichloroacetate buffer at pH 4.5 after centrifugation. 98% of lissamine green added to fresh serum was recovered by this procedure.

In order to measure the freely filtrable fraction of lissamine green, protein binding of the dye was measured as follows: the loss of extinction of a plasma sample was recorded automatically at 578 nm. The resulting curve was then extrapolated to the time at which the blood sample was taken. Knowing the reaction constants at pH 7.4, which describe the transformation of free lissamine

---

[1] II. Med. Univ.-Klinik Frankfurt a. M., West Germany.

[2] Lissamine green is an acid fuchsonimine dye i.e. a derivative of triphenylmethane. Its composition is: $C^{37}H^{34}O^{9}N_2S_3Na_2$; its structural formula as follows:

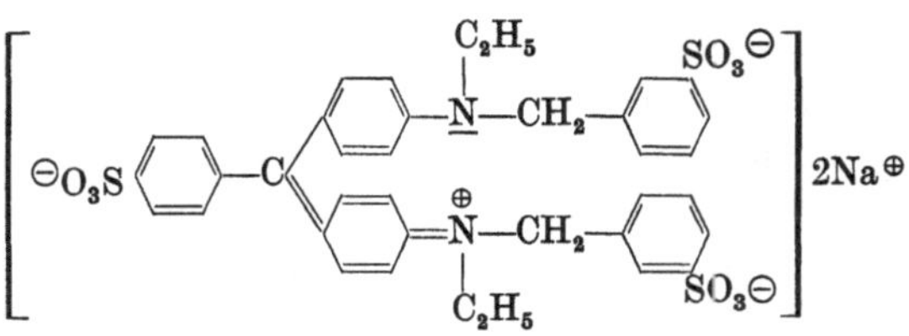

The molecular weight is 793.

green to protein-bound lissamine green and of protein-bound lissamine green to the protein-bound colorless derivative, the concentration of free lissamine green at the time at which the sample was taken, could be calculated. The reaction constants were measured as loss of extinction of a lissamine-green—serum-protein solution dialysed against a serum-chamber.

Results

1. At a constant concentration the extinction of an aqueous solution of lissamine green depends on pH and temperature. Fig. 1 shows the extinction at 578 nm as influenced by different temperatures and pH values. The wave length

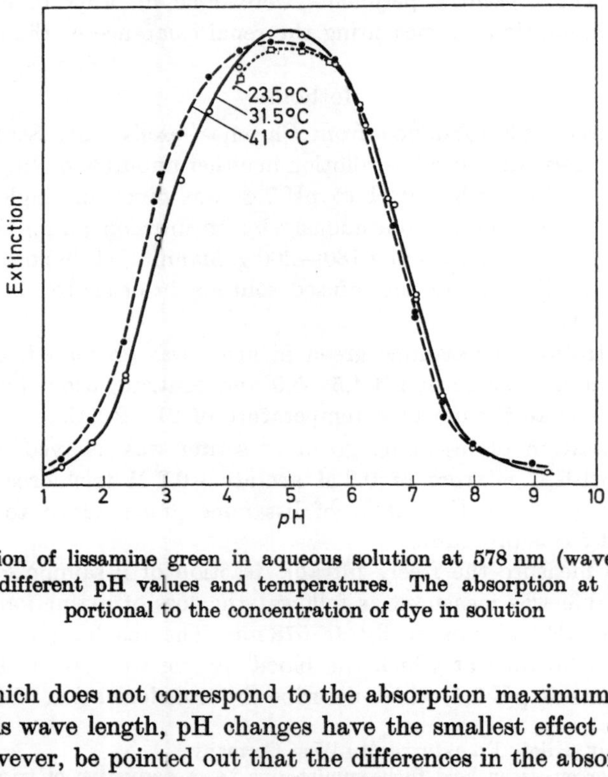

Fig. 1. Absorption of lissamine green in aqueous solution at 578 nm (wave length of Hg-vapor-line) at different pH values and temperatures. The absorption at any pH is proportional to the concentration of dye in solution

of 578 nm, which does not correspond to the absorption maximum, was selected because at this wave length, pH changes have the smallest effect on extinction. It should, however, be pointed out that the differences in the absorption spectra measured at different pH values are not considerable. Fig. 2 shows the absorption spectrum at pH 4.5. The reversible equilibrium between colored and colorless lissamine green shows 2 points of reversal as observed with pH indicator-dyes. A particular feature of the behavior of lissamine green is the rather slow conversion of one form to the other which occurs with a well defined temperature-dependent half-time. This behavior at pK 6.7 corresponds to that of triphenylmethane dyes, which form carbinol bases in alkaline solutions. Similar half-times are found by potentiometry during titration with strong acids or bases. Fig. 3 shows the half-times for the transformation of lissamine green into the colorless derivative for the range of physiologically interesting values. The slow conversion of one form of the dye to the other creates difficulties in estimating the renal clearance of lissamine green.

2. Lissamine green is strongly bound to serum proteins. The protein-bound dye is nearly colorless. Green and colorless lissamine green are bound to the same extent. It cannot be decided at present whether the protein complexes of the 2 forms of the dye are identical or differ chemically.

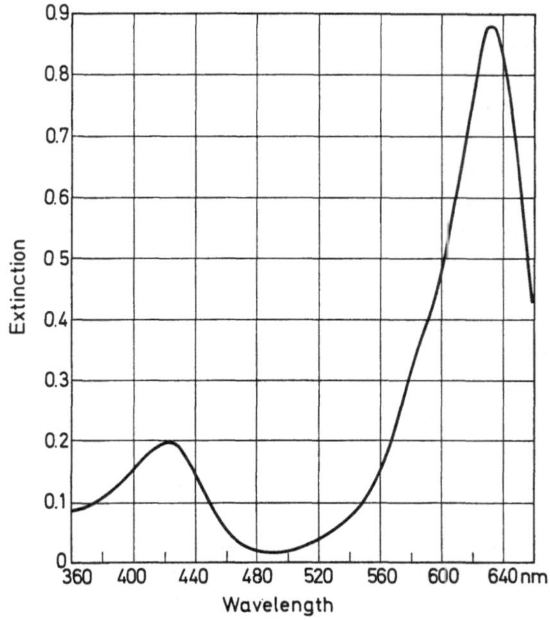

Fig. 2. Absorption spectrum of lissamine green in aqueous solution at pH 4.5. The difference in the absorption spectra in the pH-range 1—9 is negligible

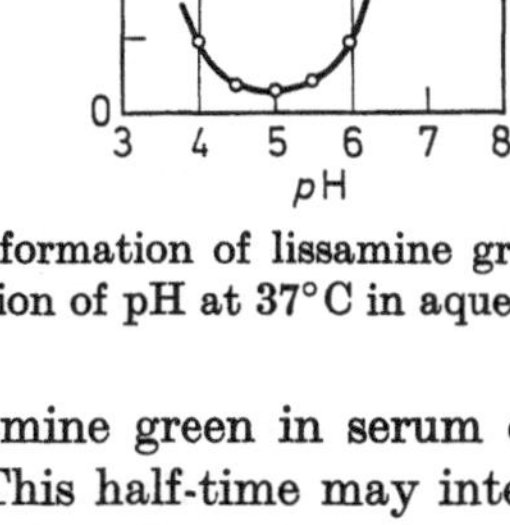

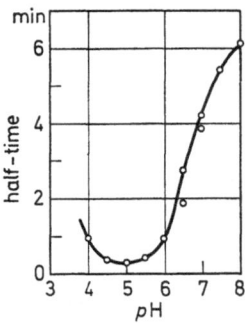

Fig. 3. Half-times of the transformation of lissamine green into the colorless derivative as a function of pH at 37° C in aqueous solution

Protein-binding of lissamine green in serum occurs slowly, the half-time at 37° C being 10.5 ± 1 min. This half-time may interfere with the half-time of the conversion of green to colorless lissamine green. If serum is mixed with dilute solutions of lissamine green in isotonic saline or in Ringer's solution (which has a very low buffering capacity as compared to a 7% solution of lissamine green,) the pH being 2—3, the half-time increased from 9.5 to 14 min in the course of one absorption experiment. A lissamine green solution preincubated at pH 7.4 gives half-times between 9.5 and 11.5 min.

At lissamine green concentrations as used in tubular passage time measurements, $95 \pm 3\%$ of the whole lissamine green present in serum is bound to protein, at equilibrium. The clearance of the unbound dye, as measured from the plasma concentration, cannot, therefore, be estimated with a high degree of certainty. Lissamine green is transformed into a colorless base in the course of a reaction of 0 order. This reaction is irreversible and does not allow the measurement of an absorption equilibrium.

3. The renal clearance of lissamine green was measured by 2 different methods. a) After single i.v. injections of lissamine green solutions, either preincubated at pH 7.4 until an equilibrium coloration was reached, or in most experiments, in Ringer's solution at a pH of 2—3. — b) With continuous infusions of one of the 2 lissamine green solutions into a tail vein. When lissamine green in Ringer's solution was used for this purpose, the rats did not survive for a long time because of unphysiologically low pH values.

Method a) gave clearance values for unbound lissamine green between 1.67 and 3.33 ml/min. Method b) gave values between 1.51 and 2.8 ml/min.

The inulin clearance of the experimental animals ranged from 1.13 to 1.5 ml/min. The urinary clearance of lissamine green, therefore, appears to fall between the clearance of inulin and its double value; in any case the clearance of lissamine green is larger than that of inulin. This finding sheds some doubt on the possibility of interpreting the velocity of the progression of a column of lissamine green in renal tubules as an expression of the rate of flow of tubular fluid.

4. Since the absorption of lissamine green solution depends on the pH and follows changes of the pH with a measurable half-time, increased intensity of coloration of tubular content cannot be interpreted as an expression of a concentration of tubular contents. Such an interpretation should be founded on a comparison with dye-solutions at the pH values found in tubular fluid. Similarly, a decrease in color intensity may be due either to an increase in pH or to a transformation into the colorless form, if the dye was not at equilibrium at pH 7.4 at the moment of injection.

Summary

1. Lissamine green exists as a colorless and as a green form. The equilibrium between the two forms depends on pH. The pK is approximately 6.7. The transformation is reversible and follows first order kinetics with pH-dependent easily measurable half-times.

2. Lissamine green is strongly bound to serum proteins under physiological conditions. The half-time of the binding reaction ranges around 10 min.

3. The renal clearance of unbound lissamine green can only be measured with considerable experimental difficulty. Its order of magnitude ranges between that of the inulin clearance and its double value.

4. Lissamine green cannot be used as an indicator of concentration or dilution of tubular fluid unless the pH values of tubular fluid and the half-times are also considered.

References

1. STEINHAUSEN, M.: Eine Methode zur Differenzierung proximaler und distaler Tubuli der Nierenrinde von Ratten in vivo und ihre Anwendung zur Bestimmung tubulärer Strömungsgeschwindigkeiten. Pflügers Arch. ges. Physiol. **277**, 23—35 (1963).

Subject Index

Universitätsdruckerei H. Stürtz AG Würzburg